Uncommon causes of stroke

This book is published as a companion to the second edition of *Stroke Syndromes*, and provides in-depth descriptions of many rare and relatively uncommon causes of stroke. Together with *Stroke Syndromes*, it emphasizes pattern recognition in the location and diagnosis of stroke.

This is the most comprehensive and authoritative text on stroke of uncommon cause. It describes various forms of angiitis, coagulation disorders, infective, paraneoplastic and metabolic disorders that may be associated with stroke, and a number of individually rare syndromes such as Eales disease, Fabry disease, and pseudoxanthoma elasticum.

For all neurologists, neurosurgeons, neuroradiologists and vascular surgeons, it is a unique scientific and clinical resource. It will provide a useful reference to help physicians diagnose and treat stroke patients who do not fit well into the usual clinical categories.

A companion volume *Stroke Syndromes, 2nd edition* completes this highly authoritative reference work, which clinicians in neurology will find essential to the understanding and diagnosis of stroke.

Julien Bogousslavsky is Professor and Chair in the University Department of Neurology, and Professor of Cerebrovascular Diseases, University of Lausanne, Switzerland. He was Co-founder of the European Stroke Conference and of the journal *Cerebrovascular Diseases* and is president-elect of the International Stroke Society.

Louis R. Caplan is Professor of Neurology at Harvard Medical School and Chief of the Stroke Service, Beth Israel Deaconess Medical Center, Boston. He is Vice-President of the American Neurological Association.

Uncommon causes of stroke

Edited by

Julien Bogousslavsky
University of Lausanne, Switzerland

and

Louis R. Caplan
Harvard Medical School and Beth Israel Deaconess Medical Center, Boston, MA, USA

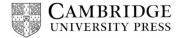

PUBLISHED BY THE PRESS SYNDICATE OF THE UNIVERSITY OF CAMBRIDGE
The Pitt Building, Trumpington Street, Cambridge, United Kingdom

CAMBRIDGE UNIVERSITY PRESS
The Edinburgh Building, Cambridge CB2 2RU, UK
40 West 20th Street, New York, NY 10011–4211, USA
10 Stamford Road, Oakleigh, VIC 3166, Australia
Ruiz de Alarcón 13, 28014 Madrid, Spain
Dock House, The Waterfront, Cape Town 8001, South Africa

http://www.cambridge.org

First published 2001

Printed in the United Kingdom at the University Press, Cambridge

Typeface Utopia (Monotype) 8.5/12pt.   *System* QuarkXPress® [SE]

A catalogue record for this book is available from the British Library

Library of Congress Cataloguing in Publication data
Uncommon causes of stroke / edited by Julien Bogousslavsky,
    Louis Caplan
        p.   cm.
Includes bibliographical references and index.
ISBN 0 521 77145 5
1. Cerebrovascular disease – Diagnosis.   2. Diagnosis, Differential.
3. Symptoms.   I. Bogousslavsky, Julien.   II. Caplan, Louis R.
RC388.5.U515 2001
616.8′1 – dc21   00-064231

ISBN 0 521 77145 5 hardback
ISBN 0 521 80258 X set (with *Stroke syndromes*, second edition)

Every effort has been made in preparing this book to provide accurate
and up-to-date information which is in accord with accepted
standards and practice at the time of publication. Nevertheless, the
authors, editors and publisher can make no warranties that the
information contained herein is totally free from error, not least
because clinical standards are constantly changing through research
and regulation. The authors, editors and publisher therefore disclaim
all liability for direct or consequential damages resulting from the use
of material contained in this book. Readers are strongly advised to pay
careful attention to information provided by the manufacturer of any
drugs or equipment that they plan to use.

To our wives
Catherine Bogousslavsky and Brenda Caplan
for their continual support and love

Contents

Contributors

Harold P. Adams Jr
Department of Neurology
Division of Cerebrovascular Diseases
University of Iowa College of Medicine
200 Hawkins Drive
Iowa City, IN 52242–1009

Jean-François Albucher
INSERM U 455
Department of Neurology
Hôpital Purpan
Place Baylac
F-31059 Toulouse
France

Irena Anselm
Department of Neurology
Children's Hospital
300 Longwood Avenue
Boston 02215 MA,
USA

Robert W. Baloh
Neurology Services
UCLA Medical Center
Reed Neurological Research Center
710 Westwood Plaza
Los Angeles, CA 920024-1769
USA

V. Barbosa
Servizio de Neurologia
Hospital Universidade Coimbra
Av. Bissaya Barreto
Coimbra 3000–075
Portugal

Ralf W. Baumgartner
Department of Neurology
University Hospital
Frauenklinikstr. 26
CH-8091 Zürich
Switzerland

José Biller
Department of Neurology
Indiana University School of Medicine
545 Barnhill Drive
Emerson Hall, Room 125
Indianapolis, IN 46202-5124
USA

Serge Blecic
Service de Neurologie
Hôpital Erasme
Université lire de Bruxelles
Route de Linnik, 808
B-1070 Bruxelles
Belgium

Julien Bogousslavsky
Department of Neurology
Centre Hospitalier Universitaire
Vaudois
Rue du Bugnon 11
CH 1011 Lausanne
Switzerland

Natan M. Bornstein
Department of Neurology
Tel Aviv Sourasky Medical Center
6 Weizmann Street
Tel Aviv 64239
Israel

Marie-Germaine Bousser
Hôpital Lariboisière
Service de Neurologie
2 Rue Anbroise Paré
75475 Paris Cedex 10
France

Robin L. Brey
Department of Medicine (Neurology)
UTHSCSA
7703 Floyd Curl Drive
San Antonio, TX 78284-7883
USA

John C.M. Brust
Harlem Hospital Center
506 Lenox Avenue
New York, NY 10037
USA

Luc Buée
INSERM U422
Place de Verdun
59045 Lille
France

Louis R. Caplan
Beth Israel Deaconess
Medical Center, 330 Brookline Avenue
Boston, MA 02215
USA

Alain Carruzzo
Department of Neurology
Centre Hospitalier Universitaire
Vaudois
Rue du Bugnon 11
CH 1011 Lausanne
Switzerland

José Castillo
Department of Neurology
Hospital Xeral de Galicia
15705 Santiago de Compostela
Spain

Hugues Chabriat
Hôpital Lariboisière
Service de Neurologie
2 Rue Anbroise Paré
75475 Paris Cedex 10
France

François Chollet
INSERM U 455
Department of Neurology
Hôpital Purpan
Place Baylac
F-31059 Toulouse
France

Chin-Sang Chung
Stroke Program Director
Department of Neurology
Samsung Medical Center
Sungkyunkwan University School of Medicine
50 ILWON-dong
Kangnam-ku
Seoul, S. Korea 135-710

Bruce M. Coull
Department of Neurology
Arizona Health Sciences Center
1501 N. Campbell Avenue
Tucson, AZ 85724-5023
USA

Luís Cunha
Servizio de Neurologia
Hospital Universidade Coimbra
Av. Bissaya Barreto
Coimbra 3000-075
Portugal

John F. Dashe
Tufts New England Medical Center
750 Washington Street
Boston, MA 02111
USA

Antoni Dávalos
Department of Neurology
Hospital Universitari Doctor Josep
Trueta
Av. de França, s/n
17007 Girona
Spain

Stephen M. Davis
Department of Neurology
Royal Melbourne Hospital
Post Office RMH
Victoria 3050
Australia

Jan L. de Bleecker
Department of Neurology
University Hospital
De Pintelaan 185
9000 Gent
Belgium

Jacques L. de Reuck
Department of Neurology
University Hospital
De Pintelaan 185
9000 Gent
Belgium

Gérald Devuyst
Department of Neurology
Centre Hospitalier Universitaire
Vaudois
Rue de Bugon
1011 Lausanne
Switzerland

Hans C. Diener
Department of Neurology
University of Essen
Hufelandstr. 55
D-45147 Essen
Germany

A. Druschky
Neurologische Klinik mit Poliklinik
Universität Erlangen-Nürnberg
Schwabachanlange 6
D-91054 Erlangen
Germany

John M. Duff
Department of Neurosurgery
Tufts New England Medical Center, #178
750 Washington Street
Boston, MA 02111
USA

Bruno Estañol
Department of Neurology
Instituti Nacional de La Nutricion – Salvador Subiran
Vasco de Quiroga 15
Delegación Tlalpan
CP 14000 Mexico DF

Nancy Futrell
Intermountain Stroke Research
5770 South 250 East, Suite 335
Murray, Utah 84107
USA

Bhuwan P. Garg
Indiana University
Department of Neurology
Riley Hospital, Room 1757
702 Barnhill Drive
Indianapolis, IN 46202-5200
USA

Thomas R. Hedges
Department of Ophthalmology
New England Medical Center
750 Washington Street
Boston MA 02111
USA

Galen V. Henderson
Department of Neurology
Brigham & Women's Hospital
75 Francis Street
Boston 02215 MA, USA

Isabel Henriques
Neurologia
Hospital do Espírito Santo
7034 Évora
Portugal

Lorenz Hirt
Massachusetts General Hospital
149 13th Street, CNY-6403
Charlestown, MA 02129
USA

Joanna C. Jen
Department of Neurology
UCLA Medical Center
Box 951769
Los Angeles, CA 920024-1769
USA

A. Joutel
INSERM U25
Faculté de Médicine Necker Enfants-Malades
Paris

Karla B. Kanis
PAREXEL International
200 West Street
Waltham, MA 02451
USA

Vadim G. Karepov
Department of Neurology
Tel Aviv Sourasky Medical Center
6 Weizmann Street
Tel Aviv 64239
Israel

W. Koroshetz
Neurological Intensive Care Unit
Harvard Medical School
Boston, MA 02114
USA

Emre Kumral
Department of Neurology
School of Medicine
Ege University
Izmir
Turkey

Tobias Kurth
Department of Neurology
University of Essen
Hufelstr. 55
D-45122 Essen
Germany

Steven R. Levine
Center for Stroke Research
Department of Neurology, K-11
Henry Ford Hospital
2799 West Grand Boulevard
Detroit MI 48220-2689
USA

Didier Leys
Clinique Neurologie – Neurologie B
Hôpital Roger Salengro
Rue Oscar Lambret
59037 Lille
France

Alfredo M. Lopez-Yunez
Department of Neurology
Indiana University School of Medicine
545 Barnhill Drive
Emerson Hall, Room 125
Indianapolis, IN 46202-5124
USA

Alexander Lossos
Department of Neurology
Hadassah University Hospital
POB 12000
Jerusalem 91120
Israel

Betsy B. Love
Department of Neurology
Indiana University School of Medicine
545 Barnhill Drive
Emerson Hall, Room 125
Indianapolis, IN 46202-5124
USA

Catherine Masson
Service de Neurologie
Hôpital Beaujon
Av. Général Leclerc
92 Lichy
France

Panayiotis Mitsias
Center for Stroke Research
Department of Neurology (K-11)
Henry Ford Hospital and Health Sciences Center
2799 West Grand Boulevard
Detroit, MI 48202-2689
USA

Bahram Mokri
Department of Neurology
Mayo Clinic
200 First Street SW
Rochester, MN 55905
USA

Bernd Neundörfer
Neurologische Klinik mit Poliklinik
Universität Erlangen-Nürnberg
Schwabachanlange 6
D-91054 Erlangen
Germany

Luis Ostrosky-Zeichner
Division of Infectious Diseases
Department of Internal Medicine
University of Texas Houston Medical School
Houston, Texas
USA

Nikolaos I.H. Papamitsakis
Center for Stroke Research
Department of Neurology (K-11)
Henry Ford Hospital and Health Sciences Center
2799 West Grand Boulevard
Detroit, MI 48202-2689
USA

Luca Regli
Department of Neurology
Centre Hospitalier Universitaire
Vaudois
Rue du Bugnon 11
CH 1011 Lausanne
Switzerland

Marc D. Reichhart
Department of Neurology
Centre Hospitalier Universitaire
Vaudois
Rue du Bugnon 11
CH 1011 Lausanne
Switzerland

E. Steve Roach
Department of Neurology
The University of Texas
Southwestern Medical School
5323 Harry Hines Blvd
Dallas, TX 75235-9036
USA

N. Paul Rosman
Department of Neurology
Floating Hospital
New England Medical Center
750 Washington Street
Boston MA 02111
USA

Robert J. Schwartzman
Hahnemann University Hospital
Broad and Vine Streets, MS 423
Philadelphia, PA 19102-1192
USA

Yukito Shinohara
Department of Neurology
Tokai University School of Medicine
Bohseidai, Isehara-shi
Kanagawa
259-1193 Japan

Peter T. Skaff
Department of Neurology
University of Arizona College of Medicine
Tucson, AZ 85724-5023
USA

Aneesh B. Singhal
Department of Neurology
VBK 802
Harvard Medical School
Boston, MA 02114
USA

Christian L. Stallworth
Department of Medicine (Neurology)
UTHSCSA
7703 Floyd Curl Drive
San Antonio, TX 78284-7883
USA

Israel Steiner
Department of Neurology
Hadassah University Hospital
PO B 12000
Jerusalem 91120
Israel

Elisabeth Tournier-Lasserve
INSERM U 25
Faculté de Médicine Necker Enfants-Malades
Paris
France

John Wade
West London Neurosciences Centre
Charing Cross Hospital
London W6 8RF
UK

Engin Y. Yilmaz
Department of Neurology
Indiana University School of Medicine
545 Barnhill Drive
Emerson Hall, Room 125
Indianapolis, IN 46202-5124
USA

Carol F. Zimmerman
Department of Ophthalmology
Southwestern Medical School
5323 Harry Hines Blvd
Dallas, TX 75235-9036
USA

Mathieu Zuber
Service de Neurologie
Centre Hospitalier Sainte-Anne
1 rue Cabanis
75674 Paris Cedex 14
France

Preface

In the years since the successful first publication of *Stroke Syndromes*, numerous comments from colleagues, ranging from trainees to international experts, have confirmed the interest and importance of this concept to clinicians. In an era of high-tech medicine, our aim remains to provide guidance on the examination and diagnosis of stroke that is deeply rooted in clinical practice.

The highest compliment for medical teachers is when their work is appreciated by students and junior colleagues. However, we recognized that there was room for improvement, and we have reshaped the books to make them more comprehensive and clinically useful.

The most substantial change has been the division of the text into two separate volumes. The first of these, *Stroke Syndromes*, 2nd edition, focuses on syndromes and their brain and vascular correlates. The second, *Uncommon Causes of Stroke*, reviews more fully the particular vascular etiologic syndromes which formed Part III of the first edition.

The books are still intended as a guide, and remain a source of information on patterns and syndromes for physicians, particularly for those who are not experts in stroke, to refer to when they encounter an unfamiliar pattern. Three main categories are covered:

 (i) patterns of symptoms and signs;
 (ii) lesion patterns found in patients with infarcts and hemorrhages in various loci and vascular territories;
(iii) patterns and syndromes that may occur in unusual conditions known to cause stroke.

We thank all our authors who have agreed to modify or rewrite their chapters from the first edition, as well as numerous new contributors. Communications and therapeutic advances are both accelerating. In the first edition we wrote that, for stroke management, 'the window of opportunity is short, probably less than 24 hours', whereas today we know that it is less than 6 hours in most instances.

Many other advances have been made, and with this in mind we hope that this completely updated and rewritten edition will continue to be of help in the care of patients with stroke.

Julien Bogousslavsky, *Lausanne*
Louis R. Caplan, *Boston*

Isolated angiitis of the central nervous system

Mathieu Zuber

Service de Neurologie, Centre Hospitalier Sainte Anne, Paris, France

Introduction

Isolated angiitis of the central nervous system (IACNS) was defined in 1959 as an idiopathic vasculitis restricted to small leptomeningeal and parenchymal arteries and veins, without apparent systemic involvement (Cravioto & Feigin, 1959). More than 40 years later, the affection remains poorly recognized and its pathogenesis mysterious, despite the growing pool of knowledge on processes responsible for CNS inflammation. The term 'primary angiitis' is sometimes preferred to 'isolated angiitis' since complete autopsy is rarely performed and minor abnormalities are occasionally observed in systemic organs of patients who died from so-called IACNS (Johnson et al., 1994). In numerous cases with no histological proof of vascular inflammation, the descriptive term 'angiopathy' would be more appropriate than 'angiitis' but the latter term has been frequently overused in the recent literature.

IACNS is a rare disorder with an incidence estimated to less than 1:2 000 000 (Moore, 1999). Although stroke may occur in the course of the disease, it appears as the initial manifestation in a minority of patients only. Because of the protean clinical symptoms and blurred diagnostic criteria, identification of IACNS is a difficult challenge for all clinicians involved in the field of cerebrovascular diseases.

Pathology and pathogenesis

Pathological picture

IACNS has been referred to by several names descriptive of the pathological findings: 'granulomatous angiitis of the CNS', 'giant cell granulomatous angiitis of the CNS' and 'cerebral granulomatous angiitis' have all been used interchangeably in the literature (Hankey, 1991; Rhodes et al.,

1995). This variable terminology partly reflects the difficulty in individualizing IACNS as a pathological entity from systemic disorders such as giant cell temporal angiitis or sarcoidosis, themselves occasionally responsible for CNS angiitis.

The non-specific pathological pattern of IACNS is characterized by infiltrations of the vascular walls with mononuclear cells including lymphocytes, macrophages and histiocytes. Fibrinoid necrosis is occasionally seen, especially in the acute phase (Cravioto & Feigin, 1959; Hankey, 1991; Lie, 1992; Rhodes et al., 1995). In about 85% of the cases, granulomas with epitheloid cells and giant Langhans cells are described. The degree of this granuloma formation is variable. In the early disease, granulomas frequently miss the histological picture and the misleading terminology 'granulomatous angiitis' should therefore no longer be used to describe IACNS. The inflammatory lesions may sometimes spread to all the vascular wall layers, but preservation of the media is the rule.

Vascular abnormalities primarily involve small- and middle-sized arteries in addition to veins and veinules. Arteries less than 500 μm in diameter may be solely affected. In most cases, leptomeningeal involvement is a dominating feature, with less consistent parenchymatous vascular involvement in white and grey matters. The segmental involvement of vessels may be responsible for false-negative histological results.

Pathogenesis

The pathogenesis of IACNS is unknown and research progress is slow because of the rarity of tissue samples acquired from carefully documented cases. It has been shown that CNS inflammation activates the brainstem noradrenergic and trigeminovascular responses, contributing to reduction of regional vascular blood flow (Moore,

1998). As an additive factor to inflammation itself, this activation could play some role in the appearance of arterial stenoses.

IACNS is now more regarded as an immunological, non-specific T cell-mediated inflammatory reaction than a specific entity (Calabrese et al., 1997; Ferro, 1998; Moore, 1998). This view is in accordance with (i) the wide spectrum of diseases described in association with IACNS (ii) the limited known responses of the CNS blood vessels to a variety of noxious stimuli (iii) the clinical and pathological heterogeneity of the disorder (although this may also reflect individual differences in the host response). Why the inflammatory response to various factors may be maladaptive and leads to disease remains mostly speculative. Chronicity of the stimuli, concurrent diseases and genetic susceptibility are probably critical parameters (Moore, 1998).

Indeed, cases of IACNS have been reported after various infections such as mycoplasma, varicella zoster or arbovirus infections (Chu et al., 1998). Both mycoplasma- and virus-like particles were identified in glial cells and cerebral blood vessels of patients with IACNS (Arthur & Margolis, 1977; Linnemann & Alvira, 1980). Moreover, histological patterns very similar to IACNS were reported as herpes zoster arteritis (Chu et al., 1998; Mackenzie et al., 1981) and a well-documented case previously published as IACNS was recently shown to be related to varicella zoster infection (Gilden et al., 1996).

When angiitis is described in association with lymphoma, it usually remains unclear whether it is due to a malignant lymphoproliferative infiltration, reactivation of some remote viral infection or to non-specific inflammatory mechanisms such as those suspected to be responsible for IACNS (Greer et al., 1988). IACNS was also found to coexist with cerebral amyloid angiopathy in several patients (Caplan & Louis, 2000; Gray et al., 1990; Riemer et al., 1999). It has been discussed whether angiitis could be an inflammatory response to beta-A4–amyloid deposits or the primary abnormality responsible for the amyloid deposition (Fountain & Eberhard, 1996; Yamada et al., 1996).

Clinical features

The clinical presentation of CNS angiitis is highly variable from one patient to the other because virtually any anatomic area of CNS may be affected by the angiitis. Angiitis (whatever its cause) may thus mimic a wide range of CNS diseases. IACNS has no specific symptoms that could help to distinguish the disease from other causes of CNS angiitis, either infectious or non-infectious (Zuber et al., 1999).

A wide range of evolution has also been reported, stretching from a quasi-indolent disease to death in a couple of months (Calabrese & Mallek, 1988; Hankey, 1991; Johnson et al., 1994). A subacute deterioration is, in fact, most frequently observed. Relapsing symptoms are episodically described.

IACNS is twice as frequent in males as in females and onset most often occurs after 40 years of age. However, the disease can affect all age categories and several cases have been reported in childhood (Moore, 1989). Headache is the most common presenting symptom (two-thirds of the patients), variable both in quality and severity (Hankey, 1991). Diffuse symptoms such as a fluctuating level of consciousness or a decrease in memory, associated with headaches, are typical of IACNS and sometimes combine in an encephalopathic clinical pattern (Calabrese et al., 1997). In some patients, headaches may suggest a chronical meningitis (Reik et al., 1983).

All types of strokes have been observed in IACNS including definite cerebral infarcts, TIAs and intraparenchymal and subarachnoid hemorrhages (Biller et al., 1987; Burger et al., 1977; Hunn et al., 1998; Koo & Massey, 1988; Kumar et al., 1997; Moore, 1989). Intracranial bleedings could be more prevalent than ischemic strokes, but this was not systematically studied. The various intracranial bleedings are supposed to result from the vessel wall weakening due to transmural inflammation. A multi-infarct status has been reported in isolated patients with IACNS (Koo & Massey, 1988).

In a recent critical review of IACNS patients, stroke was not found to be the presenting symptom in any of the histologically proved cases (Vollmer et al., 1993). Conversely, a stroke-like presentation in a patient with pre-existent diffuse cerebral symptoms should prompt one to look for radiological signs in favour of IACNS. Recently, subarachnoid haemorrhage was pointed out as the presenting manifestation in several IACNS patients (Kumar et al., 1997; Nishikawa et al., 1998; Ozawa et al., 1995).

Beside strokes, seizures and cranial neuropathies are other focal symptoms possibly related to IACNS (Hankey, 1991). A mass lesion presentation accounts for about 15% of IACNS patients. A spinal cord involvement may be inaugural with a progressive paraparesis as the most common clinical manifestation (Calabrese et al., 1997; Rawlinson & Braun, 1981). Exceptionally, the presence of spinal root pain may reveal an angiitis limited to the cauda equina (Harrison, 1976). On the whole, focal symptoms are observed in about 50% of the patients (Calabrese & Mallek, 1988). However, as previously mentioned, focal symptoms nearly always occur in the setting of diffuse higher cortical impairment.

Fever is observed in 15% of IACNS patients, and this confounding feature may be responsible for extensive extra-neurological diagnostic workups (Hankey, 1991). On the other hand, if a patient has systemic complaints in addition to the cerebral symptomatology, appropriate investigations will usually reveal some diffuse disorder responsible for a multiorgan vasculitis. It is well known that CNS angiitis, although rare, is one of the most frightful complications of connective diseases and was described in most of them (Table 1.1).

Depending on the various clinical presentations, neurological hypotheses are numerous before the diagnosis of IACNS may be considered. Meningo-encephalitis, multiple sclerosis, abscess and stroke of other mechanism are the most frequently discussed in case of acute or subacute onset. A progressive onset may suggest neoplastic disease or dementia. Specific causes may also be discussed depending on the context, such as giant cell temporal angiitis in the elderly with headaches or Behçet's disease in a young Mediterranean with subacute rhombencephalitis.

Diagnostic procedures

Because the cerebral artery has unique characteristics that serve to protect the internal environment of the CNS, biological arguments in favour of IACNS are missing in the majority of cases. The sedimentation rate is elevated in about 30% of biopsy-confirmed IACNS patients (Hankey, 1991). No immunological marker has been identified to date and antinuclear, antiphospholipid and antineutrophil cytoplasmic antibodies are invariably normal. CSF inflammation (moderate lymphocytic pleiocytosis, elevated protein and normal glucose) is observed in about 90% of patients with histologically confirmed IACNS (Calabrese et al., 1997) and is important (although highly non-specific) for the presumption of CNS vasculitis in a patient with stroke of remote origin. Oligoclonal bands are seldom reported. CSF should always be cultured, owing to possible CNS vasculitis due to viral, fungal or indolent bacterial infections (Table 1).

Perivascular inflammatory lesions may be seen in fundoscopy, and the procedure has been reported as a valuable diagnostic tool in IACNS (Ohtake et al., 1989). Optic fluorescein angiography could also be useful especially in patients with normal cerebral angiography (Scolding et al., 1997).

Cerebral imaging

Both cerebral CT scan and MRI show non-specific abnormalities in CNS angiitis. Sensitivity of CT scan is low with

Table 1.1. *Causes of cerebral angiitis*

Infectious angiitis
Varicella zoster/Herpes zoster
Cytomegalovirus infection
Human immunodeficiency virus infection
Mycotic infections
Syphilis
Borrelia burgdorferi
Tuberculosis
Purulent bacterial meningitis

Primary systemic angiitis

– Necrotizing	Polyarteritis nodosa
	Churg and Strauss angiitis
	Cogan's syndrome
– Giant cell	Temporal angiitis
	Takayasu's arteritis
– Granulomatous	Wegener's granulomatosis
	Lymphomatoid granulomatosis
– Others	Hypersensitivity angiitis, Kawasaki's arteritis, Bürger's disease, Susac's syndrome, Kohlmeier–Degos disease, acute posterior multifocal placoid pigment epitheliopathy, . . .

Angiitis secondary to systemic disease
Systemic lupus erythematosus
Sjogren's syndrome
Behçet's disease
Sarcoidosis
Rheumatoid polyarthritis
Scleroderma
Mixed connectivitis
Dermatomyositis
Ulcerative colitis
Coeliac disease

Angiitis associated with neoplasia
Hodgkin's disease and non-Hodgkin type lymphoma
Malignant histiocytosis
Hairy cell leukemia

Angiitis associated with drug abuse
Illicit drugs (cocaine, 'crack')
Sympathomimetic agents
Amphetamine and relatives

Isolated angiitis of the CNS

Source: Adapted from Zuber et al. (1999).

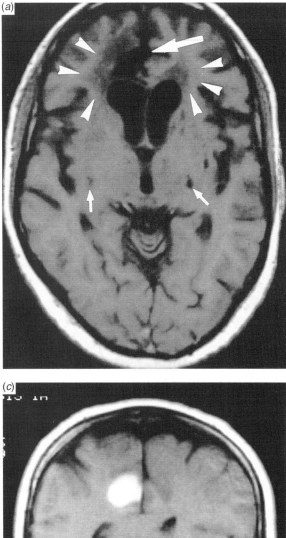

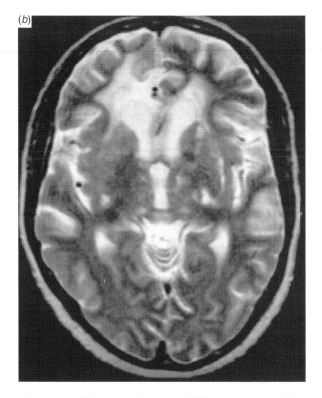

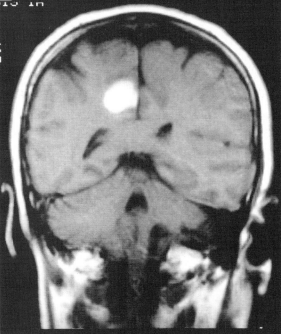

Fig. 1.1. MRI abnormalities in patients with IACNS. (*a*) and (*b*) (same patient, T_1- and T_2-weighted sequences). Large infarction in the ACA territory (large arrow) associated with deep profound infarctions (small arrows) and anterior leukoencephalopathy (arrowheads). (c). Lobar hemorrhage revealing IACNS.

about 30% (Pierot et al., 1991). MRI is more sensitive (about 80%), especially in detecting small brain lesions (Chu et al., 1998) (Fig. 1.1). The most common CT scan finding is focal or multifocal low density areas of varying sizes. Association with multiple parenchymal contrast enhancement and focal cerebral atrophy or combination of both ischemic and hemorrhagic strokes in the same patient are suggestive. Apart from signs of recent ischemic or hemorrhagic strokes, MRI frequently reveals non-specific high intensity signals on T_2-weighted sequences, sometimes responsible for leukoencephalopathy. Disseminated T_2 hypersignals in white matter with no periventricular localization could be indicative for CNS angiitis, in contrast with the hypersignals described in multiple sclerosis (Miller et al., 1987). Intracerebral hemorrhage, either in the cortex or the white matter, may occur as a result of infarction or focal necrosis of the vessel wall (Hunn et al., 1998). It is more frequent in IACNS than in infectious angiitis (Pierot et al., 1991).

Linear and punctate patterns of leptomeningeal enhancement associated with both hemispheric and penetrating vessels are said to be observed in about 60% of patients with IACNS, sometimes without significant parenchymal abnormalities (Chu et al., 1998; Negishi & Sze, 1993). Unusual CT scan and MRI presentations have been occasionally observed, including pseudotumoural lesion, repeated parenchymal or ventricular bleeding, multiple punctuate parenchymal contrast enhancement (milliary appearance) or a diffuse white matter involvement suggesting a primary demyelinating disease (Calabrese, 1995; Finelli et al., 1997; Hankey, 1991; Kristoferitsch et al., 1984).

Angiography

The angiographic features characteristic of IACNS are multifocal stenoses rendering a 'sausage-like' appearance with ectasia and occasional arterial occlusions (Fig. 1.2). If the disease is restricted to arteries less than 500 μm in diameter, angiography will be reported as normal. A normal angiographic pattern is observed in up to 50% of the patients and abnormalities may only appear on repeated procedures (Ozawa et al., 1995; Zuber et al., 1999). Intracerebral aneurysms and even multiple vanishing aneurysms have been seldom reported (Nishikawa et al., 1998). Multiple microaneurysms, a very characteristic radiological pattern in peripheral tissues with vasculitis, are invariably absent in IACNS (Chu et al., 1998). Since angiography was found to provide no excessive risk in a large number of patients with suspected CNS vasculitis (0.8% of persistent morbidity) (Hellmann et al., 1992), the technique still remains at present the 'gold standard' of the radiological procedures when CNS vasculitis is suspected.

Little is known about the usefulness of MR angiography in IACNS. The lower sensitivity of the technique for small cerebral vessels visualization compared with conventional angiography is an important drawback. Nevertheless, MR angiography is now increasingly used as the first-line radiological procedure for exploration of the intracerebral arteries, and the procedure is already useful when benign CNS angiopathy is considered as well as CNS angiitis: no conventional angiography is needed in the case of middle-sized arteries involvement with normalization on serial MR angiography associated with rapid clinical improvement, a combination highly suggestive of benign angiopathy (Fig. 1.3).

Cerebral biopsy

The diagnosis of definite IACNS relies upon the brain-leptomeningeal biopsy in all cases. It has been said that the ideal diagnostic brain biopsy is a 1 cm wedge of cortex including leptomeninges and preferably containing a cortical vessel (Moore, 1989). Including leptomeninges in the biopsy is crucial since leptomeningeal involvement is a dominating pathological feature in IACNS (see above). In a series of ten histologically confirmed IACNS patients, diagnostic changes were observed solely in leptomeningeal vessels for three patients (Chu et al., 1998). False-negative

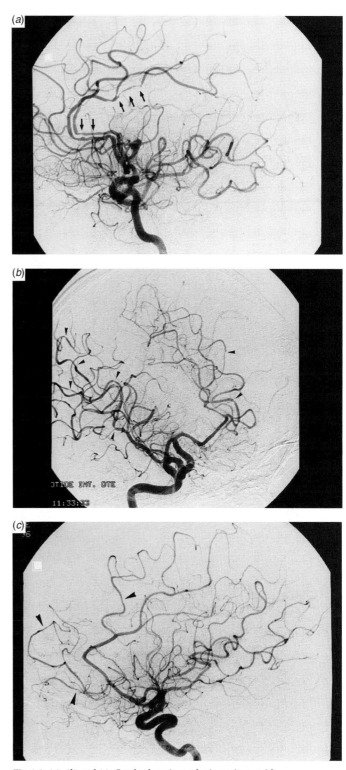

Fig. 1.2. (*a*), (*b*) and (*c*). Cerebral angiography in patients with IACNS. Note the multiple stenoses on middle- and small-sized arteries (arrows and arrowheads) delineatating 'sausage-like' appearances.

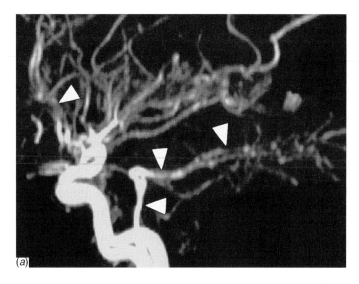

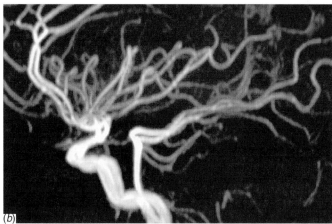

Fig. 1.3. Serial MR angiography showing (*a*) multiple stenoses and filling defects on middle-sized cerebral arteries (*b*) and complete resolution within a few weeks in a benign cerebral angiopathy.

biopsy results may be observed, and cases with pathological features typical of IACNS only on a recurrent biopsy have been reported (Kattah et al., 1987). For patients without focal lesions, the preferred biopsy site is the prefrontal area or the temporal tip of the non-dominant hemisphere. Non-specific abnormalities found on cerebral imaging should provide useful information for selecting the biopsy site. However, mismatches between the radiological abnormalities and histological predominant lesions may explain several false-negative biopsy results (Parisi & Moore, 1994). The use of stereotactic needle biopsies may account for a significant number of sampling errors since it lowers the sensitivity of biopsy to approximately 50% (Duna & Calabrese, 1995). This procedure should be confined to cases with an isolated profound pseudotumoural lesion. Cultures of brain tissue and lepto-

meninges using special stains for various microorganisms should be systematically performed. The morbidity rate of brain biopsy (0.03% to 2%) (Chu et al., 1998; Hankey, 1991) cannot be ignored but must be balanced against the risks of unnecessary immunosuppression.

Diagnostic strategy

The diagnosis of CNS angiitis may be viewed as one of the most challenging neurological diagnostic problems. The reasons for this include (i) relative rarity of the disorders, (ii) lack of specificity for clinical signs and symptoms, (iii) lack of efficient non-invasive diagnostic tests, (iv) inaccessibility of the end organ tissues for pathologic examination. The following diagnostic criteria for IACNS were proposed by Moore a decade ago (Calabrese, 1995; Calabrese & Mallek, 1988): (i) association of headaches and multiple neurological deficits which persisted for at least 6 months; (ii) segmental arterial stenoses on cerebral angiogram; (iii) exclusion of any infectious or inflammatory cause; (iv) inflammatory lesions of the vascular wall on cerebral and/or leptomeningeal biopsy or exclusion of all other causes of cerebral angiitis.

Because of lack of specificity, there is currently no consensus regarding the appropriate use of cerebral imaging, angiography and cerebral biopsy for the diagnosis of IACNS (Duna & Calabrese, 1995; Harris et al., 1994). There has been a recent trend towards diagnosing IACNS with angiography without tissue confirmation, at least in a subset of patients with a self-limited clinical course (Abu-Shakra et al., 1994). The problem is that we do not have early prognostic markers of IACNS, and the disease may rapidly kill in the absence of appropriate treatment.

Two recent studies focused on the specificity of radiological signs suggestive for IACNS and asked whether these signs were predictive of a positive biopsy (Chu et al., 1998; Duna & Calabrese, 1995). Among MRI signs useful for the diagnosis of IACNS, leptomeningeal enhancement is more sensitive than parenchymal abnormalities. It should be stressed that a combination of normal MRI and CSF test results has a strong negative predictive value and allows exclusion of CNS vasculitis in most clinical situations (Calabrese et al., 1997).

In addition to a rather low sensitivity in showing arterial abnormalities when IACNS is suspected, conventional angiography has a low positive predictive value and specificity. As shown in Table 1.2, arterial stenoses in brain may be due to various conditions among which intracranial atherosclerosis and hypertensive vasospasms are the most frequently observed. The classical 'sausage-like' segmental stenoses seem to be even more frequent in atherosclerosis or benign angiopathies than in IACNS (Chu et al., 1998).

Table 1.2. *Causes of segmental intracranial arterial narrowing*

Cerebral angiitis, either
primary or secondary
inflammatory or infectious

Intracranial dissection
traumatic
spontaneous
underlying vasculopathy (fibromuscular dysplasia)

Intracranial atherosclerosis

Recanalizing embolism

Vasospasm
acute hypertension
reversible (benign) cerebral angiopathy
migraine

Moya-moya

Cerebral radiotherapy

Tumour encasement
meningioma
chordoma
pituitary adenoma

Sickle cell anemia

Neurofibromatosis

Dysgenesis

Source: Adapted from Zuber et al. (1999).

Topographical considerations may help for the differentiation: involvement of the supraclinoid carotid arteries and of proximal MCA is usual in intracranial atherosclerosis, while more distal arteries are predominantly affected in IACNS. Variations in stenoses on serial angiography are also suggestive of IACNS, but the pattern is observed in benign cerebral angiopathy as well (Zuber et al., 1999). Given first the lack of specific clinical and radiological features of IACNS, secondly the statistical likelihood of dealing with an alternative disorder, thirdly the morbidity associated with immunosuppressive regimens involving cyclophosphamide, we believe that an early biopsic verification should be discussed in all patients with a clearly suspected CNS angiitis (Calabrese, 1995; Chu et al., 1998). In addition, the accuracy of diagnosis should be revisited periodically when the surgical procedure is delayed because of lack of evidence for CNS angiitis. In the peculiar case of stroke patients, the biopsy should be especially considered when headaches are proeminent and associated with CSF and MRI abnormalities.

Treatment and prognosis

Reports before 1980 uniformly conclude that IACNS was a more or less rapidly fatal disease. This fails to account for the fact that IACNS was invariably diagnosed late in the evolution of the disease. In addition, no treatment regimen had been proposed in most patients.

Due to the rarity of the disease, no controlled therapeutic trial has been conducted in IACNS to date, either diagnosed by leptomeningeal biopsy or by angiography. In a review of 46 patients, 19 of the 20 non-treated patients rapidly progressed either to death or to the persistence of severe sequelae, while four of the 13 patients treated by corticosteroids alone and ten of the 13 treated by a combination of corticosteroids and cyclophosphamide showed favourable progression (Calabrese & Mallek, 1988). Analysis of recent IACNS patients suggests that the prognosis of the disease is not uniformly unfavorable (Calabrese et al., 1997). Combined aggressive therapy should be reserved for those patients with histologically proven IACNS and a deteriorating clinical status. In these patients, the combination therapy should be pursued for at least 6 to 12 months after the patient is in remission (Cupps et al., 1983). To our knowledge, intravenous gammaglobulin, a treatment regimen occasionally proposed in cerebral angiitis associated with systemic diseases (Canhao et al., 2000), has not been used in IACNS patients.

The activity of the disease under treatment is appreciated using clinical, biological and radiological monitoring. Regression of CSF abnormalities may parallel clinical improvement (Oliveira et al., 1994). The successful use of serial angiography has been reported (Alhalabi & Moore, 1994). Clinical stabilization for years with discontinuation of treatment has been described in privileged cases, as well as improvement of the MRI appearance and disappearance of vessel wall inflammation years after immunosuppression (Ehsan et al., 1995; Johnson et al., 1994; Riemer et al., 1999), but a prolonged neurological supervision is necessary since relapsing episodes are possible.

In patients with a unique focal presentation such as stroke, and with IACNS suspected on the basis of angiography alone, a several-weeks' course of high-dose corticosteroids associated with a calcium channel blocker and no immunosuppressor has been proposed (Calabrese et al., 1997). Any additive vasoconstrictive stimuli including uncontrolled hypertension should be avoided.

References

Abu-Shakra, M., Khraishi, M., Grosman, H., Lewtas, J., Cividino, A. & Keystone, E.C. (1994). Primary angiitis of the CNS diagnosed by angiography. *Quarterly Journal of Medicine* **87**, 351–8.

Alhalabi, M. & Moore, P.M. (1994). Serial angiography in isolated angiitis of the central nervous system. *Neurology*, **44**, 1221–6.

Arthur, G. & Margolis, G. (1977). Mycoplasma-like structures in granulomatous angiitis of the central nervous system: case reports with light and electron microscope studies. *Archives of Pathology and Laboratory Medicine*, **101**, 382–7.

Biller, J., Loftus, C.M., Moore, S.A., Schelper, R.L., Danks, K.R. & Cornell, S.H. (1987). Isolated central nervous system angiitis first presenting as spontaneous intracranial hemorrhage. *Neurosurgery*, **20**, 310–15.

Burger, P.C., Burch, J.G. & Vogel, F.S. (1977). Granulomatous angiitis: an unusual aetiology of stroke. *Stroke*, **8**, 29–35.

Calabrese, L.H. (1995). Vasculitis of the central nervous system. *Rheumatic Diseases Clinic of North America*, **21**, 1059–76.

Calabrese, L.H. & Mallek, J.A. (1988). Primary angiitis of the central nervous system. Report of 8 cases, review of the literature and proposal for diagnostic criteria. *Medicine*, **108**, 815–23.

Calabrese, L.H., Duna, G.F. & Lie, J.T. (1997). Vasculitis in the central nervous system. *Arthritis and Rheumatism*, **40**, 1189–201.

Canhao, H., Fonseca, J.E. & Rosa, A. (2000). Intravenous gamma-globulin in the treatment of central nervous system vasculitis associated with Sjogren's syndrome. *Journal of Rheumatology*, **27**, 1102–3.

Caplan, L.R. & Louis, D.N. (2000). Case records of the Massachusetts General Hospital. Case 10–2000. *New England Journal of Medicine*, **342**, 957–65.

Chu, C.T., Gray, L., Goldstein, L.B. & Hulette, C.M. (1998). Diagnosis of intracranial vasculitis: a multi-disciplinary approach. *Journal of Neuropathology and Experimental Neurology*, **57**, 30–8.

Cravioto, H. & Feigin, I. (1959). Noninfectious granulomatous angiitis with a predilection for the nervous system. *Neurology*, **9**, 599–609.

Cupps, T.R., Moore, P.M. & Fauci, A.S. (1983). Isolated angiitis of the cerebral nervous system. Prospective diagnostic and therapeutic experience. *American Journal of Medicine*, **74**, 97–105.

Duna, G. & Calabrese, L.H. (1995). Limitations of invasive modalities in the diagnosis of primary angiitis of the central nervous system. *Journal of Rheumatology*, **22**, 662–7.

Ehsan, T., Hasan, S., Powers, J.M. & Heiserman, J.E. (1995). Serial magnetic resonance imaging in isolated angiitis of the central nervous system. *Neurology*, **45**:1462–5.

Ferro, J.M. (1998). Vasculitis of the central nervous system. *Journal of Neurology*, **245**, 766–76.

Finelli, P.F., Onyiuke, H.C. & Uphoff, D.F. (1997). Idiopathic granulomatous angiitis of the CNS manifesting as diffuse white matter disease. *Neurology*, **49**, 1696–9.

Fountain, N.B. & Eberhard, D.A. (1996). Primary angiitis of the central nervous system associated with cerebral amyloid angiopathy: report of two cases and review of the literature. *Neurology*, **46**, 190–7.

Gilden, D.H., Kleinschmidt-DeMasters, B.K., Wellish, M., Hedley-Whyte, E.T., Rentier, B. & Mahalingam, R. (1996). Varicella zoster virus, a cause of waxing and waning vasculitis: The New England Journal of Medicine case 5–1995 revisited. *Neurology*, **47**, 1441–6.

Gray, F., Viners, H.V., Le Noan, H., Salama, J., Delaporte, P. & Poirier, J. (1990). Cerebral amyloid angiopathy and granulomatous angiitis: immunohistochemical study using antibodies to the Alzheimer A4 peptide. *Human Pathology*, **21**, 1290–3.

Greer, J.M., Longley, S., Edwards, L., Elfenbein, G.J. & Panush, R.S. (1988). Vasculitis associated with malignancy. Experience with 13 patients and literature review. *Medicine*, **67**, 220–30.

Hankey, G.J. (1991). Isolated angiitis/angiopathy of the central nervous system. *Cerebrovascular Diseases*, **1**, 2–15.

Harris, K.G., Tran, D.D., Sickels, W.J., Cornell, S.H. & Yuh, W.T.C. (1994). Diagnosing intracranial vasculitis: the roles of MR and angiography. *American Journal of Neuroradiology*, **15**, 317–30.

Harrison, P.E. (1976). Granulomatous angiitis of the central nervous system. Case report and review. *Journal of the Neurological Sciences*, **29**, 335–41.

Hellmann, D.B., Roubenoff, R., Healy, R.A. & Wang, H. (1992). Central nervous system angiography: safety and predictors of a positive result in 125 consecutive patients evaluated for possible vasculitis. *Journal of Rheumatology*, **19**, 568–72.

Hunn, M., Robinson, S., Wakefield, L., Mossman, S. & Abernethy, D. (1998). Granulomatous angiitis of the CNS causing spontaneous intracerebral haemorrhage: the importance of leptomeningeal biopsy. *Journal of Neurology, Neurosurgery and Psychiatry*, **65**, 956–7.

Johnson, M.D., Maciunas, R., Creasy, J. & Collins, R.D. (1994). Indolent granulomatous angiitis. *Journal of Neurosurgery*, **81**, 472–6.

Kattah, J.C., Cupps, T.R., Di Chiro, G. & Manz, H.J. (1987). An unusual case of central nervous system vasculitis. *Journal of Neurology*, **234**, 344–7.

Koo, E.H. & Massey, E.W. (1988). Granulomatous angiitis of the central nervous system: protean manifestations and response to treatment. *Journal of Neurology, Neurosurgery and Psychiatry*, **51**, 1126–33.

Kristoferitsch, W., Jellinger, K. & Böck, F. (1984). Cerebral granulomatous angiitis with atypical features. *Journal of Neurology*, **231**, 38–42.

Kumar, R., Wijdicks, E.F.M., Brown, R.D. Jr, Parisis, J.E. & Hammond, C.A. (1997). Isolated angiitis of the CNS presenting as subarachnoid haemorrhage. *Journal of Neurology, Neurosurgery and Psychiatry*, **62**, 649–51.

Lie, J.T. (1992). Primary (granulomatous) angiitis of the central nervous system: a clinical pathologic analysis of 15 new cases and a review of the literature. *Human Pathology*, **23**, 164–71.

Linnemann, C.C. & Alvira, M.M. (1980). Pathogenesis of varicella-zoster angiitis in the CNS. *Archives of Neurology*, **37**, 239–40.

Mackenzie, R.A., Fobes, G.S. & Karnes, W.E. (1981). Angiographic findings in herpes zoster arteritis. *Annals of Neurology*, **10**, 458–64.

Matsell, D.G., Keene, D.L., Jimenez, C. & Humphrey, P. (1990). Isolated angiitis of the central nervous system in childhood. *Canadian Journal of Neurological Science*, **17**, 151–4.

Miller, D.H., Ormerod, I.E.C., Gibson, A., Du Boulay, E.P., Rudge, P. & MacDonald, W.I. (1987). MR brain scanning in patients with vasculitis: differentiation from multiple sclerosis. *Neuroradiology*, **29**, 226–31.

Moore, P.M. (1989). Diagnosis and management of isolated angiitis of the central nervous system. *Neurology*, **39**, 167–73.

Moore, P.M. (1998). Central nervous system vasculitis. *Current Opinion in Neurology*, **11**, 241–6.

Moore, P.M. (1999). The vasculitides. *Current Opinion in Neurology*, **12**, 383–8.

Negishi, C. & Sze, G. (1993). Vasculitis presenting as primary leptomeningeal enhancement with minimal parenchymal findings. *American Journal of Neuroradiology*, **14**, 26–8.

Nishikawa, M., Sakamoto, H., Katsuyama, J., Hakuba, A. & Nishimura, S. (1998). Multiple appearing and vanishing aneurysms: primary angiitis of the central nervous system. *Journal of Neurosurgery*, **88**, 133–7.

Ohtake, T., Yoshida, H., Hirose, K. & Tanabe, H. (1989). Diagnostic value of the optic fundus in cerebral angiitis. *Journal of Neurology*, **236**, 490–1.

Oliveira, V.C., Povoa, P., Costa, A. & Ducla-Soares, J. (1995). Cerebrospinal fluid and therapy of isolated angiitis of the central nervous system. *Stroke*, **25**, 1693–5.

Ozawa, T., Sasaki, O., Sorimachi, T. & Tanaka, R. (1995). Primary angiitis of the central nervous system: report of two cases and review of the literature. *Neurosurgery*, **36**, 173–9.

Parisi, J.E. & Moore, P.M. (1994). The role of biopsy in vasculitis of the central nervous system. *Seminars in Neurology*, **14**, 341–8.

Pierot, L., Chiras, J., Debussche-Depriester, C., Dormont, D. & Bories, J. (1991). Intracerebral stenosing arteriopathies. Contribution of three radiological techniques to the diagnosis. *Journal of Neuroradiology*, **18**, 32–48.

Rawlinson, D.G. & Braun, C.W. (1981). Granulomatous angiitis of the nervous system first seen as relapsing myelopathy. *Archives of Neurology*, **38**, 129–31.

Reik, L., Grunnet, M.L., Spencer, R.P. & Donaldson, J.O. (1983). Granulomatous angiitis presenting as chronic meningitis and ventriculitis. *Neurology*, **33**, 1609–12.

Rhodes, R.H., Madelaire, N.C., Petrelli, M., Cole, M. & Karaman, B.A. (1995). Primary angiitis and angiopathy of the central nervous system and their relationship to systemic giant cell arteritis. *Archives of Pathology and Laboratory Medicine*, **119**, 334–49.

Riemer, G., Lamszus, K., Zschaber, R., Freitag, H.J., Eggers, C. & Pfeiffer, G. (1999). Isolated angiitis of the central nervous system: lack of inflammation after long-term treatment. *Neurology*, **52**, 196–9.

Scolding, N.J., Jayne, D.R., Zajicek, J.P., Meyer, P.A., Wraight, E.P. & Lockwood, C.M. (1997). Cerebral vasculitis – recognition, diagnosis and management. *Quarterly Journal of Medicine*, **90**, 61–73.

Vollmer, T.L., Guarnaccia, J., Harrington, W., Pacia, S.V. & Petroff, O.A.C. (1993). Idiopathic granulomatous angiitis of the central nervous system: diagnosis challenges. *Archives of Neurology*, **50**, 925–930.

Yamada, M., Itoh, Y., Shintaku, et al. (1996). Immune reactions associated with cerebral amyloid angiopathy. *Stroke*, **27**, 1155–62.

Zuber, M., Blustajn, J., Arquizan, C., Trystram, D., Mas, J.L. & Meder, J.F. (1999). Angiitis of the central nervous system. *Journal of Neuroradiology*, **26**, 101–17.

2

Temporal arteritis

Stephen M. Davis

Department of Neurology, Royal Melbourne Hospital, Victoria, Australia

Introduction

Temporal (giant cell) arteritis is a systemic disease, involving various medium sized and larger arteries, and mostly occurring in elderly patients. In addition to the classical clinical symptoms of headache, jaw claudication and the syndrome of polymyalgia rheumatica, neurological manifestations are common. Blindness due to ischemic optic neuropathy is probably the most common and feared sinister manifestation of the disease, but stroke is a leading cause of death in patients with temporal arteritis (Caselli et al., 1988). Temporal arteritis was first described by Hutchinson in 1890 (Hutchinson, 1890) and later by Horton et al. (1934). The original clinical report described an elderly man, who was unable to wear his hat because of scalp pain. He had inflamed and hardened superficial temporal arteries on examination. The disease is variously called either temporal arteritis or giant cell arteritis. The term 'temporal arteritis' refers to the characteristic involvement of the superficial temporal arteries, while the term 'giant cell arteritis' emphasizes the systemic nature of the disease and the characteristic pathology, with giant cells being typically present in the vessel wall (see colour Figs. 2.1, 2.2).

A number of epidemiological studies have evaluated the incidence, age and gender associations of temporal arteritis (Machado et al., 1988). A Mayo Clinic study reviewed 94 residents of Olmstead County, Minnesota, diagnosed with temporal arteritis between 1950 and 1985 (Machado et al., 1988). In this study, the age and sex-adjusted incidence of the disease was 17.0 persons per 100000, in those aged 50 years or older. There was a marked increase in the incidence of temporal arteritis with age and a threefold greater incidence in women. The authors noted an apparent increase in the incidence of the disease over this 35-year period, particularly in women.

However, this change was considered likely to reflect better awareness of atypical manifestations of the disease. A Swedish necropsy study suggested that the disease might be more common than clinically apparent, with changes of giant cell arteritis found in about 1% of cases (Ostberg, 1973).

On an odd historical note, it was even suggested that the evil dictator Adolf Hitler might have had the disease in the 1940s, with recorded symptoms of headache, impaired vision, sensitivity to pressure in the temporal regions, swollen temporal arteries, constitutional symptoms and a raised erythrocyte sedimentation rate (Redlich, 1993). However, doubt has been cast on this formulation, cluster headache being considered a more likely diagnosis (Schmidt, 1994).

Pathology

Temporal arteritis is a systemic arteritis, despite its predilection for cranial vessels. Any medium or large calibre artery in the body can therefore be affected. Three cardinal histological patterns have been described (Goodman, 1979). These include first a granulomatous arteritis with prominent Langhans giant cells, typically affecting the media of the artery with smooth muscle necrosis and variable destruction of the internal elastic membrane (Fig. 2.2). Secondly, a non-specific panarteritis can affect the entire arterial wall with infiltration of inflammatory cells and eosinophils. Thirdly, an intimal fibrosis can produce occlusion of the vessel lumen. The finding of giant cells, despite the terminology of 'giant cell arteritis,' is not regarded by some pathologists as being mandatory for diagnosis. However, some authors posit that some patients considered to have temporal arteritis without giant cells on pathology, may have a form of polyarteritis (Morgan &

Harris, 1978). The presence of 'skip lesions,' indicating a segment of normal artery between other sections demonstrating active arteritis, constitutes a well-recognized problem in the diagnosis of the disease. In the Mayo Clinic series (Huston et al., 1978), skip lesions were present in 28% of 60 patients with temporal arteritis.

The condition most commonly affects the superficial temporal, occipital, facial and maxillary branches of the external carotid system, where there is high elastic content of the arterial media and adventitia (Goodman, 1979). This is thought to be the likely explanation for the preferential involvement of the ophthalmic and posterior ciliary branches of the internal carotid artery and the relative rarity of intracranial arterial involvement (Goodman, 1979; Wilkinson & Ross Russell, 1972).

However, less common sites of involvement include other medium or large-sized arteries such as the aorta, axillary, brachial and mesenteric arteries (Klein et al., 1975). Klein et al. (1975) reported a series of 248 patients with temporal arteritis, of whom 34 had evidence of involvement of the aorta or its major branches, sometimes with lethal complications. Symptoms indicating large artery involvement included intermittent claudication and Raynaud's phenomenon (Klein et al., 1975). Three of their cases had dissecting aneurysms of the aorta, and arteritis was also seen in the renal arteries. In these patients, abnormal peripheral artery pulsation and bruits over large arteries were typical. Angiography was sometimes useful in distinguishing arteritis from atherosclerosis (Klein et al., 1975).

Cardinal clinical features of temporal arteritis

Goodman (1979) reviewed the most common presenting features of temporal arteritis (Table 2.1). Headache (60%), polymyalgia rheumatica (47%), and jaw claudication (36%) were the most common clinical findings, while diaphoresis (43%), anorexia (36%) and malaise (29%) were other typical clinical manifestations. Fatigue, weight loss and other constitutional symptoms are also common (Huston et al., 1978). The headache is often severe and associated with scalp tenderness, usually in the region of the temporal arteries. Hence, the patient may have scalp pain when brushing the hair, or even resting the head on the pillow. However, the headache pattern is often atypical and the diagnosis should be considered in any elderly patient presenting with headache (Huston et al., 1978). Jaw claudication is perhaps the most specific non-neurological feature of the condition and is due to involvement of the facial artery (Goodman, 1979). Other

Table 2.1. *Cardinal symptoms of temporal arteritis*

Headache
Polymyalgia rheumatica syndrome
Jaw claudication
Constitutional symptoms (anorexia, weight loss, malaise)
Scalp necrosis
Ischemic optic neuropathy
Stroke

clinical manifestations, also due to arteritis of external carotid artery branches, can include scalp, skin and tongue necrosis (see colour Fig. 2.3).

Koorey (1984) reported an Australian series of 35 patients, average age of 71 years and a female:male ratio of 2.2:1. Headache was the most common presenting feature, in 85% of cases, with 29% patients experiencing permanent visual loss. They found that the temporal artery was clinically abnormal in two-thirds of cases. Some patients showed abnormalities in liver function tests (Koorey, 1984). In about three-quarters of their patients, temporal artery biopsy showed giant cells.

The relationship between temporal arteritis and polymyalgia rheumatica is complex, although there is an important overlap between the two conditions and they can merge under clinical observation (Goodman, 1979). In one series, 41% of cases diagnosed with polymyalgia rheumatica had pathological features of temporal arteritis (Fauchald et al., 1972).

Specific neurological and neuro-ophthalmologic manifestations of temporal arteritis

Neurological and neuro-ophthalmological complications are common in patients with temporal arteritis (Table 2.2). Caselli et al. (1988) evaluated the neurological findings in 166 consecutive patients with biopsy proven temporal arteritis. Among these, 31% had neurological features, the most common including various types of neuropathy, stroke and transient ischemic attacks, neuro-otological and neuropsychiatric syndromes, tremor, tongue numbness and myelopathy. The neuropathies include both mononeuropathies and generalised peripheral neuropathies. Among neuro-otological symptoms, vertigo is the most common. Depression is a well-recognized feature in the condition (Caselli et al., 1988; Goodman, 1979) Numbness of the tongue has been attributed to ischemia involving the lingual nerve.

Table 2.2. *Neurological manifestations of temporal arteritis*

Neuro-ophthalmological manifestations	Ischemic optic neuropathy, central retinal artery occlusion, occipital infarction, 3rd, 6th cranial nerve palsies
Neuropathy	Mononeuropathies and generalized peripheral neuropathy
Neuro-otological and neuropsychiatric syndromes	Particularly vertigo, depression, dementia
Tremor	
Tongue numbness	Due to lingual nerve ischemia
Myelopathy	Arteritis of spinal cord
Stroke	Most commonly due to vertebral arteritis

Neuro-ophthalmologic manifestations were evident in 21% of Caselli's series, including amaurosis fugax, permanent visual loss, scintillating scotoma and diplopia (Caselli et al., 1988). In Goodman's series, 'blurred vision' occurred in 16%, amaurosis and diplopia each present in 12% of patients (Goodman, 1979). Diplopia (17%) was also common in Koorey's series, typically due to third cranial nerve involvement with pupillary sparing (Koorey, 1984).

Ischemic optic neuropathy

The two most feared complications of temporal arteritis are blindness and stroke. In Caselli's series (Caselli et al., 1988), 8% of patients had permanent visual loss, and they emphasized that stroke was a leading cause of death in patients with the condition. Other series report higher rates of permanent visual loss, 29% in Koorey's Australian patients (Koorey, 1984), and an overall 36% in Goodman's pooled review of 819 temporal arteritis patients (Goodman, 1979). Visual loss is rarely preceded by a prodrome of amaurosis fugax. Blindness is usually due to anterior ischemic optic neuropathy (AION). This condition more commonly occurs in patients with vascular risk factors such as hypertension and diabetes. It typically manifests as a sudden painless loss of vision and characteristic swelling of the optic disc, sometimes with peripapillary, hemorrhages in the nerve fibre layer, and followed by disc pallor (Sawle et al., 1990) (Fig. 2.4).

The association between AION and temporal arteritis has long been recognized, usually with histological changes in the posterior ciliary arteries (Sawle et al., 1990).

In a personal experience of 300 cases of AION, Hayreh (1981) found that the condition was most commonly due to either thrombosis or embolism of the posterior ciliary arteries, or the distal arterioles feeding the anterior part of the optic nerve. Alternatively, it can be caused by perfusion failure in these nutrient vessels. In AION due to temporal arteritis, visual loss can develop in both eyes within days. Examination findings can include unilateral or bilateral optic disc edema, the Foster–Kennedy syndrome with ipsilateral optic disc edema and contralateral atrophy, or bilateral optic atrophy. In such patients, suggestive features of giant cell arteritis include headache and the characteristic systemic symptoms, with high erythrocyte sedimentation rate (ESR), in the context of severe visual loss with a chalky white appearance of the swollen optic disc (see colour Fig. 2.4). Non-filling of the optic disc and adjacent half of the choroid on fluorescein angiography is typically evident within a few days of visual loss. Temporal artery biopsy is usually confirmatory (Hayreh, 1981). Treatment of AION due to temporal arteritis is an emergency, although the prognosis for visual recovery in the involved eye is extremely poor (Hayreh, 1981). High doses of steroids are used to prevent involvement of the second eye (see below).

Other causes of visual loss in patients with temporal arteritis include ischemic retrobulbar neuritis and central retinal artery occlusion (see colour Fig. 2.5). As indicated above, ophthalmoplegia is quite common, particularly with third and sixth nerve palsies. Horner's syndrome is also well recognized (Reich et al., 1990). Rare neuro-ophthalmologic manifestations include secondary hemorrhagic glaucoma, field defects and cortical blindness due to occipital infarction (Fig. 2.6).

Cerebrovascular manifestations

Cerebral infarction is a well-recognized complication of temporal arteritis and a leading cause of death (Table 2.3). Wilkinson and Ross Russell (1972) first drew attention to the pattern of arterial involvement in patients with stroke complicating temporal arteritis. They pointed out that the distribution of the disease relates to the amount of elastic tissue in the media and adventitia of the major extracranial arteries, producing a high incidence of monocular blindness, occipital blindness and brain stem strokes in patients dying of the disease (Wilkinson & Ross Russell, 1972). The lateral medullary syndrome is a common stroke type. They described four cases with stroke and pointed out the almost invariable involvement of the superficial temporal, vertebral, ophthalmic and posterior ciliary arteries. In contrast, they emphasized the rarity of

Table 2.3. *Stroke in temporal arteritis*

The most common cause of death in patients with temporal arteritis

Related to the degree of elastic tissue in major extracranial arteries

Most commonly involves extracranial vertebral artery

Intracranial arteritis much rarer

Stroke may be presenting manifestation of the disease (even with normal ESR)

Can produce multi-infarct dementia

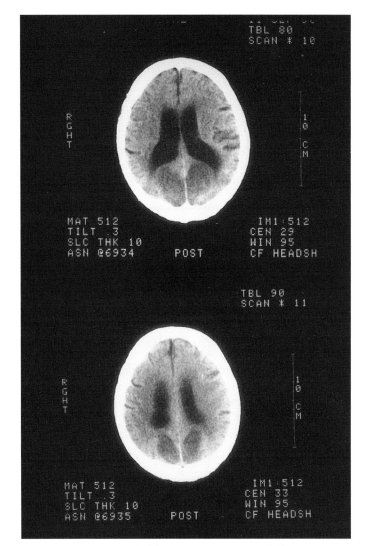

Fig. 2.6. Extensive occipital infarction on CT scan in an elderly patient presenting with cortical blindness following several weeks of severe headache and markedly elevated ESR. The diagnosis was confirmed on temporal artery biopsy.

involvement of intracranial arteries. Hence, the vertebral artery involvement has a sharply defined upper order, typically 5 mm above the point of dural perforation, correlating with the presence of the external elastic lamina. Intracranial arteries are therefore much less commonly affected. Similarly, the internal carotid arteries are often stenoses within the carotid siphon just before they penetrate the dura to enter the cranial cavity. In a necropsy series, Missen (1972) also noted that arterial obstruction in the setting of temporal arteritis was three times more frequent in the vertebral than the internal carotid arteries, correlating with the more common clinical involvement of the vertebrobasilar than the carotid circulation (Fig. 2.6). Enzmann and Scott (1977) also reported two patients with temporal arteritis with cerebrovascular involvement. In one of their patients, diagnosis was made on temporal artery biopsy and cerebral angiography showed diffuse arteritic changes, while the second was made on postmortem examination. In Caselli's series (Caselli et al., 1988), 7% of patients had transient ischemic attacks or brain infarction, including a number on steroid therapy. Contrasting with other reports, two-thirds had carotid territory ischemia, with only one-third affecting the vertebrobasilar territory. Two of their patients had 'top of the basilar' syndromes. Büttner et al. (1994) reported four patients with temporal arteritis and severe vertebrobasilar and carotid territory ischemic strokes.

The usual mechanism for stroke is an arteritis of the vertebral arteries, with secondary thrombosis and often multifocal vertebrobasilar infarction (Missen, 1972). Although arteritis appears to be the primary pathologic factor in brain ischemia, thrombocytosis due to increased production of platelets may well be another important factor (De Keyser et al., 1991). Artery to artery embolism has also been described, as has hemodynamic stroke. Bogousslavsky et al. (1985) reported a case with severe bilateral internal carotid artery stenosis due to temporal arteritis and progressive infarction in the vertebrobasilar territory, suggesting a steal phenomenon from the posterior to anterior circulations.

Intracranial arteritis is much rarer than involvement of extracranial arteries, but has been reported in patients with temporal arteritis (Gibb et al., 1985; McLean et al., 1993). McLean et al. (1993) reported a patient who had intracranial giant cell arteritis, involving the anterior inferior cerebellar and basilar arteries. They pointed out that intracranial involvement by giant cell arteritis should be distinguished from the separate entity of primary cerebral angiitis.

While stroke can occur in the setting of other clinical manifestations of temporal arteritis, it can also be the first indication of the disease, even with a normal ESR (Collado et al., 1989). More commonly, the ESR is elevated, although temporal artery biopsy can still be normal. In addition, brain infarction can develop in patients with temporal arteritis, even after institution of high dose steroid therapy. Reporting one such case, five days after initiation of steroids, the authors suggested treatment with anticoagulation during the first week of steroid therapy (Collazos et al., 1994). Michotte et al. (1986) also reported two patients with fatal brain stem infarction, occurring despite adequate steroid therapy.

Caselli (1990) emphasized the unusual occurrence of dementia in patients with temporal arteritis. Such patients have multifocal cognitive impairment typical of vascular dementia, hence representing a treatable form of the disorder. Multiple cerebral infarcts, predominantly in the posterior circulation territory were demonstrated on neuroimaging (Caselli, 1990). In this series, abrupt cognitive decline, during periods of clinically active disease, was associated with steroid reduction (Caselli, 1990).

In patients dying of temporal arteritis, stroke is the most common cause of death, recorded in five of nine patients studied by Säve-Söderbergh et al. (1986). In their series (Säve-Södebergh et al., 1986), one patient developed a vertebral artery thrombosis with cerebellar infarction following a temporal artery biopsy, but before initiation of steroids. A second patient developed bilateral vertebral thromboses with severe hindbrain ischemia. Despite an ESR of over 100, a diagnosis was not established until postmortem examination. A third patient with clinically diagnosed polymyalgia rheumatica had an exacerbation of the condition with a terminal stroke. A fourth patient developed blindness after temporal artery biopsy and 2 days later had vertebral artery thromboembolism with coma. The final patient developed brain infarction due to involvement of both internal carotid and vertebral arteries despite 40 mg of prednisolone per day. These authors concluded that most of the cerebral deaths in their series were potentially preventable by earlier higher dose steroid therapy (Säve-Söderbergh et al., 1986).

Thielen et al. (1998) reported a patient presenting with a four month history of carotid territory ischaemic attacks and later probable vertebrobasilar transient ischemic attacks. High-grade intracranial stenoses affected the internal carotid and vertebral arteries, in the extradural portions just proximal to the dural entry point. These short segment stenotic lesions should raise the possibility of temporal arteritis.

Temporal arteritis can rarely present with an acute myelopathy. In one case, a patient with active temporal arteritis developed a thoracic myelopathy due to anterior spinal artery infarction, followed 3 days later by a fatal basilar artery thrombosis (Gibb et al., 1985).

Diagnosis

The diagnosis of temporal arteritis is suggested by the presence of the cardinal clinical symptoms in an elderly patient with an elevated ESR (Table 2.4). However, patients with biopsy-proven temporal arteritis and normal ESR estimations are not unusual, occurring in up to 22.5% of cases (Wong & Korn, 1986; Ellis & Ralston, 1983). Many of these patients have ESR levels under 20 mm per hour (Wong & Korn, 1986). Furthermore, changes in the ESR do not necessarily parallel the clinical course (Ellis & Ralston, 1983). McAlindon and Ferguson (1989) described a patient with vertebrobasilar infarction and a normal ESR, with characteristic changes of giant cell arteritis on temporal artery biopsy. Despite high doses of intravenous steroids, the patient later developed an occipital infarction, and subsequent features of mononeuritis multiplex. Mason and Walport (1992) pointed out that the ESR, the most commonly used marker of disease activity, is often unreliable and that the C-reactive protein concentration could be a better index. Other typical laboratory abnormalities include a mild anemia and elevated white blood cell count.

Palpation of the temporal arteries can be helpful. In patients with temporal arteritis, the artery is often firm, difficult to compress and nodular and has no palpable pulse. Transcranial Doppler ultrasound can show thickening and abnormal signals from the arterial walls of the superficial temporal arteries. There is a general consensus that temporal artery biopsy is mandatory in the diagnosis of temporal arteritis, although this does not preclude urgent initiation of steroid therapy (Hall et al., 1983; Hall & Hunder, 1984). Because of the serious complications of temporal arteritis, there is also a consensus that high-dose steroids should be started immediately, particularly as the pathological changes take some time to resolve with steroids. Blindness has been reported where treatment had not been commenced, while waiting for temporal artery biopsy.

Hall et al. (1983) followed up 134 patients of the Olmstead County series with biopsy-proven temporal arteritis between 1965 and 1980. They pointed out the importance of temporal artery biopsy in predicting the need for subsequent steroid therapy. Biopsy should always be performed in elderly patients, before committing them to long-term steroid therapy, which is associated with a 25% risk of vertebral fractures in the elderly (Hall et al., 1983; Huston et al., 1978). In the Mayo Clinic series, the proportion of positive biopsies fell from 82% in the early 1960s to 31% in the early 1970s, indicating the need to perform biopsies in less clear cut presentations of possible temporal arteritis, because of the risk of serious complications. Overall, temporal artery biopsy correctly predicted the need for steroid therapy for temporal arteritis in 94% of cases (positive predictive value) and in 91% of those who were biopsy negative (negative predictive value).

Kattah et al. (1991) pointed out that the segmental pathology of temporal arteritis produced a significant number of false-negative biopsy results, due to the well-recognized problem of 'skip lesions' (see above). They demonstrated the usefulness of occipital artery biopsy in a patient with temporal arteritis and an initially negative superficial temporal artery biopsy. A normal biopsy does not exclude the disorder. In a significant proportion of cases, biopsy of the second side is appropriate in a case where the clinical diagnosis is strongly suspected, but not confirmed by the initial biopsy result (Hall & Hunder, 1984). Angiographic signs are sometimes present, but cerebral angiography has no advantages over biopsy, in itself a benign procedure (Huston & Hunder, 1980). There was previously some concern about the use of temporal artery biopsy in elderly patients because of the possible need for later superficial temporal-middle cerebral anastomosis in stroke prevention, but this was dispelled by the negative results of the extracranial–intracranial bypass trial (The EC/IC Bypass Study Group, 1985).

Treatment

The treatment for temporal arteritis consists of high dose corticosteroids, although there has been debate about the optimal dose to be used to both control the condition, and to prevent relapse with a minimum of adverse steroid effects (Table 2.4). Mason and Walport (1992) suggested that quite low initial doses of prednisolone, in the order of 20 mg daily could be satisfactory for the treatment of temporal arteritis, except in those patients presenting with an acute visual disturbance where a higher dose of 60–80 mg was indicated.

Other authors disagree (Kyle & Hazleman, 1989a,b) and have recommended an initial dose of at least 40 mg per day. Kyle and Hazleman (1989a,b) pointed out that whereas patients with polymyalgia rheumatica require lower doses in the range of 15–20 mg prednisolone per day, patients with giant cell arteritis generally require 40 mg prednisolone and tend to relapse on a reduction to 20 mg per day.

Table 2.4. *Diagnosis and treatment of stroke due to temporal arteritis*

Diagnosis and treatment	Comment
Diagnosis	
ESR	Normal in 22.5% of patients
C-reactive protein	May be more specific than ESR
Temporal artery biopsy	Mandatory for all patients. Skip lesions not uncommon
Treatment	
High dose steroids as acute therapy	Controversy in literature as to initial dose
Maintenance steroids	Dose adjusted for clinical symptoms, ESR, steroid side effects
Duration of treatment	Controversial. Adverse effects of steroids balanced against risk of relapse

The ESR or C-reactive protein assay do not necessarily predict relapse. They advocated 40 mg daily for at least a month, followed by 20–30 mg prednisolone daily for the second month of therapy (Kyle & Hazleman, 1989a,b).

Many authors however would recommend an initially higher dose of steroids and this is certainly the practice of most neurologists. Goodman (1979) suggested initial therapy with 60–80 mg prednisolone daily for 4–6 weeks, followed by a gradual reduction. He pointed out that after 4–6 weeks of high dose steroid therapy, a maintenance dose should be the minimum level of steroid intake required to keep the patient asymptomatic and the ESR within the normal range (Huston et al., 1978).

One of the most controversial issues has been the duration of therapy, related to uncertainties about the duration of the disease and measurement of disease activity. Goodman pointed out that there was no consensus on the duration of therapy, most patients requiring at least one year of treatment (Huston et al., 1978). Other authors (Kyle & Hazleman, 1990) have recommended treatment for at least 2 years, with most patients able to stop steroid therapy after 4–5 years. A minority of patients require long-term, low dose therapy. It has been reported that patients with a combination of both polymyalgia rheumatica and temporal arteritis are more likely to develop relapses. Concerns about complications due to temporal arteritis have to be balanced against the risks of adverse steroid effects. It has been estimated that between 20% and 50% of patients on long-term steroid therapy may have serious side effects, unless the maintenance dose is less than 7.5 mg daily (Kyle & Hazleman, 1989a,b).

In the treatment of temporal arteritis, azathioprine has been found to exert a useful steroid-sparing effect (De Silva & Hazleman, 1986). In summary, most neurologists would advocate high dose oral steroid therapy 60–80 mg daily, with initial use of parenteral high dose steroids if there are neurological complications of temporal arteritis, such as anterior ischemic optic neuropathy or cerebral infarction. Although it is dubious that acute therapy will reverse the immediate complications of the condition, the aim of therapy is to prevent further ischemic sequelae, such as blindness in the second eye or further stroke.

References

Bogousslavsky, J., Deruaz, J.P & Regli, F. (1985). Bilateral obstruction of internal carotid artery from giant-cell arteritis and massive infarction limited to the vertebrobasilar area. *European Neurology*, **24**, 57–61.

Büttner, T., Heye, N. & Przuntek, H. (1994). Temporal arteritis with cerebral complications: report of four cases. *European Neurology*, **34**, 162–7.

Caselli, R.J. (1990). Giant cell (temporal) arteritis: a treatable cause of multi-infarct dementia. *Neurology*, **40**, 753–5.

Caselli, R.J., Hunder, G.G. & Whisnant, J.P. (1988). Neurologic disease in biopsy-proven giant cell (temporal) arteritis. *Neurology*, **38**, 352–9.

Collado, A., Santamaria, J., Ribalta, T., Cinta Cid, M., Canete, J.D. & Tolosa, E. (1989). Giant-cell arteritis presenting with ipsilateral hemiplegia and lateral medullary syndrome. *European Neurology*, **29**, 266–8.

Collazos, J., Garcia-Monco, C., Martin, A., Rodriguez, J., Gomez, M.A. (1994). Multiple strokes after initiation of steroid therapy in giant cell arteritis. *Postgraduate Medical Journal*, **70**, 228–30.

De Keyser, J., De Klippel, N. & Ebinger, G. (1991). Thrombocytosis and ischaemic complications in giant cell arteritis. *British Medical Journal*, **303**, 825.

De Silva, M. & Hazleman, B.L. (1986). Azathioprine in giant cell arteritis/polymyalgia rheumatica: a double blind study. *Annals of Rheumatic Diseases*, **45**, 136–8.

Ellis, M.E. & Ralston, S. (1983). The ESR in the diagnosis and management of the polymyalgia rheumatica/giant cell arteritis syndrome. *Annals of Rheumatic Diseases*, **42**, 168–70.

Enzmann, D. & Scott, W.R. (1977). Intracranial involvement of giant-cell arteritis. *Neurology*, **27**, 794–7.

Fauchald, P., Rygvold, O. & Oystese, B. (1972). Temporal arteritis and polymyalgia rheumatica clinical and biopsy findings. *Annals of Internal Medicine*, **77**, 845–52.

Gibb, W.R., Urry, P.A. & Lees, A.J. (1985). Giant cell arteritis with spinal cord infarction and basilar artery thrombosis. *Journal of Neurology, Neurosurgery and Psychiatry*, **48**, 945–8.

Goodman, B.W. (1979). Temporal arteritis. *American Journal of Medicine*, **67**, 839–52.

Hall, S. & Hunder, G.G. (1984). Is temporal artery biopsy prudent? *Mayo Clinic Proceedings*, **59**, 793–5.

Hall, S., Persellin, S., Lie, J.T., O'Brien, P.C., Kurland, L.T. & Hunder, G.G. (1983). The therapeutic impact of temporal artery biopsy. *Lancet*, **ii**, 1217–20.

Hayreh, S.S. (1981). Anterior ischaemic optic neuropathy. *Archives of Neurology*, **38**, 675–8.

Horton, B.T., Magtath, B. & Brown, G.E. (1934). Arteritis of the temporal vessels. A previously undescribed form. *Archives of Internal Medicine*, **53**, 400–9.

Huston, K.A. & Hunder, G.G. (1980). Giant cell (cranial) arteritis: a clinical review. *American Heart Journal*, **100**, 99–105.

Huston, K.A., Hunder, G.G., Lie, J.T, Kennedy, R.H. & Elveback, L.R. (1978). Temporal arteritis. A 25 year epidemiologic, clinical and pathologic study. *Annals of Internal Medicine*, **88**, 162–7.

Hutchinson, J. (1890). Diseases of the arteries. *Archives of Surgery*, **1**, 323–33.

Kattah, J.C., Cupps, T., Manz, H.J., Khodary, A. & Caputy, A. (1991). Occipital artery biopsy: a diagnostic alternative in giant cell arteritis. *Neurology*, **41**, 949–50.

Klein, R.G., Hunder, G.G., Stanson, A.W. & Sheps, S.G. (1975). Large artery involvement in giant cell (temporal) arteritis. *Annals of Internal Medicine*, **83**, 806–12.

Koorey, D.J. (1984). Cranial arteritis. A twenty year review of cases. *Australia and New Zealand Journal of Medicine*, **14**, 143–7.

Kyle, V. & Hazleman, B.L. (1989a). Treatment of polymyalgia rheumatica and giant cell arteritis II. Relation between steroid dose and steroid associated side effects. *Annals of Rheumatic Diseases*, **48**, 662–6.

Kyle, V. & Hazleman, B.L. (1989b). Treatment of polymyalgia rheumatica and giant cell arteritis I. Steroid regimens in the first two months. *Annals of Rheumatic Diseases*, **48**, 658–61.

Kyle, V. & Hazleman, B.L. (1990). Stopping steroids in polymyalgia rheumatica and giant cell arteritis. *British Medical Journal*, **300**, 344–5.

McAlindon, T.E. & Ferguson, I.T. (1989). Mononeuritis multiplex and occipital infarction complicating giant cell arteritis. *British Journal of Rheumatology*, **28**, 257–8.

Machado, E.B.V., Michet, C.J., Ballard, D.J.et al. (1988). Trends in incidence and clinical presentation of temporal arteritis in Olmstead County, Minnesota, 1950–1985. *Arthritis and Rheumatism*, **31**, 745–9.

McLean, C.A., Gonzales, M.F. & Dowling, J.P. (1993). Systemic giant cell arteritis and cerebellar infarction. *Stroke*, **24**, 899–902.

Mason, J.C. & Walport, M.J. (1992). Giant cell arteritis. *British Medical Journal*, **305**, 68–9.

Michotte, A., de Keyser, J., Dierck, R., Impens, N., Solheid, C. & Ebinger, G. (1986). Brain stem infarction as a complication of giant-cell arteritis. *Clinical Neurology and Neurosurgery*, **88**, 127–9.

Missen, G.A.K. (1972). Involvement of the vertebro-carotid arterial system in giant-cell arteritis. *Journal of Pathology*, **106**, 2–3.

Morgan, G. Jr, & Harris, E.D. Jr. (1978). Non-giant cell arteritis. Three cases and a review of the literature. *Arthritis and Rheumatism*, **21**, 362–6.

Ostberg, G. (1973). An arteritis with special reference to polymyalgia arteritica. *Acta Pathologica Microbiologica Scandinavica*, **237**, 1–59.

Redlich, F.C. (1993). A new medical diagnosis of Adolf Hitler. Giant cell arteritis: temporal arteritis. *Archives of Internal Medicine*, **153**, 693–7.

Reich, K.A., Giansiracusa, D.F. & Strongwater, S.L. (1990). Neurologic manifestations of giant cell arteritis. *American Journal of Medicine*, **89**, 67–72.

Säve-Söderbergh, J., Malmvall, B.E., Andersson, R. & Bengtsson, B.A. (1986). Giant cell arteritis as a cause of death. Report of nine cases. *Journal of the American Medical Association*, **255**, 493–6.

Sawle, G.V., James, C.B. & Ross Russell, R.W. (1990). The natural history of non-arteritic anterior ischaemic optic neuropathy. *Journal of Neurology, Neurosurgery and Psychiatry*, **53**, 830–3.

Schmidt, D. (1994). Giant cell arteritis and Hitler. *Archives of Internal Medicine*, **154**, 930.

The EC/IC Bypass Study Group. (1985). Failure of extracranial–intracranial arterial bypass to reduce the risk of ischemic stroke. Results of an international randomized trial. *New England Journal Medicine*, **313**, 1191–200.

Thielen, K.R., Wijdicks, E.F.M. & Nichols, D.A. (1998). Giant cell (temporal) arteritis: involvement of the vertebral and internal carotid arteries. *Mayo Clinic Proceedings*, **73**, 444–6.

Wilkinson, I.M.S. & Ross Russell, R.W. (1972). Arteries of the head and neck in giant cell arteritis. A pathological study to show the pattern of arterial involvement. *Archives of Neurology*, **27**, 378–91.

Wong, R.L. & Korn, J.H. (1986). Temporal arteritis without an elevated erythrocyte sedimentation rate. Case report and review of the literature. *American Journal of Medicine*, **80**, 959–64.

3

Herpes zoster related vasculopathy and other viral vasculopathies

Ralf W. Baumgartner

Department of Neurology, University Hospital, Zurich, Switzerland

Varicella zoster virus related cerebral vasculopathy

Varicella zoster virus (VZV) is a DNA virus of the herpes family. Ten to 14 days after infection of the host, the vesicular rash characteristic of chickenpox appears (White, 1997). Subsequently, the virus migrates to the dorsal root and trigeminal ganglia, where it remains latent in neurons and satellite cells (Croen et al., 1988). It is assumed that waning of cellular immunity to VZV later in life or during immunosuppression from a variety of causes activates the virus, and herpes zoster, a unilateral, dermatomal vesicular rash ensues (White, 1997).

Epidemiology of neurological complications related to chickenpox and herpes zoster

In temperate climates such as the United States or Europe, almost all individuals are infected by VZV as they reach adulthood, whereas in tropical countries chickenpox is often a disease of young adults (White, 1997). Neurological complications of chickenpox include cerebellar ataxia and encephalitis, which are estimated to occur in 1 per 4000 (Guess et al., 1986) and in 1.7 per 100 000 (Preblud et al., 1984) children beyond 15 years of age, respectively. In addition, a few patients with ischemic strokes occurring after chickenpox were reported (Griffith et al., 1970; Hosseinipour et al., 1998; Leopold, 1993; Bodensteiner et al., 1992; Caekebeke et al., 1990; Eda et al., 1983; Ichiyama et al., 1990; Kamholz & Tremblay, 1985; Liu & Holmes, 1990; Shuper et al. 1990).

Risk factors for the development of herpes zoster are increasing age, immunosuppresssion, VZV infection acquired in utero or during the first year of life, and white compared to black race (Guess et al., 1986; Schmader et al., 1995). The estimated annual incidence rates of zoster are 74 per 100 000 children younger than 10 years of age compared to 1010 per 100 000 adults aged 80–90 years (Hope-Simpson, 1965). In the immunocompetent host, complications of the central nervous system (CNS) were 0.2% in a population-based study (Ragozzino et al., 1982). They consist of cranial neuropathy including Ramsey–Hunt syndrome (Jemsek et al., 1983), encephalomyelitis (Rose et al., 1964), optic neuritis (Jemsek et al., 1983) and leukencephalitis (Horton et al., 1981). In rare cases ischemic strokes occur several weeks after the onset of zoster. VZV infections of the CNS develop preferentially in immunocompromised individuals, especially those affected by the human immunodeficiency virus (HIV) and cancer (Jemsek et al., 1983; Dolin et al., 1978; Gray et al., 1994). CNS affection was detected in 1.5–4.4% of autopsy cases evaluating immunocompromised patients (Gray et al., 1991, 1994; Petito et al., 1986), while other neuropathological series did not mention any case (Anders et al., 1986; Budka et al., 1987; Lang et al., 1989). In the presence of HIV infection, VZV vasculopathy of the CNS occurred often late in the course of the infection, in patients with marked CD4+ depletion. This was not only true in postmortem series (Gray et al., 1994; Ryder et al., 1986; Morgello et al., 1988; Gilden et al., 1988; Rostad et al., 1989; Rosenblum, 1989; Vinters et al., 1988; McArthur, 1987; Baudrimont et al., 1994), but also in clinical observations of patients whose neurological deficits improved after antiviral treatment (Rousseau et al., 1993). The new highly active antiretroviral therapy (HAART) for patients infected with HIV substantially decreased the morbidity and mortality due to HIV infection (Egger et al., 1997; Gulick et al., 1997; Hammer et al., 1997; Palella et al., 1998; Powderly et al., 1998) (see 'Human immunodeficiency virus related vasculopathy'). Consequently, it is very likely that the incidence of VZV vasculopathy will decrease in patients treated with HAART.

Pathogenesis of cerebral vasculopathy related to chickenpox and herpes zoster

Chickenpox related cerebral vasculopathy is assumed to result from hematogenous viral invasion of vessel walls by VZV as has been shown for herpes zoster (see below). In addition, VZV-specfic IgG antibodies were identified in the cerebrospinal fluid (CSF) of two patients with strokes occurring after chickenpox (Caekebeke et al., 1990; Shuper et al., 1990). However, VZV-specific IgG antibodies can still be demonstrated several months after uncomplicated herpes zoster (Haanpää et al., 1998), and do not *per se* provide definite evidence for active infection. Furthermore, in other reports VZV-specific antibodies were either not detected (Leopold, 1993) or not mentioned (Hosseinipour et al., 1998), or the CSF/blood quotient for albumin was not given preventing an adequate interpretation of the CSF VZV-specific antibody titres (Shuper et al., 1990). Finally, no virus particles, antigen or DNA in the wall of vessels assumed to be affected by VZV after chickenpox were demonstrated (Griffith et al., 1970; Hosseinipour et al., 1998; Leopold, 1993; Bodensteiner et al., 1992; Caekebeke et al., 1990; Eda et al., 1983; Ichiyama et al., 1990; Kamholz & Tremblay, 1985; Liu & Holmes, 1990; Shuper et al., 1990). Therefore, the causal relationship of chickenpox and subsequent intracranial arteriopathy is unproven. Because chickenpox is a frequent disease, subsequent occurrence of cerebral vasculopathy and stroke may have been a coincidence.

Herpes zoster related cerebral vasculopathy is well documented in autopsy studies due to the detection of herpes-virus nucleocapsids by electron microscopy (Doyle et al., 1983; Linnemann & Alvira, 1980), VZV antigen by immunocytochemistry, and VZV DNA by *in situ* hybridization or polymerase chain reaction (PCR) (Gray et al., 1994; Morgello et al., 1988; Amlie-Lefond et al., 1995; Eidelberg et al., 1986; Gilden et al., 1996; Kleinschmidt-DeMasters et al., 1998; Melanson et al., 1996), in the walls of large and small intracranial arteries. In the pathogenesis of intracranial vasculopathy both a VZV-induced autoimmune process and viral invasion of the vessels are proposed (Melanson et al., 1996). Several possibilities for access of VZV to the cerebral vessels have been reported. (*a*) After the occurrence of HZO the virus may reach the arterial wall by direct neural passage along intracranial branches of the trigeminal nerve (Eidelberg et al., 1986; MacKenzie et al., 1981). Trigeminovascular innervation is unilateral and more dense in the middle (MCA) and anterior (ACA) than other cerebral arteries (Mayberg et al., 1980; Moskowitz, 1970). This may explain that cerebral vasculopathy occurs more frequently after ophthalmic compared to segmental herpes zoster, is frequently located on the side of the skin lesion, and is often distributed in the MCA or ACA (Eidelberg et al., 1986; MacKenzie et al., 1981). (*b*) Hematogenous seeding of intracranial vessels. A recent study indicated that VZV viremia is a frequent event in patients with herpes zoster, and that subclinical reactivations occur in immunocompetent and immunocompromised subjects (Mainka et al., 1998). Pathological studies suggest that, in some cases, VZV may enter the spinal cord and small vessels via axonal spread from dermatomal zoster (Amlie-Lefond et al., 1995). (*c*) Antero- or retrograde transaxonal and transsynaptic spread may occur within the CNS (Gray et al., 1994; Rostad et al., 1989; Amlie-Lefond et al., 1995; Cheatham, 1953).

Cerebral vasculopathy related to herpes zoster

The syndrome of HZO followed 2–6 weeks (range 1 week to 6 months) later by contralateral hemiplegia related to vasculopathy of large cerebral arteries was first recognized in 1896 (Brissaud, 1896). Since then, 68 further occurrences were reported (Gray et al., 1994; Doyle et al., 1983; Eidelberg et al., 1986; Melanson et al., 1996; MacKenzie et al., 1981; Baudouin & Lantuéjoul, 1919; Perrin et al., 1938; Gordon & Tucker, 1945; Hughes, 1951; Cope & Jones, 1954; Deitz, 1955; Minton, 1956; Anastasopoulos et al., 1958; Laws, 1960; Acers, 1964; Panchi & Romanes, 1966; Kolodny et al., 1968; Norris et al., 1970; Sato et al., 1971; Rosenblum & Hadfield, 1972; Walker et al., 1973; Gilbert, 1974; Rehurek et al., 1974; Gardner-Thorpe et al., 1976; Nishimaru & Kamei, 1976; Victor & Green, 1976; Pratesi et al., 1977; Sipe & Rosenberg, 1977; Onoda & Takahashi, 1979; Gursoy et al., 1980; Ruppenthal, 1980; Kuroiwa & Furukawa, 1981; Landi et al., 1981; Federico et al., 1982; McComas & Gutman, 1982; Vecht & Sande, 1982; Bourdette et al., 1983; Elble, 1983; Hilt et al., 1983; Menkes et al., 1983; Inoue et al., 1984; Reshef et al., 1985; Verghese & Sugar, 1986; Freedman & MacDonald, 1987; Sung et al., 1989; Sureda et al., 1989; Alvarez et al., 1990; Czlonkowska et al., 1991; Schmidbauer et al., 1992; Lexa et al., 1993; Munoz et al., 1995; Sarazin et al., 1995; Terborg & Busse, 1995) suggesting that it is the most frequent zoster related cerebral vasculopathy. More widespread neurological deficits including optical nerve infarction have been noted (Bourdette et al., 1983; Hilt et al., 1983; Reshef et al., 1985; Lexa et al., 1993; Terborg & Busse, 1995). In some cases zoster rash did not involve the trigeminal nerve (Kolodny et al., 1968; Rosenblum & Hadfield, 1972; Hilt et al., 1983), followed the CNS deficits (Jemsek et al., 1983) or was absent (Amlie-Lefond et al., 1995).

The clinical course was characterized by gradual resolution of cutaneous HZO followed by the acute onset of contralateral hemiparesis, hemisensory symptoms, or aphasia (Hilt et al., 1983; Reshef et al., 1985). The neurological manifestations were usually monophasic, but some patients had recurrent strokes (Hilt et al., 1983; Reshef et al., 1985). Transient ischemic attacks and amaurosis fugax were uncommon (Gilbert, 1974; Dalal & Dalal, 1989). In addition, Reshef et al. (1985) reported diffuse CNS symptoms in 47% of 51 patients following the onset of HZO. The symptoms occurred prior to, at, or following, the appearance of contralateral hemiparesis and consisted of stupor, somnolence, confusion, delirium, memory deficits or depression. Prognosis of stroke is guarded as mortality was 20–28% (Hilt et al., 1983; Reshef et al., 1985), and 34% had moderate or severe, and 38% mild or no neurological deficits (Hilt et al., 1983). Stroke-related death generally resulted from brain edema and herniation subsequent to an acute infarction (Doyle et al., 1983; Eidelberg et al., 1986). Immunocompromised patients probably had a greater mortality compared to patients with cerebral infarction alone (Reshef et al., 1985). This may explain that most autopsy reports of VZV vasculopathy derived from the latter group (Gray et al., 1994; Ryder et al., 1986; Morgello et al., 1988; Rosenblum, 1989; Doyle et al., 1983; Linnemann & Alvira, 1980; Amlie-Lefond et al., 1995; Eidelberg et al., 1986; Kolodny et al., 1968; Rosenblum & Hadfield, 1972; Hilt et al., 1983) compared to the scarcity of pathological descriptions in immunocompetent patients (Bourdette et al., 1983; Hilt et al., 1983; Reshef et al., 1985).

CSF studies were abnormal in 70% (Reshef et al., 1985). Most normal CSF samples were obtained only once. The most common findings were an elevated white blood cell (WBC) count consisting essentially of mononuclear cells (mean, 46; range, 0–1200 WBC/mm^3), elevated protein (mean, 90; range, 30–445 μg/dl) and normal levels of glucose (mean, 90; range, 30–445 μg/dl) (Reshef et al., 1985). Less frequently noted abnormalities included increased polymorphonuclear leukocytes (65–100% of WBC, up to 1200/mm^3) (Doyle et al., 1983; Hughes, 1951) and hypoglycorrhachia (Reshef et al., 1985). Antibodies directed against VZV, VZV antigens and DNA (PCR) can be detected in CSF to confirm the diagnosis of VZV affection of the CNS. Definite proof of a possible causal link between vasculopathy and VZV age can only be obtained by detecting viral antigen or DNA in the wall of cerebral arteries (see above). Cerebral biopsy, however, is frequently not indicated in these patients. Computed tomography (CT) or magnetic resonance imaging (MRI) of the brain showed non-specific findings consistent with ischemic infarction. Less frequently symptomatic hemorrhage complicating ischemic infarction (Elble, 1983), subarachnoid hemorrhage (Fukumoto et al., 1986) and basal meningitis (Gray et

al., 1994) were depicted. Infarcts were located in the superficial and/or deep territories of the MCA or ACA. Less frequent were infarcts located in the territories of both MCAs or ACAs, and of the posterior cerebral (PCA) or basilar (BA) arteries (Rosenblum, 1989; Baudrimont et al., 1994; Linnemann & Alvira, 1980; Eidelberg et al., 1986; Reshef et al., 1985). Cerebral catheter or magnetic resonance angiography showed abnormal findings in most cases. They included irregular beaded or segmental narrowing or occlusion of one or more basal cerebral arteries and/or their main branches including the siphon and the terminal segment of the intracranial internal carotid artery (ICA), the MCA, ACA, PCA or BA. Several authors reported obstructions of contralateral (Reshef et al., 1985) or both ACAs (Terborg & Busse, 1995) or both MCAs (Pratesi et al., 1977), and mycotic aneurysms (Gursoy et al., 1980; Fukumoto et al., 1986; O'Donohue & Enzmann, 1987).

Autopsy features of VZV vasculopathy are determined by various factors, including the phase of disease at which autopsy is performed (acute vs. chronic), host immune responsiveness, the route of viral spread to the brain from latent infection, and probably treatment (Gray et al., 1994; Gilden et al., 1996; Schmidbauer et al., 1992; Gilden & Kleinschmidt-DeMasters, 1998). Furthermore, leptomeningeal arteries showed variable abnormalities which could be present in the same brain. On one side thrombotic occlusion of large vessels with little or no inflammation or marked intimal proliferation producing severe luminal narrowing occasionally associated with thrombosis were detected (Gray et al., 1994; Eidelberg et al., 1986). On the other side granulomatous arteriitis with numerous histiocytic and fewer giant cells (Gilden et al., 1996; Hilt et al., 1983; Fukumoto et al., 1986; Blue & Rosenblum, 1983; Rosenblum et al., 1978) and rare cases with necrotizing arteriitis (Gray et al., 1994; Doyle et al., 1983) were found. One patient showed features of subarachnoid hemorrhage due to a ruptured aneurysm of the BA, which was affected by granulomatous angiitis (Fukumoto et al., 1986). There is also a more tenuous relationship between HZV infection and primary granulomatous angiitis of the nervous system (PACNS). PACNS primarily affects small penetrating and leptomeningeal vessels in a more diffuse inflammatory process associated with giant cells and granuloma formation (Kolodny et al., 1968; Cravioto & Feigin, 1959). The occasional association of PACNS with antecedent VZV infection has suggested a causal relationship (Rosenblum & Hadfield, 1972; Gilbert, 1974), and in one patient with PACNS herpesvirus nucleocapsids were detected in the wall of affected vessels (Linneman & Alvira, 1980).

In contrast to the abundance of reports of large vessel

disease due to VZV, vasculopathy of small cerebral arteries was not appreciated until Horton et al. (1981) first described fatal VZV encephalitis in patients with cancer. This was later confirmed by other groups who showed that VZV related small vessel disease occurred essentially in immunocompromised patients (Gray et al., 1994; Ryder et al., 1986; Morgello et al., 1988; Rostad et al., 1989; Rosenblum, 1989; Vinters et al., 1988; McArthur, 1987; Baudrimont et al., 1994; Linnemann et al., 1980; Amlie-Lefond et al., 1995; Gilden et al., 1996; Kleinschmidt-DeMasters et al., 1998; Kolodny et al., 1968; Rosenblum & Hadfield, 1972; Hilt et al., 1983; Blue & Rosenblum, 1983; Rosenblum et al., 1978). The neurological signs and symptoms consisted of a progressive encephalopathy with headache, mental status changes and focal neurological deficits. The neurological deficit was also determined by the fact that the vasculopathy affected essentially the cerebral hemispheres and in rare cases the brainstem (Rosenblum, 1989; Baudrimont et al., 1994). In some patients, clinical features due to concomitant large cerebral artery disease as mentioned above were present (Amlie-Lefond et al., 1995). The clinical course of small vessel disease is unknown, because no case diagnosed by brain biopsy has yet been reported. CSF findings were similar to those observed in patients with vasculopathy of the large cerebral arteries. CT and MRI of the brain showed multiple superficial and deep infarcts, either ischemic or hemorrhagic, with disproportionate involvement of white matter and a predilection for grey–white matter junctions (Amlie-Lefond et al., 1995). Cerebral angiography depicted in some cases signs of intracranial large cerebral artery disease as described above. At autopsy generally lesser degrees of blood vessel inflammation were found (Kleinschmidt-DeMasters et al., 1998). Nevertheless, cases with granulomatous (Linnemann & Alvira, 1980; Gilden et al., 1996; Kolodny et al., 1968; Rosenblum & Hadfield, 1972; Hilt et al., 1983; Blue & Rosenblum, 1983; Rosenblum et al., 1978) and necrotizing arteriitis (Gray et al., 1994; Kleinschmidt-DeMasters et al., 1998) were reported. Further findings were usually deep seated, multifocal small lesions that involved white matter more than grey matter, and that were often concentrated at grey–white matter junctions. Their mixed ischemic–demyelinative composition resulted from both vasculopathy related ischemia and from spreading of VZV into neurons, glia and especially oligodendrocytes causing focal demyelination. Some authors appreciated the additional presence of necrotic lesions (Gray et al., 1994; Amlie-Lefond et al., 1995).

Neurological deficits in patients with VZV-related cerebral vasculopathy not only result from different sizes and location of blood vessels involved, but may also be due to concomitant parenchymal penetration by VZV. Immunocompromised patients are particularly likely to develop an extension of the virus beyond the vasculature into CNS parenchyma producing combinations of large and small vessel disease, myelitis, ventriculitis, encephalitis, and leukencephalopathy (Gray et al., 1994; Amlie-Lefond et al., 1995). Finally, patients with HIV infection have other possible causes of CNS deficits (see 'Human immunodeficiency virus related vasculopathy').

It is unclear whether treatment of herpes zoster with antiviral agents prevents the development of subsequent cerebral vasculopathy and stroke. Case reports of cerebral vasculopathy and stroke following HZO treated by acyclovir suggest that this is not the case (Melanson et al., 1996; Terborg & Busse, 1995).

No proven treatment of VZV-associated intracranial vasculopathy has been described, and in most cases therapy did not noticeably alter the clinical course (Gray et al., 1994; Amlie-Lefond et al., 1995; Kleinschmidt-DeMasters et al., 1998; Hilt et al., 1983; Reshef et al., 1985). Nevertheless, patients with VZV-related cerebral vasculopathy should receive antiviral therapy. In immunocompetent patients valacyclovir (1 g orally 3 times daily for 7 days) and famacyclovir (500 mg orally every 8 h for 7 days) are preferable to acyclovir (800 mg orally 5 times daily for 7 days) (Balfour, 1999). In immunocompromised patients intravenous administration of acyclovir (10 mg per kg body weight every 8 h for 7 days) is recommended (Amlie-Lefond et al., 1995; Balfour, 1999). The role of corticosteroid therapy is controversial. Although these drugs are contraindicated in patients with acute ischemic stroke (Adams et al., 1994; The European Ad Hoc Consensus Group, 1997), many authors administered steroids due to the possible presence of granulomatous angiitis (Doyle et al., 1983; Amlie-Lefond et al., 1995; Melanson et al., 1996; MacKenzie et al., 1981; Gilbert, 1974; Pratesi et al., 1977; Hilt et al., 1983; Reshef et al., 1985; Terborg & Busse, 1995). The optimal antithrombotic therapy for acute ischemic stroke and secondary prevention are unknown. Aspirin may be appropriate in the acute ischemic stroke setting due to the low hemorrhagic risk (International Stroke Trial Collaborative Group, 1997). Anticoagulation and fibrinolytics should be administered with caution taking the possible presence of acute (necrotizing) vasculitis (Gray et al., 1994; Doyle et al., 1983; Kleinschmidt-DeMasters et al., 1998) and mycotic aneurysms (Gursoy et al., 1980; Fukumoto et al., 1986; O'Donohue & Enzmann, 1987) into consideration. Nevertheless, several patients with cerebral large artery vasculopathy were treated with anticoagulants and had 'good recovery' in two cases (MacKenzie et al.,

1981), mild (Laws, 1960) and moderate (Gilbert, 1974) disability in one case each. Secondary prevention is probably not necessary in immunocompetent patients, because no case with relapse of vasculopathy and stroke has been reported. Conversely, secondary prevention is justified in immunocompromised patients due to the frequently progressive course of vasculopathy.

Cerebral vasculopathy related to chickenpox

The association of chickenpox and ischemic stroke has been described in young adults (Griffith et al., 1970; Gibbs & Fisher, 1986; Hosseinipour et al., 1998; Leopold, 1993) and children (Bodensteiner et al., 1992; Caekebeke et al., 1990; Eda et al., 1983; Ichiyama et al., 1990; Kamholz & Tremblay, 1995; Liu & Holmes, 1990; Shuper et al., 1990). The *clinical syndrome* consisted of hemiparesis or aphasia occurring one to three months after the acute phase of chickenpox (Griffith et al., 1970; Gibbs & Fisher, 1986; Hosseinipour et al., 1998; Leopold, 1993; Bodensteiner et al., 1992; Caekebeke et al., 1990; Eda et al., 1983; Ichiyama et al., 1990; Kamholz & Tremblay, 1985; Liu & Holmes, 1990; Shuper et al., 1990). In contrast to herpes zoster related cerebral vasculopathy, no patient showed additional neurological and neuroradiological features of encephalopathy. Stroke recurrence 6 months later was reported in one child (Shuper et al., 1990). CSF findings ranged from normal to a mild monocytic pleocytosis and a raised protein content (Hosseinipour et al., 1998). In one patient WBCs contained 27% segmented neutrophils (Hosseinipour et al., 1998). Furthermore, VZV-specific antibodies were detected in the CSF of two patients (Caekebeke et al., 1990; Shuper et al., 1990). CT or MRI of the brain showed unilateral infarcts in the superficial or deep territories of the MCA (Hosseinipour et al., 1998; Leopold, 1993; Shuper et al., 1990). Cerebral catheter or MR angiography were either normal (Eda et al., 1983) or disclosed unilateral occlusion of supraclinoid ICA in four cases (Leopold, 1993; Bodensteiner et al., 1992; Caekebeke et al., 1990; Liu & Holmes, 1990), segments of narrowing and beading or focal stenoses of the MCA and ACA, and in one case of the PCA or the BA (Hosseinipour et al., 1998; Kamholz & Tremblar, 1985; Shuper et al., 1990), sometimes associated with distal occlusions (Kamholz & Tremblay, 1985). The best treatment of ischemic strokes subsequent to chickenpox is unknown. Some patients were treated without antiviral medication or steroids, other patients had intravenous acyclovir, steroids, or both (Griffith et al., 1970; Gibbs & Fisher, 1986; Hosseinipour et al, 1998; Leopold, 1993; Bodensteiner et al., 1992; Caekebeke et al., 1990; Eda et al., 1983; Ichiyama et al., 1990; Kamholz &

Tremblay, 1985; Liu & Holmes, 1990; Shuper et al., 1990). Antithrombotic therapy was either not given or consisted of aspirin (plus low molecular weight heparin in one case) (Griffith et al., 1970; Gibbs & Fisher, 1986; Hosseinipour et al., 1998; Leopold, 1993; Bodensteiner et al., 1992; Caekebeke et al., 1990; Eda et al., 1983; Ichiyama et al., 1990; Kamholz & Tremblay, 1985; Liu & Holmes, 1990; Shuper et al., 1990). No antithrombotics for secondary stroke prevention were administered (Griffith et al., 1970; Gibbs & Fisher, 1986; Hosseinipour et al., 1998; Leopold, 1993; Bodensteiner et al., 1992; Caekebeke et al., 1990; Eda et al., 1983; Ichiyama et al., 1990; Kamholz & Tremblay, 1985; Liu & Holmes, 1990; Shuper et al., 1990).

Human immunodeficiency virus related cerebral vasculopathy

Treatment of patients infected with HIV has changed enormously in the last few years. In 1996, a combination of two nucleosides became the recommended initial regimen as several trials have shown that this therapy is superior to zidovudine alone (Carpenter et al., 1996). More recently, HAART consisting of a protease inhibitor and two non-nucleoside analogue reverse transcriptase inhibitors led to suppression of plasma HIV concentrations and repletion of CD4+ cell counts, translating into substantial decreases of morbidity and mortality due to AIDS (Egger et al., 1997; Gulick et al., 1997; Hammer et al., 1997; Palella et al., 1998), and reduction in the incidence of AIDS (Powderly et al., 1998). Therefore the incidence of HIV-related cerebral vasculopathy might decrease in patients treated with HAART. Unfortunately, of the more than 30 million patients worldwide who are living with the HIV infection, only a tiny proportion will have access to HAART, and it is thus unlikely that the overall incidence of HIV-related cerebral vasculopathy will decrease.

Before the introduction of HAART, CNS dysfunction frequently complicated the course of HIV infection. Involvement of the CNS occurred due to primary HIV infection or to secondary complications of immunodeficiency such as infection with opportunistic microorganisms and neoplasm. In a recent review Pinto (1996) concluded that it remained unclear whether there is an association between stroke and AIDS in adults. Subsequently, Qureshi et al. (1997) found in a retrospective case-control study that HIV infection was associated with an increased risk of stroke. However, their patients had a mean age of 35 years, used cocaine in 40%, were HIV seropositive in 22% and had AIDS in 9% (Qureshi et al., 1997). Besides the possibility of cocaine-related strokes, the latter patients do not reflect the average stroke patient and the issue of an association between HIV infection and stroke remains unanswered.

The incidence of symptomatic cerebrovascular disease in pediatric AIDS is 1.3%, but at autopsy cerebrovascular lesions were present in 25% (Burns, 1992; Husson et al., 1992). The pathomechanisms include cardiac embolism, hypoperfusion, thrombocytopenia, and vasculopathy related to VZV, mycobacterial or fungal infections. Reports on 13 cases suggest that children with AIDS may rarely develop cerebral aneurysmal arteriopathy, which may cause ischemic and hemorrhagic strokes (Husson et al., 1992; Dubrovsky et al., 1998; Park et al., 1990; Philippet et al., 1994; Shah et al., 1996; Lang et al., 1992). Strokes in AIDS patients with VZV vasculopathy are given in the chapter 'VZV-related cerebral vasculopathy'.

Cerebral granulomatous angiitis related to HIV infection

An actual review of the literature for the presence of HIV/AIDS related vasculopathy resulted in the detection of two adult patients, who had autopsy proven cerebral arteriitis possibly related to HIV infection (Yankner et al., 1986; Scaravilli et al., 1989). In the first case HIV infection was probably limited to the CNS at the time of evaluation (Yankner et al., 1986), whereas the second patient had AIDS (Scaravilli et al., 1989). The patients developed a progressive encephalopathic syndrome with short-term memory deficits, disorientation to time and place, inappropriate behaviour, and focal neurological deficits. CT of the brain showed bilateral, non-enhancing, hypodense lesions with supra- and infratentorial location and cerebral atrophy. Cerebral catheter angiography was done in the first patient and revealed diffuse and segmental narrowing of both ACAs, MCAs, PCAs and superior cerebellar arteries. Autopsy showed granulomatous arteriitis of large and medium-sized intracerebral and leptomeningeal arteries with severe luminal narrowing and thrombosis with vessel occlusion, and infarcts located in the cortex, white matter and basal ganglia of both cerebral hemispheres, and the pons. However, no viral material was detected in the wall of intracranial vessels, and the causal relationship between cerebral vasculopathy and HIV remains unproven.

Cerebral aneurysmal arteriopathy in childhood AIDS

Cerebral aneurysmal arteriopathy (CAA) is characterized by diffuse dilatation of the large intracranial cerebral arteries (Husson et al., 1992; Dubrovsky et al., 1998; Park et al., 1990; Shah et al., 1996; Philippet et al., 1994; Lang et al., 1992). Dubrovsky et al. (1998) recently described clinical and radiological features of 13 children with CAA. Cerebrovascular disease was detected 2 to 11 years following HIV infection and, on average, 2½ years after the diagnosis of AIDS. All children had a severely depressed immune system with a history of multiple opportunistic infections, and the mean CD4+ count was 23 (range, 0 to 107) at the time of CAA diagnosis. Three children were asymptomatic, ten had strokes due ischemic infarction in eight and fatal subarachnoid and intracerebral hemorrhage in two cases. Five children presented with unilateral ischemic strokes affecting the basal ganglia or the thalamus, and three had bihemispheric ischemic infarcts. A second ischemic stroke occurred in three patients. The mean survival time after diagnosis of CAA was 8 months and shortened to 5.5 months after cerebrovascular accidents. The few performed CSF studies were normal. Cerebral CT, MRI, catheter or magnetic resonance angiography showed uni- or bilateral ectasia and aneurysmal dilatation of the large intracranial cerebral arteries. Three patients with ischemic strokes had catheter angiography, which showed in addition segmental stenoses (Park et al., 1990) or thrombotic occlusions (Philippet et al., 1994) of small cortical branches distal to the dilated cerebral arteries. These findings suggest that ischemic strokes may have resulted from arterio-arterial thromboembolism originating in the dilated large cerebral arteries, a well-known phenomenon in cerebral aneurysms of adult patients. Autopsy studies were done in four children and confirmed vascular ectasia and aneurysmal dilatation limited to the large basal cerebral arteries, whereas leptomeningeal and intraparenchymal arteries and arterioles were spared. Typical findings were medial fibrosis with loss of muscularis, destruction of the internal elastic lamina, and intimal hyperplasia suggesting the prior presence of vasculitis. The very unusual presentation of the vasculopathy and the detection of HIV protein or genomic material in two autopsy cases argue in favour of an HIV-related arteriitis as a possible causative factor (Dubrovsky et al., 1998; Kure et al., 1989). Unilateral involvement of the cerebral arteries in three children and the presence of ipsilateral HZO in one of the three children suggest also that VZV may have played a pathogenetic role.

Other viruses and cerebral vasculopathy

Several observations suggest that infection with cytomegalovirus (CMV) or herpes simplex virus (HSV) plays a role in the pathogenesis of atherosclerosis. Clinical studies reported an increased prevalence of CMV and HSV infections among individuals with accelerated atherosclerosis in the extracranial carotid arteries (Melnick et al., 1990; Nieto et al., 1996; Sorlie et al., 1994). In addition, histopathological studies have detected CMV and HSV particles within atherosclerotic vessels (Benditt et al., 1983; Gyorkey et al., 1984; Hendrix et al., 1990), and infection with HSV-induced atherosclerosis in avian models (Minick et al., 1979). Furthermore, prior infection with CMV has been shown to be a strong independent risk factor for restenosis after coronary atherectomy (Zhou et al., 1996). Conversely, two prospective studies including a nested case-control study of apparently healthy American men followed up over a 12-year period found no evidence of a positive association between baseline IgG antibodies directed against CMV or HSV and the development of future thromboembolic stroke and myocardial infarction (Fagerberg et al., 1999; Ridker et al., 1998). CMV was present in smooth-muscle cells from restenotic lesions of patients who have undergone coronary angioplasty, and can express immediate early gene products, which can inhibit the p53 tumour-suppressor gene product (Speir et al., 1994). In conclusion, infection with CMV, HSV or both may play a role in the pathogenesis of atherosclerosis of the extracranial and probably also intracranial cerebral arteries.

Cerebral arteriitis in other viral infections

A patient treated with immunosuppressive therapy for a lymphoma developed a progressive neurological deficit characterized by decreasing alertness, epileptic seizures, blindness, deafness and paraplegia (Koeppen et al., 1981). Autopsy showed multiple infarcts in the brain and spinal cord due to occlusive arteriitis, and electron microscopy of brain and retinal tissue revealed particles compatible with CMV. Another patient with progressive focal neurologic deficit showed granulomatous vasculitis affecting the leptomeninx and reaching into cerebral tissue, and PCR revealed HSV type 1 as the cause of inflammation (Schmidt et al., 1992). Brain biopsy in a case with stealth viral encephalopathy delineated also focal perivascular lymphocytic inflammation in the leptomeninges and brain parenchyma (Martin, 1996). In all presumed viral vasculitides of the brain mentioned above no CMV, HSV type 1 or stealth virus material was detected in the wall of cerebral arteries. Therefore, the cause of the vasculitis remains unclear.

References

Acers, T.E. (1964). Herpes zoster ophthalmicus complicated by contralateral hemiplegia. *Archives of Ophthalmology*, **63**, 273–80.

Adams, H.P.J., Brott, T.G., Crowell, R.B. et al. (1994). Guidelines for the management of patients with acute ischemic stroke. A statement for healthcare professionals from a special writing group of the stroke council, American Heart Association. *Stroke*, **25**, 1901–14.

Alvarez, R., Graus, F., Abos, J. et al. (1990). Postherpetic vasculopathy. A study of 3 cases in immunosuppressed patients. *Medical Clinics*, **95**, 782–4.

Amlie-Lefond, C., Kleinschmidt-DeMasters, B.K., Mahalingam, R., Davis, L.E. & Gilden, D.H. (1995). The vasculopathy of varicella zoster virus encephalitis. *Annals of Neurology*, **37**, 784–90.

Anastasopoulos, G., Routsonis, K. & Ierodiakonou, C.S. (1958). Ophthalmic zoster with contralateral hemiplegia. *Journal of Neurology, Neurosurgery and Psychiatry*, **21**, 210–12.

Anders, K.H., Guerra, W.F., Tomiyasu, U., Verity, M.A. & Vinters, H.V. (1986). The neuropathology of AIDS. UCLA experience and review. *American Journal of Pathology*, **124**, 537–58.

Balfour, H.H. Jr. (1999). Antiviral drugs. *New England Journal of Medicine*, **340**, 1255–68.

Baudouin, E. & Lantuéjoul, P. (1919). Les troubles moteurs dans le zona. *Gazette des Hopitaux*, **82**, 1293–5.

Baudrimont, M., Mou`lignier, A., Huerre, M. & Dupont, B. (1994). Varicella-zoster virus (VZV) brain stem encephalitis: report of one case [abstract]. *Neuropathology and Applied Neurobiology*, **20**, 313.

Benditt, E.P., Barrett, T. & McDougall, J.K. (1983). Viruses in the etiology of atherosclerosis. *Proceedings of the National Academy of Sciences, USA*, **80**, 6386–9.

Blue, M.C. & Rosenblum, W.C. (1983). Granulomatous angiitis of the brain with herpes zoster and varicella encephalitis. *Archives of Pathology and Laboratory Medicine*, **107**, 126–8.

Bodensteiner, J.B., Hille, M.R. & Riggs, J.E. (1992). Clinical features of vascular thrombosis following varicella. *American Journal of Diseases in Children*, **146**, 100–2.

Bourdette, D.N., Rosenberg, N.L. & Yatsu, F.M. (1983). Herpes zoster ophthalmicus and delayed ipsilateral cerebral infarction. *Neurology*, **33**, 1428–32.

Brissaud. E. (1896). Du zona ophthalmique avec hémiplégie croisée. *Journal de Medicak Chirurgie*, **3**, 209–25.

Budka, H., Costanzi, G., Cristina, S., Lechi, A., Parravicini, C. & Trabattoni, R. (1987). Brain pathology induced by infection with the human immunodeficiency virus (HIV). A histological, immunocytochemical, and electron microscopical study of 100 autopsy cases. *Acta Neuropathologica*, **75**, 185–98.

Burns, D.K. (1992). The neuropathology of pediatric acquired immunodeficiency syndrome. *Journal of Child Neurology*, **7**, 332–46.

Caekebeke, J.F.V., Boudewyn, O.F., Peters, A.C., Vandvik, B., Brower, O.F. & de Bakker, H.M. (1990). Cerebral vasculopathy associated with primary varicella infection. *Archives of Neurology*, **47**, 1033–5.

Carpenter, C.C.J., Fischl, M.A., Hammer, S.M. et al. (1996). Antiretroviral therapy for HIV infection in 1996. *Journal of the American Medical Association*, **276**, 146–54.

Cheatham, W.J. (1953). The relation of heretofore unreported lesions to pathogenesis of herpes zoster. *American Journal of Pathology*, **29**, 401–11.

Cope, C. & Jones, A.Y. (1954). Hemiplegia complicating herpes zoster. *Lancet*, **2**, 898–9.

Cravioto, H. & Feigin, I. (1959). Noninfectious granulomatous angiitis with a predilection for the nervous system. *Neurology*, **9**, 599–609.

Croen, K.D., Ostrove, J.M., Dragovic, L.J. & Straws, S.E. (1988). Patterns of gene expression and sites of latency in human nerve ganglia are different for varicella-zoster and herpes simplex viruses. *Proceedings of the National Academy of Sciences, USA*, **85**, 9773–7.

Czlonkowska, A., Kruszewska, J., Szpakowa, G., Tarnowska-Dziduszko, E. & Kryst-Widzgowska, T. (1991). Two cases of ophthalmic zoster followed by hemiplegia. *Neurological and Neurochirurgical Policy*, **25**, 95–100.

Dalal, P.M. & Dalal, K.P. (1989). Cerebrovascular manifestations of infectious disease. In *Handbook of Clinical Neurology*, ed. P. Vinken & C.J.F. Bruyn, pp. 411–41. Amsterdam: Elsevier.

Deitz, H. (1955). Periarteritis nodosa zosterica des Gehirns mit Zoster ophthalmicus. *Nervenarzt*, **26**, 170–1.

Dolin, R., Reichman, R.C., Mazur, M.H. & Whitley, R.J. (1978). Herpes zoster-varicella infections in immunosuppressed patients. *Annals of Internal Medicine*, **89**, 375–88.

Doyle, P.W., Gibson, G. & Dolman, C.L. (1983). Herpes zoster ophthalmicus with contralateral hemiplegia: identification of cause. *Annals of Neurology*, **14**, 84–5.

Dubrovsky, T., Curless, R., Scott, G. et al. (1998). Cerebral aneurysmal arteriopathy in childhood AIDS. *Neurology*, **51**, 560–5.

Eda, I., Takashima, S. & Takeshia, K. (1983). Acute hemiplegia with lacunar infarct after varicella infection in childhood. *Brain Development*, **5**, 358–60.

Egger, M., Hirschel, B., Francioli, P. et al. (1997). Impact of new antiretroviral combination therapies in HIV infected patients in Switzerland: prospective multicentre study. *British Medical Journal*, **315**, 1194–9.

Eidelberg, D., Sotrel, A., Horoupian, D.S., Neumann, P.E., Pumarola-Sune, T. & Price, R.W. (1986). Thrombotic cerebral vasculopathy associated with herpes zoster. *Annals of Neurology*, **19**, 7–14.

Elble, R.J. (1983). Intracerebral hemorrhage with herpes zoster ophthalmicus. *Annals of Neurology*, **14**, 591–2.

Fagerberg, B., Gnarpe, J., Gnarpe, H., Agewall, S. & Wikstrand, J. (1999). *Chlamydia pneumoniae* but not cytomegalovirus antibodies are associated with future risk of stroke and cardiovascular disease: a prospective study in middle-aged to elderly men with treated hypertension. *Stroke*, **30**, 299–305.

Federico, F., Pedone, D., Lamberti, P. et al. (1982). Ophthalmic herpes zoster with contralateral hemiparesis: a case report. *Journal of Neurology*, **228**, 283–7.

Freedman, M.S. & MacDonald, R. (1987). Herpes zoster ophthalmicus with delayed cerebral infarction and meningoencephalitis. *Canadian Journal of Neurological Science*, **14**, 312–14.

Fukumoto, S., Kinjo, M., Hokamura, K. & Tanaka, K. (1986). Subarachnoid hemorrhage and granulomatous angiitis of the basilar artery: demonstration of the varicella-zoster virus in the basilar artery lesions. *Stroke*, **17**, 1024–8.

Gardner-Thorpe, C., Foster, J.B. & Barwick, D.D. (1976). Unusual manifestations of herpes zoster: a clinical and electrophysiological study. *Journal of Neurological Science*, **28**, 427–47.

Gilbert, G.J. (1974). Herpes zoster ophthalmicus and delayed contralateral hemiparesis. *Journal of the American Medical Association*, **229**, 302–4.

Gilden, D.H. & Kleinschmidt-DeMasters, B.K. (1998). Reply from the authors. *Neurology*, **51**, 324–5.

Gilden, D.H., Murray, R.S., Wellish, M., Kleinschmidt-DeMasters, B.K. & Vafai, A. (1988). Chronic progressive varicella-zoster virus encephalitis in an AIDS patient. *Neurology*, **38**, 1150–3.

Gilden, D.H., Kleinschmidt-DeMasters, B.K., Wellish, M., Hedley-White, E.T., Rentier, B. & Mahalingam, R. (1996). Varicella zoster virus, a cause of waxing and waning vasculitis: *The New England Journal of Medicine*, case 5 – 1995 revisited. *Neurology*, **47**, 1441–6.

Gibbs, M.A. & Fisher, M. (1986). Cerebral infarction in an adult with disseminated varicella. *Bulletin of Clinical Neuroscience*, **51**, 65–7.

Gordon, I.R.S. & Tucker, J.F. (1945). Lesions of the central nervous system in herpes zoster. *Journal of Neurology, Neurosurgery and Psychiatry*, **8**, 40–6.

Gray, F., Geny, C., Lionnet, F. et al. (1991). Etude neuropathologique de 135 cas adultes de syndrome d'immuno-déficience acquise (SIDA). *Annals of Pathology*, **11**, 236–47.

Gray, F., Bélec, L., Lescs, M.C. et al. (1994). Varicella-zoster virus infection of the central nervous system in the acquired immune deficiency syndrome. *Brain*, **117**, 987–99.

Griffith, J.F., Salam, M.V. & Adams, R.D. (1970). The nervous system diseases associated with varicella. *Acta Neurologica Scandinavica*, **46**, 279–300.

Guess, H.A., Broughton, D.D. Melton, L.J.III & Kurland, L.D. (1986). Population-based studies of varicella complications. *Pediatrics*, **78**(Suppl), 723–7.

Gulick, R.M., Mellor, J.W., Havlir, D. et al. (1997). A controlled trial of two nucleoside analogues plus indinavir in persons with human immunodeficiency virus infection and prior antiretroviral therapy. *New England Journal of Medicine*, **33**, 734–9.

Gursoy, G., Aktin, E., Bahar, S., Tolun, R. & Ozden, B. (1980). Postherpetic aneurysm in the intrapetrosal portion of the internal carotid artery. *Neuroradiology*, **19**, 279–82.

Gyorkey, F., Melnick, J.L., Guinn, G.A., Gyorkey, P. & DeBakey, M.E. (1984). Herpes viridiae in the endothelial and smooth muscle cells of the proximal aorta of atherosclerotic patients. *Experimental Molecular Pathology*, **40**, 328–39.

Haanpää, M., Dastidar, P., Weinberg, A. et al. (1998). CSF and MRI findings in patients with acute herpes zoster. *Neurology*, **51**, 1405–11.

Hammer, S.M., Squires, K.E., Hughes, M.D. et al. (1997). A controlled trial of two nucleosid analogues plus indinavir in persons with human immunodeficiency virus and CD4 cell counts of 200 per cubic millimeter or less. *New England Journal of Medicine*, **337**, 725–33.

Hendrix, M.G., Salimans, M.M., van Boven, C.P. & Bruggemann, C.A. (1990). High prevalence of latently present cytomegalovirus in arterial walls of patients suffering from grade III atherosclerosis. *American Journal of Pathology*, **136**, 23–28.

Hilt, D.C., Buchholz, D. & Krumholz, A. (1983). Herpes zoster ophthalmicus and delayed contralateral hemiparesis caused by cerebral angiitis: diagnosis and management approaches. *Annals of Neurology*, **14**, 543–53.

Hope-Simpson, R.E. (1965). The nature of herpes zoster: a long-term study and a new hypothesis. *Proceedings of the Royal Society of Medicine*, **58**, 9–20.

Horton, B., Price, R.W. & Jimenez, D. (1981). Multifocal varizella-zoster virus leukoencephalitis temporally remote from herpes zoster. *Annals of Neurology*, **9**, 151–266.

Hosseinipour, M.C., Smith, N.H., Simpson, E.P., Greenberg, S.B., Armstrong, R.M. & White, A.C. Jr. (1998). Middle cerebral artery vasculitis and stroke after varicella in a young adult. *South Medical Journal*, **91**, 1070–2.

Hughes, W.N. (1951). Herpes zoster of the right trigeminal nerve with left hemiplegia. *Neurology*, **1**, 167–9.

Husson, R.N., Salni, R., Lewis, L.L., Butler, K.M., Patronas, N. & Pizzo, P.A. (1992). Cerebral artery aneurysms in children infected with human immunodeficiency virus. *Journal of Pediatrics*, **121**, 927–30.

Ichiyama, T., Houdou, S., Kisa, T., Ohno, K. & Takeshita, K. (1990). Varicella with delayed hemiplegia. *Pediatric Neurology*, **6**, 279–81.

Inoue, N., Shirai, S., Tsuda, T. et al. (1984). Herpes zoster ophthalmicus with contralateral hemiplegia and normal pressure hydrocephalus. *Journal of Neurology*, **231**, 96–8.

International Stroke Trial Collaborative Group. (1997). The International Stroke Trial (IST): a randomised trial of aspirin, subcutaneous heparin, both, or neither, among 19 435 patients with acute ischemic stroke. *Lancet*, **349**, 1569–81.

Jemsek, J., Greenberg, S.B., Taber, L., Harvey, D., Gershon, A. & Couch R.B. (1983). Herpes zoster-associated encephalits: clinicopathologic report of 12 cases and review of the literature. *Medicine*, **62**, 81–97.

Kamholz, J. & Tremblay, G. (1985). Chickenpox with delayed contralateral hemiparesis caused by cerebral angiitis. *Annals of Neurology*, **18**, 358–60.

Kleinschmidt-DeMasters, B.K., Mahalingam, R., Shimek, C. et al. (1998). Profound cerebrospinal pleocytosis and Froin's syndrome secondary to widespread necrotizing vasculitis in a HIV-positive patient with varicella zoster virus encephalomyelitis. *Journal of Neurological Science*, **159**, 213–18.

Koeppen, A.H., Lansing, L.S., Peng, S.K. & Smith, R.S. (1981). Central nervous system vasculitis in cytomegalovirus infection. *Journal of Neurological Science*, **51**, 395–401.

Kolodny, K.H., Rebeiz, J.J., Caviness, V.S. & Richardson, E.P. (1968). Granulomatous angiitis of the central nervous system. *Archives of Neurology*, **19**, 510–24.

Kure, K., Park, Y.D., Kim, T.S. et al. (1989). Immunohistochemical localization of an HIV epitope in cerebral aneurysmal arteriopathy in pediatric acquired immunodeficiency syndrome (AIDS). *Pediatric Pathology*, **9**, 655–67.

Kuroiwa, Y. & Furukawa, T. (1981). Hemispheric infarction after herpes zoster ophthalmicus: computed tomography and angiography. *Neurology*, **31**, 1030–2.

Landi, G., Calloni, M.V. & Scarlato, G. (1981). Transient contralateral hemiplegia after ophthalmic zoster: therapeutic problems in elderly patients. *Journal of Neurology*, **224**, 297–300.

Lang, W., Miklossy, J., Deruaz, J.P., Pizzolato, G.P., Probst, A. & Schaffner, T. (1989). Neuropathology of the acquired immune deficiency syndrome (AIDS): a report of 135 consecutive autopsy cases from Switzerland. *Acta Neuropathologica*, **77**, 379–90.

Lang, C., Jacobi, G., Kreuz, W. et al. (1992). Rapid development of giant aneurysm at the base of the brain in an 8-year-old boy with perinatal HIV infection. *Acta Histochemica*, **57**(Suppl), 83–90.

Laws, H.W. (1960). Herpes zoster ophthalmicus complicated by contralateral hemiplegia. *Archives of Ophthalmology*, **63**, 273–80.

Leopold, N.A. (1993). Chickenpox stroke in an adult. *Neurology*, **43**, 1852–3.

Lexa, F., Galetta, S.L., Yousem, D.M., Farber, M., Oberholtzer, J.C. & Atlas, S.W. (1993). Herpes zoster ophthalmicus with orbital pseudotumor syndrome complicated by optic nerve infarction and cerebral granulomatous angiitis: MR-pathologic correlation. *American Journal of Neuroradiology*, **14**, 185–90.

Linnemann, C.C. & Alvira, M. (1980). Pathogenesis of the varicella-zoster angiitis in the CNS. *Archives of Neurology*, **37**, 239–40.

Liu, G.T. & Holmes, G.L. (1990). Varicella with delayed contralateral hemiparesis detected by MRI. *Pediatric Neurology*, **6**, 131–4.

McArthur, J.C. (1987). Neurologic manifestations of AIDS. *Medicine*, **66**, 407–37.

McComas, C.F. & Gutman, L. (1982). Hemispheric infarction after herpes zoster ophthalmicus (letter). *Neurology*, **32**, 914–15.

MacKenzie, R.A., Forbes, G.S. & Karnes, W.E. (1981). Angiographic findings in herpes zoster arteritis. *Annals of Neurology*, **10**, 458–64.

Mainka, C., Fuss, B., Geiger, H., Hofelmayr, H. & Wolff, M.H. (1998). Characterization of viremia at different stages of varicella-zoster virus infection. *Journal of Medical Virology*, **56**, 91–8.

Martin, W.J. (1996). Stealth viral encephalopathy: report of a fatal case complicated by cerebral vasculitis. *Pathobiology*, **64**, 59–63.

Mayberg, M., Langer, R. & Moskowitz, M.A. (1980). Perivascular connections from the trigeminal ganglia of the cat: a possible neuroanatomical substrate for vascular headaches in humans. *Annals of Neurology*, **8**, 120.

Melanson, M., Chalk, C., Georgevich, L. et al. (1996). Varicella-zoster virus DNA in CSF and arteries in delayed contralateral hemiplegia: evidence for viral invasion of cerebral arteries. *Neurology*, **47**, 569–70.

Melnick, J.L., Adam, E. & DeBakey, M.E. (1990). Possible role of cytomegalovirus in atherogenesis. *Journal of the American Medical Association*, **263**, 2204–7.

Menkes, D.B., Bishara, S.N. & Corbett, A.J. (1983). Hemispheric infarction after herpes zoster ophthalmicus. *Journal of Neurology, Neurosurgery and Psychiatry*, **46**, 786–7.

Minick, C.R., Fabricant, C.R., Fabricant, J. & Litrenta, M.M. (1979). Atherosclerosis induced by infection with herpes virus. *American Journal of Pathology*, **96**, 673–706.

Minton, J. (1956). A case of left herpes zoster ophthalmicus followed by viral encephalitis with right-sided anesthesia, paresthesia and hemiplegia. *Transactions of the Ophthalmology Society UK*, **76**, 227–33.

Morgello, S., Block, G.A., Price, R.W. & Petito, C.K. (1988). Varicellazoster virus leukoencephalitis and cerebral vasculopathy. *Archives of Pathology and Laboratory Medicine*, **112**, 173–7.

Moskowitz, M.A. (1970). The neurobiology of vascular head pain. *Annals of Neurology*, **16**, 157–68.

Munoz, A., Vinuela, F., Mesa, A., Fernandez, J.M., Garcia Moreno, J.M. & Izquierdo, G. (1995). CNS vasculitis after ophthalmic herpes zoster infection. *Revista e Neurologia*, **23**, 1063–6.

Nieto, F.J., Adam, E., Sorlie, P. et al. (1996). Cohort study of cytomegalovirus infection as a risk factor for carotid intimal-medial thickening, a measure of subclinical atherosclerosis. *Circulation*, **94**, 922–7.

Nishimaru, K. & Kamei, H. (1976). Herpes zoster ophthalmicus with contralateral hemiplegia. *Rinsho Shinkeigaku*, **16**, 649–53.

Norris, F.H., Leonards, R., Calanchini, P.R. & Calder, C.D. (1970). Herpes zoster meningoencephalitis. *Journal of Infectious Diseases*, **122**, 335–8.

O'Donohue, J.M. & Enzmann, D.R. (1987). Mycotic aneurysm in angiitis associated with herpes zoster ophthalmicus. *American Journal of Neuroradiology*, **8**, 615–19.

Onoda, M. & Takahashi, A. (1979). Herpes zoster ophthalmicus followed by contralateral hemiparesis. *Rinsho Shinkeigaku*, **19**, 496–503.

Palella, F.J. Jr, Delaney, K.M., Moorman, A.C. et al. (1998). Outpatient Investigators. Declining morbidity and mortality among patients with advanced human immunodeficiency virus infection. *New England Journal of Medicine*, **338**, 853–60.

Panchi, D.N. & Romanes, G.J. (1966). Ophthalmological herpes zoster complicated by hemiplegia. *British Journal of Ophthalmology*, **50**, 610–11.

Park, Y.D., Belman, A.L., Kim, T.S. et al. (1990). Stroke in pediatric acquired immunodeficiency syndrome. *Annals of Neurology*, **28**, 303–11.

Perrin, M., Kissel, P., Pierquin, L. & Gayet, P. (1938). Hémiplégie post-zonateuse. *Revue Medicale de Nancy*, **66**, 309–14.

Petito, C.K., Cho, E-S., Lemann, W., Navia, B.A. & Price, R.W. (1986). Neuropathology of acquired immunodeficiency syndrome (AIDS): an autopsy review. *Journal of Neuropathology and Experimental Neurology*, **45**, 635–46.

Philippet, P., Blanche, S., Sebag, G., Rodesch, G., Griscelli, C. & Tardieu, M. (1994). Stroke and cerebral infarcts in children infected with human immunodeficiency virus. *Archives of Pediatric and Adolescent Medicine*, **148**, 965–70.

Pinto, A.N. (1996). AIDS and cerebrovascular disease. *Stroke*, **27**, 538–43.

Powderly, W.G., Landay, A. & Lederman, M.M. (1998). Recovery of the immune system with antiretroviral therapy. *Journal of the American Medical Association*, **280**, 72–7.

Pratesi, R., Freemon, F.R. & Lowry, J.L. (1977). Herpes zoster ophthalmicus with contralateral hemiplegia. *Archives of Neurology*, **34**, 640–1.

Preblud, S.R., Orenstein, W.A. & Bart, K.J. (1984). Varicella: clinical manifestations, epidemiology and health impact in children. *Pediatric Infectious Diseases*, **3**, 505–9.

Qureshi, A.I., Janssen, R.S., Karon, J.M. et al. (1997). Human immunodeficiency virus infection and stroke in young patients. *Archives of Neurology*, **54**, 1150–3.

Ragozzino, M.W., Melton, L.J., Kurland, L.T., Chu, C.P. & Perry, H.O. (1982). Population-based study on herpes zoster and its sequelae. *Medicine*, **61**, 310–16.

Rehurek, J., Hanak, L. & Rehurekova, M. (1974). Rare cerebral complications in herpes zoster ophthalmicus. *Ceskoslovenska Oftalmologie*, **5**, 370–4.

Reshef, E., Greenberg, S.B. & Jankovic, J. (1985). Herpes zoster ophthalmicus followed by contralateral hemiparesis: report of two cases and review of the literature. *Journal of Neurology, Neurosurgery and Psychiatry*, **48**, 122–7.

Ridker, P.M., Hennekens, C.H., Stampfer, M.J. & Wang, F. (1998). Prospective study of herpes simplex virus, cytomegalovirus, and the risk of future myocardial infarction and stroke. *Circulation*, **98**, 2796–9.

Rose, F.C., Brett, E.M. & Burston, J. (1964). Zoster encephalomyelitis. *Archives of Neurology*, **11**, 155–72.

Rosenblum, M.K. (1989). Bulbar encephalitis complicating trigeminal zoster in the acquired immune deficiency syndrome. *Human Pathology*, **20**, 292–5.

Rosenblum, W.L. & Hadfield, M.G. (1972). Granulomatous angiitis of nervous system in cases of herpes zoster and lymphosarcoma. *Neurology*, **22**, 348–54.

Rosenblum, W.I., Hadfield, M.G. & Young, H.F. (1978). Granulomatous angiitis of the brain with herpes zoster and varicella encephalitis. *Annals of Neurology*, **3**, 374–5.

Rostad, S.W., Olson, K., McDougall, J., Shaw, C-M. Alvord, E.C.J. (1989). Transsynaptic spread of varicella zoster virus through the visual system: a mechanism of viral dissemination in the central nervous system. *Human Pathology*, **20**, 174–9.

Rousseau, F., Perronne, C., Rauguin, G., Thouvenot, D., Vidal, A. & Leport, C. (1993). Necrotizing retinitis and cerebral vasculitis due to varicella-zoster virus in patients infected with the human immunodeficiency virus [letter]. *Clinical Infectious Diseases*, **17**, 943–4.

Ruppenthal, M. (1980). Changes of central nervous system in herpes zoster. *Acta Neuropathologica*, **52**, 59–68.

Ryder, J.W., Croen, K., Kleinschmidt-DeMasters, B.K., Ostrove, J.M., Straus, J.M. & Cohn, D.L. (1986). Progressive encephalitis three months after resolution of cutaneous zoster in patients with AIDS. *Annals of Neurology*, **19**, 182–8.

Sarazin, L., Duong, H., Bourgouin, P.M. et al. (1995). Herpes zoster vasculitis: demonstration by MR angiography. *Journal of Computer Assisted Tomography*, **19**, 624–7.

Sato, M., Nabeyama, T. & Ikeda, H. (1971). A case of herpes zoster encephalitis complicated by sensory aphasia and contralateral hemiparesis. *Rinsho Shinkeigaku*, **11**, 365–72.

Scaravilli, F., Daniel, S.E., Harcourt-Webster, N. & Guiloff, R.J. (1989). Chronic basal meningitis and vasculitis in acquired immunodeficiency syndrome. A possible role for human immunodeficiency virus. *Archives of Pathological Laboratory Medicine*, **113**, 192–5.

Schmader, K., George, L.K., Burchett, B.M., Pieper, C.F. & Hamilton, J.D. (1995). Racial differences in the occurrence of herpes zoster. *Journal of Infectious Diseases*, **171**, 701–4.

Schmidbauer, M., Budka, H., Pilz, P., Kurata, T. & Hondo, R. (1992). Presence, distribution and spread of productive varicella zoster virus infection in nervous tissues. *Brain*, **115**, 383–98.

Schmidt, J.A., Dietzmann, K., Müller, U. & Krause, P. (1992). Granulomatous vasculitis – an uncommon manifestation of herpes simplex infection of the central nervous system. *Zentralblatt Pathologie*, **138**, 298–302.

Shah, S.S., Zimmerman, R.A., Rorke, L.B. & Vezina, L.G. (1996). Cerebrovascular complications of HIV in children. *American Journal of Neuroradiology*, **17**, 1913–17.

Shuper, A., Vining, E.P. & Freeman, J.M. (1990). Central nervous system vasculitis after chickenpox – cause or coincidence? *Archives of Diseases of Childhood*, **65**, 1245–8.

Sipe, J.C. & Rosenberg, J.H. (1977). Granulomatous giant arteriitis of the central nervous system – Neurological Clinicopathological Conference. *West Journal of Medicine*, **127**, 215–20.

Speir, E., Modali, R., Huang, E.S. et al. (1994). Potential role of human cytomegalovirus and p53 interaction in coronary restenosis. *Science*, **265**, 391–4.

Sorlie, P.D., Adam, E., Melnick, S.L. et al. (1994). Cytomegalovirus/herpes virus and carotid atherosclerosis: the ARIC study. *Journal of Medical Virology*, **42**, 33–7.

Sung, K.B., Kim, S.H., Kim, J.H., Chung, K.C. & Kim, M.H. (1989). Herpes zoster ophthalmicus and delayed contralateral hemiparesis. *Journal of Korean Medical Science*, **3**, 79–82.

Sureda, Ramis, B., Bautista, J. & Martinez Navarro, M.L. (1989). Herpes zoster ophthalmicus with contralateral hemiplegia. *Annales Medicale Internale*, **6**, 639–40.

Terborg, C. & Busse, O. (1995). Granulomatous vasculitis of the CNS as a complication of herpes zoster ophthalmicus. *Fortschrift Neurologie Psychiatrie*, **63**, 383–7.

The European Ad Hoc Consensus Group. (1997). Optimizing intensive care in stroke: a European perspective. A report of an *ad hoc* consensus group meeting. *Cerebrovascular Disorders*, **7**, 113–28.

Vecht, C.J. & Sande, C.C. (1982). Hemispheric infarction after herpes zoster ophthalmicus (letter). *Neurology*, **32**, 914.

Verghese, A. & Sugar, A.M. (1986). Herpes zoster ophthalmicus and granulomatous angiitis. An ill-appreciated cause of stroke. *Journal of the American Geriatric Society*, **34**, 309–312.

Victor, D.I. & Green, W.R. (1976). Temporal artery biopsy in herpes zoster ophthalmicus with delayed arteritis. *American Journal of Ophthalmology*, **82**, 428–30.

Vinters, H.V., Guerra, W.F., Eppolito, L. & Keith, P.E. (1988). Necrotizing vasculitis of the nervous system in a patient with AIDS-related complex. *Neuropathology and Applied Neurobiology*, **14**, 417–24.

Walker, R.J., Gammal, T. & Allen, M.B. (1973). Cranial arteritis associated with herpes zoster. *Neuroradiology*, **107**, 109–10.

White, C.J. (1997). Varicella-zoster virus vaccine. *Clinical Infectious Diseases*, **24**, 753–64.

Yankner, B.A., Skolnik, P.R., Shoukimas, G.M., Gabuzda, D.H., Sobel, R.A. & Ho, D.D. (1986). Cerebral granulomatous angiitis associated with isolation of human T-lymphotropic virus type III from the central nervous system. *Annals of Neurology*, **20**, 362–4.

Zhou, Y.F., Leon, M.B., Waclawiw, M.A. et al. (1996). Association between prior cytomegalovirus infection and the risk of restenosis after coronary atherectomy. *New England Journal of Medicine*, **335**, 624–30.

4

Polyarteritis nodosa and Churg–Strauss syndrome

Marc D. Reichhart and Julien Bogousslavsky

Department of Neurology, University of Lausanne, Switzerland

Polyarteritis nodosa (PAN)

In 1866, Kussmaul and Maier (Freiburg, Germany) observed two young patients who died from asthenia, weight loss, abdominal pain, fever, renal failure and severe neuromuscular disease (Kussmaul & Maier, 1866). They found abnormal segmental thickening (macroscopic nodes) and inflammation of medium/small-sized arteries in many organs, hence describing the disease 'periarteritis nodosa'. Now called polyarteritis nodosa (PAN), it remains the archetype of necrotizing vasculitis. Since the availability of antineutrophil cytoplasmic antibodies (ANCA), new classifications (Jenette et al., 1994; Jenette & Falk, 1997) have been proposed to discriminate PAN (classic; without glomerulonephritis) from microscopic polyangiitis (MPA), the latter being characterized by involvement of arterioles, capillaries, or venules, the absence of granuloma, and its association with focal segmental necrotizing glomerulonephritis (Lhote et al., 1996). Positive p-ANCA (antimyeloperoxidase of the perinuclear staining pattern) can be found in 75% of patients with MPA (Lhote et al., 1996). However, the distinction between PAN and MPA is difficult and has not always been made (Watts et al., 1996), so that we will still apply the American College of Rheumatology criteria for PAN (Lightfoot et al., 1990). PAN can be diagnosed when three or more of the following criteria are present: weight loss (4 kg); livedo reticularis; testicular pain or tenderness; myalgias, weakness or leg tenderness; mononeuropathy or polyneuropathy; diastolic blood pressure >90 mmHg; elevated BUN or creatinine; hepatitis B virus; arteriographic abnormality; biopsy of small- or medium-sized artery containing polymorphonuclear neutrophils. PAN affects (in order of decreasing frequency) the peripheral nerves, muscles, joints, skin, kidney, gastrointestinal tract, heart and eyes, and manifests itself by weight loss, fever, asthenia, and hypertension, and biological signs of inflammation, i.e., anemia, leukocytosis, thrombocytosis, elevated C-proteins and sedimentation rate (Lhote et al., 1995; Conn, 1990; Moore, 1995). Formerly classically associated with B-type Hepatitis Virus (HV; see Guillevin et al., 1995) infection (one-third before the vaccines era in France; in decreasing frequency since then), PAN also occurs after infection with A and C HV, HTLV-I, CMV, parvovirus B19 (Lhote & Guillevin, 1995), and HIV (Font et al., 1996), and may complicate rheumatoid arthritis, Gougerot–Sjögren's syndrome, mixed cryoglobulinemia, and hairy cell leukemia (Conn, 1990). Although rare (annual prevalence rate 6.3 per 100 000), PAN affects middle-aged patients (average age 40–60 years, male/female sex ratio 2:1), and all racial groups.

PAN-associated strokes

In contrast with peripheral nervous system complications, which are frequent (50–75% of patients) and often inaugural, central nervous system (CNS) involvement occurs in 20 to 40% of patients with PAN and 2 to 3 years after the initial diagnosis is made (Moore & Fauci, 1981; Moore & Cupps, 1983). Two subgroups of CNS complications have been recognized: a diffuse encephalopathy with cognitive dysfunction, stupor, and seizures, and a focal pattern (ischemic/hemorrhagic stroke, subarachnoidal hemorrhage). However, the mechanisms, – i.e., CS- or hypertension-induced atherosclerosis vs. arteritic occlusions, and patterns of PAN-associated strokes are less well known (Moore & Fauci, 1981; Cohen et al., 1980; Moore, 1995; Moore & Cupps, 1983; Conn, 1990).

PAN is mediated by immune complex deposition (circulating and *in situ*), but endothelial cells play the most important role in the mechanisms of inflammation. They express immunoglobulin (Fc), complement, Class 2 antigens receptors, and release IL-1, and PAF. Conversely, the endothelial production of dilator substances (prostacyclin, adenosine, nitric oxide) is impaired, while the underlying diseased smooth muscle cells show reduced mechanical properties (Conn, 1990). Furthermore, as studied in Kawasaki disease, the production of thromboxane A2 (TXA2, vasoconstrictor, stimulator of platelet activation/ aggregation) may be increased. Thus, the final effect of endothelial inflammation is luminal occlusion (vasoconstriction, platelet aggregation, clot formation). In many ways, these mechanisms resemble those of atherosclerosis, and the mechanisms of arterial occlusion are complicated by the occurrence of associated hypertension in PAN (40% of patients; Lhote & Guillevin, 1991). Less is known as regards the CNS immunopathogenic mechanisms of PAN. Indeed, the CNS endothelium levels of lymphocyte adhesion and MHC expression are lower than in other organs, but how the lymphocytes interact after inflammation (probably mediated by IL-1 and 6 and TNF-alpha) with lymphocytes and perivascular microglia cells remains obscure (Moore, 1995).

In 1965, Ford and Siekert described ischemic or hemorrhagic stroke as late CNS manifestations in 19% of patients (total 114 patients) with PAN (Ford & Siekert, 1965). Among 14 patients with hemispheric infarcts, pure ischemic, ischemic and hemorrhagic, and hemorrhagic strokes occurred in near one-third each. Five patients showed multiple deep small ischemic or petechial hemorrhagic infarcts involving the basal ganglia, internal capsule, or the thalamus. Clinical evidence (one necropsy) for brainstem strokes was found in seven patients.

A more recent series (Cohen et al., 1980) of 53 patients with PAN found cerebrovascular disease as the cause of death in five cases, with a mean latency after the onset of the vasculitis of 2 years. Because all strokes occurred while the vasculitis was controlled by immunosupressive therapy (CS with/without cyclophosphamide or azathioprine), they hypothesized atherosclerosis-like mechanisms (promoted by long-term use of CS) as the cause of arterial occlusion in PAN. Another series (Moore & Fauci, 1981) described five PAN patients with clinical evidences of focal deficits occurring at either the cerebral, brainstem, or cerebellar level (CT abnormalities in three patients only). Again, all strokes occurred on CS therapy (with a mean latency of 2 years). Three patients showed hypertension. Thus, they suggested that vascular scarring was responsible for those late CNS complications of PAN.

To study the relationship between PAN-associated strokes and the use of CS, and trying to delineate a specific stroke syndrome in PAN, we analysed the data of 11 patients with PAN and stroke from literature (Mayo et al., 1986; Wildhagen et al., 1989; Koppensteiner et al., 1989; Kasantikul et al., 1991; Harlé et al., 1991; Iaconetta et al., 1994; Squire et al., 1993; Hirohata et al., 1993; Long & Dolin, 1994; de la Fuente Fernandez & Grana Gil, 1994; Stahl et al., 1995), together with four similar patients from Lausanne (period 1982–98, Reichhart et al., 2000). The details of the source, patient age and sex, clinical and neuroradiological features, latencies (between the onset of PAN and the cerebrovascular insult), and current immunosuppressive therapy at onset, i.e. methylprednisolone (MP), corticosteroids (CS), prednisone (P), prednisolone (PL), with/without cyclophosphamide (CY) or azathioprine (AZA), for the 15 PAN-associated strokes are listed in Table 4.1. Here below, the case history of one typical patient with PAN and stroke who was admitted in our Department is detailed.

Case history (Patient 3, 1996, Reichhart et al., 2000)

A 55-year-old Italian woman developed over 2 months asthenia, weight loss (five kg), night fever (38.5 °C), hypertension, large joints arthritis, myalgia, lower limbs livedo reticularis, and Raynaud's phenomena. Admitted for a bilateral asymmetric peroneal mononeuritis (confirmed electrophysiologically), there were biological signs of inflammation (ESR, 90 mm/h; WBC, 13.4 G/l; eosinophiles, 15%) and renal failure with nephrotic syndrome. The diagnosis of PAN was confirmed by sural nerve and renal biopsy (although positive p-ANCA were found). MP (250 mg) was promptly initiated, but eight hours later she developed a left-side sensorimotor syndrome without hemineglect (two adjacent right-side deep small infarcts, anterior choroidal artery, Fig. 4.1). Echocardiography and Doppler studies of the carotids were normal, and tests for coagulation (including antithrombin III and anticardiolipin antibodies, aCL) were normal or negative. CSF immunoelectrophoresis showed signs of blood–brain barrier rupture (p-ANCA could therefore also be detected in the CSF). Following treatment with iv MP (5×500 mg), then prednisone (1 mg/kg/d), together with antiplatelet drug (ASA, 200 mg), and i.v. pulsed CY therapy (750 mg/m^2/month), the clinical course improved. During a 3-year follow-up, there was no stroke recurrence.

The present study (Reichhart et al., 2000) of 15 PAN-associated strokes (Table 4.1) shows similar population characteristics as previously published series (male/female ratio, 1.5; mean age, 49 years). Lacunar syndromes seem to be the specific and most frequent (73%, 11/15) stroke pattern associated with PAN. More than half of them (55%, 6/11) developed either pure (four patients), sensori(one patient)- motor strokes or ataxic hemiparesis (one patient), which correlated with typical small deep infarcts (internal

Table 4.1. *Clinical and neuroradiological features, latencies (disease-onset-to stroke) and current corticosteroid (CS) therapy at stroke onset (latencies between stroke and CS initiation) for the 15 PAN-associated strokes*

N°/source	Age Y/Sex	Clinical features	CT	MRI	Latency (months)	CS (latencies)
1, Reichhart et al. (1982)	49/F	Blt blindness	Blt temporo-occipital infarcts	Not available	2½	P (2 m)
2, Reichhart et al. (1994)	44/M	R hemiparesis		Blt centrum semiovale lacunes	2	P (3 days)
3, Reichhart et al. (1996)	55/F	L sensorimotor syndrome		R capsular lacune	2	MP (8 hours)
4, Reichhart et al. (1998)	67/M	Wernicke's aphasia, R hemianopia	L temporo-parietal hematoma	R caudate petechial infarct	1	None
5, Mayo et al. (1986)	68/M	Parkinsonian syndrome	L striatum lacune		3 weeks	None
		R hemiparesis	L capsular lacune		11 days	MP, P + CY (11 days)
6, Wildhagen et al. (1989)	55/M	R ataxic hemiparesis		Blt centrum semiovale lacunes	12	CS + AZA (6 months)
7, Koppensteiner et al. (1989)	35/M	Seizures, R hemiparesis		Multiple white matter T_2-weighted signals	5	None
8, Kasantikul et al. (1991)	35/F	L hemiparesis, pseudo-bulbar syndrome		R pontine lacune	Inaugural	None
9, Harlé et al. (1991)	64/M	Dementia, incontinence, pyramidal tract signs	Leukoaraiosis	Multiple white matter T_2-weighted signals	13	MP + CY (13 months)
10, Iaconetta et al. (1994)	38/F	Dysarthria, L hemiparesis	R temporo-parietal hematoma		1	Unknown
11, Squire et al. (1994)	43/M	Dysarthria, L hemiparesis	R basal ganglia lacune		14	None
		Hemiparesis deterioration	New R basal ganglia lacune		3 weeks later	P + CY (3 weeks)
		Hemiparesis deterioration	R temporo-parietal infarct		5 days later	P + CY (5 days)
12, Hirohata et al. (1993)	26/M	L sensorimotor syndrome		Pontine lacune	32	Prednisolone (32 months)
13, Long & Dolin (1994)	23/F	Bilateral blindness		Blt parieto-occipital infarcts	2	P (10 days)
14, de la Fuente Fernandez & Grana (1994)	58/F	L INO, L III and R VII nerve palsy		Multiple lacunes (pons, basal ganglia, thalamus)	8	P (6 months)
15, Stahl et al. (1995)	70/M	R crural paresis	L caudate lacune		1	None

Notes:

L = left; R = right; Blt = bilateral; P = prednisone; MP = methylprednisolone; CY = cyclophosphamide; AZA = azathioprine.

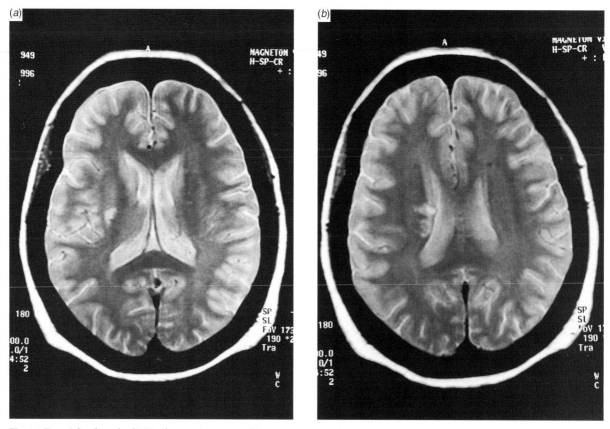

Fig. 4.1. T$_2$-weighted cerebral MRI of our patient 3 (case history): Lacunar infarcts involving (*a*) the posterior limb of the right internal capsule and (*b*) adjacent corona radiata.

capsule, lenticulate and caudate nucleus, centrum semi-ovale or corona radiata). Pontine lacunes (together with asymptomatic small deep infarcts in one case) were found in three patients (27%, 3/11), and the remaining patients disclosed leukoaraiosis (18%, 2/11). This distribution of lacunes is similar to that described by Fischer (see corresponding chapter) and confirms a predominantly small- and medium-sized artery involvement in PAN, inducing multiple small penetrating artery occlusions at the subcortical or pontine level. This preponderance of lacunar stroke may be partially explained by PAN-associated hypertension, seen in 40% (Lhote & Guillevin, 1991) to more than half of patients (Moore & Cupps, 1983). The short time interval between disease onset and subsequent cerebrovascular complications in the present series allows hypertension to be considered only as a risk factor for stroke in PAN, rather than the main etiology. In fact, stroke developed within 14 months in all but one patients (mean latency, 6.5 months; range, 3 weeks to 32 months), within 8 months in 73% of patients (11/15), and was either inaugural or occurred within 1 month of the onset of PAN in one-third of patients (33%, 5/15). The earlier initiation and

universal use of corticosteroid (CS) treatment in the recent cases of vasculitis probably explain the discrepancy between the previously late stroke occurrence (2–3 years) and the shorter latencies found in the present study. A close relationship between the use of CS and stroke exists in PAN. All strokes in the aforementioned series occurred while patients received adequate CS treatment. In the present study, most of the 77% of all first-time or recurrent ischemic strokes that developed despite CS therapy appeared within 6 months (80%) and 3 weeks (50%) of starting CS treatment (associated with other immunosuppressive therapy in only three patients). Although it must be concluded that CS alone failed to prevent stroke (or recurrent stroke, see patients 5 and 11) in PAN (concomitant immunosuppressive treatment being not yet active), the previously suspected promoting effect of CS in the mechanisms of arterial occlusion seems to be confirmed in the present study. In fact, two of our patients (patient 2 and 3) developed lacunar strokes within 8 hours and 3 days of CS therapy initiation, respectively, while two other patients (patient 5 and 11) showed recurrent (two consecutive in patient 11) new lacunes within 11 days and 3 weeks of the beginning of CS therapy. CS acts on the primary inflammatory stage of PAN, without preventing the occurrence of later arteritic changes (intimal proliferation, granulation and scarring; Conn, 1990). Pathological studies of systemic arteries in two patients with PAN treated with CS showed no signs of active inflammation but multiple arterial occlusions (predominantly intimal fibrosis), within 3 weeks and 3 months of initiation of cortisone acetate, respectively (Bagenstoss et al., 1951). However, cerebral histological studies were normal, except in one patient (atheromatous small MCA aneurysm, medullar small infarct). In our study, four patients (one-fourth) with PAN and stroke showed at autopsy. In one patient (patient 8; inaugural pontine infarct) who died despite a short-term CS therapy, although histological studies showed signs of necrotizing vasculitis of the medium- and small-sized arteries of the leptomeninges, there were only thromboses of small pontine penetrating arteries. On the other hand, of the three remaining patients who died, despite a minimal 3-month CS therapy, no signs of active vasculitis were found. Furthermore, it is relevant to note that cerebral histological studies of our patient 1, performed 3 months after CS initiation, showed arterial wall fibrosis of deep white matter arterioles (see colour Fig. 4.2(a)).

While CS should equally decrease the production of both prostacyclin (PGI2, vasodilator, platelet aggregation inhibitor) and TXA2 by inhibiting phospholipase A2 (see Oates et al., 1988b), in vitro studies showed that the generation of PGI2 was more depressed at pharmacological doses (Conn, 1990). Furthermore, TXA2 synthesis in platelets is CS resistant due to their inability to induce lipocortin (phospholipase A2 inhibitor), because they are anucleated. As aforementioned, TXA2 may be increased in PAN (as in Kawasaki disease). Finally, one recent study (Ellison et al., 1993) showed cerebral medium-sized artery platelet fragment deposition in PAN by immunochemistry analysis. In conclusion, there is evidence that (penetrating) medium-/small-sized artery occlusions in PAN, producing deep small or pontine lacunar infarcts, are related to atherosclerosis-like mechanisms, which in turn may be promoted by both associated hypertension and mainly the use of CS, and are caused by uncontrolled (TXA2–mediated) platelet aggregation with further thrombus formation. From a therapeutic point of view, antiplatelet drugs, which also inhibit platelet TXA2 production, might reduce the risk of CS-induced arterial occlusion in PAN (once hemorrhagic stroke is excluded, see below). The association of ASA and CS prospectively prevented stroke recurrence in two patients in the present study (patient 3 and 14, Table 4.1).

Hemorrhagic strokes are rare in PAN (20% of all patients). Patients with pure lobar hematoma (two cases)

had no signs of microaneurysm on MRI-/angiography. Because both hematomas involved the temporo-parietal lobes, they could not be related to PAN-induced hypertension, but rather to rupture of the internal elastic lamina in the arterial wall (Bagenstoss et al., 1951). The two other patterns of hemorrhagic strokes in PAN-ie, hemorrhagic transformation of an ischemic infarct, and tiny petechial hemorrhage(s) (Ford & Siekert, 1965), were found in only one case each.

Although echocardiographic studies were performed in only one-third of patients with PAN-associated ischemic strokes in this study, half of them showed signs consistent with a cardio-embolic origin, which is closely similar to the frequency of cardiac involvement in PAN (40% of patients, Lhote & Guillevin, 1991). However, whereas only one patient showed a large ischemic (bilateral parieto-occipital) stroke of cardio-embolic origin (patient 13), the sole patient with an identified left intra-atrial thrombus developed a lacunar stroke syndrome (patient 15).

Livedo reticularis (LR), which is common in PAN (Lhote & Guillevin, 1991), could be observed in near one-fourth of patients with PAN and stroke, but was only weakly correlated with positive aCL (one-fourth of patients with LR). On the other hand, aCL, which when tested (one-third of cases) were found positive in 20% of patients with PAN and stroke, may play a role in the genesis of (small vessel) thrombotic stroke in PAN. The role of antiendothelial cell antibodies (not tested in any patients of this study), which have been reported in 28% of patients with active PAN without stroke and in 35% of patients with Sneddon's syndrome (cerebrovascular accidents and LR), respectively (Frances et al., 1995), requires further evaluation.

Conclusions

Early lacunar stroke syndrome (73% of cases), caused by thrombotic small/medium-sized penetrating artery occlusions rather than by vasculitic arterial changes, was the paramount PAN-associated stroke pattern, followed by pure lobar hematoma (two cases), and ischemic/secondary hemorrhagic infarct (one case each). The roles of cardio-embolic stroke, anticardiolipin (livedo reticularis present in 25% of cases) and antiendothelial antibodies need further evaluation. The shorter stroke latencies (mean 6.5 months) found, as compared with the previously reported late stroke occurrence (2–3 years), correlated well with the use of CS in PAN, i.e. most of the 77% of all first-time or recurrent ischemic strokes that developed despite CS therapy appeared within 6 months (80% of cases: within 3 weeks in 50% of cases). Indeed, CS may promote small-/medium-sized artery occlusion by enhancing the platelet TXA2 production/activity in PAN. Because these mechanisms (and stroke patterns) resemble those of atherosclerosis, and because platelets (together with endothelial cells) play a central role in the genesis of this PAN-associated thrombotic microangiopathy, antiplatelet drugs in association with CS may be advisable.

Churg–Strauss syndrome (CSS)

In 1951, Jacob Churg and Lotte Strauss (Churg & Strauss, 1951) reported 13 patients who developed a clinical vasculitic syndrome (allergic granulomatosis and angiitis) that showed different clinical and pathologic features as compared with PAN. It was characterized by severe asthma with a 'strikingly uniform clinical picture', including fever, hypereosinophilia, and multisystem vascular involvement (Churg & Strauss, 1951). They delineated three major histologic criteria from pathological examination and postmortem studies: tissue infiltration by eosinophils, necrotizing vasculitis, and extravascular granulomas.

CSS is rare, representing only 20% of the systemic necrotizing vasculitis of the PAN group (Lhote & Guillevin, 1991). The male-to-female ratio ranges from 1.1 to 3, and the mean age at onset is younger in CSS (47.5; range, 14–75) than in PAN (54.2; range, 20–80; Guillevin et al., 1996). The pathologic features of CSS are extravascular necrotizing granulomas (palisading epitheloid histiocytes surrounding eosinophilic infiltrates/central necrosis) and necrotizing vasculitis involving the pulmonary and systemic arteries and veins. Extrapulmonary lesions are found in the gastrointestinal tract, heart, and skin. CSS develops in three clinical phases: the prodromal period (allergic rhinitis/nasal polyposis and asthma) precedes for many years the peripheral blood/tissue eosinophilia phase, that is followed by the vasculitic phase. The systemic vasculitis appears within a mean latency of 3 years after the onset of asthma and is characterized by cutaneous lesions (purpura, nodules; two-thirds of patients), peripheral neuropathy (mononeuritis multiplex; 64 to 75% of patients), cardiac (congestive heart failure, pericardial effusions), gastrointestinal (abdominal pain, diarrhoea, bleeding; 37 to 62% of patients), renal (focal segmental glomerulonephritis with necrotizing features) and musculoskeletal (arthritis, 28 to 51% of patients) involvements. In contrast with PAN, two biological markers are strongly associated with (if together not specific) CSS: eosinophilia and ANCA. Eosinophilia (>10% of WBC) is constant and above 10^9/l in 97% of cases (mean eosinophil count, 12.9×10^9/l; range, 1.5–29 $\times 10^9$/l). Approximately 70% of patients with CSS show positive 'perinuclear' p-ANCA (Cohen Taervert & Kallenberg, 1993), which recognize different myeloid proteins such as myeloperoxidase (MPO-ANCA). According to the ACR 1990 (Masi et al., 1990), a patient with vasculitis is said to have CSS (sensitivity, 85%; specificity, 99.7%) when four or more of the six following criteria are present: asthma, eosinophilia (>10% of WBC), mononeuropathy (including multiplex) or polyneuropathy, non-fixed pulmonary infiltrates (radiography), paranasal sinus abnormality, and biopsy containing a blood vessel with extravascular eosinophils. The combination of only asthma (or documented allergy including allergic rhinitis) and eosinophilia discriminates correctly CSS from other vasculitis (sensitivity, 90%; specificity, 99.7%).

CSS-associated strokes

Recently, Chinese authors (Liou et al., 1994) reported a young patient with a history of chronic paranasal sinusitis and asthma who developed mononeuritis multiplex and demyelinating optic neuritis with eosiniphilia (74% of 49 600 WBC/mm³) and positive p-ANCA. Whereas CSS was confirmed by transbronchial, bone marrow, and sural nerve biopsies, cerebral MRI showed asymptomatic multiple and bilateral small periventricular ischemic infarcts, together with a tiny petechial cerebellar hemorrhage. The clinical course improved only after prednisolone together with cyclophosphamide immunosuppressive therapy were initiated.

More recently, Sehgal et al. (1995) reviewed the medical records of 47 consecutive patients with CSS from the Mayo Clinic (1974–1992). Of the 29 patients (62%) with neurologic involvement, the majority (25) had peripheral neuropathy (multiple mononeuropathy, 17; symmetric polyneuropathy, 7; asymmetric polyneuropathy, 1). Three patients with CSS developed stroke (6.4%); of the two patients with MCA ischemic infarcts, one showed a left ventricular thrombus at echocardiography; the third patient had a thalamic stroke. Hence, the mechanism of stroke was known in only one patient (cardioembolism). The time interval between the diagnosis of CSS and the onset of stroke ranged from 2 to 15 years, but it was not specified which stroke patients received CS therapy. Early onset intracerebral/subarachnoidal hemorrhages have also been reported in CSS (Cohen Tervaert & Kallenberg, 1993; Ferro, 1998).

Although there are only a few reported patients with CSS and stroke, it is relevant to note that half of ischemic strokes (2/4) were small deep infarcts: the patient reported by Liou et al. (Liou et al., 1994) showed leukoaraiosis whereas one patient in the series of Sehgal et al. (1995) had a thalamic infarct.

Conclusion

CSS-associated strokes show probably the same patterns, i.e. small deep infarcts and leukoaraiois, large ischemic infarcts, intracerebral (and subarachnoidal) hemorrhages, as those studied in PAN, and certainly share the same mechanisms. Confirmation of these hypotheses is restricted by the even greater rarity of this vasculitic syndrome.

Prognosis and treatment of PAN and CSS

In a prospective study of 342 patients (260 with PAN and 82 with CSS), Guillevin et al. (1996) established a five-factor prognostic score (FFS) in which each item underwent univariate and multivariate analysis. Of the FFS, i.e., renal failure with creatininemia (Cr) >1.58 mg/dl, CNS involvement, cardiomyopathy, the presence of proteinuria (>1 g/d) and gastrointestinal tract involvement were significantly associated with a high mortality rate in a multivariate analysis.

Before the use of CS, only 13% of patients with PAN remained alive at 5 years (Guillevin et al., 1996), and only 50% of patients with CSS survived 3 months after the onset of the vasculitis (Sehgal et al., 1995). Since their initial use in 1950, CS alone have increased the 5-year survival rate of patients with PAN from 10% (untreated) to 55%, and the adjunction of either cyclophosphamide or azathioprine enhances this rate at 82% (Lhote & Guillevin, 1995).

In PAN and CSS, the initial CS therapy (prednisone 1mg/kg per day), giving frequently dramatic response in CSS, should begin with methylprednisolone pulses (15 mg/kg over 60 minutes repeated at 24-h intervals for 1–3 days; Guillevin et al., 1996). The association of cyclophosphamide (preferred pulse therapy with 0.6 g/m² delivered monthly for 1 year) should be considered in patients with PAN and CSS presenting with proteinuria, renal insufficiency (especially with Cr >1.58 mg/dl), cardiomyopathy or CNS involvement, and for those with relapse of vasculitis. The major side effects associated with daily cyclophosphamide administration (2 mg/kg per day) include hemorrhagic cystitis, bladder fibrosis, bone marrow suppression, ovarian failure, and neoplasm (bladder cancer and hematologic malignancies). In HBV-related PAN, the preferred treatment is antiviral agents (vidarabine or interferon-alpha 2b).

Whether antiplatelet drug treatment should be associated with CS for the prevention of stroke in patients with PAN will need further evaluation.

References

Bagenstoss, A.H., Shick, R.M. & Polley, H.F. (1951). The effect of cortisone on the lesions of periarteritis nodosa. *American Journal of Pathology*, **27**, 537–59.

Churg, J. & Strauss, L. (1951). Allergic granulomatosis, allergic angiitis, and periarteritis nodosa. *American Journal of Pathology*, **27**, 277–301.

Cohen, R.D., Conn, D.L. & Ilstrup, D.M. (1980). Clinical features, prognosis, and response to treatment in polyarteritis. *Mayo Clinic Proceedings*, **55**, 146–55.

Cohen Tervaert, J.W. & Kallenberg, C. (1993). Neurologic manifestations of systemic vasculitides. *Rheumatic Diseases Clinics of North America*, **19**, 913–40.

Conn, D.L. (1990). Polyarteritis. *Rheumatic Diseases Clinics of North America*, **16**, 341–62.

De La Fuente Fernandez, R. & Grana Gil, J. (1994). Anticardiolipin antibodies and polyarteritis nodosa. *Lupus*, **3**, 523–4.

Ellison, D., Gatter, K., Heryet, A. & Esiri, M. (1993). Intramural platelet deposition in cerebral vasculopathy of systemic lupus erythematosus. *Journal of Clinical Pathology*, **46**, 37–40.

Ferro, J.M. (1998). Vasculitis of the central nervous system. *Journal of Neurology*, **245**, 766–76.

Font, C., Miro, O., Pedrol, E. et al. (1996). Polyarteritis nodosa in human immunodeficiency virus infection: report of four cases and review of the literature. *British Journal of Rheumatics*, **35**, 796–9.

Ford, R.G. & Siekert, R.G. (1965). Central nervous system manifestations of periarteritis nodosa. *Neurology*, **15**, 114–22.

Frances, C., Le Tonqueze, B.S., Salohzin, K.V. et al. (1995). Prevalence of anto-endothelial cell antibodies in patients with Sneddon's syndrome. *Journal of the American Academy of Dermatology*, **33**, 64–8.

Guillevin, L., Lhote, F., Cohen, P. et al. (1995). Polyarteritis nodosa related to hepatitis B virus. A prospective study with long-term observation of 41 patients. *Medicine*, **74**, 238–53.

Guillevin, L., Lhote, F., Gayraud, M. et al. (1996). Prognostic factors in polyarteritis nodosa and Churg–Strauss syndrome. A prospective study in 342 patients. *Medicine*, **75**, 17–28.

Harlé, J.R., Disdier, P., Ali Cherif, A., Figarella-Branger, D., Pellissier, J.F. & Weiller, P.J. (1991). Démence curable et panartérite noueuse. *Revue Neurologie (Paris)*, **147**, 148–50.

Hirohata, S., Tanimoto, K. & Ito, K. (1993). Elevation of cerebrospinal fluid interleukin-6 activity in patients with vasculitides and central nervous involvement. *Clinical Immunology and Immunopathology*, **66**, 225–9.

Iaconetta, G., Benvenuti, D., Lamaida, E., Gallicchio, B., Signorelli, F. & Maiuri, F. (1994). Cerebral hemorrhagic complication in polyarteritis nodosa. *Acta Neurologica (Napoli)*, **16**, 64–9.

Jenette, J.C. & Falk, R.J. (1997). Small-vessel vasculitis. *New England Journal of Medicine*, **337**, 1512–23.

Jenette, J.C., Falk, R.J., Andrassy, K. et al. (1994). Nomenclature of systemic vasculitides. Proposal of an international consensus conference. *Arthritis and Rheumatism*, **37**, 187–92.

Kasantikul, V., Suwanwela, N. & Pongsabutr, S. (1991). Magnetic resonance images of brain stem infarct in periarteritis nodosa. *Surgical Neurology*, **36**, 133–6.

Koppensteiner, R., Base, W., Bognar, H., Kiss, A., Al Mubarak, M. & Tscholakoff, D. (1989). Course of cerebral lesions in a patient with periarteritis nodosa studied by magnetic resonance imaging. *Klinik Wochenschrift*, **67**, 398–401.

Kussmaul, A. & Maier, R. (1866). Ueber eine bisher nicht beschriebene eigenthuemliche Arterienkrankung (Periarteritis nodosa), die mit Morbus Brightii und rapid fortschreitender allgemeiner Muskellaehmung einhergeht. *Deutsch Archiv Klinik Medicin*, **1**, 484–518.

Lhote, F. & Guillevin, L. (1991). Polyarteritis nodosa, microscopic polyangiitis, and Churg–Strauss syndrome: clinical aspects and treatment. *Rheumatic Disease Clinics of North America*, **21**, 911–47.

Lhote, F., Cohen, P., Genereau, T., Gayraud, M. & Guillevin, L. (1996). Microscopic polyangiitis: clinical aspects and treatment. *Annales Medicales Internes (Paris)*, **147**, 165–77.

Lightfoot, R.W.J., Michel, A.B., Bloch, D.A. et al. (1990). The American College of Rheumatology 1990 criteria for the classification of polyarteritis nodosa. *Arthritis and Rheumatism*, **33**, 1088–93.

Liou, H-H., Yip, P-K., Chang, Y-C. & Liu, H-M. (1994). Allergic granulomatosis and angiitis (Churg–Strauss syndrome) presenting as prominent neurologic lesions and optic neuritis. *Journal of Rheumatology*, **21**, 2380–4.

Long, S.M. & Dolin, P. (1994). Polyarteritis nodosa presenting as acute blindness. *Annals of Emergency Medicine*, **24**, 523–5.

Masi, A.T., Hunder, G.G., Lie, J.T. et al. (1990). The American College of Rheumatology 1990 criteria for the classification of Churg–Strauss syndrome (allergic granulomatosis and angiitis). *Arthritis and Rheumatism*, **33**, 1094–100.

Mayo, J., Arias, M., Leno, C. & Berciano, J. (1986). Vascular parkinsonism and periarteritis nodosa, *Neurology*, **36**, 874–5.

Moore, P.M. (1995). Neurological manifestations of vasculitis: update on immunopathogenic mechanisms and clinical features. *Annals of Neurology*, **37**(S1), S131–41.

Moore, P.M. & Cupps, T.R. (1983). Neurological complications of vasculitis. *Annals of Neurology*, **14**, 155–67.

Moore, P.M. & Fauci, A.S. (1981). Neurologic manifestations of systemic vasculitis: a restrospective and prospective study of the clinicopathologic features and responses to therapy in 25 patients. *American Journal of Medicine*, **71**, 517–24.

Oates, J.A., Fitzgerald, G.A., Branch, R.A., Jackson, E.K., Knapp, H.R. & Roberts, L.J.X. (1988a). Clinical implications of prostaglandins and thromboxane A2 formation (part one). *New England Journal of Medicine*, **319**, 689–98.

Reichhart, M.D., Bogousslavsky, J. & Janzer, R.C. (2000). Early lacunar strokes complicating polyarteritis nodosa: thrombotic microangiopathy. *Neurology*, **54**, 883–9.

Sehgal, M., Swanson, J.W., Deremee, R.A. & Colby, T.V. (1995). Neurologic manifestations of Churg–Strauss syndrome. *Mayo Clinic Proceedings*, **70**, 337–41.

Squire, I.B., Grosset, D.G. & Lees, K.R. (1993). Immunosupressive treatment in stroke and renal failure. *Annals of Rheumatic Diseases*, **52**, 165–8.

Stahl, H., Mihatsch, M.J., Orantes, M. & Lehmann, F. (1995). Pneumonia, biclonal gammopathy, paresis of the fibular nerve and cerebrovascular insult. *Schweiz Rund Medicin*, **84**, 1071–8.

Watts, R.A., Jolliffe, A.V., Carruthers, D.M., Lockwood, M. & Scott, D. (1996). Effect of classification on incidence of polyarteritis nodosa and microscopic polyangiitis. *Arthritis and Rheumatism*, **39**, 1208–12.

Wildhagen, K., Stoppe, G., Meyer, G.J., Heintz, P., Hundeshagen, H. & Deicher, H. (1989). Bildgebende Diagnostik der zentralnervoesen Beteiligung der Panarteriitis nodosa. *Zeitschrift Rheumatologie*, **48**, 323–5.

5

Takayasu disease

Yukito Shinohara

Department of Neurology, Tokai University School of Medicine Bohseidai, Kanagawa, Japan

Introduction

The clinical signs and symptoms caused by stenosing and obstructing processes in the aortic arch and the origin of its major vessels, the innominate arteries, the carotid arteries and the subclavian arteries, have an enormous variety of nomenclatures. These include Takayasu disease (Pahwa et al., 1959), Takayasu's syndrome (Ask-Upmark, 1956), Takayasu's arteritis (Hirsch et al., 1964), Takayasu–Ohnishi's disease (Hirose & Baba, 1963), aortic arch syndrome (Frövig, 1946), aortic arch arteritis (Koszewski, 1958), aortitis syndrome, pulseless disease (Shimizu & Sano, 1951), pulseless syndrome (Lessoff & Glynn, 1959), reversed coarctation (Giffin, 1939), carotis-subclavia arteritis, brachiocephalic arteritis, chronic subclavian-carotid obstruction syndrome (Bustamante et al., 1954), chronic subclaviocarotid syndrome, syndrome of obliteration of supraaortic branches (Martorell et al., 1944), obliterative brachiocephalic arteritis Gibbons & King, 1957), thromboarteritis obliterans subclaviocarotica, thromboangitic obliterans of the branches of the aortic arch (Kalmanson & Kalmansohn, 1957), panarteritis branchiocephalica (Gilmour, 1941), idiopathic medial aortopathy and arteriopathy (Marquis et al., 1968), Martorell syndrome and so on. Among them, aortic arch syndrome and Takayasu disease or Takayasu's arteritis are most frequently used to describe the overall clinical picture of this syndrome or disease. However, the term aortic arch syndrome can be used to describe many conditions including arteriosclerosis, syphilitic aortitis, young female arteritis of unknown etiology and other pathological conditions (traumatic, congenital, thrombotic, neoplastic, embolic and so on) (Ross & McKusick, 1953; Thurlbeck & Currens, 1959; Judge et al., 1962). On the other hand, Takayasu disease usually means an arteritis of unknown origin, involving the aortic arch, with inflammatory narrowing or obstruction of the proximal portion of the major branches, and occurring predominantly in young women. Therefore, Takayasu disease is one of the causes of aortic arch syndrome and should be defined separately from other types of aortic arch syndrome.

Historical review

At the Annual Meeting of the Japanese Ophthalmological Society in 1905, Takayasu (1908), a Japanese ophthalmologist, presented a 21-year-old woman with peculiar eye ground findings in both eyes. She had a wreath-like anastomosis surrounding the optic disc at a distance of 2 or 3 mm and surrounding this was another circular anastomosis. There were anastomotic shunts of arterioles and venules. Both the surrounding vessels and their branches had lumps which were seen to move from day to day. Although Takayasu did not understand the etiology of the disease, this was the first description of the so-called Takayasu retinopathy (Ito, 1995). At the same meeting, Ohnishi mentioned a similar patient who had circular anastomosis and aneurysma-like lumps in the optic fundi, with no palpable radial pulses. Immediately afterwards, Kagoshima also mentioned a similar pulseless patient with cataracta. Those presentations and discussions were the origin of the term Takayasu disease or Takayasu–Ohnishi's disease. However, according to Judge et al. (1962), Pokrovsky et al. (1980) and Bleck (1989), the first description of this kind of disorder, i.e. Takayasu disease, observed usually in young women, was not by Takayasu and Ohnishi, but by Davy (1939) in 1839 and independently by Savory (1856) and by Kussmaul (1873) in 1856. But, since the term Takayasu disease is now most commonly used, we have adopted it in this chapter.

Table 5.1. (a) *Age distribution and* (b) *estimated age of onset of Takayaru disease in Japan*

Year examined:	(a) Age distribution			(b) Estimated age of onset		
	1973–5	1982–4	1991	1973–5	1982–4	1991
Age < 9	22	3	2	11	19	10
10<19	180	128	47	285	333	182
20<29	637	397	168	453	625	342
30<39	527	714	213	253	408	281
40<49	448	601	387	96	233	187
50<59	218	512	357	39	138	100
60<69	84	203	228	13	22	35
70<79	20	46	72	3	10	10
Unknown	12	2	1	233	818	328
Total number of patients	2148	2606	1475	1386	2606	1475

Epidemiology

Koide (1992) and his colleagues performed epidemiological studies in Japan from 1973 to 1991. The age distribution of the aortic arch syndrome, mainly Takayasu disease, is shown in Table 5.1. The female to male ratio was 11 to 1, and the great majority of patients developed their initial symptoms in their third or fourth decade; more recent results delineate slightly different manifestations in an older population, probably due to the upward shift of the average age of the female population in Japan. As shown on the right of Table 5.1, the estimated age of onset was rather similar in all the studies.

In China, Deyu et al. (1992) reported 530 cases of Takayasu disease. The age distribution was quite similar to that in Japan, but the female to male ratio was 2.9 to 1, which is very different from Japan. Hall et al. (1985) suggested that the North American incidence of this disease was 2.6 per million per year.

These results suggest that, while this disease has an unexplained predilection for Orientals, it occurs in all racial groups.

Pathogenesis

The etiology of this disease is unknown. An autoimmune pathogenesis is often suggested, but so far there is no direct evidence for this. Coexistent tuberculosis was also suspected to be one of the causes, but no direct evidence has been found, including the case of Takayasu (1908).

Since Takayasu disease seems to occur predominantly in Asian countries and twin patients with this disease are sometimes observed, there is a possibility that hereditary factors may participate in its pathophysiology. Dong et al. (1992) examined HLA-DP antigen in 64 patients with Takayasu disease and 317 healthy individuals in the Japanese population, and found that the combination or haplotype of HLA–Bw52-DRB1*1502-DRB5*0102-DQA1*0103-DQB1*0601-DPA1*02-DPB1*0901 may confer susceptibility to this disorder, while another combination or haplotype of HLA Bw54-DRB1*0405-DRB4*0101-DQA1*0301-DQB1*0401 may confer resistance to the disease.

Pathology and hemodynamics

In Takayasu disease, the aortic arch with its main arterial trunks and the descending aorta, as well as renal arteries, are the main site of inflammation. The lymphoplasmacytic inflammation affects primarily the tuna media, causing destruction of the elastic lamellae (acute phase). In the intermediate stage the inflammatory infiltrate subsides, and the partially necrotic media is revascularized by new branches of the vasa vasorum. Secondary fibrosis of all layers causes thickening and loss of compliance of the vessel walls. The involved arteries are finally transformed into rigid, thick-walled tubes with severe narrowing or occlusion by superimposed thrombosis. Saccular aneurysms may also arise during this phase (sclerosing stage).

Cerebral blood flow (CBF) studies were done in some patients by using SPECT (Grosset et al., 1992) and PET (Takano et al., 1993). However, the results were different depending on the patients and on their stages. In some cases, CBF was reduced in the watershed territories of the brain (Grosset et al., 1992). In others, CBF and cerebral oxygen extraction fraction were well maintained (Takano et al., 1993), but the hemodynamic reserve, as well as oxygen metabolism, was impaired in cases with cerebral infarction (Takano et al., 1993).

Classification of Takayasu disease

Four types of aortic arch involvements in Takayasu disease are known. In type 1, involvement is limited to the ascending aorta and the aortic arch, type 2 to the infradiaphragmatic aorta, type 3 to the supra- and infradiaphragma and type 4 to the pulmonary arteries (Nakao et al., 1967; Lupi-Herrera et al., 1979).

Clinical manifestations and prognosis

Initial manifestations

Takayasu disease is thought to begin clinically with symptoms of systemic inflammation (Bleck, 1989) or with eye symptoms (Takayasu, 1908). Bleck (1989) described myalgias, arthralgias, fatigue, fever and weight loss as prominent early symptoms. He also mentioned that the occurrence of neurological symptoms such as claudication, transient ischemic attack, and stroke-like symptoms can seldom be categorized into early or late phenomena. However, Kerr et al. (1994) mentioned that only 33% of their patients had systemic symptoms. In a large study of more than 1000 patients in Japan (Koide, 1992), the most frequent chief complaints at the first visit in patients with Takayasu disease were symptoms related to ischemia of the extremities, such as paresthesia, cold sensation, pulselessness, claudication and so on (72.3%, 969/1341), followed by systemic symptoms such as fever, easy-fatiguability or lassitude (66.8%, 885/1324) and symptoms related to cerebral ischemia such as dizziness, headache, syncope and so on (64.6%, 837/1351 patients), although some headache may not have been related to cerebral ischemia.

Neurological symptoms related to stroke

It is known that serious illness and death in younger patients with Takayasu disease is often due to central nervous system involvement. Cerebral vascular disease is usually a consequence of severe hypertension, or carotid or brachiocephalic obstruction. Among his 81 patients with Takayasu disease, Ishikawa (1981) reported that five of 16 deaths were due to stroke. These 16 patients also experienced serious morbidity, including two subarachnoid hemorrhages, one intracerebral hemorrhage, two cases of acute unilateral blindness, and two bilateral blindness.

On the other hand, Rose and Sinclair-Smith (1980) reported that three of 16 deaths with a mean age of 20 years were due to hypertensive intracerebral hemorrhages. In a large study in Japan (Koide, 1992), eight out of 69 deaths were due to stroke in 1972 to 1975, while five of 59 deaths were due to stroke in a study which was done in 1991. In the latter study, only three out of five stroke deaths were due to intracerebral hemorrhage. Among the above 59 deaths, 21 were due to cardiac disorders and 12 were due to rupture of aortic aneurysma. However, in a Chinese study (Deyu et al., 1992), cerebral hemorrhage was the most common cause of death. 23.6% of deaths (13 of 55 among 530 patients) were due to cerebral hemorrhage and

3.6% (2 of 55 among 530) to cerebral infarction (Deyu et al., 1992).

Because the subclavian artery proximal to the origin of the vertebral artery is often involved earlier, diversion of blood from the vertebro-basilar territory into the subclavian artery via retrograde flow through the ipsilateral vertebral artery may occur. This steal phenomenon of the blood from the posterior circulation of the brain, if symptomatic, is called the 'subclavian steal syndrome' (Reivich et al., 1961).

Diagnosis and laboratory data

It is well known that the erythrocyte sedimentation rate (ESR) is elevated in most patients, particularly in the stage of exacerbation. At the first visit to the hospital, the laboratory abnormalities usually found were elevation of ESR, positive CRP, anemia, elevated serum gamma globulin, leucocytosis and so on, in that order.

Usually, physical examinations reveal weakness or right-to-left difference of radial pulsation, weakness of femoral arterial pulsation, asymmetry of blood pressure, hypertension, cardiac murmur, bruit especially on the neck, supraclavicula, anterior chest, abnormal ocular findings, and so on.

If such physical abnormalities and abnormal laboratory data are found, especially in young women, angiography should be performed to confirm the diagnosis. Angiography still remains the cornerstone of diagnosis (Fig. 5.1). MR-angiography may also be a useful tool for diagnosing Takayasu disease (Fig. 5.2).

Differential diagnosis

Disorders which should be differentiated from Takayasu disease include arteriosclerosis, Buerger's disease, congenital vessel anomalies, coarctation of aorta, dissecting aneurysm, collagen disease, and Behcet's disease.

Complications

Major complications of this disease include aortic regurgitation (33%), dilatation of aortic arch (27%), and renovascular hypertension (21%) (Koide, 1992). Others include coarctation of the aorta, pulmonary infarction, myocardial infarction and so on.

As regards stroke, 16 patients with intracranial aneurysma were reported and among them 13 were ruptured

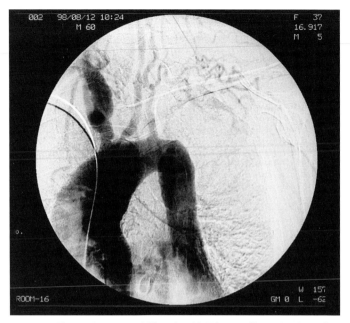

Fig. 5.1. A 57-year-old female with Takayasu disease (estimated age of onset: 23-years). Note occlusion of the left subclavian artery and collateral circulation through left vertebral artery, although this patient did not show symptomatic subclavian steal syndrome.

and three were unruptured (Asaoka et al., 1998). Intracranial aneurysmas arose predominantly along the course of collateral flow, especially in the vertebrobasilar system, and a high incidence of multiplicity has been reported.

Therapy

Concerning the treatment and management for Takayasu disease patients with stroke, one has to consider the treatment of Takayasu disease and stroke separately. Intracerebral hemorrhage in Takayasu disease can be managed in the same way as usual hypertensive intracerebral hemorrhage. Since the patients may have aortic regurgitation, aortic arch dilation or intracranial aneurysmas, the control of high blood pressure is essential, especially in patients with hemorrhagic stroke. In patients with subarachnoid hemorrhage, immediate detection of the site of ruptured aneurysma is necessary and immediate surgery should be performed. In patients with ischemic stroke, systemic blood pressure should not be reduced abruptly, but attention must always be paid to the control of extremely high blood pressure in order to prevent the development of cardiac failure. The use of antiplatelet drugs such as aspirin

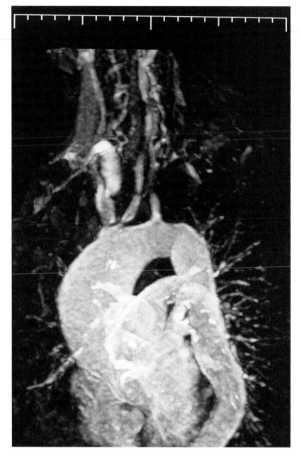

Fig. 5.2. MR angiography of the same patient.

(80 to 350 mg/day) or ticlopidine (100–300 mg/day) is recommended in ischemic stroke if blood pressure is not so high. In cerebral thrombosis, thromboxane A2 inhibitor may be used in the acute stage.

Together with the management of stroke, treatment for Takayasu disease itself is also necessary in the active stage of the disease. Although there has been no randomized controlled study regarding the efficacy of medical and surgical treatments of Takayasu disease, it is generally believed that corticosteroids are effective in controlling the inflammatory symptoms. The dose of steroid is initially in the 0.5–1.5 mg/kg/day or 20 to 75 mg/day predonisolone-equivalent range. Usually, the dose of steroid should be reduced by 5 to 10 mg every 2 to 3 weeks. Five to 10 mg should be continued until the ESR drops below 20 mm/h and CRP becomes negative. During the acute stage, surgical procedures, angiography with contrast media or percutaneous angioplasty should be avoided. In this connection, MR angiography (Fig. 5.2) is a useful tool for diagnosing this disease atraumatically. Immunosuppressants such as cyclophosphamide, azathioprine or 6–mercaptoprine are not used so often recently, but may be used if steroid therapy is not effective. Anticoagulants such as heparin or warfarin have been employed in the hope of preventing thrombosis distal to the stenosis or occlusions, but so far no data concerning efficacy are available.

Surgical procedures, including intravascular technique, are necessary in some cases with severe aortic regurgitation, aortic coarctation or reno-vascular hypertension. But, these procedures should not be undertaken in the acute stage of inflammation or stroke. Aneurysma or aneurysma-like dilation may be observed in the territories of brachiocephalic artery, subclavian artery, descending aorta or carotid artery as well as cerebral artery. If the aneurysma increases in size during observation, surgical treatment should be done before rupture. Subclavian steal syndrome or moderate carotid stenosis, as well as renal artery stenosis (Sharma et al., 1992), may be an indication for angioplasty.

References

Asaoka, K., Houkin, K., Fujimoto, S., Ishikwa, T. & Abe, H. (1998). Intracranial aneurysmas associated with aortitis syndrome: case report and review of the literature. *Neurosurgery*, **42**, 157.

Ask-Upmark, E. & Fajers C-M. (1956). Further observations on Takayasu's syndrome. *Acta Medica Scandinavica*, **155**, 275.

Bleck, T.P. (1989). Takayasu's disease. In *Handbook of Clinical Neurology* vol. 11: Part III chap. 20, ed. J.F. Toole, p. 335. Elsevier Science Publ.

Bustamante, R.A., Milanes, B., Casas, M. & De-La Torre, A. (1954). The chronic subclavian-carotid obstruction syndrome (pulseless disease). *Angiology*, **5**, 479.

Davy, J. (1839). Researches, Physiological and Anatosiscal. Vol. 1 pp.426, London: Smith Elder and Co. (quoted from Judge et al., 1962).

Deyu, Z., Dijun, F. & Lisheng, L. (1992). Takayasu arteritis in China: a report of 530 cases. *Heart Vessels*, Suppl 7: 32.

Dong, R-P., Kimura, A., Numano, F. et al. (1992). HLA-DP antigen and Takayasu arteritis. *Tissue Antigens*, **39**, 106.

Frøvig, A.G. (1946). Bilateral obliteration of the common caroid artery. Thrombangitis obliterans? *Acta Phychiatrica Neurologica Scandinavica*, Suppl, **39**.

Gibbons, T.B. & King, R.L. (1957). Obliterative brachiocephalic arteritis: pulseless disease of Takayasu. *Circulation*, **15**, 845.

Giffin, H.M. (1939). Reversed coarctation and vasomotor gradient: report of a cardiovascular anomaly with sympotoms of brain tumor. *Proceedings of the Mayo Clinic*, **14**, 561.

Gilmour, J.R. (1941). Giant-cell arteritis. *Journal of Pathology and Bacteriology*, **53**, 263.

Grosset, D.G., Patterson, J. & Bone, I. (1992). Intracranial hae-modynamics in Takayasu's arteritis. *Acta Neurochirurgica*, **119**, 161.

Hall, S., Barr, W., Lie, J.T., Stanson, A.W., Kazmier, F.J. & Hunder, G.G. (1985). Takayasu arteritis. *Medicine*, **94**, 89.

Hirose, K. & Baba, K. (1963). A study of fundus changes in the early stages of Takayasu–Ohnishi (pulseless) disease. *American Journal of Ophthalmology*, **55**, 293.

Hirsch, M.S., Aikat, B.K. & Basu, A.K. (1964). Takayasu arteritis. *Bulletin Johns Hopkins Hospital*, **115**, 29.

Ishikawa, K. (1981). Survival and morbidity after diagnosis of occlusive thromboaortopathy (Takayasu's disease). *American Journal of Cardiology*, **47**, 1026.

Ito, I. (1995). Aortitis syndrome (Takayasu's arteritis). A historical perspective. *Japan Heart Journal*, **36**, 273.

Judge, R.D., Currier, R.D., Gracie, W.A. & Figley, M.M. (1962). Takayasu's arteritis and the aortic arch syndrome. *American Journal of Medicine*, **32**, 379.

Kalmanson, R.B. & Kalmansohn, R.W. (1957). Thrombotic obliteration of the branches of the aortic arch. *Circulation*, **15**, 237.

Kerr, G.S., Hallahan, C.W., Gierdant, J. et al. (1994). Takayasu arteritis. *Annals of Internal Medicine*, **120**, 919.

Koide, K. (1992). Aortitis syndrome. *Nihon Rinsho*, **50**, 343 (in Japanese).

Koszewski, B.J. (1958). Branchial arteritis or aortic arch arteritis. A new inflammatory arterial disease (pulseless disease). *Angiology*, **9**, 180.

Kussmaul, A. (1873). Zwei Falle von spontaner allmaliger Verschliessung grosser Halsarterienstamme. *Deutsche Klinik*, **24**, 461.

Lessoff, M.H. & Glynn, L.E. (1959). Pulseless syndrome. *Lancet*, 799.

Lupi-Herrera, E., Sanchez-Torres, G., Marcushamer, J., Mispireta, J., Hornitz, S. & Espinovela, J. (1979). Takayasu's arteritis. Clinical study of 107 cases. *American Heart Journal*, **73**, 94.

Marquis, J., Richardson, J.B., Ritchie, A.C. & Wigle, E.D. (1968). Idiopathic medial aortopathy and arteriopathy. *American Journal of Medicine*, **44**, 939.

Martorell, F. &, Fabbé Tersol, J. (1944). El síndrome de obliteración de los troncos supraaorticos. *Medicina Clínica (Barcelona)*, **2**, 26.

Nakao, K., Ikeda, M., Kimata, S. et al. (1967). Takayasu's arteritis. Clinical report of eighty-four cases and immunological studies of seven cases. *Circulation*, **35**, 1141.

Pahwa, J.M., Pandey, M.P. & Gypha, D.P. (1959). Pulseless disease, or Takayasu's disease. *British Medical Journal*, **2**, 1439.

Pokrovsky, A.V., Tsereshkin, D.M. & Golossovskaya, M.A. (1980). Pathology of non-specific aortoarteritis. *Angiology*, **31**, 549.

Reivich, M., Holling, H.E., Roberts, B. & Toole, J.F. (1961). Reversal of blood flow through the vertebral artery and its effects on cerebral circulation. *New England Journal of Medicine*, **265**, 878.

Rose, A.G. & Sinclair-Smith, C.C. (1980). Takayasu's arteritis; a study of 16 autopsy cases. *Archives of Pathology and Laboratory Medicine*, **104**, 231.

Ross, R.S. & McKusick, V.A. (1953). Aortic arch syndromes. Diminished or absent pulses in arteries arising from arch of aorta. *Archives of Internal Medicine*, **92**, 701.

Savory, W.S. (1856). Case of a young woman in whom the main

arteries of both upper extremities and of the left side of the neck were throughout completely obliterated. *Transactions Medical-Chirurgical Society (London), London,* **39**, 205, (quoted from Judge et al., 1962).

Sharma, S., Saxena, A., Talwar, K.K., Kaul, U., Mehta, S.N. & Rajani, M. (1992). Renal artery stenosis caused by nonspecific arteritis (Takayasu disease): Results of treatment with percutaneous transluminal angioplasty. *American Journal of Radiology,* **158**, 417.

Shimizu, K. & Sano, K. (1951). Pulseless disease. *Journal of Neuropathology and Experimental Neurology,* **1**, 37.

Takano, K., Sadoshima, S., Ibayashi, S., Ichiya, Y. & Fujishima, M. (1993). Altered cerebral hemodynamics and metabolism in Takayasu's arteritis with neurological deficits. *Stroke,* **24**, 1501.

Takayasu, M. (1908). A case with peculiar changes of the central retinal vessels. *Acta Societatis Ophthalmologicae Japonicae,* **12**, 554, (in Japanese).

Thurlbeck, W.M. & Currens, J.H. (1959). The aortic arch syndrome (pulseless disease): a report of ten cases with three autopsies. *Circulation,* **19**, 499.

6

Bürger's disease (Thrombangiitis obliterans)

Hans C. Diener and Tobias Kurth

Department of Neurology, University of Essen, Germany

Introduction

Bürger's disease or thrombangiitis obliterans (TAO) is a non-atherosclerotic segmental inflammatory obliterative vascular disease that affects medium- and small-sized arteries as well as superficial veins. Distal vessels of the legs and arms are mainly involved. TAO rarely affects cerebral and visceral vessels and even more rarely deep veins. It was first described by von Winiwarter in 1879 and later by Bürger in 1908. The pathological examination may show two phases of the disease. In the acute phase, arteries or veins are occluded by a fresh thrombus (Crawford, 1977). The intima is inflamed. Endothelial cells proliferate, lymphocytes can be observed in the intima and fibrinoid necorisis of the intima (Leu, 1969; Leu & Brunner, 1973). In the chronic phase, pathological changes are unspecific and include recanalization of the organized thrombus and perivascular fibrosis.

According to Zülch and Pilz (1989), Bürger's disease manifested in the brain has the following morphologic characteristics:

(i) arterial occlusions caused by thrombosis in small arteries without arteriosclerosis,

(ii) spatial predilection for the cerebral surface in the watershed region between the middle cerebral artery and the anterior and posterior cerebral arteries, respectively.

Lindenberg and Spatz (1940) described two neuropathologically distinct forms of cerebral thrombangiitis obliterans (TAO):

(i) one form with changes of the arteries with a diameter below 1 mm; and

(ii) another form with thrombosis of the large basal arteries (internal carotid artery or middle cerebral artery) in combination with involvement of distal small arteries.

The cerebral form of TAO was criticized by Fisher (1957) who doubted that a cerebral form of TAO existed. The vascular changes could be caused by pial artery occlusion in the presence of systemic arterial hypotension (Romanuel & Abramowitz, 1964).

Epidemiology

The incidence of TAO in white men under the age of 45 years is 8–12/100000/year (DeBakey & Cohen 1963; Lie, 1989). It is more common in Eastern Europe, the Middle East and Asia than in Western countries (Reny & Cabane, 1998). In recent years a decrease of prevalence rates has been reported (Matsushita et al., 1998); Mills and Porter reported a male-to-female ratio variation between 8:1 and 3.3:1 (Mills & Porter, 1991; Olin et al., 1990). Recent studies showed a ratio up to 14:1 or even more (Jimenez-Paredes et al. 1998; Puchmayer, 1996). The median age at the time of diagnosis is between 35 and 45 years. The cerebral form of TAO accounts for about 2% of all cases of TAO (Zülch & Pilz, 1989; Lippmann, 1952). Inzelberg et al. identified, in a cumulative follow-up period of 833 patient–years of 46 patients with TAO, only one patient with no other risk factor for stroke who suffered from transient aphasia and right hemiparesis (Inzelberg et al., 1989). The rarity of the cerebral manifestation makes it difficult to conclude that cerebrovascular manifestations are part of this disease.

Pathogenesis

The pathogenesis of TAO is still poorly understood and there is no specific marker of the disease. TAO in the limbs is seen almost exclusively in smokers. Cessation of smoking leads to regression of the vessel lesions and finally to remission. Recent studies indicate that autoimmune mechanisms act via a cell-mediated immune response to human artery type specific collagens (Papa et al., 1992; Adar et al., 1983). A tobacco antigen has been suggested as a cause of vascular reactivity in cigarette smokers. A study by Papa et al. (1992) in 13 patients with TAO, 16 healthy smokers and 12 non-smokers found identical cellular responses to tobacco glycoprotein in smokers and patients with TAO. Patients with TAO had a significantly higher frequency of HLA-DR4 and a lower frequency of HLA-DRW6 antigens. Other studies report a significant increase in other HLA antibodies (HLA-B40, HLA-B35 and HLA-DR2) and anticollagen antibodies in patients with TAO (Fernandez-Miranda et al., 1993; Jaini et al., 1998). These results indicate that an autoimmune mechanism is involved. Pietraszek found an increased blood level of free serotonin and a decreased maximal platelet serotonin uptake velocity. This may lead to platelet activation via 5–HT2 receptors (Pietraszek et al., 1993).

Clinical features

TAO is characterized by claudication or ischemia of both legs and less so of the arms. The disease begins distally and progresses more proximally. With disease progression Raynaud's phenomenon (34%), upper extremities involvement (34%) and superficial phlebitis (37%) occur (Mills & Porter, 1991). Two limbs are affected in 16%, three in 41% and all limbs in 43% (Shionoya, 1989). Later during the disease, gangrene, ulcerations and rest pain are the leading symptoms. Leg amputation is required in 5–15% and finger amputations in 15–20% of patients (Joyce, 1990). Diagnostic criteria are shown in Table 6.1.

The clinical picture of neurological disturbances is nonspecific: monoparesis, hemiparesis, visual field defects, aphasia, dysarthria and cerebellar symptoms may occur (Zülch & Pilz 1989). One case with involvement of the external carotid artery showing vascular lesions in the oral cavity was described by Farish et al. (1990).

The diagnosis of TAO requires the exclusion of an embolic source, autoimmune disease, diabetes, hyperlipidemia. Arteriography should show the distal involvement with normal arterial lumen proximal to the popliteal or distal brachial level and the absence of atheromatous changes in the large vessels.

Therapy

Abstinence from tobacco will halt disease progression and sometimes result in regression of vascular changes. Ex-

Table 6.1. *Diagnostic criteria*

A. Onset distal extremity ischemic symptoms before 45 years of age
B. Normal arteries proximal to the popliteal or distal brachial level
C. Distal occlusive disease documented by distinctive plethysmographic, arteriographic, or pathological findings
D. Absence of any of the following conditions:
1. proximal embolic source
2. trauma
3. autoimmune disease
4. diabetes
5. hyperlipidemia

Source: From Mills and Porter (1991).

smokers have a significantly smaller frequency of amputations than smokers. It is not known whether immunosuppressive therapy with azathioprine is helpful. Corticosteroids, reserpine, calcium channel blockers, alpha-blockers, antiplatelet drugs and anticoagulants are not effective (Olin et al., 1990). There are no reports of a specific therapy for the cerebral form of TAO.

References

Adar, R., Papa, M.Z., Halpern, Z. et al. (1983). Cellular sensitivity of collagen in thrombangitis obliterans. *New England Journal of Medicine*, **308**, 1113–16.

Bürger, L. (1908). Thrombo-angiitis obliterans: a study of the vascular lesion leading to pre-senile spontaneous gangrene. *American Journal of Medical Sciences*, **136**, 567–80.

Crawford, T. (1977). Blood and lymphatic vessels, thrombangiitis obliterans (Buerger's disease). In *Pathology* Vol. 1, ed. W.A.D. Anderson & J.M. Kissane, pp. 897–927. Mosby: St Louis.

DeBakey, M.E. & Cohen, B. (1963). *Buerger's Disease: Follow-up Study of World War II Army Cases.* Springfield, Ill: Charles C. Thomas Publishing.

Farish, S.E., el Mofty, S.K. & Colm, S.J. (1990). Intraoral manifestation of thromboangiitis obliterans (Buerger's disease). *Oral Surgery, Oral Medicine, and Oral Pathology*, **69**, 223–6.

Fernandez-Miranda, C., Rubio, R., Vicario, J.L. et al. (1993) [Thromboangiitis obliterans (Buerger's disease). Study of 41 cases (comment)]. *Medical Clinics (Barcelona)*, **101**, 321–6.

Fisher, M.C. (1957). Cerebral thromboangiitis obliterans (including a critical review of the literature). *Medicine*, 36, 169–209.

Inzelberg, R., Bornstein, N.M. & Korczyn, A.D. (1989). Cerebrovascular symptoms in thromboangiitis obliterans. *Acta Neurologica Scandinavica*, **80**, 347–50.

Jaini, R., Mandal, S., Khazanchi, R.K. & Mehra, N.K. (1998).

Immunogenetic analysis of Buerger's disease in India. *International Journal of Cardiology*, **66** Suppl. 1, S283–5.

Jimenez-Paredes, C.A., Canas-Davila, C.A., Sanchez, A. et al. (1998). Buerger's disease at the 'San Juan De Dios' Hospital, Santa Fe De Bogota, Colombia. *International Journal of Cardiology*, **66** Suppl 1, S267–72.

Joyce, J.W. (1990). Buerger's disease (thromboangiitis obliterans). *Rheumatological Disease Clinics of North America*, **16**, 463–70.

Leu, H.J. (1969). Die entzündlichen Arterien- und Venenerkrankungen. *Zentralblatt für Phlebologie*, **8**, 164–4.

Leu, H.J. & Brunner, U. (1973). Zur pathologisch-anatomischen Abgrenzung der Thrombangiitis obliterans von der Arteriosklerose. *Deutsche Medizinische Wochenschrift*, **98**, 158–61.

Lie, J.T. (1989). The rise and fall of resurgence of thrombangiitis obliterans (Buerger's disease). *Acta Pathologica Japan*, **39**, 153.

Lindenberg, R. & Spatz, H. (1940). Über die Thrombendarteriitis obliterans der Hirngefäße (cerebrale Form der Winiwarter-Buergerschen Krankheit). *Virchow's Archiv für Pathologische Anatomie*, **305**, 531–57.

Lippmann, H.I. (1952). Cerebrovascular thrombosis in patients with Buerger's disease. *Circulation*, **5**, 680–92.

Matsushita, M., Nishikimi, N., Sakurai, T. & Nimura, Y. (1998). Decrease in prevalence of Buerger's disease in Japan. *Surgery*, **124**, 498–502.

Mills, J.L. & Porter, J.M. (1991). Buerger's disease (Thrombangiitis obliterans). *Annals of Vascular Surgery*, **5**, 570–2.

Olin, J.W., Young, J.R., Graor, R.A., Ruschhaupt, W.F. & Bartholomew, J.R. (1990). The changing clinical spectrum of thromboangiitis obliterans (Buerger's disease). *Circulation*, **82**, Suppl. IV, IV3–8.

Papa, M., Bass, A., Adar, R. et al. (1992). Autoimmune mechanisms in thromboangiitis obliterans (Buerger's disease): the role of tobacco antigen and the major histocompatibility complex. *Surgery*, **111**, 527–31.

Pietraszek, M.H., Choudhury, N.A., Baba, S. et al. (1993). Serotonin as a factor involved in pathophysiology of thromboangiitis obliterans. *Internal Angiology*, **12**, 9–12.

Puchmayer, V. (1996). [Clinical diagnosis, special characteristics and therapy of Buerger's disease]. *Bratislava Lek Listy*, **97**, 224–9.

Reny, J.L. & Cabane, J. (1998). [Buerger's disease or thromboangiitis obliterans]. *Revue Medicine Interne*, **19**, 34–43.

Romanuel, F.C.A. & Abramowitz, A. (1964). Changes in brain and pial vessels in arterial boundary zones. *Archives of Neurology*, **11**, 40–65.

Shionoya, S. (1989). Buerger's disease (thrombangitis obliterans). In *Vascular Surgery*, ed. R.B. Rutherford, pp. 207–17. Philadelphia: W.B. Saunders.

von Winiwarter, F. (1879). Über eine eigentümliche Form von Endarteritis und Endophlebitis mit Gangrän des Fußes. *Archiv für Klininische Chirurugie*, **23**, 202–26.

Zülch, K-J. & Pilz, P. (1989). Thrombangitis obliterans (von Winiwarter-Buerger). In *Handbook of Clinical Neurology*, ed. J.F. Toole, pp. 307–16. Amsterdam: Elsevier Science Publishers.

7

Cerebral vasculitis and stroke in patients with cerebral cysticercosis, tuberculosis and mycosis

Bruno Estañol[1] and Luis Ostrosky-Zeichner[2]

[1]Department of Neurology, Instituti Nacional de la Nutricion – Salvador Subiran, Mexico
[2]Department of Internal Medicine, University of Texas Houston Medical School, USA

Vasculitis in cerebral cysticercosis

Introduction

Cerebral cysticercosis (CC) is a common parasitic cerebral infestation around the world. Extensive travel has made this infestation common in highly developed countries (Estañol et al., 1983; Solvillo et al., 1992; Ehnert et al., 1992). It is a highly heterogeneous disease from the clinical, pathogenic and prognostic standpoints (Rabiela et al., 1979; Estañol et al., 1983; Couldwell & Apuzzo, 1992; Monteiro et al., 1992; Bills & Symon 1992; Collister & Dire, 1991; Puri et al., 1991; Jimenez et al., 1992; Sanchetee et al., 1991; Vazquez & Sotelo, 1992; Estañol et al., 1986; Sotelo et al., 1985; Del Brutto, 1992; TerPfenning et al., 1992; Alarcón et al., 1992a; Estañol, 1983).

CC may be parenchymal, intraventricular or subarachnoid, although some patients have a combination of lesions (Rodríguez-Carvajal et al., 1977). Symptomatology in CC depends upon the following factors (i) number, size and type of parasites; (ii) location of the parasites; (iii) presence of an inflammatory reaction in the surrounding tissue, such as arachnoiditis, granuloma, focal cerebral edema or arteritis; and (iv) obstruction to the CSF flow (Rabiela et al., 1979; Estañol et al., 1983; Estañol, 1983). An important number of infected people have asymptomatic CC (Rabiela et al., 1979).

Parenchymal cysticercosis

Most people with asymptomatic CC, if not all, have parenchymal cysticercosis (Rabiela et al., 1979). This has been shown in postmortem studies in Mexico (Rabiela et al., 1979, 1982) by Rabiela, Rivas and Rodríguez, in an analysis of CC as a cause of death. They found that all of the patients who died as a consequence of CC had hydrocephalus (Rabiela et al., 1979, 1982), whereas in an important number of cases it was a fortuitous or an incidental autopsy finding. The asymptomatic cases were mostly parenchymal cysts or calcifications. Patients with parenchymal cysticercosis may have active or inactive disease. Active disease is characterized by cysts that may be seen with or without surrounding inflammatory reaction. The cysts may be multiple or singular. The cysts undergo colloid changes and at that particular time the surrounding brain tissue may show an inflammatory reaction. Then a granuloma usually develops. During the period of inflammatory reaction the patients may have partial seizures or have headaches. The patients may or may not have a seizure disorder as a sequel of parenchymal cysticercosis. The patients with parenchymal cysticercosis do not develop hydrocephalus. The cysts may disappear or may become calcified. Patients with calcified lesions may or may not have epilepsy as a sequel of the infestation. It is not clear that patients with parenchymal cysticercosis have cerebral vasculitis. It is possible, however, if the cysts are near a cerebral artery that they may undergo a vasculitic reaction. As some patients with CC have small vessel disease and lacunar syndromes (Collister & Dire, 1991; Puri et al., 1991; Jimenez et al., 1992; Barinagarrementeria & Del Brutto, 1989, 1998; Barinagarrementaria, 1990) it is probable that small parenchymal cysts may cause focal arteritis.

Subarachnoid cysticercosis

In contrast to parenchymal cysticercosis, subarachnoid infestation is a highly complex disease. It is frequently associated with hydrocephalus. We have found that the location of the parasite at the subarachnoid space is the most important factor that determines the clinical manifestations and is also of prime prognostic importance.

Three other very important factors are the presence or absence of focal arachnoiditis, CSF obstruction flow with or without hydrocephalus, and the presence of arteritis. The majority of the patients with CC who die or are left disabled by the infestation have hydrocephalus (Rabiela et al., 1979; Estañol et al., 1986). Hydrocephalus in CC may be secondary to subarachnoid or intraventricular blockade, although this last form of CC is relatively rare accounting in some series for less of five per cent of the cases (Rabiela et al., 1979). On the other hand subarachnoid obstruction at the base of the brain or Sylvian cisterns is the main cause of hydrocephalus in CC (Rabiela et al., 1979; Rodriguez-Carvajal et al., 1977; Estañol et al., 1983).

The clinical syndromes observed by us in subarachnoid cysticercosis were: (i) syndrome of subarachnoid cysticercosis of the convexity of the cerebral hemispheres, (ii) syndrome of the Sylvian cistern, (iii) syndrome of optochiasmatic arachnoiditis, (iv) syndrome of cysticercosis of the cistern of the great cerebral vein; (v) syndrome of subarachnoid cysticercosis of the brainstem cisterns (pre-pontine, interpeduncular, cerebellopontine angle, ambiens); (vi) syndrome of cysticercosis of the cisterna magna; (vii) spinal subarachnoid cysticercosis.

Symptoms in subarachnoid cysticercosis depend upon four main factors: (i) blockade or sealing of the subarachnoid space leading to hydrocephalus; (ii) presence of an arachnoiditis; (iii) development of arteritis and ischemic damage to the cranial nerves, the brain stem and the cerebral hemispheres; (iv) number and size of the parasites. The transformation of a cystic parasite in the subarachnoid space into a focal arachnoiditis is the cause of the hydrocephalus and the arterial damage. When a great number of parasites or a large racemous cyst invades several cisterns the symptoms are more severe and the prognosis poorer. Giant cysts may also compress adjacent structures and produce increased intracranial pressure due to a mass effect. A parasite can be easily removed surgically at a cystic stage before an inflammatory reaction develops. At this stage subarachnoid cysticercosis may be a curable illness.

Vasculitis in CC of the subarachnoid type is probably more common than heretofore recognized. Several syndromes have been described and recent reviews have appeared (Del Brutto, 1992; Alarcón et al., 1992a; Alarcón et al., 1992b; Barinagarrementeria & Del Brutto, 1989; McCormick et al., 1983; Barinagarrementeria & Cantú, 1992; Rodríguez-Carvajal et al., 1989; Levy et al., 1995; Barinagarrementeria & Del Brutto, 1998; Barinagarrementeria, 1990). Large arteries, including the carotid and the middle cerebral arteries, have been reported to be involved (Del Brutto, 1992; TerPfenning et al.,

1992; Alarcón et al., 1992a; Alarcón et al., 1992b; McCormick et al., 1983; Rodríguez-Carvajal et al., 1989; Levy et al., 1995). Bilateral middle cerebral arteries occlusion has been observed (TerPfenning et al., 1992). In Ecuador, Alarcón, found that CC is an independent risk factor for stroke particularly in young people (Alarcón et al., 1992a,b). Several lacunar syndromes have been described including ataxic hemiparesis, pure motor hemiparesis and blepharoespasm (Collister & Dire, 1991; Puri et al., 1991; Jimenez et al., 1992; Barinagarrementeria & Del Brutto, 1989; Levy et al., 1995; Barinagarrementeria & Del Brutto, 1998; Barinagarrementeria, 1990). The lacunar syndromes are due to arteritis and occlusion of small penetrating arteries (Barinagarrementeria & Del Brutto, 1989; Levy et al., 1995). The arteritis has been evaluated with conventional cerebral angiography, MRI angiography and by transcranial doppler (TerPfenning et al., 1992; Alarcón et al., 1992a,b; Cantú & Barinagarrementeria, 1996; Cantú et al., 1998; Barinagarrementeria & Del Brutto, 1989; McCormick et al., 1983; Rodríguez-Carbajal et al., 1989; Levy et al., 1995). Transcranial doppler may be useful for inexpensive follow up of these patients (Cantú et al., 1998). The CSF shows inflammatory changes and the glucose may be low (Cantú & Barinagarrementeria, 1996). The prognosis appears to be better in patients with small vessel arteritis than in those with large vessel arteritis and hydrocephalus (Cantú et al., 1998). The vasculitis of the nervous system, as well as other pathological manifestations may be the consequence of the immune response of the host (Ostrosky-Zeichner & Estañol, 1999).

Clinical descriptions
Cysticercosis of the subarachnoid space of the convexity of the brain
With the advent of the CT and MRI technologies we became aware that infestation of the subarachnoid space at the convexity of the cerebral hemispheres by the cysticercus is perhaps the most common form of CC in endemic countries. Clinically, most of the patients present with the sudden onset of partial motor seizures, usually starting in the face or with head rotation, sometimes with a classical Jacksonian progression. Some of the patients present with transient hemiparesis that follows the seizure (Collister & Dire, 1991; Rolak et al., 1992). We have seen ten patients presenting with this syndrome which appears to be fairly stereotyped. Neurological examination of these cases is usually normal or a mild hemiparesis is found. The optic fundi are normal. The CSF shows a mild pleocytosis with slightly elevated total protein. The CT or the MRI scan demonstrates most of the time a solitary round cyst that is located at the surface of the cortex or just underneath it.

The cyst itself has a colloidal appearance. By CT the cyst is hyperdense and in the MRI T_2-weighted images appears hyperintense. The cyst is surrounded by an area of edema, sometimes annular and other times triangular. Pathological studies have shown that at this stage a granuloma develops (Rabiela et al., 1979, 1982). The cysts may disappear spontaneously (Miller et al., 1983; Goldberg, 1984) with the administration of steroids alone or with steroids and albendazol or praziquantel in a mean time of four months. Occasionally the cyst becomes a granuloma and calcifies. The prognosis for the seizure disorder is generally good (Sanchetee et al., 1991; Vazquez & Sotelo, 1992) although Del Brutto has found that some patients may develop an intractable seizure disorder (Del Brutto et al., 1992). From the pathogenic standpoint, it is likely that the symptoms are due to the edema surrounding the cyst because when the edema disappears the symptoms subside. The majority of these patients do not develop hydrocephalus or cerebral infarction. We think that several cases considered in the literature as parenchymal or cortical cysticercosis are in fact cases of subarachnoid cysticercosis of the convexity of the brain (Rabiela et al., 1982). The cyst may actually be located deep in a sulcus of the cortex (Rabiela et al., 1982). Solitary cysts of the convexity of the brain without inflammatory changes are usually asymptomatic and are an incidental or fortuitous finding by CT or MRI. Albendazol therapy to a patient with a cyst without inflammatory changes may precipitate colloidal changes in the cyst, periparasite edema and partial seizures. Giant cysts of the subarachnoid space of the convexity of the hemispheres are rare and may be confused with congenital arachnoid cysts; we have seen only one case and they usually require surgical excision (Estañol et al., 1986).

Cysticercosis of the Sylvian cisterns

This type of CC has been relatively poorly studied. Patients may present with seizures, stroke, or a syndrome of increased intracranial pressure with headache or a low grade papilledema. Stroke as the initial presentation is more common in this form than in any other; occlusion of the main trunk or branches of the middle cerebral artery is fairly common (Del Brutto, 1992; TerPfenning et al., 1992; Alarcón et al., 1992a,b). Hemiparesis, focal seizures, aphasia, apraxia, or visuo-spatial disorientation may be seen. Hydrocephalus is common in this condition. We have found that hydrocephalus is always present when both Sylvian cisterns are affected. The case of bilateral middle cerebral artery occlusion probably had bilateral occupation of the Sylvian cisterns (TerPfenning et al., 1992). When there is unilateral occupation of a Sylvian cistern, hydrocephalus may be absent or it may be moder-

ate. In the autopsied cases large racemose cysts or arachnoiditis are found in one or both Sylvian cisterns. CT or MRI discloses a large racemose cyst in one or both Sylvian cisterns. The cysts are irregular and may extend to the cisterns of the base of the brain, particularly to the chiasmatic cisterns. In some cases there is no arachnoiditis and the administration of contrast media by CT or gadolinum DTPA does not show enhancement of the lesion. If an arachnoiditis has developed the CT may show a high density in and around the Sylvian cortex that overlies the cyst. Isotope cisternography discloses a blockade of the circulation of the CSF in the affected cisterns (Estañol et al., 1983; Gordon & Estañol, 1985). The EEG may show focal slowing or spiking. There is an increased number of lymphocytes, eosinophils and plasma cells in the CSF (Punzo-Bravo et al., 1990). Glucose may be low and the IgG and the IgG index are usually elevated. The albumin index in these cases is usually elevated indicating rupture of the CSF barrier (Estañol et al., 1989a,b). The IgG and the IgG index are elevated which indicates de novo synthesis in the CSF (Estañol et al., 1989a,b). In post-mortem studies IgG and plasma cells are seen surrounding the cysts (Mancilla et al., 1987). The treatment of this form of cysticercosis is controversial. Our experience is that if a racemose cyst is present without much evidence of an inflammatory reaction, all attempts should be made to excise it surgically. We also believe that patients with this type of cysticercosis should not receive albendanzol or praziquantel therapy because of the danger of producing a severe arachnoiditis and vasculitis. We have seen several cases in whom the administration of albendazol or praziquantel resulted in cerebral infarction. If there is no cyst but only an arachnoiditis and a hydrocephalus is present, these patients should be shunted and receive oral steroids for a prolonged period of time and hope that a vasculitis will not develop. The duration of the treatment could be assessed by serial lumbar punctures. Postmortem studies have shown that patients with CC who develop hydrocephalus have a severe illness with a high mortality rate (Rabiela et al., 1979; Estañol et al., 1986). The natural history of this form of CC shows that the prognosis is generally poor, leading to premature death or disability, due to stroke or hydrocephalus, unless the parasite could be removed during its cystic stage.

Optochiasmatic arachnoiditis

The clinical manifestations of optochiasmatic arachnoiditis are well known in the neurological literature. Optochiasmatic arachnoiditis may be secondary to any type of chronic meningitis. It is a relatively rare form of subarachnoid cysticercosis, particularly in an isolated form. We have seen only one case. The patient presented with decreased peripheral visual fields with a tunnel vision. Optic atrophy was present. It has a poor prognosis because of the vascular involvement of the optic chiasm. We believe that early surgery is indicated if the symptoms have been present for less than six months, but its value remains uncertain. In patients with advanced disease, steroids should be given for a prolonged period of time. In our case the CSF showed pleocytosis with a positive Elisa test. There was no hydrocephalus.

Cysticercosis of cistern of the great cerebral vein

The clinical syndrome produced by the location of the parasite at the great cerebral vein cistern has been described by Zenteno-Alanis (1982). This type of cysticercosis has been poorly studied. This cistern extends downwards to the quadrigeminal and supracerebellar cisterns and laterally to the ambiens cistern. This syndrome appears to be a particularly malignant form of CC. It may present with hydrocephalus and increased intracranial pressure, a Parinaud syndrome or an organic mental syndrome with hypersomnolence. CT or MRI shows a cyst or arachnoiditis of the aforementioned cisterns. Zenteno-Alanís thinks that the syndrome is due in part to vasculitis and obstruction of the great cerebral vein with venous infarction of diencephalic structures (Zenteno-Alanis, 1982). If a cyst without evidence of arachnoiditis is present it should be excised surgically. However, surgery of this area may be difficult. The CSF shows increased protein, IgG, high IgG index, and pleocityosis due to increased lymphocytes, eosinophil and plasma cells. The EEG shows diffuse slowing. If there are CT or MRI signs of arachnoiditis, steroids should be given. It is a relatively uncommon form. We have only seen two cases. Zenteno-Alanís (1982) has seen several of these cases. The prognosis of these cases is poor, although more information regarding clinical presentation, natural history and treatment is needed.

Cysticercosis of the basal cisterns around the brainstem

This type of cysticercosis is fairly common and over the years has been considered the sole form of subarachnoid cysticercosis. It usually presents with signs and symptoms of increased intracranial pressure without focal signs. The parasite is usually racemous and may occupy the prepontine, the cerebellopontine angle or interpeduncular cisterns. Sometimes the cysts may occupy all the basal cisterns and may even protrude into the supratentorial Sylvian cisterns. At other times, the parasite may occupy only the interpeduncular or pontine cisterns. As the disease evolves and arachnoiditis appears, focal brainstem signs become prominent. The patient may present with a syndrome of increased intracranial pressure long before focal signs come into the picture. The patient may, however, present with focal ischemic syndromes of the brain stem as the initial presentation. These focal syndromes are likely to be due to arteritis of the circumferential arteries of the brainstem. Lesions of the cranial nerves are frequent in this type of cysticercosis including the third, fourth and sixth cranial nerves (Rabiela et al., 1982). A cerebello-pontine angle syndrome may be seen in this condition. Blepharospasm and myoclonic movements have been reported (Puri et al., 1991; Jimenez et al., 1992). The MRI is the diagnostic method of choice for this condition as the CT scan does not visualize the subarachnoid cysts of the basal cisterns well. As in other forms of subarachnoid cysticercosis, if the lesion is discovered in the cystic stage, surgical excision should be made by a competent neurosurgeon. Again, as in other forms of subarachnoid cysticercosis, if an arachnoiditis is present, surgery should be avoided and little can be done except to put in a shunt and give steroids. Prognosis is poor in this condition because most of the patients see the physician when an arachnoiditis has been fully established. Praziquantel and albendazol are contraindicated in this form of cysticercosis. Long-term prognosis is poor because of the damage to the cranial nerves and the brainstem and because the shunts have a tendency to become obstructed, and therefore frequent surgeries are performed to change the shunt devices. This is probably due to the high protein content of the CSF and remains one of the main problems in the treatment of subarachnoid cysticercosis with hydrocephalus.

Cysticercosis of the cisterna magna

It is perhaps one of the most common locations of subarachnoid cysticercosis (Rodríguez-Carvajal et al., 1977; Estañol et al., 1983; Loyo et al., 1980). It is frequently associated with cysticercosis of the fourth ventricle (Loyo et al., 1980). Most patients with fourth ventricle cysticercosis also have large racemose cysts at the cisterna magna. The patients usually present with a syndrome of acute intracranial pressure or a Bruns syndrome. Positional vertigo may be a prominent sign. Some patients find relief of the symptoms kneeling with the head down. When an operation is performed, it is found that the large racemose cyst at the cisterna magna communicate freely with the fourth ventricle. When the parasite is still cystic and no inflammatory reaction is present, it can be surgically removed easily and the patient is cured. This form of cysticercosis has been studied by Loyo et al. (1980). If an arachnoiditis develops an intense inflammatory reaction ensues and a thick arachnoiditis is the result. At this point, however, and in contrast to other forms of subarachnoid cysticercosis sur-gical removal of the inflammatory debris may be useful. In non-surgical cases steroids should be given.

Spinal cysticercosis
Cysticercosis of the spinal subarachnoid space has been described previously in several anecdotal cases (Rodríguez-Carvajal et al., 1977). It usually presents with a syndrome of acute or subacute dysfunction of the spinal cord. It is a rare condition. We have only seen one case. To our knowledge, a systematic study of this form of sub-arachnoid cysticercosis has not been made. We believe the diagnostic method of choice is MRI of the spine that may disclose the cyst or a focal arachnoiditis. During surgical exploration, a parasite is found. An arachnoiditis is the most frequent finding, although sometimes a parasite in the cystic form can be removed. The prognosis depends upon the vascular damage to the cord and the presence of arachnoiditis. More research is needed into this form of the disease.

Intraventricular cysticercosis

Intraventricular CC (IVCC) is the one form of CC that may present to the clinician or the neurosurgeon as a neurolog-ical emergency. Many patients, develop acute hydroceph-alus with a catastrophic syndrome of acute increase in the intracranial pressure (Cuetter et al., 1997; Martínez et al., 1995). This is likely to occur in patients with a cyst in the fourth ventricle, the sylvian aqueduct or the third ventricle. The acute increase in the intracranial pressure may be intermittent when the cysts acts as a valve mechanism. Bruns, first described, at the beginning of the century, a syndrome characterized by transient postural vertigo and headache in patients with cysticercal cysts located at the fourth ventricle. Cysts located in the third ventricle have been shown to migrate to the fourth ventricle through the sylvian aqueduct (Kramer et al., 1992; Martínez et al., 1995). Cysts located at the fourth ventricle frequently extrude through the Luschka and Magendie foramina to the cisterna magna. Cysts located in the Monro foramen may present with unilateral ventricular dilatation and this may present with symptoms of chronic increase in intra-cranial pressure without focal signs or mild hemiparesis (Zee et al., 1993; Ginier & Porier, 1992; Bellard et al., 1990). Some patients with cysts located in the lateral ventricles may be asymptomatic because the cyst does not obstruct the CSF circulation inside the ventricular system. Other patients may develop acute increase in the intracranial pressure due to a 'trapped' fourth ventricle (Bellard et al., 1990; Bhoopat et al., 1989; Teitelbaum et al., 1989; Spickler

et al., 1989; Zee et al., 1988; Hanlan et al., 1988; Duplessis et al., 1988). In this condition the fourth ventricle is obstructed in the upper part due to a cyst or ependimitis, and there is also obstruction at the level of the outlets of the fourth ventricle due to arachnoiditis.

When the obstruction to the CSF circulation within the ventricular system is incomplete, the patient may present with a syndrome of increased intracranial pressure with headache and papilledema with or without focal signs. When a cyst is present in the fourth ventricle, the patients usually have gaze-evoked nystagmus, ataxic pursuit, a wide based ataxic gait. Cysts located in the Sylvian aque-duct may present with a Parinaud syndrome with lid retraction. With complete obstruction of the CSF circula-tion, the patients may present in a comatose or stuporous state with bradycardia, hypertension and ataxic breathing, the so-called Cushing reaction. We have seen intermittent bradycardia and tachycardia in this condition. The brady-cardia presents usually when the patient is stimulated noc-iceptively. We have also observed that the cardiovascular reactions may be drastically relieved by shunting and alle-viation of the increased intracranial pressure. It is unknown whether ventricular cysticercosis produces small vessel angiitis but it is possible.

When a cysts dies or degenerates inside the ventricular system, there is a change in the morphology of the cyst that may become hyperintense in T_1 and T_2 images and the ependymal lining surrounding the cyst may become also hyperintense in T_1 particularly with gadolinium enhance-ment.

Vasculitis in tuberculosis

Tuberculous meningitis is found in aproximately 3% of fatal cases of tuberculosis in adults (Auerbach, 1951). Incidence is thought to rise with the rise of the general inci-dence of tuberculosis in some populations. Developed countries are experiencing a re-emergence of the disease, often based on migrant populations and the emergence of diseases such as AIDS.

One of the most severe complications of the disease is vascular involvement, which often causes death or severe disability. Cerebrovascular involvement was first described in the indexed literature by Collomb et al. (1967). Since then, multiple studies have been performed for better understanding of this complication and to find the means for early diagnosis and treatment.

Vasculitis involving vessels in the base of the brain is one of the landmark histopathological features of tuberculous meningitis. It is also thought to be a central point in the pathogenesis and clinical features of the disease. It may involve small, medium and large arteries and veins, and occlusion in several degrees may be found. Histopathology is characterized by mononuclear infiltrates, caseating necrosis and fibrinoid changes. The most commonly involved arteries are the middle and anterior cerebral arteries. Involvement of veins ocurrs in veins going through inflammatory zones and typically results in phlebitis with or without thrombosis and occlusion (Molavi & Le Frock, 1985). The mechanism by which all of these changes happen is not completely understood, but direct vessel/endothelial damage by the microorganisms is thought to be involved, rather than cytokines, coagulation dysfunction and immune complexes (Somer & Finegold, 1995).

Clinical features are preceded by a 2-week period of malaise, and have been traditionally divided in three stages: (i) Prodromal phase with no definite neurological symptoms, (ii) signs of meningeal irritation with slight or no clouding of consciousness and minor or no focal defects, and (iii) severe clouding of consciousness, stupor or coma, seizures and weakness (Medical Research Council, 1948). Cerebrovascular symptoms usually manifest as sudden onset motor deficits as a result of ischemia early or late in the course of the disease (Osuntokun et al., 1971). Hemiplegia usually correlates with ischemia or infarction in the middle cerebral or internal carotid territories. Quadriplegia, while rare, is associated with bilateral infarction in advanced cases (Udani et al., 1971). Diagnosis of cerebrovascular complications has evolved with technology. While neuroimaging techniques and procedures are non-diagnostic for tuberculous meningitis, they have become the standard for diagnosing its complications. CT scan is readily available but lacks the sensitivity that MRI has, and digital subtraction angiography has shown promise as an invaluable tool for early diagnosis of vascular involvement (Rojas-Echeverri et al., 1996).

Despite the availability of excellent antimycobacterial agents in different combinations, morbidity and mortality remain high, especially in patients that seek treatment late in the course of the disease, when complications have already developed. Aside from chemotherapy, complicated tuberculous meningitis is one of the few infectious diseases in which use of corticosteroids appears to be useful for improving the clinical condition acutely and lowering mortality and morbidity (McGowan et al., 1992). Although evidence is not very solid, prednisone 1–3 mg/kg/day tapered over 4–6 weeks, is recommended for patients with elevated intracranial pressure, focal neurologic deficit, altered conciousness and cerebrospinal fluid blockage (Molavi & LeFrock, 1985).

Specific prognosis for vascular involvement has not been studied, but mortality rates for cases with advanced disease range between 50 and 70%.

Vasculitis in cerebral mycosis

Although fungal infections of the central nervous system are more common in immunocompromised hosts, they should be part of the differential diagnosis in patients with chronic infections of the central nervous system, regardless of the immune status of the host. Careful epidemiological history should be obtained, for many of these mycoses are endemic or related to some particular exposure. Risk factors include: neurological and cardiovascular surgery, mycotic endocarditis and disseminated infection. Cerebrovascular involvement is usually associated with large vessel vasculitis, and thought to be caused by direct vessel damage by invasion or embolization (Somer & Finegold, 1995).

Fungal infections that are known to have cerebrovascular involvement are: Aspergillosis, Candidiasis, Coccidiodomycosis, Cryptococcosis, Hystoplasmosis and Mucormycosis. We will briefly discuss particular features of these infections.

Aspergillosis
Invasive large vessel cerebral vascultis associated to *Aspergillus* infection ocurrs mainly in granulocytopenic hosts, and is characterized by necrosis, edema, infarction and tissue hyphae (Bennett, 1992). Vascular invasion and embolization are common. Mortality is high (over 40%), and a neurosurgical consultation is often required to perform embolectomy, which often leads the way to diagnose the infection by histopathological analysis.

Candidiasis
Candida meningitis and brain microabscesses are usually the result of disseminated infection in infants and immunocompromised adults (Salaki et al., 1984). Vascular involvement is a rare complication, and includes large vessel arteritis, which may be complicated by subarachnoid hemorrhage (Rabah et al., 1998).

Coccidiodomycosis
Coccidiodomycosis is an endemic fungal infection, common to desert areas. It may have an asymptomatic course or present as a rapidly fatal disease with central nervous system involvement, which accounts for most of the fatalities. Focal neurologic signs are uncommon. Vascular involvement, as a complication, is rare and

usually consists of *endarteritis obliterans* and infarcts (Mischel & Vinters, 1995).

Cryptococcosis

Perhaps the most common fungal infection of the central nervous system, Cryptococcosis also occurs in both immunocompromised and immunocompetent hosts. Immunocompetent hosts respond better to antifungal treatment, while the immunocompromised often have a harsh course with a fatal outcome. Vascular involvement is very rare, and it may include large vessel cerebral vasculitis (Scalzini et al., 1990).

Histoplasmosis

An endemic fungal infection, it is often related to places such as caves. Infection is primarily pulmonary, with the possibility of dissemination. It may cause meningitis and large vessel vasculitis in the central nervous system (Somer & Finegold, 1995).

Mucormycosis

Mucormycosis is a fungal infection caused by the Mucorales *Mucor*, *Rhizopus* and *Absidia*, which is associated to immunocompromised states, such as diabetes and leukemia (Sugar, 1992). It often involves several cranial structures and the central nervous system. Its most dreaded complications are of vascular nature: cavernous sinus and internal carotid thrombosis (Lowe & Hudson, 1975) This infection has a high mortality rate, despite appropriate chemotherapy and extensive surgical debridment.

Mainstream therapy for all of these infections is intravenous Amphotericin B, with early neurosurgical consultation for vascular events, debridement and treatment of increased intracranial pressure. Corticosteroids have not proved to be beneficial for these diseases so far.

References

Alarcon, F., Hidalgo, F., Moncayo, J., Vinan, I. & Dueñas, G. (1992a). Cerebral cysticercosis and stroke. *Stroke*, **123**, 224–8.

Alarcón, F., Vanormeligen, K., Moncayo, J. & Vinan, I. (1992b). Cerebral cysticercosis as a risk factor for stroke in young and middle-aged people. *Stroke*, **23**, 1563–5.

Auerbach, O. (1951). Tuberculous meningitis: correlation of therapeutic results with the pathogenesis and pathologic changes. I. General considerations and pathogenesis. *American Reviews of Tuberculosis*, **64**, 408–18.

Barinagarrementeria, F. (1990). Non vascular etiologies of lacunar syndromes. *Journal of Neurology, Neurosurgery and Psychiatry*, **53**, 1111.

Barinagarrementeria, F. & Cantú, C. (1992). Neurocysticercosis as a cause of stroke. *Stroke*, 23, 224–8.

Barinagarrementeria, F. & Del Brutto, O.H. (1989). Lacunar syndrome due to neurocysticercosis. *Archives of Neurology*, **46**, 415–17.

Barinagarrementeria, F & Del Brutto, O.H. (1998). Neurocysticercosis and pure motor hemiparesis. *Stroke*, **19**, 1156–8.

Barinagarrementería, F., Del Bruto, O.H. & Otero, E. (1988). Ataxic hemiparesis from cysticercosis. *Archives of Neurology*, **45**, 246.

Bellard, S., Vincentelli, F., Rabehanta, P., Polydor, J.P. & Caruso, G. (1990). Hydrocephalus and cerebral cysticercosis. A case report. Review of the literature. *Neurochirurgie*, **36**, 185–90.

Bennett, J.E. (1992). Apergillus species. In *Principles and Practice of Infectious Diseases*, 3rd edn. ed. G.L. Mandell, R.G. Douglas Jr & J.E. Bennett, pp. 1958–62. New York: Churchill Livingstone.

Bhoopat, W., Poungvarin, N., Issaragrisil, R., Suthipongchai, S. & Khanjanastihiti, P. (1989). CT diagnosis in cerebral cysticercosis. *Journal of the American Association of Thailand*, **72**, 673–81.

Bills, D.C. & Symon, L. (1992). Cysticercosis producing various neurogical presentations in a patient: case report. *British Journal of Neurosurgery*, **6**, 365–9.

Cantú, C. & Barinagarrementeria, F. (1996). Cerebrovascular complications of Neurocysticercosis. *Archives of Neurology*, **53**, 233–9.

Cantú, C., Villarreal, J., Soto, J.L. & Barinagarrementeria, F. (1998). Cerebral cysticercotic arteritis: detection and follow-up by transcranial doppler. *Cerebrovascular Diseases*, **8**, 2–7.

Collister, R.E. & Dire, D.J. (1991). Neurocysticercosis presenting to the emergency department as a pure motor hemiparesis. *Journal of Emergency Medicine*, **9**, 425–9.

Collomb, H., Lemercier, G., Virieu, R. & Dumas, M. (1967). (Multiple cerebrovascular thrombosis due to arteritis associated with tuberculous meningitis). *Bulletin Societé Medécin Africa Noire Langue Français*, **12**, 813–22.

Couldwell, W.T. & Apuzzo, M.L. (1992). Cysticercosis cerebrii. *Neurosurgery Clinics of North America*, **3**, 471–81.

Cuetter, A.C., García-Bobadilla, J., Guerra, L.G., Martínez, F.M. & Kaim, B. (1997). Neurocysticercosis: focus on intraventricular disease. *Clinical Infectious Diseases*, **24**, 157–64.

Del Brutto, O.H. (1992). Cysticercosis and cerebrovascular disease: a review. *Journal of Neurology, Neurosurgery and Psychiatry*, **55**, 252–4.

Del Brutto, O.H., Santibañes, R., Noboa, C.A., Aguirre, R., Dias, E. & Alarcon, T.A. (1992). Epilepsy due to neurocysticercosis. Analysis of 203 patients. *Neurology*, **142**, 389–92.

Duplessis, E., Dowling-Carter, D., Vidaillet, M., Piette, J.C. & Phillipon, J. (1988). Intraventricular cysticercosis. A propos of 3 cases. *Neurochirugie*, **34**, 275–9.

Ehnert, K.L., Roberto, R.R., Barrett, L., Solvillo, F.J. & Rutherford, G.W. (1992). Cysticercosis. First 12 months of reporting in California. *Bulletin of the Pan Health Organisation*, **26**, 165–72.

Estañol, B. (1983). Controversias en cisticercosis cerebral. *Gaceta Medica de Mexico*, **119**, 461–6.

Estañol, B., Kleriga, E., Loyo, M., Mateos, J.H., Lombardo, L. &

Saguchi, F. (1983). Mechanisms of hydrocephalus in cerebral cysticercosis: implications for therapy. *Neurosurgery*, **13**, 119–23.

Estañol, B., Corona, T. & Abad, P. (1986). A prognostic classification of cerebral cysticercosis. Therapeutic implications. *Journal of Neurology, Neurosurgery and Psychiatry*, **86**, 43–53.

Estañol, B., Juárez, H., Irigoyen, M.C., González Barranco, D. & Corona, T. (1989a). Humoral immune response in patients with cerebral parenchymal cysticercosis treated with praziquantel. *Journal of Neurology, Neurosurgery and Psychiatry*, **52**, 254–7.

Estañol Vidal, B., Díaz Granados, J. & Corona Vázquez T. (1989b). Integridad de la barrera hematoencefálica y síntesis intratecal de IgG en la cisticercosis subaracnoidea y parenquimatosa. *Revista de Investigacion Clinica*, **41**, 327-30.

Fandino, J., Botana, C., Fandino, C., Rodríguez, D. & Gomez-Bueno, J. (1991). Clinical and radiographic response of fourth ventricle cysticercosis to praziquantel therapy. *Archives of Neurochirurgie*, **111**, 135–7.

Ginier, B.L. & Porier, V.C. (1992). MR imaging of intraventricular cysticercosis. *American Journal of Neuroradiology*, **13**, 1247–8.

Goldberg, M.A. (1984). Praziquantel for cysticercosis of the brain parenchyma. *New England Journal of Medicine*, **311**, 733–4.

Gordon, F. & Estañol, B. (1985). La cisternografía radioisotópica en el diagnóstico de la hidrocefalia por cisticercosis. *Revista Médica del IMSS*, **23**, 267–70.

Hanlan, K.A., Vern, B.A., Tan, W.S., Passen, E. & Jafar, J.J. (1988). MRI in intraventricular cysticercosis: a case report. *Infection*, **16**, 242–4.

Jimenez, F.J., Molina, J.A., Roldan, A., Aguila, A., Santos, J. & Fernandez, A. (1992). Blepharospasm associated with neurocysticercosis. *Acta Neurologie Napoli*, **14**, 56–9.

Kramer, J., Carrazana, E.J., Cosgrove, G.R., Kleefield, J. & Edelman, R.R. (1992). Transaqueductal migration of a neurocysticercus cyst. Case report. *Journal of Neurosurgery*, **6**, 956–8.

Levy, A.S., Lileher, K.O., Rubenstein, D. & Stears, J.C. (1995). Subarachnoid neurocysticercosis with occlusion of the major intracranial arteries:case report. *Neurosurgery*, **36**, 183–8.

Lowe, J.T. Jr & Hudson, W.R. (1975). Rhinocerebral phycomycosis and internal carotid artery thrombosis. *Archives of Otolaryngology*, **101**, 100–3.

Loyo, M., Klériga, E. & Estañol, B.V. (1980). Cysticercosis of the fourth ventricle. *Neurosurgery*, **7**, 456–8.

McCormick, G.F., Giannota, S., Zee, C.S. & Fisher, M. (1983). Carotid occlusion in cysticercosis. *Neurology*, **33**, 1078–80.

McGowan, Jr. J.E., Chesney, P.J., Crossley, K.B. & LaForce, F.M. (1992). Guidelines for the use of systemic glucocorticosteroids in the management of selected infections. *Journal of Infectious Diseases*, **165**, 1–13.

Mancilla, R.J., Szymanski, G. & Estañol, B.V. (1987). Demonstración de inmunoglobulinas y complemento en la interfase huésped-parásito en cisticercosis del sistema nervioso central. *Patología*, **25**, 83–9.

Martínez, H.R., Rangel-Guerra, R., Arredondo-Estrada, J.H., Marfil, A. & Onofre, J. (1995). Medical and surgical treatment in neurocysticercosis a magnetic resonance study of 161 cases. *Journal of Neurological Science*, **130**, 25–34.

Medical Research Council. (1948). Streptomycin treatment of tuberculous meningitis: report of the committee on Streptomycin in tuberculosis trial. *Lancet*, **1**, 582–96.

Miller, B., Grinnell, V., Goldberg, M.A. & Heiner, D. (1983). Spontaneous radiographic disappearance of cerebral cysticercosis: three cases. *Neurology*, **33**, 1377–9.

Mischel, P.S. & Vinters, H.V. (1995). Coccidiodomycosis of the central nervous system: neuropathological and vasculopathic manifestations and clinical correlates. *Clinical Infectious Diseases*, **20**, 400–5.

Molavi, A. & LeFrock, J.L. (1985). Tuberculous meningitis. *Medical Clinics of North America*, **69**, 315–31.

Monteiro, L., Coetho, T. & Stocker, A. (1992). Neurocysticercosis – a review of 231 cases, *Infection*, **20**, 61–5.

Ostrosky-Zeichner, L. & Estañol, B. (1999). Immunopathogenesis of neurocysticercosis: is damage mediated by the host immune response? *International Journal of Parasitology*, **29**, 649–50.

Osuntokun, B.O., Adeuja, A.O. & Familusi, J.B. (1971). Tuberculous meningitis in Nigerians. A review of 194 patients. *Tropical Geo Medicine*, **23**, 225–31.

Punzo-Bravo, G., Corona-Vázquez, T., Polanco-Morales, M., Godínez-Quesada, R. & Estañol-Vidal, B. (1990). Células plasmáticas en el líquido cefalorraquídeo en pacientes con cisticercosis cerebral. *Revista Investigacion de Clinica*, **42**, 23–8.

Puri, V., Chowdhury, V. & Gulati, P. (1991). Myoclonus. a manifestation of neurocysticercosis, *Postgraduate Medical Journal*, **67**, 68–9.

Rabah, R., Kupsky, W.J. & Haas, J.E. (1998). Arteritis and fatal subarachnoid hemorrhage complicating occult Candida meningitis: unusual presentation in pediatric acquired immunodeficiency syndrome. *Archives of Pathology and Laboratory Medicine*, **122**, 1030–3.

Rabiela, M.T., Rivas, H.A. & Rodríguez, I.J. (1979). Consideraciones anatomopatológicas sobre cisticercosis cerebral como causa de muerte. *Patologia (México)*, **17**, 119–36.

Rabiela, M.T., Rivas, A., Castillo, S. & Cancino, F. (1982). Anatomopathological aspects of human brain cysticercosis. In *Cysticercosis. Present State of Knowledge and Perspectives*, ed. A. Flisser, K. Wilms, J.P. Laclette, C. Larralde, C. Ridaura & F. Beltran, pp. 179–200. New York: Academic Press.

Rodríguez-Carvajal, J., Palacios, E. et al. (1977). Radiology of cysticercosis of the nervous system including CT. *Radiology*, **125**, 127–31.

Rodríguez-Carbajal, J., Del Brutto, O.H., Penagos, P., Huebe, J. & Escobar, A. (1989). Occlusion of the middle cerebral artery due to cysticercotic angiitis. *Stroke*, **20**, 1095–8.

Rojas-Echeverri, L.A., Soto-Hernandez, J.L., Garza, S. et al. (1996). Predictive value of digital subtraction angiography in patients with tuberculous meningitis. *Neuroradiology*, **38**, 20–4.

Rolak, L.A., Rutecki, P., Ashizawa, T. & Harati, Y. (1992). Clinical features of Todd's post-epileptic paralysis. *Journal of Neurology, Neurosurgery and Psychiatry*, **55**, 63–4.

Salaki, J.S., Louria, D.B. & Chmel, H. (1984). Fungal and yeast infections of the central nervous system. A clinical review. *Medicine*, **63**, 108–32.

Sanchetee, P.C., Venkataraman, C.S., Dhamija, R.M. & Roy, A.K.

(1991). Epilepsy as a manifestation of neurocysticercosis. *Journal of the Association of Physicians India*, **39**, 325–8.

Scalzini, A., Castelnuovo, F., Puoti, M. & Cristini, G. (1990). A case of cryptococcal meningoencephalitis and focal cerebral vasculitis with transient immunodeficiency. *Acta Neurologica*, **12**, 301–4.

Solvillo, F.J., Waterman, S.H., Richard, F.D. & Shantz, P.M. (1992). Cysticercosis surveillance: locally acquired and travel related infections and detection of intestinal tapeworm carriers in Los Angeles County. *American Journal of Tropical Medicine and Hygiene*, **47**, 365–71.

Somer, T. & Finegold, S.M. (1995). Vasculitides associated with infections, immunization and antimicrobial drugs. *Clinical Infectious Diseases*, **20**, 1010–46.

Sotelo, J., Escobedo, F., Rodríguez Carbajal, J. et al. (1984). Therapy of parenchymal brain cysticercosis with praziquantel. *New England Journal of Medicine*, **310**, 1001–7.

Sotelo, J., Guerrero, V. & Rubio, F. (1985). Neurocysticercosis. A new classification based on active and inactive forms. A study of 730 cases. *Archives of Internal Medicine*, **145**, 442–6.

Spickler, E.M., Lufkin, R.B., Teresi, L., Lanman, T., Levesque, M. & Bentson, J.R. (1989). High signal intraventricular cysticercosis on T_1-weighted MR imaging. *American Journal of Neurology and Radiology*, **10**, Suppl, S64.

Sugar, A.M. (1992). Agents of mucormycosis and related species. In *Principles and Practice of Infectious Diseases*. 3rd edn, ed. G.L. Mandell, R.G. Douglas & J.E. Bennett, pp. 1962–72. New York: Churchill Livingstone.

Teitelbaum, G.P., Otto, R.J., Lin, M. et al. (1989). MR imaging of neurocysticercosis. *American Journal of Radiology*, **153**, 857–66.

TerPfenning, B., Litchman, C.D. & Heiner, L. (1992). Bilateral middle cerebral artery occlusions in neurocysticercosis. *Stroke*, **23**, 280–3.

Udani, P.M., Parekh, U.C. & Dastur, D.K. (1971). Neurological and related syndromes in CNS tuberculosis: clinical features and pathogenesis. *Journal of Neurological Science*, **14**, 341–57.

Vazquez, V. & Sotelo, J. (1992). The course of seizures after treatment for cerebral cysticercosis. *New England Journal of Medicine*, **327**, 696–701.

Zee, C.S., Segall, H.D., Boswell, W., Ahmadi, J., Nelson, M. & Colletti, P. (1988). MR imaging of neurocysticercosis. *Journal of Computer Assisted Tomography*, **12**, 927–34.

Zee, C.S., Segall, H.D., Destian, S., Ahmadi, J. & Apuzzo, M.L. (1993). MRI of intraventricular cysticercosis: surgical implications. *Journal of Computer Assisted Tomography*, **17**, 932–9.

Zenteno-Alanis, G. (1982). A classification of human cysticercosis. In *Cysticercosis. Present State of Knowledge and Perspectives*, ed. A. Flisser, K. Willms, J.P. Laclette, C. Larralde, C. Ridaura & F. Beltran, pp. 107. New York: Academic Press.

8

Systemic lupus erythematosus

Nancy Futrell

Intermountain Stroke Research, Murray, UT, USA

Introduction

Patients with systemic lupus erythematosus (SLE) have an increased risk of stroke.(Futrell & Millikan, 1989). As these patients are relatively young compared to other stroke patients, SLE is generally considered in the evaluation of stroke in the young. SLE is actually a relatively uncommon etiology of stroke, even in the young, being found in only 3.5% of patients presenting with stroke before the age of 45 (Adams et al., 1995). The risk of recurrence of stroke in patients with SLE is much higher than other stroke patients, and the preventative treatment is influenced by the underlying systemic disease. This, along with the need to determine when to order expensive diagnostic tests to rule out SLE in young stroke patients, makes an understanding of the systemic disease of SLE and many unique features of stroke in SLE an important part of the general knowledge base for the management and prevention of stroke.

Background

Systemic lupus erythematosus (SLE) was initially described as a skin disorder in the mid-ninteenth century, with recognition of the systemic, multiorgan involvement by Kaposi in 1872. Although Kaposi included descriptions of patients with brain dysfunction, including headache, delirium and coma, the first description of focal neurological deficits was by Osler, who reported a patient with episodes of right hemiparesis and aphasia in 1904. The presence of systemic 'thrombosis' (more likely cardiogenic emboli) was recognized as early as 1935, with a report of lupus patients with renal infarcts and endocarditis at autopsy (Baehr et al., 1935). Multiple cerebral infarcts were described at autopsy in lupus patients with Libman–Sacks endocarditis in 1947 (von Albertini & Alb, 1947) and lupus presenting with stroke

was reported in 1963 (Silverstein, 1963)and in 1971 (Jentsch et al., 1971). Widespread recognition of stroke as a complication of SLE began in the early 1980s (Delaney, 1983; Haas, 1982; Hart & Miller, 1983; Harris et al., 1984).

Diagnosis of SLE

A diagnosis of SLE includes documentation of 4 of 11 potential abnormalities (Tan et al., 1982) (Table 8.1). In young stroke patients an appropriate history should be taken to determine whether any clinical manifestations of SLE have been present, or whether there is a family history of SLE or other autoimmune disorders. Review of systems should include questions about arthritis, skin rashes, photosensitivity, pleurisy, seizures and psychotic episodes, which will screen for 6 of the 11 potential lupus criteria. The physical examination should include evaluation of the skin, mucous membranes and joints, along with auscultation for pericardial or pleural rubs, screening for 5 of the 11 criteria. The usual admitting laboratory panel for stroke patients includes a CBC, chemistry panel, prothrombin time (PT), partial thromboplastin time (PTT) and urinalysis. This serves as a screen for the two additional lupus criteria, and also screens for the lupus anticoagulant (elevated PTT). An echocardiogram (standard portion of the stroke evaluation), would screen for a pericardial effusion if present.

If the admitting history, physical examination and laboratory results do not suggest lupus, specific tests for SLE (ANA, ds-DNA), or for lupus anticoagulant (Russell's Viper Venom Time) are not warranted.

Frequency

The are no accurate data on the percentage of patients with lupus who will develop stroke, due to bias in the

Table 8.1. *Criteria for the diagnosis of systemic lupus erythematosus*[a]

(i) Malar rash
(ii) Discoid rash
(iii) Photosensitivity
(iv) Oral ulcers (generally painless)
(v) Arthritis (two or more joints, with swelling – arthralgias not sufficient)
(vi) Serositis
(a) Pleuritis (pleurisy, pleural effusion, pleural rub)
(b) Pericarditis (pericardial effusion or rub, or typical EKG changes)
(vii) Renal
(a) 3+ proteinuria
(b) Cellular casts
(viii) Neurological
(a) Seizures
(b) Psychosis
(ix) Hematological
(a) Hemolytic anemia
(b) Leukopenia (<4000/mm^3 on two or more occasions)
(c) Lymphopenia (<1500/mm^3 on two or more occasions)
(d) Thrombocytopenia (<100000/mm^3)
(x) Immunological
(a) Positive LE prep (rarely performed now)
(b) False-positive syphilis test
(c) Anti-DNA antibodies
(xi) Antinuclear antibody
1:320 or greater

Note:

[a] The diagnosis of SLE requires positivity in 4 of the 11 categories. 'Seronegative' lupus is described as lupus patients without a positive ANA or Anti-DNA. There is disagreement as to whether seronegative lupus is bonafide systemic lupus erythematosus.

Source: Tan et al. (1982).

published series. Stroke frequency was likely underestimated in series before 1975, due to the failure to recognize focal neurological events as stroke in these relatively young patients. One report of consecutive patients in a university based rheumatology clinic reports 4% of lupus patients having stroke, but some likely stroke patients with diplopia, gaze palsy and/or vertigo were classed as 'brainstem syndrome' rather than stroke (Sibley et al., 1992). As no neurologist is involved in many of the series from rheumatology clinics, the diagnosis of stroke may be incomplete. Series selected from consecutive hospital admissions overestimate the frequency of stroke, as they are biased toward patients with more severe SLE.

The frequency of recurrent stroke in patients with SLE is better documented, with over 50% of SLE patients who have a stroke going on to have multiple infarcts if preventative treatment is not instituted (Futrell & Millikan, 1989; Asherson et al., 1987).

Microinfarcts and microhemorrhages (Johnson & Richardson, 1968; Hanly et al., 1991) are seen frequently in autopsy specimens of SLE patients. Asymptomatic microinfarcts are common, and are now diagnosed due to the high sensitivity of MRI (Ishikawa et al., 1994). Occlusions of large arteries (Trevor et al., 1972) and major strokes also occur in lupus patients (Fig. 8.1).

Etiology of stroke in patients with SLE

Vasculitis, an overestimated association

Lupus patients are known to have systemic vasculitis, most commonly in the kidney or the skin. This led Osler to postulate in 1903 that similar vascular lesions could be causing stereotyped TIAs in one of his patients (Osler, 1904). Unfortunately, this concept has persisted in the absence of verification. 'Cerebral vasculitis' has been reported as the etiology of stroke in series of patients who did not have neuropathological confirmation, but used indirect evidence such as concomitant vasculitis in the skin. Other errors in diagnosis come from series with an angiographic diagnosis of vasculitis, which has low specificity. Major autopsy studies have failed to provide evidence for cerebral vasculitis as the cause of stroke in SLE patients (Johnson & Richardson, 1968; Devinsky et al., 1988; Hanly et al., 1991). The more common pathology is a vasculopathy, with perivascular inflammatory infiltrates (Johnson & Richardson, 1968), perivascular hemorrhages (Smith et al., 1994) and proliferation of blood vessels (Lie, 1989), which includes vascular occlusion with multiple channels of recanalization (Futrell & Asherson, 1993) (Fig. 8.2).

In spite of the lack of pathological evidence of CNS vasculitis in SLE, vasculitis is commonly a strong consideration in these patients. This may be due to widespread multifocal hyperintensity of white matter on T_2-weighted MRI scans, as seen in a patient who presented with mild confusion and apraxia (Fig. 8.3). This patient underwent biopsy and tissue was sampled from four separate areas. One was normal, two were consistent with edema in otherwise normal brain tissue and one showed subacute ischemia. There was no vasculitis. Apparently this patient had multifocal ischemic lesions with an unusually large amount of white matter edema. It is possible that cytokine

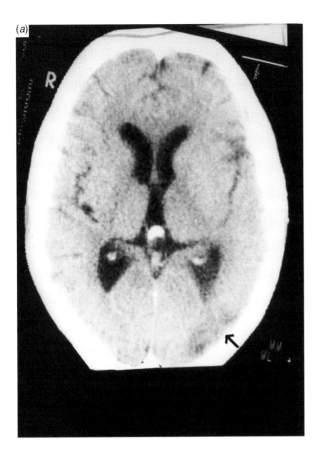

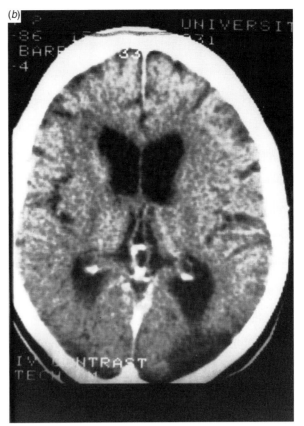

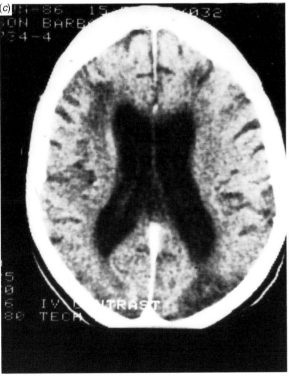

Fig. 8.1 Patient with SLE, lupus anticoagulant and 16 spontaneous abortions. (*a*) Head CT scan following a left parietal stroke (arrow). Major atrophy was not present at that time. Anticoagulant therapy was not initiated, as the patient was hospitalized for a major GI bleed. (*b*),(*c*) Head CT scan 2 years later, following multiple cerebral infarcts. Multiple areas of low density are present, along with significant interval enlargement of the ventricles. Anticoagulant was started because of a pulmonary embolus. The patient had no clinical strokes over the subsequent year.

abnormalities in patients with SLE could contribute to unusually severe white matter changes in these patients.(Al-Janadi et al., 1993; Gilad et al., 1997)

In cases with inflammatory changes within brain tissue and brain blood vessels, infection rather than primary inflammatory vasculitis is an important consideration (Fig. 8.4). Infections are common in patients with SLE, being a common cause of death. These can produce infected emboli. There can also be basilar meningitis from aspergillus (Futrell et al., 1992) which is indeed a 'vasculitis', but is a secondary rather than a primary inflammatory process. The treatment would obviously be based on antimicrobial therapy, as opposed to immunosuppression.

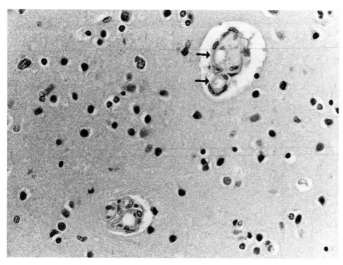

Fig. 8.2. Typical vascular changes in the brain of an SLE patient with lupus anticoagulant, who died of multiple organ involvement with SLE. She had multiple cerebral infarcts. Occluded vessels with recanalization are seen in this section (small arrows).

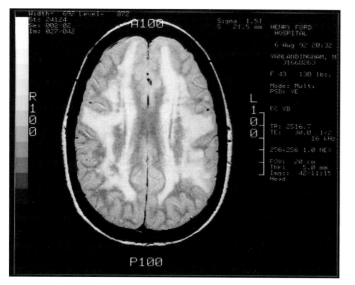

Fig. 8.3. MRI of the brain from a patient with SLE. Diffuse multifocal white matter disease led to a presumptive diagnosis of vasculitis. Biopsy revealed subacute infarcts and normal tissue with edema. No vasculitis was present. The overdiagnosis of 'vasculitis' based on multiple lesions on MRI is an important pitfall.

Without biopsy proof, cerebral vasculitis should not be considered the etiology of a stroke in a patient with SLE. Careful evaluation for cardiogenic emboli, hypercoagulable states and atherosclerosis should be performed.

Cardiogenic emboli

There are multiple cardiac abnormalities in patients with SLE. Libman–Sacks endocarditis is a varrucous endocarditis with deposition of hyalinized blood and platelet thrombus, not covered by endothelium (Libman & Sacks, 1924). These lesions can involve cardiac valves as well as the endocardium, and they can produce emboli. As many as 75% of SLE patients may have cardiac abnormalities on echocardiography, with valvular lesions in 37.5% (Ong et al., 1992). The most commonly diseased valve is the mitral valve. Cardiac valvular abnormalities are associated with anticardiolipin antibodies(Metz et al., 1994; Stein et al., 1994). Based on autopsy material, cardiogenic sources of emboli appear to be the most common etiology in patients with stroke (Devinsky et al., 1988).

Hypercoagulable states

The lupus anticoagulant includes a heterogeneous group of antibodies that interfere with phospholipid coagulation tests in vitro (Espinoza & Hartmann, 1986). The lupus anticoagulant (LA) and anticardiolipin (ACL) antibodies are partially overlapping autoantibodies (Branch et al., 1987) associated with venous thrombosis (Asherson et al., 1989), multiple spontaneous abortions (Branch et al., 1985) and stroke (Fields et al., 1990). They were initially described in patients with SLE, but also occur in individuals without SLE (Asherson et al., 1989; Love & Santoro, 1990). There is evidence that the lupus anticoagulant may convey a higher risk for thrombosis than anticardiolipin antibodies (Derksen et al., 1988). The thrombogenic tendency of both LA and ACL is multifactorial, with contributions from defects in protein C (Amer et al., 1990) and protein S(Amster et al., 1993), both endogenous anticoagulants, may contribute to this thrombogenic tendency, along with low functional levels of antithrombin III (Cosgriff & Martin, 1981).

Endothelial dysfunction (Byron et al., 1987) and fibrinolytic defects (Glas-Greenwalt et al., 1984) have also been reported in patients with SLE, with decreased endogenous t-PA activity and inhibition of plasminogen activation (Awada et al., 1988). Endothelial cell dysfunction has been correlated with the lupus anticoagulant (Byron et al., 1987), and specific antibodies against the endothelial cell are also reported (Vismara et al., 1988).

Atherosclerosis

Atherosclerosis may be more frequent in SLE than in the general population. Steroids, which are frequently administered to lupus patients, are associated with the development of a lipid profile which is atherogenic (MacGregor et al., 1992). This becomes even more important due to an atherogenic effect of LDL-containing immune complexes in lupus patients (Kabakov et al., 1992). The combination of increased triglycerides with anticardiolipin antibodies in these patients also has increased atherogenic potential (MacGregor et al., 1992).

Thrombogenic cytokines

Multiple cytokine abnormalities are present in patients with SLE, with significant variability between patients (Al-Janadi et al., 1993). Tumor necrosis factor (TNF) is a thrombogenic cytokine (van der Poll et al., 1990). Baseline TNF levels are higher in patients with SLE, but levels may not elevate normally following stimulation (Malavé et al., 1989). The exact implications of abnormal cytokines and thrombogenicity in SLE are not yet clear.

Prevention of stroke in lupus patients

Warfarin

As the major causes of stroke in lupus are cardiogenic emboli and hypercoagulable (including hypofibrinolytic) states, the mainstay of stroke prevention is long term Warfarin, with an INR of approximately 3.0 (Khamashta et al., 1995). This is based on a study of 147 patients having a history of thrombosis who were positive for antiphospholipid antibodies. SLE was present in 66 of these patients. The risk/benefit ratio of long term Warfarin must be carefully weighed in patients with SLE. As many of them have serious underlying disorders, including anemia, GI bleeding (from vasculitic lesions or gastric irritation from steroids and non-steroidal antiinflammatory agents), seizures and psychosis, anticoagulation may carry increased risk. In addition these patients are sometimes more difficult to manage on Warfarin, as their Warfarin requirement can vary significantly with changes of disease activity. On the other hand, the risk of recurrent stroke is over 50% (Futrell & Millikan, 1989), justifying the use of Warfarin in a large proportion of these patients.

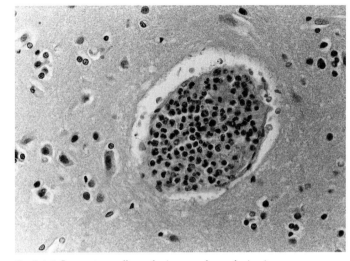

Fig. 8.4. Inflammatory cells producing vascular occlusion in an SLE patient who died with pneumococcal pneumonia and positive blood cultures for pneumococcus. This is most likely an infected embolus.

Heparin

Even with an INR of 3.0–3.5, some lupus patients continue to have ischemic events. Also, during pregnancy Warfarin cannot be used as it crosses the placenta. In both of these situations, full dose subcutaneous heparin is a reasonable alternative. The 24-hour dose of heparin can be estimated from weight based nomograms. TID dosage can then be administered in three equal doses. As many of these patients are young women, the possibility of heparin induced osteoporosis is important. Low molecular weight heparins are an alternative, with less predisposition to osteoporosis. The major drawback is high cost.

Ancrod

Ancrod is extracted from the Malayan pit viper. It functions as an anticoagulant by decreasing fibrinogen levels, and there is also an indirect fibrinolytic effect (Reid et al., 1963). It also may decrease blood viscosity (Hossmann et al., 1983).

Ancrod has been used in patients with SLE and renal disease. Patients with fibrinolytic defects responded with improved fibrinolysis, improved prostacyclin production and improved renal function (Kant et al., 1982). Those patients who did not respond had an α-2 antiplasmin (Kant et al., 1985).

The use of Ancrod at the present time may not be practical, as it is not widely available. The long term role of

Ancrod in SLE requires further studies, but theoretical considerations and preliminary data in patients with SLE are promising.

Platelet inhibition

The role of the platelet in thrombosis in SLE has not received as much attention as fibrin formation and lysis. It is clear that intramural platelet deposition is seen in occluded vessels in the brain (Ellison et al., 1993), along with being present in the heart in patients with verrucous endocarditis (Libman & Sacks, 1924).

The matter of platelet inhibition is more complicated, as patients with lupus may have thrombycytopenia and many of them are already on maximum doses of nonsteroidal antiinflammatory medications, making aspirin therapy undesirable. Ticlopidine or clopidogril are alternate medications, with the advantage of less direct GI irritation than aspirin. Both appear superior to aspirin in secondary stroke prevention in the general population, but there is increased expense and important side effects. Ticlopidine produces neutropenia and skin rashes, which may complicate the management of the patient with SLE. Lupus patients seem to have more hematological and allergic reactions to anticonvulsant medications. There are no data on whether similar increased complications occur with ticlopidine. An alternative possibility is clopidogril, which does not have as many hematological complications but is associated with skin rash.

Steroid or immunosuppression

The failure of steroids alone to prevent stroke in lupus patients has been documented (Appan et al., 1987). Steroids decrease lupus anticoagulant prothrombotic activity, but effects on anticardiolipin antibody levels are variable (Derksen et al., 1986). Steroids have been successful in preventing recurrant spontaneous abortions in patients with SLE or the primary antiphospholipid antibody syndrome. As SLE patients have lifetime risk of stroke, and long term steroids produce serious side effects, steroids should not be the first line treatment for preventing stroke in patients with SLE. Steroids or immunosuppression are recommended only as temporary measures, particularly if strokes or TIAs occur despite therapeutic anticoagulation.

Conclusions

Lupus patients have a higher risk of stroke than the general population. Of greatest concern is the very high risk of multiple recurrent strokes if aggressive preventative treatment is not given. This must be balanced with the higher risk of treatments in this complicated, multisystem disease. As the major causes of stroke are cardiogenic emboli and hypercoagulable states, both of which are treated with warfarin, this is the mainstay for stroke prevention in lupus patients. Platelet inhibition may also be desirable and steroids or immunosuppression should be reserved for limited periods of time in patients with incomplete responses to anticoagulation and platelet inhibition. Previous dogma that stroke is caused by vasculitis and should be treated with steroids or immunosuppression cannot be validated by autopsy studies or biopsy data.

Although stroke is an important problem in lupus patients, leading to significant morbidity in young patients, SLE is relatively uncommon in young patients presenting with strokes or TIAs. Laboratory evaluation for SLE can be reserved for those patients with evidence of SLE by history, physical exam or standard laboratory tests used in all stroke patients.

References

Adams, H.P., Kappelle, L.J., Biller, J. et al. (1995). Ischemic stroke in young adults; experience in 329 patients enrolled in the Iowa registry of stroke in young adults. *Archives of Neurology*, **52**, 491–5.

Al-Janadi, M., Al-Balla, S., Al-Dalaan, A. & Raziuddin, S. (1993). Cytokine profile in systemic lupus erythematosus, rheumatoid arthritis, and other rheumatic diseases. *Journal of Clinical Immunology*, **13**(1), 58–67.

Amer, L., Kisiel, W., Searles, R.P. & Williams, R.C., Jr. (1990). Impairment of the protein C anticoagulant pathway in a patient with systemic lupus erythematosus, anticardiolipin antibodies and thrombosis. *Thrombosis Research*, **57**, 247–58.

Amster, M.S., Conway, J., Zeid, M. & Pincus, S. (1993). Cutaneous necrosis resulting from protein S deficiency and increased antiphospholid antibody in a patient with systemic lupus erythematosus. *Journal of the American Academy of Dermatology*, **29**, 853–7.

Appan, S., Boey, M.L. & Lim, K.W. (1987). Multiple thromboses in systemic lupus erythematosus. *Archives of Diseases in Children*, **62**, 739–41.

Asherson, R.A., Khamashta, M.A., Gil, A. et al. (1987). Cerebrovascular disease and antiphospholipid antibodies in systematic lupus erythematosus, lupus-like disease, and the primary antiphospholipid syndrome. *American Journal of Medicine*, **86**, 391–9.

Asherson, R.A., Khamashta, M.A., Ordi-Ros, J. et al. (1989). The 'primary' antiphospholipid syndrome: major clinical and serological features. *Medicine*, **68**, 366–74.

Asherson, R.A., Mercey, D., Phillips, G. et al. (1987). Recurrent stroke and multi-infarct dementia in systemic lupus erythematosus: association with antiphospholipid antibodies. *Annals of Rheumatic Diseases*, **46**, 605–11.

Awada, H., Barlowatz-Meimon, G., Dougados, M., Masionneuve, P., Sultan, Y. & Amor, B. (1988). Fibrinolysis abnormalities in systemic lupus erythematosus and their relation to vasculitis. *Journal of Laboratory and Clinical Medicine*, **111**, 229–36.

Baehr, G., Klemperer, P. & Schifrin, A. (1935). A diffuse disease of the peripheral circulation (usually associated with lupus erythematosus and endocarditis). *Transactions of the Association of American Physicians*, **50**, 139–55.

Branch, D.W., Rote, N.S., Dostal, D.A. & Scott, J.R. (1987). Association of lupus anticoagulant with antibody against phosphatidylserine. *Clinical Immunology and Immunopathology*, **42**, 63–75.

Branch, D.W., Scott, J.R., Kochenour, N.K. & Hershgold, E. (1985). Obstetric complications associated with the lupus anticoagulant. *New England Journal of Medicine*, **313**, 1322–6.

Byron, M.A., Allington, M.J., Chapel, H.M., Mowat, A.G. & Cederholm-Williams, S.A. (1987). Indications of vascular endothelial cell dysfunction in systemic lupus erythematosus. *Annals of Rheumatic Diseases*, **46**, 741–5.

Cosgriff, T.M. & Martin, B.A. (1981). Low functional and high antigenic antithrombin III level in a patient with the lupus anticoagulant and recurrent thrombosis. *Arthritis and Rheumatism*, **24**, 94–6.

Delaney, P. (1983). Neurologic complications of systemic erythematosus. *AFP* **28**, 191–3.

Derksen, R.H.W.M., Beisma, D., Bouma, B.N., Meyling, F.H.J. & Kater, L. (1986). Discordant effects of prednisone on anticardiolipin antibodies and the lupus anticoagulant [letter]. *Arthritis and Rheumatism*, **29**, 1295–6.

Derksen, R.H.W.M., Hasselaar, P., Blokzijl, L., Gmelig-Meyling, F.H.J. & De Groot, P.G. (1988). Coagulation screen is more specific than the anticardiolipin antibody ELISA in evaluating a thrombotic subset of lupus patients. *Annals of Rheumatic Diseases*, **47**, 364–71.

Devinsky, O., Petito, C.K. & Alonso, D.R. (1988). Clinical and neuropathological findings in systemic lupus erythematosus: the role of vasculitis, heart emboli and thrombotic thrombocytopenic purpura. *Annals of Neurology*, **23**, 380–4.

Ellison, D., Gatter, K., Heryet, A. & Esiri, M. (1993). Intramural platelet deposition in cerebral vasculopathy of systemic lupus erythematosus. *Journal of Clinical Pathology*, **46**, 37–40.

Espinoza, L.R. & Hartmann, R.C. (1986). Significance of the lupus anticoagulant. *American Journal of Hematology*, **22**, 331–7.

Fields, R.A., Sibbitt, W.L., Toubbeh, H. & Bankhurst, A.D. (1990). Neuropsychiatric lupus erythematosus, cerebral infarctions, and anticardiolipin antibodies. *Annals of Rheumatic Diseases*, **49**, 114–17.

Futrell, N. & Asherson, R.A. (1993). Probable antiphospholipid syndrome with recanalization of occluded blood vessels mimicking proliferative vasculopathy. *Clinical and Experimental Rheumatology*, **11**, 230.

Futrell, N. & Millikan, C. (1989). Frequency, etiology, and prevention of stroke in patients with systemic lupus erythematosus. *Stroke*, **20**, 583–91.

Futrell, N., Schultz, L.R. & Millikan, C. (1992). Central nervous system disease in patients with systemic lupus erythematosus. *Neurology*, **42**, 1649–57.

Gilad, R., Lampl, Y., Eshel, Y., Barak, V. & Sarova-Pinhas, I. (1997). Cerebrospinal fluid soluble interleukin-2 receptor in cerebral lupus. *British Journal of Rheumatology*, **36**, 190–3.

Glas-Greenwalt, P., Kant, K.S., Allen, C. & Pollak (1984). Fibrinolysis in health and disease: severe abnormalities in systemic lupus erythematosus. *Journal of Laboratory and Clinical Medicine*, **104**, 962–76.

Haas, L.F. (1982). Stroke as an early manifestation of systemic lupus erythematosus. *Journal of Neurology, Neurosurgery and Psychiatry*, **45**, 554–6.

Hanly, J.G., Walsh, N.M.G. & Sangalang, V. (1991). Brain pathology in systemic lupus erythematosus. *Journal of Rheumatology*, **71**, 416–22.

Harris, E.N., Gharavi, A.E., Asherson, R.A., Boey, M.L. & Hughes, G.R.V. (1984). Cerebral infarction in systemic lupus: association with anticardiolipin antibodies. *Clinical and Experimental Rheumatology*, **2**, 47–51.

Hart, R.G. & Miller, V.T. (1983). Cerebral infarction in young adults: a practical approach. *Stroke*, **14**, 110–14.

Hossmann, V., Heiss, W.D., Bewermeyer, H. & Wiedemann, G. (1983). Controlled trial of ancrod in ischemic stroke. *Archives of Neurology*, **40**, 803–8.

Ishikawa, O., Ohnishi, K., Miyachi, Y. & Ishizaka, H. (1994). Cerebral lesions in systemic lupus erythematosus detected by magnetic resonance imaging. Relationship to anticardiolipin antibody. *Journal of Rheumatology*, **21**, 87–90.

Jentsch, H.J., Haas, H., Haffner, B. & Berger, H. (1971). Fokale Anfälle und hemiplegie als Erstmanifestation eine systemicher Lupus erythematodes. *Therapiewoche*, **29**, 1187–94.

Johnson, R.T. & Richardson, E.P. (1968). The neurological manifestations of systemic lupus erythematosus: a clinical-pathological study of 24 cases and review of the literature. *Medicine (Baltimore)*, **47**, 337–69.

Kabakov, A.E., Tertov, V.V., Saenko, V.A., Poverenny, A.M. & Orekhov, A.N. (1992). The atherogenic effect of lupus sera: systemic lupus erythematosus-derived immune complexes stimulate the accumulation of cholesterol in cultured smooth muscle cells from human aorta. *Clinical Immunology and Immunopathology*, **63**, 214–20.

Kant, K.S., Doeskun, A.K., Chandran, K.G.P., Glas-Greenwalt, P., Weiss, M.A. & Pollak, V.E. (1982). Deficiency of a plasma factor stimulating vascular prostacyclin generation in patients with lupus nephritis and glomerular thrombi and its correction by ancrod: in-vivo and in-vitro observations. *Thrombosis Research*, **27**, 651–8.

Kant, K.S., Pollak, V.E., Dosekum, A., Glas-Greenwalt, P., Weiss, M.A. & Glueck, H.I. (1985). Lupus nephritis with thrombosis and abnormal fibrinolysis: effect of ancrod. *Journal of Laboratory and Clinical Medicine*, **105**, 77–88.

Kaposi, M.K. (1872). Neue Beiträge zur Kenntniss des Lupus ery-thematosus. *Archives of Dermatitis and Syphilis*, 4, 36–78.

Khamashta, M.A., Cuadrado, M.J., Mujic, F., Taub, N.A., Hunt, B.J. & Hughes, G.R.V. (1995). The management of thrombosis in the antiphospholipid-antibody syndrome. *New England Journal of Medicine*, **332**, 993–1027.

Libman, E. & Sacks, B. (1924). A hitherto undescribed form of val-vular and mural endocarditis. *Archives of Internal Medicine*, **33**, 701–37.

Lie, J.T. (1989). Vasculopathy in the antiphospholipid syndrome: thrombosis or vasculitis, or both? [editorial]. *Journal of Rheumatology*, **16**, 713.

Love, P.E. & Santoro, S.A. (1990). Antiphospholipid antibodies: anticardiolipin and the lupus anticoagulant in systemic lupus erythematosus (SLE) and in non-SLE disorders. *Annals of Internal Medicine*, **112**, 682–98.

MacGregor, A.J., Dhillon, V.B., Binder, A. et al. (1992). Fasting lipids and anticardiolipin antibodies as risk factors for vascular disease in systemic lupus erythematosus. *Annals of Rheumatic Diseases*, **51**, 152–5.

Malavé, I., Searles, R.P., Montano, J. & Williams Jr, R.C. (1989). Production of tumor necrosis factor/cachectin by peripheral blood mononuclear cells in patients with systemic lupus ery-thematosus. *International Archives Allergy and Applied Immunology*, **89**, 355–61.

Metz, D., Jolly, D., Graciet-Richard, J. et al. (1994). Prevalence of val-vular involvement in systemic lupus erythematosus and associ-ation with antiphospholipid syndrome: a matched echocardiographic study. *Cardiology*, **85**, 129–36.

Ong, M.L., Veerapen, K., Chambers, J.B., Lim, M.N., Manivasagar, M. & Wang, F. (1992). Cardiac abnormalities in systemic lupus erythematosus: prevalence and relationship to disease activity. *International Journal of Cardiology*, **34**, 69–74.

Osler, W. (1904). On the visceral manifestations of the erythema group of skin diseases. *American Journal of Medicine Science*, **127**, 1–23.

Reid, H., Chan, K. & Thean, P. (1963). Prolonged coagulation defect (defibrination syndrome) in the Malayan viper bite. *Lancet*, **i**, 621–6.

Sibley, J.T., Olszynski, W.P., Decoteau, W.E. & Sundaram, M.B. (1992). The incidence and prognosis of central nervous system disease in systemic lupus erythematosus. *Journal of Rheumatology*, **19**, 47–52.

Silverstein, A. (1963). Cerebrovascular accidents as the initial major manifestation of lupus erythematosus. *NY State Journal of Medicine*, **5**, 2942–8.

Smith, R.W., Ellison, D.W., Jenkind, E.A., Gallagher, P.J. & Cawley, M.I.D. (1994). Cerebellum and brainstem vasculopathy in sys-temic lupus erythematosus: two clinico-pathological cases. *Annals of Rheumatic Diseases*, **53**, 327–30.

Stein, P.D., Hull, R.D. & Raskob, G. (1994). Risks for major bleeding from thrombolytic therapy in patients with acute pulmonary embolism. *Annals of Internal Medicine*, **121**, 313–17.

Tan, E.M., Cohen, A.S., Fries, J.F. et al. (1982). The 1982 revised cri-teria for the classification of systemic lupus erythematosus. *Arthritis and Rheumatism*, **25**, 1271–7.

Trevor, R.P., Sondheimer, F.K., Fessel, W.J. & Wolpert, S.M. (1972). Angiographic demonstration of major cerebral vessel occlusion in systemic lupus erythematosus. *Neuroradiology*, **4**, 202–7.

Van Der Poll, T., Buller, H.R., Ten Gate, H. et al. (1990). Activation of coagulation after administration of tumor necrosis factor to normal subjects. *New England Journal of Medicine*, **322**, 1622–7.

Vismara, A., Meroni, P.L., Tincani, A. et al. (1988). Relationship between anti-cardiolipin and anti-endothelial cell antibodies in systemic lupus erythematosus. *Clinical and Experimental Immunology*, **74**, 247–53.

Von Albertini, V.A. & Alb, O. (1947). Ueber die atypische verrucoese endocarditis Libman-Sacks und ihr beziehungen zum lupus ery-thematodes acutus. *Cardiologica*, **12**, 133–69.

9

Antiphospholipid antibody syndrome

Christian L. Stallworth and Robin L. Brey

Department of Medicine (Neurology), San Antonio, TX, USA

Introduction

The Antiphospholipid Syndrome (APS) was first described in 1983. The major clinical features consist of arterial (APASS, 1990; Rosove & Brewer 1992; Brey et al., 1990; Levine et al., 1995; Nojima et al., 1997) and venous (Wahl et al., 1998) thrombosis leading to tissue ischemia and placental thrombosis resulting in recurrent fetal loss (Rand et al., 1997; Levy et al., 1998), and thrombocytopenia in the presence of anti-phospholipid antibodies (aPL) (Hughes, 1983) (see Table 9.1). aPL antibodies form a heterogeneous family that can be detected using a number of immunoreactivity assays (see Table 9.2) (McNeil et al., 1991; Inanc et al., 1997). Thrombotic episodes in patients with APS are primarily venous, but if the thrombosis occurs on the arterial side, the brain is affected most often (Hughes, 1983). APS is classified as secondary if it occurs in an individual with systemic lupus erythematosus (SLE) or another collagen disease and primary in the absence of SLE. However, primary and secondary APS are indistinguishable (Shah et al., 1998; Krnic-Barrie et al., 1997) with regard to the types of thromboses and the risk of recurrent thrombosis.

Phospholipids (PL) are ubiquitous in the plasma membranes of all cells, and can form complexes with phospholipid-binding proteins under certain conditions that may involve cellular activation or injury (Arnout & Vermylen, 1998; Arnout, 1996). aPL antibodies associated with thrombosis are characterized by the requirement of a phospholipid-binding protein for detection, the ability to prolong phospholipid dependent coagulation tests *in vitro*, and the IgG-2 isotype (Brey & Escalante, 1998). Although originally assumed to be directed solely against negatively charged PL, it is now well recognized that autoimmune aPL are actually directed against antigens made up of these phospholipid/phospholipid-binding protein complexes (Sheng et al., 1998a). aPL's definitive role in thrombogenesis con-

tinues to elude investigators, however, and not all patients with aPL develop thrombosis. aPL associated with infection or certain medications are usually transient, contain a more restricted range of phospholipid immunoreactivity, and are not associated with clinical symptoms (Drouvalakis & Buchanan, 1998). In addition, aPL may be found in otherwise normal people. A prospective blood bank study found that approximately 6.5% of normal subjects had ELISA detected aPL IgG (Vila et al., 1994). Many aPL levels normalized with time, though, and no thrombotic events occurred in aPL+ patients over a 12-month period. Krnic-Barrie and colleagues (Krnic-Barrie et al., 1997) described recurrent thromboses after a lengthy quiescent period of many years in some aPL+ patients, however; thus a 12-month follow-up period may not be long enough to determine thrombosis risk. Here, we review the history, clinical features, potential pathogenic mechanisms, screening techniques, and treatment of neurological disorders currently associated with APS.

Historical perspectives

Following the description of APS in the early 1980s, the aPL screening tests consisted of solid-phase and later enzyme-linked immunosorbent assay (ELISA) techniques that utilized cardiolipin as the detecting antigen (Loizou et al., 1985). This negatively charged phospholipid, found primarily in the plasma membranes of mitochondria (McNeil et al., 1991), was assumed to be the antigen aPLs were directed against. However, it was soon recognized that other anionic phospholipid antigens could better serve in the detection of aPL. Phosphatidylserine, for instance, seemed better at identifying antibodies associated with fetal loss (Rote et al., 1990; Levy et al., 1998) and thrombosis (Inanc et al., 1997; Tuhrim et al., 1998). Biologically, the

Table 9.1. *Classification criteria of APS*[a]

Clinical criteria

Vascular thrombosis

(i) One or more clinical episodes of arterial, venous or small vessel thrombosis in any tissue or organ. Thrombosis must be confirmed via imaging, Doppler studies or histopathology, with the exception of superficial venous thrombosis.

Pregnancy morbidity

(i) One or more unexplained deaths of a morphologically normal fetus at or beyond the tenth week of gestation with normal fetal morphology documented by ultrasound or exam

Or

(ii) One or more premature births or a morphologically normal neonate at or before the 34th week of gestation because of preeclampsia, or severe placental insufficiency

Or

(iii) three or more unexplained consecutive spontaneous abortions before the tenth week of gestation with maternal anatomic, or hormonal abnormalities and exclusion of maternal and paternal chromosomal causes.

Laboratory criteria

(i) Anticardiolipin antibody (aCL) of IgG and/or IgM isotype in blood, present in medium or high titer, on two or more occasions, 6 weeks or more apart, and measured by a standardized ELISA for β_2GPI-dependent aCL.

(ii) Lupus anticoagulant (LA) present in plasma on two or more occasions 6 weeks or more apart and detected according to the guidelines of the International Society of Thrombosis and Hemostasis, in the following steps:

  (a) Demonstration of a prolonged phospholipid-dependent coagulation screening test, e.g. APTT, KCT, dRVVT, dPT, Textarin time

  (b) Failure to correct the prolonged screening test by mixing with normal platelet poor plasma.

  (c) Shortening or correction of the prolonged screening test by the addition of excess phospholipid.

  (d) Exclusion of other coagulopathies as appropriate, e.g. factor VIII inhibitor, heparin.

Note:

[a] Adopted from the International Consensus Statement On Preliminary Classification Criteria for Definite Antiphospholipid Syndrome: Report of an International Workshop (Wilson et al., 1999).

Table 9.2. *Immunoreactivity assays utilized for aPL antibody detection*

Those whose antigens are
  Anionic phospholipids alone
    cardiolipin
    phosphatidylserine
    phosphatidylinositol

  β_2GP-I or other protein co-factors alone
    prothrombin
    annexin V

  anionic phospholipids *and* β_2GP-I or other protein co-factors

or phospholipid-dependent coagulation assays
  lupus anticoagulants (LA)

concept that these antibodies might target phosphatidylserine in vivo seemed more plausible since it is found in the plasma membrane of all cells and is commonly displayed on the extracellular surface in response to cell injury, activation, and re-modelling (McNeil et al., 1991). This was theoretically problematic, though, considering the poor immunogenic properties of lipids (Gharavi & Pierangeli, 1998). Several groups identified the need for a cooperative phospholipid binding protein in order to detect most, but not all aPL antibodies (McNeil et al., 1990; Galli et al., 1990; Matsuura et al., 1990; Meroni et al., 1998). Considering the substantial immunogenic quality of proteins, the involvement of a phospholipid-binding protein was more biologically sound. Shortly thereafter, co-precipitation and subsequent protein sequencing identified one serological co-factor to be beta-2-glycoprotein-I (β_2GP-I) (Galli et al., 1990; Matsuura et al., 1990). Proteins such as prothrombin, annexin V, protein C, protein S, low molecular weight kininogens and factor XI (Arnout et al., 1998) have also been shown to bind phospholipids, but β_2GP-I is by far the most common and well-characterized protein with this ability (McNeil et al., 1991; Inanc et al., 1997).

β_2GP-I, or apolipoprotein H, is a cationic plasma glycoprotein with a molecular mass of 50 kD (Schlutze et al., 1961) and a plasma concentration of approximately 200 μg/ml. Approximately 40% of the circulating protein may be associated with any number of various classes of lipoproteins (Polz & Kostner 1979). The gene for β_2GP-I is located on chromosome 17 (Haagerup et al., 1991) and encodes 326 amino acids preceded by a 19-amino acid leader sequence. Mammalian species, including bovine, mouse, and rat, display significant conservation of these sequences and maintain an approximate 84% homology with the human β_2GP-I amino acid sequence (Sheng et al., 1998a). Structurally, β_2GP-I contains five definitive domains (Steinkasserer et al., 1991; Reid & Day, 1989). The fifth domain contains two internal loops, the first of which contains a positively charged region of amino acids (Lys^{282}–Asn–Lys–Glu–Lys–Lys^{287}) that is responsible for PL-binding (Hunt et al., 1993; Hunt & Krilis, 1994; Hagihara et al., 1995; Sheng et al., 1996). Furthermore, work suggests that residues Lys^{284}, Lys^{286} and Lys^{287} are critical for β_2GP-I binding to anionic phospholipids (Sheng et al., 1996). However, antibody binding is not limited to this domain (George et al., 1998).

Collectively, recent data strongly suggest that phospholipid membranes serve as a binding surface for the sequestration of the primary antigen, β_2GP-I, in vivo (Sheng et al., 1998a). While most autoimmune aPL antibodies target a β_2GP-I -bound cardiolipin antigen, and not cardiolipin itself, in immunoassay systems (McNeil et al., 1990), antibodies can also be detected in the presence of β_2GP-I alone in the absence of phospholipid (Roubey et al., 1996). However, the phospholipid-binding protein must be attached to a negatively charged surface in order for these assays to work (Matsuura et al., 1994; Roubey et al., 1995, 1996). Some aPL antibodies exhibit preferential binding of immobilized β_2GP-I on anionic phospholipid membranes or certain synthetic surfaces as well (Matsuura et al., 1994; Roubey, 1998). This led to the theory that aPL antibodies might bind a cryptic epitope on β_2GP-I that is only exposed after interaction with a negatively charged phospholipid or appropriately treated surface. The conformational change of β_2GP-I upon phospholipid binding would then permit an otherwise improbable interaction with aPL. For these reasons it is assumed that negatively charged synthetic surfaces mimic the environment with which β_2GP-I will interact in vivo. In order to characterize further the binding behaviour of β_2GP-I, Sheng and colleagues created mutant forms of the protein with truncated C-terminal tails, leaving an exposed Cys288 residue, thereby permitting spontaneous dimer formation. They found anti-β_2GP-I antibodies to have a significantly higher affinity for the spontaneous dimer-forming proteins than for the native, wild-type proteins, implying an importance for bivalent binding of these autoantibodies in the ELISA system (Sheng et al., 1998b). Ultimately, these data support the hypothesis that autoantibodies to monovalent β_2GP-I have an intrinsically low affinity.

Clinical manifestations

Cerebral ischemia

Case-control studies of aPL-associated stroke in young people have been uniformly positive (Brey et al., 1990;

Table 9.3. *Factors associated with increased thrombotic risk*

Elevated, persistent aCL-IgG titre
Presence of β_2GP-I aPL antibodies
Increased lupus anticoagulant

Nencini et al., 1992; Angelini et al., 1994). Some (Kushner, 1990; Chakravarty et al., 1991; Hess et al., 1991; APASS, 1993), but not all (Muir et al., 1994; Metz et al., 1998) case-control studies among older adults have found aPL antibodies to be associated with ischemic stroke. Case-control studies have been criticized because of the difficulty of establishing the temporal relationship. However, studies that obtained blood within 7 days of the event (APASS, 1993), or even within 6 hours of onset (Camerlingo et al., 1995) have had positive findings. While these time periods may be too short to allow the development of measurable IgG levels due to a primary or amnestic immune response (Barrett, 1983), they do not preclude the possibility of antibodies induced by a recent prior febrile illness. Indeed, infection-associated cerebral infarction is not only quite common, but is also associated with higher levels of anticardiolipin antibodies of the IgG isotype (Ameriso et al., 1991) (see Table 9.3).

Three prospective studies of antiphospholipid antibodies and stroke have been performed. Two of these were negative (Ginsburg et al., 1992; Sletnes et al., 1992). However, both were limited in statistical power and had technical limitations. The first study to show a prospective association between anticardiolipin antibodies and ischemic stroke evaluated patients enrolled in the Honolulu Heart Program (Brey et al., 1999). The overall risk factor-adjusted odds ratio for aCL of the IgG class was 1.5 (95% CI 1.0–2.3), which was increased for the age group 56–70 at baseline (OR 2.1, 95% CI 1.3–3.4). When the association with stroke over the 20-year follow-up period was examined by 5-year intervals, the odds ratio for the last 5 year interval was significantly lower than each of the first three 5-year intervals. This suggests that the antibodies may be changing over time or that they may be a reflection of a similarly changing physiologic state. However, we still do not recommend screening all patients who have strokes for aPL. Instead, we feel an evaluation for aPL is warranted based on the factors summarized in Table 9.4.

Recurrent stroke and thromboembolic events in patients with aPL have been reported to occur both early (within the first year of an index episode of cerebral ischemic) (Levine et al., 1993, 1995) and late (5 to 10 years) (Krnic-Barrie et al., 1997; Shah et al., 1998). The initial type

Table 9.4. *Factors warranting evaluation of aPL presence in stroke*

Patient <40 years of age

Stroke is recurrent

Thrombocytopenia, fetal loss or venous thrombosis have been documented

Lupus or other connective disease is present

of the thromboembolic event (i.e. arterial, venous, miscarriage) appears to be the most likely type of event to recur in a given patient in some (Rosove & Brewer, 1992) but not all studies (Triplett et al., 1988; Krnic-Barrie et al., 1997). Shah and colleagues studied patients with both primary and secondary APS over a 10-year period and found recurrent thromboembolic events to be common in both groups (Shah et al., 1998). In their series of 52 patients with aPL, 9/31 (29%) patients with APS developed recurrent thrombotic episodes and 11/21 (52%) patients with aPL but without clinical manifestations developed them over the follow-up period. Krnic-Barrie and colleagues (Krnic-Barrie et al., 1997) retrospectively evaluated 61 patients with primary and secondary APS for an average of 6.4 years to identify risk factors for the development of recurrent thrombosis. There was no difference between patients with primary and secondary APS regarding recurrent arterial or venous events (arterial: 55% vs. 38%; venous: 47% vs. 50%). In patients with primary and secondary APS recurrent arterial events were associated with Caucasian race and venous events with the puerperium or oral contraceptive use. High titers of aCL have been associated with recurrent events in patients with primary (Levine et al., 1993, 1995, 1997) and secondary APS (Alarcon-Segovia et al., 1989; Escalante et al., 1995). In a study of 141 patients with secondary APS related to SLE the presence of both aCL and LA were associated with thrombotic events (Nojima et al., 1997). In this study 84% of patients with an abnormal aCL IgG level and LA had at thrombotic event as compared to 16% with an abnormal aCL IgG only, 9.1% with LA only, and 3.8% with neither. All patients with high levels of aCL and LA and none of the patients without LA had an arterial thrombosis. The correlation between a high level of aCL and LA has been previously reported, however, Verro and colleagues did not find a similar relationship between very high titer and risk for recurrent thrombotic events (Verro et al., 1995). Specker and colleagues have shown that cerebral microemboli detected by transcranial Doppler are found in patients with APS and that they correlate with a history

of cerebral ischemia (Specker et al., 1997). If this technique is validated prospectively, it may provide a powerful new approach to assess cerebrovascular thrombosis risk.

There are no data to suggest that the severity of the thromboembolic event, including stroke, influences aCL titre. aCL do not appear to be a result of the thrombotic event in the brain (Brey et al., 1990; Levine et al., 1995) or elsewhere (Alarcon-Segovia et al., 1989). In a case-control study of patients with giant cell arteritis the prevalence of abnormal aCL levels was higher in patients with temporal arteritis than in controls (20.7% vs. 2.9%). The prevalence was even higher in patients who also had positive temporal artery biopsies than in temporal arteritis patients with normal biopsies (31.2% vs. 16.7%) (Duhaut et al., 1998). Both aCL and a positive biopsy were associated with thrombosis in univariate analyses, however, only a positive biopsy remained predictive of thrombosis in multivariate analyses. Further, nearly half of biopsy positive patients with high aCL levels at the time of diagnosis had normal levels when retested after 10 days of corticosteroid treatment. The authors speculate that in giant cell arteritis, the aCL produced may be a consequence of severe endothelial damage and have no relationship to thrombosis. No further analysis of aCL subtype or other phospholipid specificities were performed, thus it is possible that non-pathogenic antibodies are formed in this situation, similar to those found in response to drugs or infections (Drouvalakis et al., 1998).

Stroke mechanisms in patients with aPL

Cerebral ischemic events can occur in any vascular territory (Coull et al., 1992). Cerebral angiography typically demonstrates intracranial branch or trunk occlusion or is normal in about one-third of patients so studied (APASS, 1990). Data from in vitro studies, from experimental animal models, and clinical studies showing an association of aPL with placental infarction, peripheral and cerebral venous thrombosis strongly suggest that these antibodies cause stroke through induction of a prothrombotic state. A higher than expected frequency of coronary artery (Klemp et al., 1988) and peripheral arterial (Ciocca et al., 1995) graft occlusion has been noted in patients with aPL, as well. These clinical observations coupled with recent findings of endothelial cell activation by aPL (Del Papa et al., 1997a, 1997b) support the hypothesis that aPL may act in concert with other vascular risk factors which damage endothelial cells.

A variety of cardiac valvular lesions have been associated with aPL making cardiac emboli a possible stroke mechanism in some patients. Echocardiography (primarily 2-dimensional, transthoracic) is abnormal in one-third of patients, typically demonstrating non-specific left-sided valvular (predominantly mitral) lesions, characterized by valve thickening (Ford et al., 1989; Khamashta et al., 1990). These may represent a potential cardiac source of stroke (Ford et al., 1989; Khamashta et al., 1990; Badui et al., 1995; Nesher et al., 1997). In a large consecutive autopsy series, a higher incidence of cardiac valvular abnormalities and 'bland' (non-vasculitic) thromboembolic lesions were found in patients with aPL (Ford et al., 1994).

Classic Libman–Sacks verrucous valvular lesions may also be attributable to phenomena associated with APS. In 1924, Libman and Sacks originally described a 'hitherto undescribed form of valvular and mural endocarditis' (Libman & Sacks, 1924), which would later be attributed to SLE (Gross, 1940; Ziporen et al., 1996). These valvular lesions are typically clinically silent and are frequently associated with thickened, functionally impaired cardiac valves that are prone to hemodynamic deterioration. The causative mechanisms for this pathology have yet to be defined (for review see Ziporen et al., 1996).

The origins of atherosclerosis comprise a multifaceted histopathological process. It has been proposed that the oxidative modification of LDL in vivo may be a central contributor to atherogenesis. Therefore, aPL may play a role in atherosclerosis because of a cross-reactivity with oxidized aPL (Matsuura et al., 1998, Vaarala, 1998).

Venous sinus thrombosis

A recent review suggests that aPL may be an important factor contributing to cerebral venous sinus thrombosis (CVT) even in the presence of other potential risk factors for thrombosis (Carhuapoma et al., 1997) including the syndrome of activated protein C resistance due to Factor V Leiden mutation (Deschiens et al., 1996). The onset of CVT in patients with aPL occurs at a younger age and has more extensive superficial and deep cerebral venous system involvement than CVT without aPL. Headache, papilloedema, seizures, focal deficits, coma and death contribute to the clinical classification of CVT, along with pathological identification of hemorrhagic infarction (Ameri & Bousser, 1992). Patients who present with CVT typically have headache (85%), long tract signs (35%), cognitive disturbances (25%) and visual dysfunction (40%). In addition, a higher rate of post CVT migraine and more infarctions on brain imaging studies are seen in patients with aPL than in those without them (Carhuapoma et al., 1997).

Sneddon's syndrome and other vascular dementia

Recurrent stroke in patients with livedo reticularis (Sneddon's syndrome) has been associated with aPL (Kalashnikova et al., 1990). The frequency of aPL in patients with Sneddon's syndrome has ranged from 0 to 85% (Kalashnikova et al., 1990; Zelzer et al., 1993; Tourbah et al., 1997). This syndrome is also frequently accompanied by dementia, most likely on the basis of multiple infarctions. Sneddon's original patients all had focal neurological deficits which he considered to be 'limited and benign', leaving little residual disability (Sneddon, 1965). Subsequent descriptions of the syndrome have revealed a spectrum of clinical neurological manifestations. Zelger and colleagues described three stages of neurological involvement: (i) 'prodromal' symptoms such as dizziness or headache preceding focal neurological deficits by years; (ii) recurrent focal neurologic deficits due to recurrent cerebral ischemia, also lasting years; and (iii) progressive cognitive impairment leading to severe dementia (Coull et al., 1987). Tourbah and colleagues retrospectively studied 26 Sneddon's Syndrome patients and correlated magnetic resonance imaging (MRI) abnormalities with disability, the presence of cardiovascular risk factors, cardiac valvular abnormalities on ECHO and titer of aPL (Tourbah et al., 1997). Disability (defined by memory disturbance or ability to perform activities of daily living) was found in 50% of patients and was severe (consisting of dementia) in over half of patients with disability. Systemic hypertension was present in 65%, cardiac valvular abnormalities in 61% and aPL in 42% of patients with no correlation found between any of these and MRI abnormalities. The presence of disability was correlated with increasing severity of MRI lesions. An aPL-associated dementia without the other features of Sneddon's Syndrome has also been described. In many patients this appears to be due to multiple cerebral infarctions (Coull et al., 1987). In addition, the catastrophic APS can occasionally present with an acute organic brain syndrome characterized by fulminant encephalopathy (Chinnery et al., 1997).

Schmidt and colleagues found that subtle neuropsychological dysfunction without evidence of anatomic abnormalities on MRI are also increased in otherwise normal elderly people with aCL IgG (Schmidt et al., 1995). de Moerloose and colleagues recently evaluated the prevalence of aCL in 192 elderly patients. The overall prevalence of aCL was 10.9% and decreased by decade in patients 70–99 years of age from 18% to 10% to 7%, whereas the prevalence of ANA positivity increased by decade from 22% to 32% to 42% (de Moerloose et al., 1997). There was no association between the presence of aCL and decreased survival. In contrast, and in keeping with previous findings, Cesbron found a trend towards an increased prevalence of aCL by decade in 1042 elderly subjects between the ages of 60 and 99 years (Cesbron et al., 1997). In addition, high aCL levels were associated with increased physical disability in this population independent of age, gender, visual or hearing abnormalities, Mini-Mental Status Exam score, or history of cerebro- or cardiovascular disease (OR = 2.24, $P < 0.001$). Depression and psychosis have been associated with aPL, but it has not been clear whether this finding is simply related to the development of medication-induced aPL (Schwartz et al., 1998). Schwartz and colleagues demonstrated an association between aCL and LA and psychosis in 34 unmedicated patients without known autoimmune disorder admitted to the hospital with a first acute episode of psychosis (Schwartz et al., 1998). Thirty-four percent of patients had aCL IgG and 9% had LA. Neither was present in 20 normal control subjects. Patients were treated with a variety of neuroleptics and reassessed for the presence of these antibodies three to nine months later. One patient developed aCL IgM, and four developed aCL IgG after treatment, however, three patients who previously had aCL IgG were negative after treatment. There was no relationship between the presence of aCL or LA and thrombotic manifestations, response to antipsychotic therapy or type of antipsychotic used. The authors speculate that aPL may be causally related to the development of psychosis in some patients on an autoimmune basis and conclude that their presence cannot be assumed to simply be the result of antipsychotic treatment.

Progressive sensorineural hearing loss

Toubi and colleagues studied the association between aCL and sudden or progressive sensorineural hearing loss in 30 patients and matched normal controls. None of the control group had aCL, whereas 27% of the patient group had aCL in low-moderate titers (Toubi et al., 1997). Of the patients with aCL, five of eight had sudden deafness. In addition, two of five patients with sudden deafness and aCL relapsed as compared with none of six patients without them. Naarendorp and Spiera reported six patients with SLE or a lupus-like syndrome with sudden sensorineural hearing loss, all of which had aCL or LA (Naarendorp & Spiera, 1998). The authors suggest that sudden sensorineural hearing loss may be a previously unrecognized manifestation of APS, that the mechanism is likely to be vascular and speculate that the appropriate treatment for these patients may be anticoagulant therapy.

Transient global amnesia

Transient global amnesia, a syndrome of sudden, unexplained memory loss has been associated with aPL immunoreactivity (Montalban et al., 1989). The etiology of transient global amnesia in patients without aPL is controversial and thought to be related to ischemia or epileptiform activity in bilateral hippocampal areas. As both cerebral ischemia and epilepsy have been associated with aPL, either could play a role in aPL-associated TGA.

Ocular manifestations

Many reports of stroke and transient ischemic attack associated with aPL include some patients with ocular ischemia as well (Rafuse & Canny, 1992; Labutta, 1996). The ophthalmologic ischemic manifestations commonly associated with aPL include anterior ischemic optic neuropathy, branch and central retinal artery occlusions, cilioretinal artery occlusions, combined artery and vein occlusions and amaurosis fugax (Labutta, 1996). These manifestations are found in patients with both primary and secondary APS.

Neuroimaging studies

Brain magnetic resonance imaging studies in patients with APS (primary or secondary) have revealed small foci of high signal in subcortical white matter scattered throughout the brain (Molad et al., 1992; Provenzale et al., 1994; Toubi et al., 1995). This type of pattern is seen in many other disease processes and is, as such, non-specific. The correlation between MRI lesions in patients with aPL and clinical nervous system symptoms is reported to be high by some investigators (Molad et al., 1992; Provenzale et al., 1994; Toubi et al., 1995; Tietjen et al., 1998) and not by others (Schmidt et al., 1995; Sailer et al., 1997). Fig. 9.1 illustrates multiple cerebral infarction on brain imaging in a 23-year-old woman with aPL and SLE.

Toubi and colleagues (Toubi et al., 1995) found aPL immunoreactivity in 53/96 (55%) SLE patients with CNS manifestations as compared too 20/100 (20%) of SLE patients without them. In this study, 53 patients with CNS manifestations underwent MRI imaging and 33 showed high-density lesions that were interpreted as 'suggestive of vasculopathy'. MRI abnormalities were seen more frequently in patients with aPL immunoreactivity as compared to those without. Some of these patients with MRI abnormalities had seizures or psychiatric disturbances but

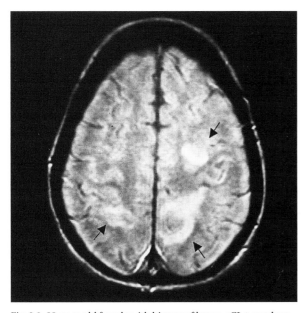

Fig. 9.1. 23-year-old female with history of lupus, aCL+ serology and stroke. Image obtained on 1.5 tesla mRI scanner (TR = 2000, TE = 30). Note two lesions in the patient's left parietal region and one small lesion in the right parietal region.

not stroke. This suggests that in some cases, aPL-associated neurologic manifestations may be due to an aPL–brain phospholipid interaction whereas in others the underlying pathogenic feature may be thrombotic.

Sailer and colleagues (Sailer et al., 1997) studied 35 SLE patients with inactive SLE using brain MRI and PET imaging, neuropsychological testing, a neurological examination and serum testing for aPL antibodies and anti-neuronal antibodies. Twenty patients had neurological deficits, three had psychiatric symptoms and ten had cognitive impairment. No differences in global glucose utilization by PET imaging were seen between SLE patients with as compared to those without neurological or cognitive abnormalities. On MRI imaging, the number and size of the white matter lesions correlated with the presence of neurological deficit, but were unrelated to the severity of cognitive impairment. Large lesions (8 mm or greater) were associated with high aCL IgG levels. Tietjen also found an association between MRI lesions and aCL levels in young patients with migraine-associated transient focal neurologic events (Tietjen et al., 1998). In a study evaluating the association between neuropsychological abnormalities and aPL in an elderly population no association between aCL and MRI lesions was found, supporting Sailer's findings in the group with cognitive impairment only (Schmidt et al., 1995). Hachulla and colleagues performed brain MRI in patients with primary and secondary APS (Hachulla et

al., 1998). Both cerebral atrophy and white matter lesions were more common in both groups with respect to control subjects. The number and volume of white matter lesions were increased in patients with primary and secondary APS who also had neurological symptoms. Only a weak correlation was found between the presence of a LA and cerebral atrophy.

In addition to MRI, Specker and colleagues (Specker et al., 1998) report the use of transcranial Doppler technique for the assessment of stroke risk in patients with aPL. Transcranial Doppler has been used to identify microembolic signals, which have been detected in the intracranial circulation of patients with carotid artery disease (Babikian & Wechsler, 1994; Babikian et al., 1997; Del Sette et al., 1997), artificial heart valves (Georgiadis et al., 1997) and coagulopathy (Babikian & Wechsler 1994; Del Sette et al., 1997), but are infrequently associated with small vessel disease (Del Sette et al., 1997). They are thought to arise from vascular air bubbles, formed elements, and experimentally induced emboli (Padayachee et al., 1987; Spencer et al., 1990; Russell et al., 1991), and are detected based on the site, degree, extent and surface of stenosis (Sitzer et al., 1995). Two of their patients with the highest event rates were aPL positive, and the rate of microembolic signals correlated with the titer of IgG-aCL, arguing for a pathophysiological association between aPL and microembolic signals. The use of transcranial Doppler to detect microembolic signals in APS is an inexpensive, non-invasive method. It may offer a new approach in risk stratification and possibly therapy monitoring in patients with aPL (Brey & Carolin, 1997).

Potential mechanisms for aPL induced thrombosis

The range of clinical manifestations in APS might be explained by the breadth of autoantibodies and their characteristics (specificity, affinity/avidity, valency, titre). Consequently, mechanisms may be widely characterized by those involving antibody interference with hemostatic reactions and those involving cell-mediated events (for review see Roubey, 1998).

One of the most promising aspects of the discovery of β_2GP-I as a target antigen for aPL is the possibility that aPL interfere with the function of β_2GP-I in vivo, thereby conferring a prothrombotic diathesis in APS (Sheng et al., 1998a). β_2GP-I, a minor natural anticoagulant, competes in vitro for available phospholipid surface area needed for assembly of the prothrombinase complex, thereby inhibiting prothrombinase activity (Roubey et al., 1992). This inhibitory capacity is weak under normal physiological conditions. However, aPL may cross-link membrane-bound β_2GP-I and increase β_2GP-I's inhibitory abilities (Willems et al., 1996; Arnout et al., 1998). Also, β_2GP-I mobility remains high on phospholipid surfaces due to ionic binding interactions. Once complexed with aPL, however, there could be a higher affinity for phospholipids that would impede coagulation by competing with coagulation factors for the available catalytic surface. Therefore, bivalency would be essential for cross-linking two β_2GP-I molecules and inducing a correct spatial orientation of their phospholipid binding domains, thereby markedly increasing their affinity for the phospholipid surface (Arnout et al., 1998). aPL can also interfere with the Protein C pathway by inhibiting thrombin formation, interfering with thrombomodulin expression, and inhibiting the degradation of Factor Va by activated Protein C (activated protein C resistance) (for review see McNeil et al., 1991). APL-related activated Protein C resistance does not appear to be associated with a mutation in the coagulation factor V gene (Bokarewa et al., 1995; Deschiens et al., 1996).

A variety of effects on platelets, coagulation proteins and endothelial cells have been ascribed to aPL, making them not only serological markers for APS, but direct contributors to the development of thrombosis and other clinical manifestations. β_2GP-I binding to phosphatidylserine may serve in the identification of apoptotic cells, since cells undergoing apoptosis are known to redistribute PL to expose phosphatidylserine on the extracellular surface (Casciola-Rosen et al., 1996). In vitro opsonization of apoptotic cells by β_2GP-I antibodies enhances scavenger macrophages binding. With respect to platelet–antibody interactions, Arnout has drawn attention to the similarities between the pathogenic mechanism for heparin-induced thrombocytopenia and a potential mechanism for aPL-induced thrombosis (Arnout, 1996). Heparin-induced thrombocytopenia involves antibody binding of a protein (mainly platelet factor 4) that is bound to heparin, which then interacts with the cellular Fc-gamma receptor to induce activation of a prothrombotic process. There is emerging evidence that aPL binding to phospholipid complexes on various cells, including platelets and vascular endothelium, also results in their activation through the Fc-gamma receptor (Meroni et al., 1998). Campbell has demonstrated the induction of a dose-dependent increase in the activation and aggregation of human platelets using aPL from patients with APS (Campbell et al., 1995). This effect appears to be mediated through binding to phosphatidylserine (Vasquez-Mellado et al., 1994) or β_2GP-I (Inanc et al., 1997; Duhaut et al., 1998). The feasibility of β_2GP-I binding to endothelial cells is more controversial

since they infrequently express large amounts of negatively charged structures at the cell surface. Recent evidence suggests that β_2GP-I may be involved in lipid metabolism and serves as an endothelial growth factor. Meroni and colleagues have demonstrated that β_2GP-I probably binds to endothelial cells through heparin-sulphate (HS) proteoglycan, which plays a role in the function of vascular endothelial growth factors (Meroni et al., 1998).

Both passive and active immunization of normal laboratory mice with either aPL or with β_2GP-I results in the induction of an experimental APS, including thrombocytopenia, placental infarction and fetal loss, myocardial infarction and neurological dysfunction (for review see Ziporen & Shoenfeld, 1998). Brey and colleagues were able to accelerate neurological dysfunction in an autoimmune mouse strain by immunization with β_2GP-I (Brey *et al.*, 1995). Immunization with β_2GP-I in both normal and autoimmune mouse strains leads to the development of antibodies to both β_2GP-I and phospholipids (for review see Ziporen & Shoenfeld, 1998).

Some aPL may arise due to infection by common viruses and bacteria (for review see Gharavi & Pierangeli, 1998). Gharavi and colleagues demonstrated that pathogenic aPL and anti-β_2GP-I antibody production can be induced following immunization with mutant forms of β_2GP-I containing the aPL binding site alone (Gharavi et al., 1995). A subsequent Genebank screen yielded seven proteins with sequence homology to the mutant proteins. Four of the peptides were identified as part of viruses or bacteria to which humans are commonly exposed (human cytomegalovirus and *Bacillus subtilus*). Interestingly, these peptides had a greater ability to bind PL than the mutants they generated. Normal mice immunized with these viral protein fragments developed aPL and suffered intrauterine fetal death, spinal cord infarction and thrombosis (Gharavi et al., 1996) suggesting that infection may well be the trigger for pathogenic aPL antibody production (Gharavi & Pierangeli, 1998). A recent report describing APS associated with cytomegalovirus infection illustrates that infection-induced aPL may occasionally be associated with thrombosis (Labarca et al., 1997). In support of this proposal, Vermylen provides corroborative evidence for infective origins of aPL. Varicella-associated neutralizing antibodies against Protein S present clinical resemblance to purpura fulminans (reviewed in Vermylen et al., 1998), a congenital homozygous protein S deficiency that may exhibit widespread cutaneous thrombosis and necrosis shortly following birth (Marlar & Neumann, 1990). Similar symptoms may arise from IgG and IgM antibodies to protein S in children recovering from varicella infection. Ultimately, common bacterial or viral infection might incite similar mechanisms in humans and yield aPL production in APS.

Many investigators favour a 'two hit' hypothesis to explain how aPL might lead to thrombosis; (i) continually circulating aPL and phospholipid-binding proteins require (ii) a local trigger (i.e. infection, injury, EC activation) to induce site specific thrombosis or amplify the thrombotic process (Vaarala, 1997). This hypothesis proposes aPL induction of a prothrombotic state in which thrombosis is triggered by an otherwise insufficient local trigger (Roubey, 1998). Thrombosis would require a second triggering factor, so explaining why patients with persistent serum autoantibodies display clotting events only occasionally and in the absence of detectable Ig deposits (Meroni et al., 1998). Although there is some evidence that aPL antibodies may actually lead to accelerated atherosclerosis (George et al., 1997), the majority of evidence favours a prothrombotic mechanism that amplifies thrombosis in certain settings. Pierangeli and Harris demonstrated larger clot size with a longer time to dissolution in mice treated with human aPL compared to control IgG using a pinch clamp injury model (Pierangeli & Harris, 1998). Taken together, these studies provide important evidence that antibodies to phospholipids and phospholipid-binding proteins like β_2GP-I can cause thrombosis and other antibody-mediated clinical manifestations.

Treatment

General treatment issues

Treatment of the APS can be directed at thrombo-occlusive events using antithrombotic medications or at modulating the immune response with immunotherapy. In the case of thrombotic manifestations, both approaches have been used (Babikian & Levine, 1992; Brey & Coull, 1992; Coull et al., 1992; Brey, 1994; Feldmann & Levine, 1995; Krnic-Barrie et al., 1997; Brey & Escalante, 1998; Shah et al., 1998). Because the mechanism by which aPL lead to thrombosis is probably heterogeneous, it is likely that the most appropriate therapeutic choice for a given patient may depend on which of these the patient's thrombo-occlusive episode was due to. For platelet or prostaglandin abnormalities aspirin or ticlopidine might be expected to be beneficial whereas for thrombomodulin, Protein C, or Protein S abnormalities, anticoagulation might be needed. This may provide a partial explanation for the discrepant findings in the aPL treatment literature on thrombo-embolic manifestations.

Therapies aimed at modulating the immune-response in preventing both thrombotic and non-thrombotic neurologic manifestations of APS also have variable success (Babikian & Levine, 1992; Brey, 1994; Feldmann & Levine, 1995). As with aPL-associated thrombosis, a more precise definition of the nature of the aPL-target tissue interaction would help guide more rational therapeutic decision-making.

Treatment of aPL-associated cerebrovascular ischemia

Primary prevention

The strong association between aPL and incident ischemic stroke suggests that primary prevention strategies should be sought, however, it is unclear what, if any, treatment should be offered when aPL is discovered in a patient with no prior thrombotic episodes. Many patients with aPL-associated stroke also have other cardiovascular disease risk factors such as smoking and hyperlipidemia (Levine et al., 1990, 1993; Verro et al., 1998). It is possible that primary preventative strategies may be more important in asymptomatic patients who also have other cardiovascular disease risk factors. Conventional risk factor reduction strategies should not be neglected in this group, however. Many patients with the various manifestations of the APS tend to have repeated episodes of the same manifestations (Levine et al., 1995). It is unclear, for example, whether young women with recurrent fetal loss due to aPL require primary preventative therapy for stroke or other arterial or venous thrombotic manifestations. The prevalence of aPL is highest in patients with SLE than in any other population (Love & Santoro, 1990), and aPL increases the risk of thrombosis from twofold to ninefold in patients with SLE. This suggests that a primary prevention strategy may be important in this group more than any other (Love & Santoro, 1990; Escalante et al., 1995).

Secondary prevention

Prevention of recurrent disease in a patient found to have aPL at the time of a thrombo-occlusive event is the source of great concern and anxiety for both patients and physicians. The same factors for determining the risk of a first aPL-associated thrombo-occlusive event described above are important in determining the risk for recurrence, e.g. antibody characteristics and the presence of other cardiovascular disease risk factors. A variety of treatment modalities have been suggested to prevent recurrent events in patients with aPL-associated thrombosis (Babikian & Levine, 1992; Brey & Coull, 1992; Coull et al., 1992; Brey, 1994; Feldmann & Levine, 1995; Krnic-Barrie et al., 1997; Brey & Escalante 1998; Shah et al., 1998). These are based on case reports and selected or retrospective series, and are therefore, all limited in their clinical applicability and generalizability. These studies provide guidance in an area where no prospective data exist and are very important. However, there are limitations to utility of these data that should not be over-stepped. Standardized treatment recommendations for stroke associated with aPL cannot be made or extrapolated.

In their long-term follow-up study of 61 patients with aPL, Krnic-Barrie and colleagues found that there was no difference in the number of recurrent thrombotic events between patients who were taking aspirin and those who were taking warfarin (Krnic-Barrie et al., 1997). Both of these had fewer events than groups who were on no therapy or who were taking corticosteroid therapy. Patients taking corticosteroid therapy, in general, had SLE and were likely to have other medical problems that could have predisposed them to developing thrombosis. Nonetheless, these data underscore the notion that corticosteroid therapy is not effective in preventing thrombosis in patients with aPL.

One important problem that is difficult to overcome is that 'natural history' data regarding the risk for recurrent thrombosis either with no medication or with standardized treatment is unavailable for aPL-associated stroke. Controlled epidemiological studies are needed which assess the risk of recurrent thrombo-occlusive events in an ischemic stroke population. In addition, more basic work is needed to identify unique characteristics of pathogenic aPL. Assays need to be developed which consistently allow us to differentiate pathogenic from non-pathogenic aPL and which allow us to discriminate among the many pathogenic mechanisms for thrombosis. This knowledge would permit separation of aPL-positive stroke patients into groups that need (i) no treatment; (ii) antiplatelet therapy; (iii) warfarin; or (iv) other immune-modulating therapy.

References

Alarcon-Segovia, D., Deleze, M. & Oria, C.V. (1989). Antiphospholipid antibodies and the antiphospholipid syndrome in systemic lupus erythematosus: a prospective analysis of 500 consecutive patients. *Medicine*, **68**(6), 353–65.

Ameri, A. & Bousser, M.G. (1992). Cerebral venous thrombosis. *Neurology Clinics*, **10**, 87–111.

Ameriso, S.F., Wong, V.L., Quismorio, F.P. Jr & Fisher, M. (1991). Immunohematologic characteristics of infection-associated cerebral infarction. *Stroke*, **22**, 1004–9.

Angelini, L., Ravelli, A., Caporali, R., Rumi, V., Nardocci, N. & Martini, A. (1994). High prevalence of antiphospholipid antibodies in children with idiopathic cerebral ischemia. *Pediatrics*, **94**(*4 Pt 1*), 500–3.

Antiphospholipid Antibodies in Stroke Study (APASS) Group. (1990). Clinical and laboratory findings in patients with antiphospholipid antibodies and cerebral ischemia. *Stroke*, **21**, 1268–73.

Antiphospholipid Antibodies in Stroke Study Group (APASS). (1993). Anticardiolipin antibodies are an independent risk factor for first ischemic stroke. *Neurology*, **43**, 2069–73.

Antiphospholipid Antibody in Stroke Study Group (APASS). (1997). Anticardiolipin antibodies and the risk of recurrent thrombo-occlusice events and death. *Neurology*, **48**, 91–4.

Arnout, J. (1996). The pathogenesis of antiphospholipid antibody syndrome: hypothesis based on parallelisms with heparin-induced thrombocytopenia. *Thrombosis and Haemostasis*, **75**, 536–41

Arnout, J. & Vermylen, J. (1998). Mechanism of action of Beta-2-glycoprotein-1-dependent lupus anticoagulants. *Lupus*, **7**, S23–8.

Arnout, J., Wittevrongel, C., Vanrusselt, M., Hoylaerts, M. & Vermylen, J. (1998). β_2GP-I dependent lupus anticoagulants form stable bivalent antibody-β_2GP-I complexes on phospholipid surfaces. *Thrombosis and Haemostasis*, **79**, 79–86.

Babikian, V.L. & Levine, S.R. (1992). Therapeutic considerations for stroke patients with antiphospholipid antibodies. *Stroke*, **23**(Suppl. 2), 33–7.

Babikian, V. & Wechsler, L. (1994). Recent developments in transcranial Doppler sonography. *Journal of Neuroimaging*, **4**, 159–63.

Babikian, V.L., Wijman, C.A., Hyde, C. et al. (1997). Cerebral microembolism and early recurrent cerebral or retinal ischemic events. *Stroke*, **28**, 1314–18.

Badui, E., Solorio, S., Martinez, E. et al. (1995). The heart in the primary antiphospholipid syndrome. *Archives of Medical Research*, **26**, 115–120.

Barrett, J.T. (1983). Natural resistance and acquired immunity. In *Textbook of Immunology*, ed. S.E. Harshberger, pp. 203–22. St. Louis: CV Mosby.

Bokarewa, M.I., Bremme, K., Falk, G., Sten-Linder, M., Egberg, N. & Blomback, M. (1995). Studies on antiphospholipid antibodies, APC-resistence and associated mutation in the coagulation factor V gene. *Thrombosis Research*, **78**, 193–200.

Brey, R.L. (1994). Stroke prevention in patients with antiphospholipid antibodies. *Lupus*, **3**, 299–302.

Brey, R.L. & Carolin, M.K. (1997). Detection of cerebral microembolic signals by transcranial Doppler may be a useful part of the equation in determining stroke risk in patients with antiphospholipid antibody syndrome. *Lupus*, **6**, 621–4.

Brey, R.L. & Coull, B.M. (1992). Antiphospholipid antibodies: origin, specificity and mechanism of action. *Stroke*, **23**(Suppl. 2), 15–18.

Brey, R.L. & Escalante, A. (1998). Neurological manifestations of antiphospholipid syndrome. *Lupus*, **7**, S67–S74.

Brey, R.L. & Levine, S.R. (1996). Treatment of neurologic complications of the antiphospholipid syndrome. *Lupus*, **5**(5), 473–6.

Brey, R.L., Hart, R.G., Sherman, D.G. & Tegeler, C.T. (1990). Antiphospholipid antibodies and cerebral ischemia in young people. *Neurology*, **40**, 1190–6.

Brey, R.L., Cote, S., Barohn, R., Jackson, C., Crawley, R. & Teale, J.M. (1995). Model for the neuromuscular complications of systemic lupus erythematosus. *Lupus*, **4**(3), 209–12.

Brey, R.L., Abbott, R.D., Sharp, D.S. et al. (1999). Beta-2-glycoprotein 1-dependent (B2GP1-dep) anticardiolipin antibodies are an independent risk factor for ischemic stroke in the Honolulu Heart Cohort. *Stroke*, **39**, 252 (Abstract).

Camerlingo, M., Casto, L., Censori, B. et al. (1995). Anticardiolipin antibodies in acute non-hemorrhagic stroke seen within six hours after onset. *Acta Neurologica Scandinavica*, **92**, 60–71.

Campbell, A.L., Pierangeli, S.S., Wellhausen, S. & Harris, E.N. (1995). Comparison of the effects of anticardiolipin antibodies from patients with the antiphospholipid antibody syndrome and with syphilis on platelet activation and aggregation. *Thrombosis and Haemostatics*, **73**, 529–34.

Carhuapoma, J.R., Mitsias, P. & Levine, S.R. (1997). Cerebral venous thrombosis and anticardiolipin antibodies. *Neurology*, **28**, 2363–9.

Casciola-Rosen, L., Rosen, A., Petri, M. & Schlissel, M. (1996). Surface blebs on apoptotic cells are sites of enhanced procoagulant activity implications for coagulation events and antigenic spread in systemic lupus erythematosus. *Proceedings of the National Academy of Sciences, USA*, **93**:1624–9.

Cesbron, J-Y., Amouyel, Ph. & Masy, E. (1997). Anticardiolipin antibodies and physical disability in the elderly. *Annals of Internal Medicine*, **126**, 1003.

Chakravarty, K.K., Al-Hillawi, A.H., Byron, M.A. & Durkin, C.J. (1990). Anticardiolipin antibody associated ischemic strokes in elderly patients without system lupus erythematosus. *Age and Aging*, **19**(2), 114–18.

Chakravarty, K.K., Byron, M.A., Webley, M. et al. (1991). Antibodies to cardiolipin in stroke: association with mortality and functional recovery in patients without systemic lupus erythematosus. *Quarterly Journal of Medicine*, **79**, 397–405.

Chinnery, P.F., Shaw, P.I., Ince, P.G., Jackson, G.H. & Bishop, R.I. (1997). Fulminant encephalopathy due to the catastrophic primary antiphospholipid syndrome. *Journal of Neurology, Neurosurgery and Psychiatry*, **62**, 300–1.

Ciocca, R.G., Choi, J. & Graham, A.M. (1995). Antiphospholipid antibodies lead to increased risk in cardiovascular surgery. *American Journal of Surgery*, **170**, 198–200.

Coull, B.M., Bourdette, D.N., Goodnight, S.H., Briley, D.P. & Hart, R. (1987). Multiple cerebral infarctions and dementia associated with anticardiolipin antibodies. *Stroke*, **18**, 1107–12.

Coull, B.M., Levine, S.R. & Brey, R.L. (1992). The role of antiphospholipid antibodies and stroke. *Neurology Clinics*, **10**, 125–43.

de Moerloose, P., Boehlen, F. & Reber, G. (1997). Prevalence of anticardiolipin and antinuclear antibodies in an elderly hospitalized population and mortality after a 6-year follow-up. *Age and Aging*, **27**, 319–21.

Del Papa, N., Raschi, E.R., Catelli, L. et al. (1997a). Endothelial cells as a target for antiphospholipid antibodies: role of anti-beta-2-glycoprotein 1 antibodies. *American Journal of Radiological Imaging*, **38**, 212–17.

Del Papa, N., Guidali, L., Sala, A. et al. (1997b). Endothelial cells as target for antiphospholipid antibodies. *Arthritis and Rheumatology*, **40**, 551–61.

Del Sette, M., Angeli, S., Stara, I., Finocchi, C. & Gandolfo, C. (1997). Microembolic signals with serial transcranial Doppler monitoring in acute focal ischemic deficit: a local phenomenon? *Stroke*, **28**(7), 1311–13.

Deschiens, M-A., Conard, J., Horellou, M.H. et al. (1996). Coagulations studies, factor V Leiden, and anticardiolipin antibodies in 40 cases of cerebral venous sinus thrombosis. *Stroke*, **27**, 1724–30.

Drouvalakis, K.A. & Buchanan, T.T.C. (1998). Phospholipid specificity of autoimmune and drug induced lupus anticoagulants; association of phosphatidylethanolamine reactivity with thrombosis in autoimmune disease. *Journal of Rheumatology*, **25**, 290–5.

Duhaut, P., Berruyer, M., Pinede, L. et al. (1998). Anticardiolipin antibodies and giant cell arteritis: a prospective, multicenter case-control study. *Arthritis and Rheumatology*, **41**, 701–9.

Escalante, A., Brey, R.L., Mitchell, B.D. & Dreiner, U. (1995). Accuracy of anticardiolipin antibodies in identifying a history of thrombosis among patients with systemic lupus erythematosus. *American Journal of Medicine*, **98**, 559–67.

Feldmann, E. & Levine, S.R. (1995). Cerebrovascular disease with antiphospholipid antibodies: immune mechanisms, significance and therapeutic options. *Annals of Neurology*, **37**(Suppl), S114–30.

Ford, S.E., Lillicrap, D.M., Brunet, D. & Ford, P.M. (1989). Thrombotic endocarditis and lupus anticoagulant, a pathogenetic possibility for idiopathic rheumatic type valvular heart disease. *Archives of Pathological Laboratory Medicine*, **113**, 350–3.

Ford, S.E., Kennedy, L.A. & Ford, P.M. (1994). Clinico-pathological correlations of antiphospholipid antibodies. *Archives of Pathological Laboratory Medicine*, **118**, 491–5.

Galli, M., Comfurius, P., Maassen, C. et al. (1990). Anticardiolipin antibodies (ACA) directed not to cardiolipin but to a plasma protein cofactor. *Lancet*, **335**, 1544–7.

George, J., Afek, A., Gilburd, B. et al. (1997). Atherosclerosis in LDL-receptor knock-out mice is accelerated by immunization with anticardiolipin antibodies. *Lupus*, **6**, 723–9.

George, J., Gilburd, B., Hojnik, M. et al. (1998). Target recognition of β2-glycoprotein I (β2-GPI)-Dependent anticardiolipin antibod-

ies: evidence for involvement of the fourth domain of β2-GPI in antibody binding. *Journal of Immunology*, **160**, 3917–23.

Georgiadis, D., Preiss, M., Lindner, A., Gybels, Y., Zierz, S. & Zerkowski, H.R. (1997). Doppler microembolic signals in children with prosthetic cardiac valves. *Stroke*, **28**, 1328–9.

Gharavi, A.E. & Peirangeli, S.S. (1998). Origin of antiphospholipid antibodies: induction of aPL by viral peptides. *Lupus*, **7**, S52–4.

Gharavi, A.E., Tang, H., Gharavi, E.E., Wilson, W.A. & Espinoza, L.R. (1995). Induction of aPL by immunization with a 15 amino acid peptide. *Arthritis and Rheumatism*, **38**, S296 (Abstract).

Gharavi, A.E., Tang, H., Gharavi, E.E., Espinoza, L.R. & Wilson, W.A. (1996). Induction of antiphospholipid antibodies by immunization with a viral peptide. *Arthritis and Rheumatism*, **39**, S319 (Abstract).

Ginsburg, K.S., Liang, M.H., Newcomer, L. et al. (1992). Anticardiolipin antibodies and the risk for ischemic stroke and venous thrombosis. *Annals of Internal Medicine*, **117**, 997–1002.

Gross, L. (1940). The cardiac lesion in Libman-Sacks disease with a consideration of its relationship to acute diffuse lupus erythematosus. *American Journal of Pathology*, **16**, 375–408.

Haagerup, A., Kristensen, T. & Kruse, T.A. (1991). Polymorphism and genetic mapping of the gene encoding human β2-glycoprotein I to chromosome 17. *Cytogenetics and Cell Genetics*, **58**, 2004–10.

Hachulla, E., Michon-Pasturel, U., Leys, D. et al. (1998). Cerebral magnetic imaging in patients with or without antiphospholipid antibodies. *Lupus*, **7**, 124–31.

Hagihara, Y., Goto, Y., Ksao, H. & Yoshimura, T. (1995). Role of the N- and C-terminal domains of bovine β2-glycoprotein I in its interaction with cardiolipin. *Journal of Biochemistry (Tokyo)*, **118**, 129–36.

Hess, D.C., Krauss, J., Adams, R.J., Nichols, F.T., Zhang, D. & Rountree, H.A. (1991). Anticardiolipin antibodies: a study of frequency in TIA and stroke. *Neurology*, **41**, 525–8.

Hughes, G.R.V. (1983). Thrombosis, abortion, cerebral disease and lupus anticoagulant. *British Medical Journal*, **187**, 1088–91.

Hunt, J.E. & Krilis, S.A. (1994). The fifth domain of β2-glycoprotein I contains a phospholipid binding site (Cys281–Cys288) and a region recognized by anti-cardiolipin antibodies. *Journal of Immunology*, **152**, 653–9.

Hunt, J.E., Simpson, R.J. & Krilis, S.A. (1993). Identification of a region of β2-glycoprotein I critical for lipid binding and anti-cardiolipin antibody co-factor activity. *Proceedings of the National Academy of Sciences USA*, **90**, 2141–5.

Inanc, M., Radway-Bright, E.L. & Isenberg, D.A. (1997). Beta-2-glycoprotein 1 and anti-beta-2-glycoprotein 1 antibodies: where are we now? *British Journal of Rheumatology*, **36**, 1247–57.

Kalashnikova, L.A., Nasonov, E.L., Kushekbaeva, A.E. & Gracheva, L.A. (1990). Anticardiolipin antibodies in Sneddon's syndrome. *Neurology*, **40**, 464–7.

Khamashta, M.A., Cervera, R., Asherson, R.A. et al. (1990). Association of antibodies against phospholipids with valvular heart disease in patients with systemic lupus erythematosus. *Lancet*, **335**(8705), 1541–4.

Khamashta, M.A., Cuadrado, M.J., Mujic, F., Taub, N.A., Hunt, B.J. &

Hughes, G.R.V. (1995). The management of thrombosis in the antiphospholipid antibody syndrome. *New England Journal of Medicine*, **332**, 993–7.

Klemp, P., Cooper, R.C., Strauss, F.J., Jordaan, E.R., Przybojewski, J.Z. & Nel, N. (1988). Anticardiolipin antibodies in ischemic heart disease. *Clinical Experimental Immunology*, **74**(2), 254–7.

Krnic-Barrie, S., Reister, O., Connor, C., Looney, S.W., Pierangeli, S.S. & Harris, E.N. (1997). A retrospective review of 61 patients with antiphospholipid syndrome. *Archives of Internal Medicine*, **157**, 2101–8.

Kushner, M.J. (1990). Prospective study of anticardiolipin antibodies in stroke. *Stroke*, **21**(2), 295–8.

Labarca, J.A., Rabaggliati, R.M., Radrigan, F.J. et al. (1997). Antiphospholipid syndrome associated with cytomegalovirus infection: case report and review. *Clinical and Infectious Diseases*, **24**, 197–200.

Labutta, R.J. (1996). Ophthalmic manifestations in the antiphospholipid syndrome. *The Antiphospholipid Syndrome*, ed. R.A. Asherson, R. Cervera, J.C. Piette & Y. Shoenfeld, pp. 213–18, CRC Press.

Levine, S.R., Deegan, M.J., Futrell, N. & Welch, K.M.A. (1990). Cerebrovascular and neurologic disease associated with antiphospholipid antibodies: 48 cases. *Neurology*, **40**, 1190–6.

Levine, S.R., Brey, R.L., Salowich-Palm, L., Sawaya, K.L. & Havstad, S. (1993). Antiphospholipid antibody associated stroke: prospective assessment of recurrent event risk. *Stroke*, **24**, 188.

Levine, S.R., Brey, R.L., Sawaya, K.L. et al. (1995). Recurrent stroke and thrombo-occlusive events in the antiphospholipid syndrome. *Annals of Neurology*, **38**, 119–24.

Levine, S.R., Salowich-Palm, L., Sawaya, K.L. et al., (1997). IgG anticardiolipin antibody titer >40 GPL and the risk of subsequent thrombo-occlusive events and death. *Stroke*, **28**, 1660–5.

Levy, R.A., Avvad, E., Olivera, J. & Porto, L.C. (1998). Placental pathology in antiphospholipid syndrome. *Lupus*, **7**, S81–5.

Libman, E. & Sacks, B. (1924). A hitherto undescribed form of valvular and mural endocarditis. *Archives of Internal Medicine*, **33**, 701–37.

Loizou, S., McCrea, J.D., Rudge, A.C., Reynolds, R., Boyle, C.C. & Harris, E.N. (1985). Measurement of anticardiolipin antibodies by an enzyme linked immunosorbent assay (ELISA): standardization and quanitation of results. *Clinical and Experimental Immunology*, **62**, 738–45.

Love, P.E. & Santoro, S.A. (1990). Antiphospholipid antibodies: Anticardiolipin and the lupus anticoagulant in systemic lupus erythematosus (SLE) and in non-SLE disorders. *Annals of Internal Medicine*, **112**, 682–98.

Marlar, R.A. & Neumann, A. (1990). Neonatal purpura fulminans due to homozygous protein C or protein S deficiencies. *Seminars in Thrombosis and Hemostasis*, **16**(4), 299–309.

Matsuura, E., Igarashi, Y., Fujimoto, M., Ichikawa, K. & Koike, T. (1990). Anticardiolipin cofactors and the differential diagnosis of autoimmune disease. *Lancet*, **336**(8708), 177–8.

Matsuura, E., Igarashi, Y., Yasuda, T., Triplett, D.A. & Koike, T. (1994). Anticardiolipin antibodies recognize beta-2-glycoprotein-I structure altered by interacting with an oxygen-modified solid phase surface. *Journal of Experimental Medicine*, **179**(2), 457–62.

Matsuura, E., Kobayashi, K., Yasuda, T. & Koike, T. (1998). Antiphospholipid antibodies and atherosclerosis. *Lupus*, **7**(Suppl. 2), S135–9.

McNeil, H.P., Simpson, R.J., Chesterman, C.N. & Krilis, S.A. (1990). Antiphospholipid antibodies are directed to a complex antigen that includes a lipid-binding inhibitor of coagulation: β2-glycoprotein I (apolipoprotein H). *Proceedings of the National Academy of Sciences USA*, **87**, 4120–4.

McNeil, H.P., Chesterman, C.N. & Krilis, S.A. (1991). Immunology and clinical importance of antiphospholipid antibodies. *Advances in Immunology*, **49**, 193–280.

Meroni, P.L., Del Papa, N., Raschi, E. et al. (1998). β2 glycoprotein 1 as a co-factor for antiphospholipid reactivity with endothelial cells. *Lupus*, **7**(Suppl. 2), S44–7.

Metz, L.M., Edworthy, S., Mydlarski, R. & Fritzler, M.J. (1998). The frequency of phospholipid antibodies in an unselected stroke population. *Canadian Journal of Neurological Science*, **25**, 64–9.

Molad, Y., Sidi, Y., Gornish, M., Lerner, M., Pinkhas, J. & Weinberger, A. (1992). Lupus anticoagulant: correlation with magnetic resonance imaging of brain lesions. *Journal of Rheumatology*, **19**, 556–61.

Montalban, J., Arboix, A., Staub, H. et al. (1989). Transient global amnesia and antiphospholipid antibodies. *Clinical and Experimental Rheumatology*, **7**, 85–7.

Muir, K.W., Squire, I.B., Alwan, W. & Lees, K.R. (1994). Anticardiolipin antibodies in an unselected stroke population. *Lancet*, **344**, 452–6.

Naarendorp, M. & Spiera, H. (1998). Sudden sensorineural hearing loss in patients with systemic lupus erythematosus or lupus-like syndromes and antiphospholipid antibodies. *Journal of Rheumatology*, **25**, 589–92.

Nencini, P., Baruffi, M.C., Abbate, R., Massai, G., Amaducci, L. & Inzitari, D. (1992). Lupus anticoagulant and anticardiolipin antibodies in young adults with cerebral ischemia. *Stroke*, **23**(2), 189–93.

Nesher, G., Ilany, J., Rosenmann, D. & Abraham, A.S. (1997). Valvular dysfunction in antiphospholipid syndrome: prevalence, clinical features and treatment. *Seminars in Arthritis and Rheumatism*, **27**, 27–35.

Nojima, J., Suehisa, E., Akita, N. et al. (1997). Risk of arterial thrombosis in patients with anticardiolipin antibodies and lupus anticoagulant. *British Journal of Haematology*, **96**, 447–450.

Padayachee, T.S., Parsons, S., Theobold, R., Linley, J., Gosling, R.G. & Deverall, P.B. (1987). The detection of microemboli in the middle cerebral artery during cardiopulmonary bypass: a transcranial Doppler ultrasound investigation using membrane and bubble oxygenators. *Annals of Thoracic Surgery*, **44**(3), 298–302.

Pierangeli, S.S. & Harris, E.N. (1998). Antiphospholipid antibodies in an in vivo thrombosis model in mice. *Lupus*, **3**, 247–51.

Polz, E. & Kostner, G.M. (1979). The binding of beta 2-glycoprotein I to human serum lipoproteins: distribution among density fractions. *FEBS Letters*, **102**, 183–6.

Provenzale, J.M., Heinz, E.R., Ortel, T.L., Macik, B.G., Charles, L.A. & Alberts, M.J. (1994). Antiphospholipid antibodies in patients without systemic lupus erythematosus: neuroradiologic findings. *Radiology*, **192**, 531–7.

Rafuse, P.E. & Canny, C.L.B. (1992). Initial identification of antinuclear antibody-negative systemic lupus erythematosus on ophthalmic examinaton: a case report with discussion of the ocular significance of anticardiolipin (antiphospholipid) antibodies. *Canadian Journal of Ophthalmology*, **27**, 189–93.

Rand, J.H., Wu, X.X., Andree, H.A. et al. (1997). Pregnancy loss in the antiphospholipid antibody syndrome-a possible thrombogenic mechanism. *New England Journal of Medicine*, **337**(3), 154–60.

Reid, K.B.M. & Day, A.J. (1989). Structure-function relationships of the complement components. *Immunology Today*, **10**, 177–80.

Rosove, M.H. & Brewer, P.M.C. (1992). Antiphospholipid thrombosis:clinical course after the first thrombotic event in 70 patients. *Annals of Internal Medicine*, **117**, 303–8.

Rote, N.S., Dostal-Johnson, D. & Branch, D.W. (1990). Antiphospholipid antibodies and recurrent pregnancy loss: correlation between the activated partial thromboplastin time and antibodies against phosphatidylserine and cardiolipin. *American Journal of Obstetrics and Gynecology*, **163**, 575–84.

Roubey, R.A.S. (1998). Mechanisms of autoantibody-mediated thrombosis. *Lupus*, **7**(Suppl. 2), S114–19.

Roubey, R.A.S., Pratt, C.W., Buyon, J.P. & Winfield, J.B. (1992). Lupus anticoagulant activity of autoimmune antiphospholipid antibodies is dependent upon β_2GP-I. *Journal of Clinical Investigation*, **90**, 1100–4.

Roubey, R.A.S., Eisenberg, R.A., Harper, M.F. & Winfield, J.B. (1995). 'Anticardiolipin' autoantibodies recognize β2-glycoprotein-I in the absence of phospholipids: importance of antigen density and bivalent binding. *Journal of Immunology*, **154**(2), 954–60.

Roubey, R.A.S., Maldonado, M.A. & Byrd, S.N. (1996). Comparison of an enzyme-linked immunosorbent assay for antibodies to β2-glycoprotein-I and a conventional cardiolipin immunoassay. *Arthritis and Rheumatism*, **39**(9), 1606–7.

Russell, D., Madden, K.P., Clark, W.M., Sandset, P.M. & Zivin, J.A. (1991). Detection of arterial emboli using Doppler ultrasound in rabbits. *Stroke*, **22**, 253–8.

Sailer, M., Burchert, W., Ehrenheim, C. et al. (1997). Positron emission tomography and magnetic resonance imaging for cerebral involvement in patients with systemic lupus erythematosus. *Journal of Neurology*, **244**, 186–93.

Schlutze, H.E., Heide, K. & Haupt, H. (1961). Uber einbisher unbekanntes niedermole kulares β2 globulin des human serums. *Naturwissens-Schaften*, **48**, 719.

Schmidt, R., Auer-Grumbach, P., Fazekas, F., Offenbacher, H. & Kapeller, P. (1995). Anticardiolipin antibodies in normal subjects. Neuropsychological correlates and MRI findings. *Stroke*, **26**, 749–54.

Schwartz, M., Rochas, M., Weller, B. et al. (1998). High association of anticardiolipin antibodies with psychosis. *Journal of Clinical Psychiatry*, **59**, 20–3.

Shah, N.M., Khamashta, M.A., Atsumi, T. & Hughes, G.R.V. (1998). Outcome of patients with anticardiolipin antibodies: a 10 year follow-up of 52 patients. *Lupus*, **7**, 3–6.

Sheng, Y., Sali, A., Herzog, H., Lahnstein, J. & Krilis, S.A. (1996). Site-directed mutagenesis of recombinant human β2-glycoprotein I identifies a cluster of lysine residues that are critical for phospholipid binding and anti-cardiolipin antibody activity. *Journal of Immunology*, **157**(8), 3744–51.

Sheng, Y., Kandiah, D.A. & Krilis, S.A. (1998a). Beta-2-glycoprotein-1: target antigen for antiphospholipid antibodies. Immunological and molecular aspects. *Lupus*, **7**, S5–S9.

Sheng, Y., Kandiah, D.A. & Krilis, S.A. (1998b). Anti-β2-glycoprotein-I autoantibodies from patients with the antiphospholipid syndrome bind to β2-glycoprotein-I with low affinity. Dimerisation of β2-glycoprotein-I induces a significant increase in anti-β2-glycoprotein-I antibody affinity. *Journal of Immunology*, **161**(4), 2038–43.

Sitzer, M., Muller, W., Siebler, M. et al. (1995). Plaque ulceration and lumen thrombus are the main sources of cerebral microemboli in high-grade internal carotid artery stenosis. *Stroke*, **26**(7), 1231–3.

Sletnes, K.E., Smith, P., Abdolnoor, M., Arnosen, H. & Wisloff, F. (1992). Antiphospholipid antibodies after myocardial infarction and their relation to mortality, reinfarction, and non-haemorrhagic stroke. *Lancet*, **339**, 451-3.

Sneddon, I.B. (1965). Cerebral vascular lesions in livedo reticularis. *British Journal of Dermatology*, **77**, 180–5.

Specker, C.H., Perniok, A., Brauckmann, U., Siebler, M. & Schneider, M. (1998). Detection of cerebral microemboli in APS – Introducing a novel investigation method and implications of analogies with carotid artery disease. *Lupus*, **7**, S75–S80.

Spencer, M.P., Thomas, G.I., Nicholls, S.C. & Sauvage, L.R. (1990). Detection of middle cerebral artery emboli during carotid artery endarterectomy using transcranial Doppler ultrasonography. *Stroke*, **21**, 415–23.

Steinkasserer, A., Estaller, C., Weiss, E.H., Sim, R.B. & Day, A.J. (1991). Complete nucleotide and deduced amino acid sequence of human β2-glycoprotein I. *Biochemical Journal*, **277**, 387–91.

Tietjen, G.E., Day, M., Norris, L. et al. (1998). Role of anticardiolipin antibodies in young persons with migraine and transient focal neurologic events. *Neurology*, **50**, 1433–40.

Toubi, E., Khamashta, M.A., Panarra, A. & Hughes, G.R.V. (1995). Association of antiphospholipid antibodies with central nervous system disease in systemic lupus erythematosus. *American Journal of Medicine*, **99**, 397–401.

Toubi, E., Ben-David, J., Kessel, A., Podoshin, L. & Golan, T.D. (1997). Autoimmune aberration in sudden sensorineural hearing loss: association with anticardiolipin antibodies. *Lupus*, **6**, 540–2.

Tourbah, A., Peitte, J.C., Iba-Zizen, M.T., Lyon-Caen, O., Godeau, P. & Frances, C. (1997). The natural course of cerebral lesions in sneddon syndrome. *Archives of Neurology*, **54**, 53–60.

Triplett, D.A., Brandt, J.T., Musgrave, K.A. & Orr, C.A. (1988). The relationship between lupus anticoagulants and antibodies to phospholipids. *Journal of the American Medical Association*, **259**, 550–4.

Tuhrim, S., Rand, J.H., Godbold, J.H., Weinberger, J., Horowitz, D.R. & Goldman, M. (1998). Elevated antiphosphatidylserine antibodies are a risk factor for ischemic stroke. *Neurology*, **50**, A246 (abstract).

Vaarala, O. (1997). Atherosclerosis in SLE and Hughes syndrome. *Lupus*, **6**, 489–90.

Vaarala, O. (1998). Antiphospholipid antibodies and myocardial infarction. *Lupus*, **7**(Suppl. 2), S132–4.

Vasquez-Mellado, J., Llorente, L., Richaud-Patin, Y. & Alarcon-Segovia, D. (1994). Exposure of anionic phospholipids upon platelet activation permits binding of beta-2-glycoprotein 1 and through it that of IgG antiphospholipid antibodies. *Journal of Autoimmunity*, **7**, 335–48.

Vermylen, J., Van Geet, C. & Arnout, J. (1998). Antibody-mediated thrombosis: relation to the antiphospholipid syndrome. *Lupus*, **7**, S63–6.

Verro, P., Levine, S.R. & Tietjen, G.E. (1998). Cerebrovascular ischemic events with high positive anticardiolipin antibodies. *Stroke*, **29**, 2245–53.

Vila, P., Hernandez, M.C., Lopez-Fernandez, M.F. & Batlle, J. (1994). Prevalence, follow-up and clinical significance of the anticardiolipin antibodies in normal subjects. *Thrombosis and Haemostasis*, **72**, 209–13.

Wahl, D.G., Guillemin, F., de Maistre, E., Perret-Guillaume, C., Lecompte, T. & Thibaut, G. (1998). Meta-analysis of the risk of venous thrombosis in individuals with antiphospholipid antibodies without underlying autoimmune disease or previous thrombosis. *Lupus*, **7**, 15–22.

Willems, G.M., Janssen, M.P., Pelsers, M.M. et al. (1996). Role of divalency in the high-affinity binding of anticardiolipin antibody-β_2GP-I complexes to lipid membranes. *Biochemistry*, **35**(43), 13833–42.

Wilson, W.A., Gharavi, A.E., Koike, T. et al. (1999) & other workshop members. International Consensus Statement On Preliminary Classification Criteria for Definite Antiphospholipid Syndrome: Report of an International Workshop. *Arthritis and Rheumatism*, **42**(7), 1309–11.

Zelzer, B., Sepp, N., Stockhammer, G. et al. (1993). Sneddon's syndrome; a long term follow-up of 21 patients. *Archives of Dermatology*, **129**, 437–44.

Ziporen, L. & Shoenfeld, Y. (1998). Antiphospholipid syndrome: from patient's bedside to experimental animal models and back to the patient's bedside. *Hematological Cell Therapy*, **40**, 175–82.

Ziporen, L., Goldberg, I., Arad, M. et al. (1996). Libman-Sacks endocarditis in the antiphospholipid syndrome: immunopathologic findings in deformed heart valves. *Lupus*, **5**, 196–205.

10

Disseminated intravascular coagulation

Robert J. Schwartzman

Hahnemann University Hospital, Philadelphia, PA, USA

Disseminated intravascular coagulation

Acute generalized bleeding complicates the course of many diseases and is often secondary to disseminated intravascular coagulation (DIC). This process is characterized by excessive quantities of thrombin and plasmin within the circulation that results in the consumption of platelets, coagulation factors, and plasma inhibitors (Rocha et al., 1998). It initiates secondary hyperfibrinolysis and profound changes in endothelial cells and cytokine cascades. This complex process leads to diffuse hemorrhage and microthrombosis of all major organ systems. The systemic hemorrhagic syndrome is its most impressive clinical manifestation but associated generalized intravascular thrombosis occurs that causes ischemia and generalized organ damage. The process may rarely remain organ-specific (Bick, 1992). DIC is primarily seen in a setting of: (i) sepsis (Gando et al., 1998b); (ii) malignancy (Caroll & Binder (1999); (iii) trauma (Gando et al., 1999); and obstetric catastrophes (Sterchele, 1969). It may also complicate liver disease, burns (Garcia-Avello et al., 1998), hip replacement (Breakwell et al., 1999), intravascular hemolysis (Kravans et al., 1957), viremia (Persoons et al., 1998), prosthetic devices (Bick, 1991), Kasabach–Merritt syndrome (Shoj et al., 1998), malignant pheochromocytoma (Arai et al., 1998), Klippel–Trenaunay–Weber syndrome (Katsaros & Grundfest-Broniatowski, 1998), status epilepticus (Felcher et al., 1998), catastrophic antiphospholipid syndrome (Anderson, 1998), stroke in the setting of a medical intensive care unit (Wijdicks & Scott, 1998).

Some systemic clinical signs and symptoms of DIC are dependent on the specific organ system most affected. The combination of DIC and sustained systemic inflammatory response syndrome (SIRS) and its duration predict multiple organ dysfunction (MOD) after trauma. The organ system most severely involved in this setting, the lung, causes acute respiratory distress syndrome or heart and renal failure which determine the major clinical manifestations (Gando et al., 1999). Most patients demonstrate wide spread bleeding, petechiae, purpura, acral cyanosis, hemorrhagic bullae, wound bleeding and oozing from venipuncture sites and arterial lines (Baker, 1989). The patients are frequently in shock with fever, hypotension, acidosis and hypoxia in an intensive care unit setting (Bick, 1992). Those rare patients with low grade or compensated DIC present with subacute bleeding and microthrombosis rather than hemorrhage (Bick, 1992). Low-grade DIC patients demonstrate modest thrombocytopenia, increased turnover and decreased survival of their clotting factors with increased levels of fibrin degradation products (Bick, 1988).

Initiating mechanisms that trigger DIC

Activation of coagulation is a fundamental component of the acute inflammatory response. Release of cytokines from macrophages, monocytes and lymphocytes at the site of tissue damage initiates local coagulation by converting the antithrombotic blood vessel endothelium to a prothrombotic surface. This is achieved by: (i) inducing the production of tissue factor (TF) that, in turn, activates both the extrinsic and intrinsic coagulation systems; (ii) inducing platelet activating factor release; (iii) acutely activating the fibrinolytic system (Weiss & Rashid, 1998). This complex cascade results in an imbalance of coagulation and fibrinolysis that results in a procoagulant state. DIC results when thrombin generation and platelet activation overwhelm inhibitory mechanisms.

Septicemia, particularly with gram negative organisms, is a very important cause of DIC (Gando et al., 1998b). One triggering mechanism that has been extensively studied in several animal models is the initiating of the clotting cascade by bacterial-coat lipopoly-saccharide (LPS) (Gando et al., 1998a). A major mechanism for the induction of DIC in patients with severe sepsis and shock is the activation of the extrinsic coagulation pathway as demonstrated by increased concentrations of tissue factor antigen prothrombin fragments F1 and 2, fibrinopeptide A and D dimer. It has also been demonstrated that the thrombin generated is not fully neutralized by antithrombin III (Gando et al., 1998a). A direct interaction between LPS and platelets through P-selectin has also been demonstrated (Malhotra et al., 1998). DIC may be triggered by endothelial damage caused by the viremia of CMV, HIV, hepatitis and varicella. These infections cause antigen–antibody reactions that activate factor XII and the consequent endothelial damage exposes subendothelial arterial collagen or basement membrane which initiates the clotting cascade (Persoons et al., 1998; McKay & Margaretten, 1967).

Intravascular hemolysis triggers DIC by direct release of reduced adenosine diphosphate (ADP) or membrane phospholipoprotein into the circulation which activates the clotting cascade (Inceman & Tangun, 1969). Similar mechanisms may be operative in Klippel–Trenaunay–Weber and Kasabach–Merritt Syndrome as well as other vascular varices (Katsaros et al., 1998).

All collagen vascular diseases such as Sjogren's syndrome, severe rheumatoid arthritis, scleroderma, dermatomyositis and SLE may present with low grade or compensated DIC (Baker, 1989). The common mechanism underlying DIC in these diseases may be damage to the endothelial cell membrane. Thrombomodulin (TM) is a high affinity thrombin receptor on the endothelial cell membrane that is a natural anticoagulant. It is a cofactor for thrombin-catalysed activation of protein C and inhibits the procoagulant actions of thrombin. Endothelial TM is enzymatically cleaved in the presence of cytokines, activated neutrophiles and macrophages which release soluble fragments (pTM). These fragments are a molecular marker that reflect endothelial cell injury and have been correlated with disease activity in DIC and systemic inflammatory disease (Boffa & Karmochkine, 1998).

The obstetrical complication of amniotic fluid embolism, the retained fetus syndrome and placental abruption are less common than formerly. Placental enzymes, thromboplastin-like material and tissue factor may activate both the intrinsic and extrinsic pathway under these conditions (Bick, 1992). Burn patients and those with crush injuries and tissue damage from severe infarction release tissue factor into the circulation that initiates the clotting cascade through the external pathway (Garcia-Avello et al., 1998).

The relationship between clotting disorders and metastatic malignancy is well known. These patients may demonstrate unusual sites of deep vein thrombosis (upper extremities), warfarin resistance and thromboembolic disease. Antihemostatic agents may suppress experimental tumours. Metastatic malignant cells express tissue factor and urokinase receptors that may be important for neovascularization as well as clotting abnormalities (Francis et al., 1998). The plasminogen activation system may also play a pivotal role in the hemorrhagic events that are common in cancer patients (Caroll & Binder, 1999). DIC may be initiated in cancer patients by hyperfibrinolysis (Weltermann et al., 1998), elevated serum concentrations of hepatocyte growth factor (Hjorth-Hansen et al., 1999) complications of chemotherapy in patients with acute myeloid leukemia with hyperleukocytosis (Wurthner et al., 1999) and disseminated adenocarcinoma (Meijer et al., 1998).

Unusual causes of DIC are paroxysmal nocturnal hemoglobinuria, polycythemia vera, agnogenic myeloid metaplasia, allergic vasculitides, amyloid and hyperlipoproteinemias (Bick, 1992).

Pathophysiology of DIC

DIC is initiated by pathology that activates both coagulation and fibrinolytic cascades to a degree that overwhelms the body's ability to inhibit and limit the process for its intended physiologic purpose. Massive amounts of thrombin and plasmin circulate systemically. Earlier studies have demonstrated the cleavage by thrombin of fibrinogen to fibrinopeptides A, B and fibrin monomer which polymerizes into fibrin clots in the microcirculations of the kidney, lung, mesenteric vessels and CNS. Platelets are activated, trapped in the multiple microthrombi and depleted from the systemic circulation (Bick, 1992; Muller-Berghous, 1989). The systemically circulating plasmin cleaves fibrinogen into X, Y, D and E fragments which complex with fibrin monomers (soluble fibrin monomer) before they polymerize into a stable clot (Bick & Baker, 1992).

The fibrin degradation products (FDP) interfere with fibrin monomer polymerization (stable clot formation) with subsequent hemorrhage. Fibrin fragments D and E adhere to platelet membranes making them dysfunctional causing further hemorrhage (Niewiarowski et al., 1972).

Plasmin further degrades fibrinogen, clotting factos V, VIII, IX and XI. The degradation of cross-linked fibrin by plasmin releases the D-dimer into the circulation. Plasmin actives the complement cascade that lyses RBCs and platelets which releases adenosine diphosphate (ADP), membrane phospholipids and procoagulant material. This further activates the clotting cascades and depletes remaining circulating platelets (Bick, 1988; Bick & Baker, 1992). DIC activates the kinin system by generating factor XIIa which converts prekallikrein to kallikrein. This cleaves kinogens to kinin which directly increases vascular permeability leading to hypotension and shock (Bick, 1992).

Recent experimental and clinical studies have demonstrated a proinflammatory vascular cytokine response to coagulation activation (Johnson et al., 1998). Utilizing cell separation techniques it was found that thrombin stimulated the release of interleukins IL-6 and IL-8 that are proinflammatory cytokines from CD14+ monocytes. A similar cytokine response was elicited from cultured blood vessel endothelial cells. The endothelial cell IL-6 and IL-8 response to thrombin could also be produced by the thrombin receptor agonist peptide (TRAP) thus implicating this receptor in proinflammatory vascular response (increased permeability) to coagulation activation (Johnson et al., 1998).

In patients with severe sepsis, tissue factor Ag, prothrombin fragments F1 and 2, fibrinopeptide A and D dimer are significantly increased as compared to control patients. Antithrombin III complex was also lower in septic patients as compared to control patients (Gando et al., 1998a). Thus there is clear evidence that the extrinsic coagulation pathway is activated in severe sepsis which generates excessive activated thrombin and fibrin formation (Gando et al., 1998b). Multiple organ failure (multiple organ dysfunction syndrome) is a common component of DIC in septic shock patients. The inducing agent for this syndrome is frequently the lipopolysaccharide component (LPS) of the bacterial wall of the invading organism. Recently, the P-selectin of the platelet has been shown to be the receptor for the bacterial LPS (Malhotra et al., 1998). The binding of LPS to P-selectin is dramatically increased in platelets pretreated with thrombin (Malhotra et al., 1998). Accumulation of platelets and neutrophils in the target organs of DIC patients can thus generate thrombin (extrinsic pathway) and activate a local proinflammatory vascular response (Malhotra et al., 1998). Recent molecular studies have demonstrated down-regulation of LPS-induced monocyte tissue factor (TF) expression by the nuclear hormone all-transretinoic acid (ATRA). This inhibition is selective in that LPS induction of TNF-alpha and interleukin-8 (IL-8) are not affected. This inhibition of TF expression occurs at the level of transcription and does not involve repression of AP-1 or NF-Kappa mediated transcription (Oeth et al., 1998).

Tissue factor expression in lipopolysaccharide stimulated endothelial cells reaches a maximum in 6 hours. TF is also secreted by small vesicles on endothelial cells and reaches maximum expression 12 hours after LPS stimulation. Immunoelectron microscopy revealed that small vesicles produced by endothelial cells express TF. Tissue factor functional activity may be correlated to Factor X activation mediated by VIIa and TF. The time course of factor X activation closely matched the twelve hour peak period of small vesicle TF expression and suggests that this may be the source of TF that triggers DIC under specific clinical circumstances (Kagawa et al., 1998).

The role of the endothelial cell membrane and its high affinity thrombin receptor thrombomedulin (TM) is pivotal in those pathologic processes affecting blood vessels that initiate DIC (angiitides, vasculitis, sepsis, microangiophilic hemolytic anemia, and viremia) (Boffa & Karmochkine, 1998). TM is expressed on keratinocytes, osteoblasts and macrophages the latter cell being a link to thrombin generation and cytokine expression. Activated macrophages and cytokines enzymatically cleave TM to a soluble fragment (pTM) that is a molecular marker for widespread endothelial cell damage. It is frequently elevated in DIC, CNS blood vessel infections (plasmodium malaria) and hypertensive complications of pregnancy (Boffa & Karmochkine, 1998).

Recent research on structural and functional aspects of endothelial cells has elucidated the location and signaling mechanisms of thrombin-thrombomodulin interaction. Thrombomodulin is located on the apical endothelial cell surface and the caveolae in close approximation to tissue factor, tissue factor pathway inhibitor (TFPI), thrombin receptor and urokinase receptor which suggests that this structure (caveolae)is important for regulation of coagulation and the fibrinolytic system on the endothelial cell surface (Maruyama, 1998).

Thrombin cleaves the N-terminus of its receptor that exposes a new N-terminus which is a ligand that activates platelets, endothelial cells and vascular smooth muscle cells. Thrombin receptor activation initiates a protein C kinase, tyrosine kinase and MAP kinase cascade that activates NF-Kappa B with consequent proliferation of endothelial cells (Maruyama, 1998).

Recent studies in patients with DIC, thrombotic thrombocytopenic purpura (TTP) and hemolytic uremic syndrome (HUS) have demonstrated high soluble Fas levels. Fas is a member of the tumour necrosis receptor super family that contains a 36kD surface protein with one single transmembrane region that induces apoptosis by Fas-Fas binding. Soluble Fas loses the transmembrane domain. Plasma Fas and sFas ligand in active TTP/HUS and DIC patients were noted to be higher than in non-DIC patients without organ failure. Plasma TM (thrombomodulin levels) were also significantly elevated in these patients. These results suggest that sFas–sFas ligand induced apoptosis of endothelial cells may be a common pathological pathway for vascular endothelial cell injury in TTP/HUS and DIC (Hori et al., 1999).

Neurological complications of DIC

Many patients with DIC are suffering multiorgan system failure and present in coma with a non-focal exam.

The neurological complications of DIC are: (i) large-vessel occlusion; (ii) coma; (iii) lethargy, obtundation and stupor; (iv) small vessel stroke and concomitant SAH; (v) embolic infarction from nonbacterial thrombotic vegetations; (vi) subarachnoid hemorrhage (SAH); (vii) multiple anterior and posterior circulation hemorrhages and infarction (Schwartzman & Hill, 1982).

Embolic stroke in the prescence of a malignancy, particularly an adenocarcinoma is most suggestive of nonbacterial thrombotic embolus (NBTE) or marantic endocarditis (Kearsley & Tattersall, 1982; Ojeda et al., 1985; Rosen & Armstrong, 1973). Most strokes occur in large vessels and are in the middle cerebral artery territory although they have been described in the spinal cord (Ojeda et al., 1985). The most common malignancies associated with marantic endocarditis are adenocarcinomas of the lung, stomach and pancreas (Bryan, 1969). Marantic emboli may also be seen with other solid tumours as well as with leukemia and lymphoma. Marantic endocarditis may also occur with diabetic ketoacidosis, tuberculosis, chronic liver disease, SLE, and the antiphospholipid syndrome (Maulight et al., 1972; Timperley et al., 1974; Verstraete et al., 1974; Fulham et al., 1994).

The verrucous valve lesions of marantic endocarditis consist of a coagulated fibrin and platelet mass usually on the aortic and mitral valves. These lesions embolize frequently (10–30% of cases to the kidneys, spleen and heart as well as the CNS). The heart lesions are often silent but may be a cause of death in these patients (Chomette et al., 1980). McKay and Rodriquez were the first to suggest that the association of pancreatic carcinoma, venous thrombosis and NBTE was secondary to DIC (Schwartzman & Hill, 1982). The vegetations of marantic endocarditis are unassociated with cardiac murmurs and are often only found at autopsy (Schwartzman & Hill, 1982).

A recent survey of the occurrence of acute onset stroke in critically ill patients admitted to the medical intensive care unit identified DIC as a major cause and it is noted as a complication of a terminally ill patient (Wijdicks & Scott, 1998).

Differential diagnosis

Acute generalized widespread bleeding is most often related to DIC but must be differentiated from primary hyperfibrinolysis, thrombotic thrombocytopenic purpura, hemalytic uremic syndrome and SLE with or without the catastrophic antiphospholipid syndrome (Rocha et al., 1998; Asherson, 1992, 1998). TTP may be seen in the setting of SLE which presents special problems in diagnosis as they have similar clinical presentations that include thrombotic microangiopathy (Musio et al., 1998).

The vascular occlusions in SLE are often multiple and recurrent and may involve any vessel or organ system. The kidneys, central and peripheral nervous system are most frequently involved. Multiple small cortical pial artery infarction, seizures, psychosis, proximal myopathy, transverse myelitis, mononeuritis multiplex and sensorimotor neuropathy are the most common nervous system presentations (Johnson & Richardson, 1968). Patients that present with recurrent abortion, venous and arterial occlusions and elevated titres of a PL (lupus anticoagulant and anticardiolipin antibodies) have the antiphospholipid syndrome (APS). This is usually a single event that responds to anticoagulation therapy (Asherson et al., 1992). The compensated form of DIC that manifests as a diffuse thrombosis with mild bleeding is most often seen with SLE (Schwartzman & Hill, 1982).

In contradistinction to patients with simple antiphospholipid syndrome (APS) in which large vessel venous or arterial occlusions are seen, the catastrophic antiphospholipid syndrome (CAPS) involves major organ systems. The mortality of the syndrome is 50% with most patients dying of concomitant cardiac and pulmonary failure (Asherson, 1998). Approximately 30% of these patients suffer DIC which compounds the multiorgan thrombotic microangiopathy. The systemic inflammatory response syndrome (SIRS) is often associated with CAPS and may cause adult respiratory distress syndrome (ARDS) (Asherson, 1998).

Primary fibrinolytic states often present during surgery as a fulminant hemorrhagic syndrome from excessive fibrinolytic activity (Perouansky et al., 1999). Patients ooze from all wounds and the fibrinolysis is so rapid that whole blood appears incoaguable. The patient's plasma is clotted by thrombin but then redissolves in minutes. Platelets may be normal in the face of a prolonged thrombin, prothrombin time and partial thromboplastin time, depletion of clotting factors and elevated fibrinogen related antigens.

The episode may reflect an episode of diffuse DIC in which fibrinolysis rather than thrombosis predominates (Perouansky et al., 1999; Cehaan & Van Oeveren, 1998).

The primary fibrinolytic state from the use of urokinase and tissue plasminogen activators will increase as more centres start using both agents for treatment of stroke (Jichici & Frank, 1997; Brandt et al., 1996). In primary fibrinolytic states, plasmin formation overwhelms serum tissue plasma inhibitor activity (TPI activity), there is a decrease of clotting factors and fibrinogen without a fall of platelets. Hemorrhagic complications are common (Albers et al., 1998).

The TTP-HUS is a syndrome characterized by microangiopathic hemolytic anemia, severe thrombocytopenia with purpura fever, renal failure, neurological involvement and a fluctuating course (George et al., 1998). TTP most frequently presents neurologically with hallucinations, mental status fluctuations, delerium, seizures, and focal deficits (Silverstein, 1968). Hemolytic uremic syndrome primarily is organ specific to the kidney but clinical symptoms may overlap with TTP. HUS may be triggered by a verotoxin-producing serotype of *Escherichia coli* (poorly cooked meat) or *Shigella* infection in children while in adults it may occur after chemotherapy, mitomycin or cyclosporin administration.

SLE, TTP, HUS and DIC all damage the endothelial cell which activates both coagulation pathways and the fibrinolytic pathway as noted above. Thrombomodulin, vonWillebrand antigen and multimers are all elevated in TTP, aPL and active SLE suggesting widespread endothelial cell damage (Maruyama, 1998; Hori et al., 1999; Asherson, 1998; Musio et al., 1998).

Laboratory diagnosis of DIC

A peripheral blood smear in patients with DIC reveals shistocytes and fragmented RBCs in 50% of patients that are formed by fibrin RBC interactions. Most patients demonstrate large immature platelets, thrombocytopenia (less than 80000 per mm^3), reticulocytosis and a shift to immature leukocytes (Bick, 1992).

The prothrombin and activated partial thromboplastin time (aPTT) are prolonged in 80% of patients with DIC. In 20% of patients, the PT and a PTT may be normal or fast due to circulating activated clotting factors (thrombin and activated X) or clottable early degradation products from fibrinolysis (Bick, 1992).

Platelet count and function is abnormal in the overwhelming majority of DIC patients. It varies from 2000 per mm^3 to greater than 100000 per mm^3 (Schwartzman & Hill, 1982). Most patients bleed when their platelet count nears 20000 per mm^3. Functional abnormalities of platelets are caused by FDP coating and their release of procoagulant substances. Measures of platelet reactivity such as β-thromboglobulin and platelet factor 4 are frequently elevated in DIC although both markers may be elevated in other thrombotic microangiopathic diseases (Bick, 1992).

Massive levels of thrombin are seen in the systemic circulation of DIC patients. The conversion of prothrombin to thrombin generates intermediate prethrombin 2 and inactive prothrombin fragments (F1 and 2). Thrombin cleaves fibrinogen to fibrin or is inactivated by antithrombin III (AT III) which forms an inactive enzyme inhibitor complex: thrombin-antithrombin III (TAT). The AT-III determination is an excellent test to detect excessive thrombin generation. Fibrinopeptide A levels in the circulation is diagnostic of thrombin's enzymatic conversion of fibrinogen to fibrin but is a non-specific marker for thrombosis (Bick, 1992). Thrombin cleaves fibrinopeptide B and the amino acid sequence 1–14 from the B-chain of fibrinogen. These B-peptides 1–42, 1–118, and 15–42 derived from the B-chain of fibrinogen are further degraded by plasmin and can be measured by radioimmunoassay (Fareed et al., 1983). These assays aid in the diagnosis of DIC versus primary fibrinolysis. In primary fibrinolysis concentrations of B-peptide 15–42 and related peptides are elevated but fibrinopeptide A is normal. In DIC both fibrinopeptide A and B and peptide 15–42 concentrations are elevated (Bick, 1992).

Fibrinolytic-system activation is monitored by measurement of plasminogen and plasmin serum concentrations (Bick, 0000). Once generated, circulating plasmin is regulated by complexing with α_2 antiplasmin or α_2 macroglobulin (Bick, 1992). There are several reliable techniques to measure the concentration of α_2 antiplasmin or α_2 plasmin inhibitor (α_2 – PI) that provide direct evidence of plasmin generation and are elevated in DIC (Bick, 1992).

The D-dimer is a neoantigen that is formed when thrombin converts fibrinogen to fibrin which activates factor XIII that cross links the newly generated fibrin. Plasmin cleavage of cross-linked fibrin generates D-dimer and monoclonal antibodies against DD-3B6/22 are specific for cross-linked fibrinogen degradation products (FDPs) (Bick, 1992). This test differentiates the specific D-dimer formed from thrombin generation from other FDP X, Y, D or E fragments that may be generated from the massive plasmin activation of the fibrinocytic system.

Recent research has concentrated on the measurement of prethrobmotic markers in the assessment of acquired hypercoaguable states (Lopez et al., 1999). An evaluation of hemostatic molecular markers 1–7 days prior to the onset of DIC in leukemic patients revealed increased levels of plasma thrombin antithrombim complex (TAT), plasmin-plasmin inhibitor complex (PPIC), D-dimer and soluble fibrinomonomer (SFM). Plasma soluble fibrin monomers (SFM) levels were significantly increased 5 days prior to DIC, TAT increased three days prior to DIC and D-dimer levels were increased 1 day prior to DIC onset (Lopez et al., 1999). Plasma thrombomodulin levels were significantly increased while antithrombin and protein C activities were markedly decreased in those patients that died during DIC (Wada et al., 1988). A study evaluating changes in plasma tissue factor pathway inhibitor levels during the clinical course of DIC revealed that plasma tissue factor levels as well as plasma total tissue factor inhibitor (TFPI) and lipoprotein-associated factor tissue inhibitors (LP-TFPI) were significantly higher in DIC patients than in pre-DIC or non DIC patients. During the course of the illness, plasma levels of tissue factor (TF) increased to their highest levels one day prior to the onset of DIC and then gradually declined while those of the tissue factor inhibitors gradually increased (Yamamuro et al., 1998). Increased levels of truncated TFPI (proteolysis of the intact protein) have also been noted in active DIC patients as DIC progresses (Shimura et al., 1999). Measurement of the platelet count, D-dimer TPFIs and AT-III are being used more widely for the diagnosis and monitoring of patients with DIC (Shimura et al., 1999).

Treatment

The cornerstone for the treatment of DIC is the optimal management of the underlying disorder (De Jonge et al., 1998). Plasma and platelet transfusion may be utilized for those patients who are bleeding or at risk for hemorrhage and who demonstrate low levels of coagulation factors and platelets (Ozier, 1998). Heparin and low molecular weight heparin are frequently used in active DIC but this practice is controversial (De Jonge et al., 1998). There is some evidence to support the use of low molecular heparin rather than unfractionated heparin because of a lower risk of bleeding. Antithrombin III (AT III) may be effective at higher doses (supranormal plasma levels of 100% or greater) (Cohendy et al., 1998; Balk et al., 1998; Fourrier, 1998). Present studies on the use of prtein C concentrate, thrombomodulin and tissue factor inhibitors are under way (Fourrier et al., 1998). DIC remains a difficult problem to treat with high morbidity and mortality particularly if neurological complications are present (Schwartzman & Hill, 1982).

References

Albers, W., Easton, D.J., Sacco, R. et al. (1998). Antithrombotic and thrombolytic therapy for ischemic stroke. *Chest*, (Suppl. 114), 683S–97S.

Anderson, R.A. (1998). The catastrophic antiphospholipid syndrome. A review of the clinical features, possible pathogenesis and treatment. *Lupus*, (Suppl. 7), **2**, S55–62.

Arai, A., Naruse, M., Naruse, K. et al. (1998). Cardiac malignant pheochromocytoma with bone metastases. *Internal Medicine*, **37**(11), 940–4.

Asherson, R.A. (1992). The catastrophic antiphospholipid syndrome. *Journal of Rheumatology*, **19**, 508–12.

Asherson, R.A. (1998). The catastrophic antiphospholipid syndrome. A review of the clinical features, possible pathogenesis and treatment. *Lupus*, (Suppl. 7) **2**, S55–62.

Asherson, R.A., Cervera, R. & Font, J. (1992). Multiorgan thrombotic disorders in systemic lupus erythematosus: a common link? *Lupus*, **1**, 199–203.

Baker, W.F. (1989). Clinical aspects of disseminated intravascular coagulation: a clinician's point of view. *Seminars in Thrombosis and Hemostasis*, **15**, 1.

Balk, R., Emerson, T., Fourrier, F. et al. (1998). Therapeutic use of antithrombin concentrate in sepsis. *Seminars in Thrombosis and Hemostasis*, **24**, 183–94.

Bick, R.L. (1988). Disseminated intravascular coagulation and related syndromes. *Seminars in Thrombosis and Hemostasis*, **14**, 299.

Bick, R.L. (1991). Alterations of hemostasis associated with surgery, cardiopulmonary bypass surgery and prosthetic devices. In *Disorders of Hemostasis*, ed. O.D. Ratnoff & C. Forbes, p. 382. Philadelphia: WB Saunders.

Bick, R.L. (1992). Disseminated intravascular coagulation. In *Disorder of Thrombosis and Hemostasis: Clinical and Laboratory Practice*, ed. R.L. Bick, p. 137. Chicago: ASCP Press.

Bick, R.L. & Baker, W.F. (1992). Disseminated intravascular coagulation. *Hematological Pathology*, **6**, 1.

Boffa, M.C. & Karmochkine, M. (1998). Thrombomodulin: an overview and potential implications in vascular disorders. *Lupus*, **7**(Suppl. 2), S120–5.

Brandt, T., Kummer, R., Muller-Kupers, M. et al. (1996). Thrombolytic therapy of acute basilar artery occlusion. Variables affecting recanalization and outcome. *Stroke*, **27**, 875–80.

Breakwell, L.M., Getty, C.J. & Austin, C. (1999). Disseminated intravascular coagulation in elective primary total hip replacement. *Journal of Anthroplasty*, **14**(2), 239–42.

Bryan, C.S. (1969). Non-bacterial thrombotic endocarditis with malignant tumors. *American Journal of Medicine*, **46**, 787.

Caroll, V.A. & Binder, B.R. (1999). The role of the plasminogen activation system in cancer. *Seminars in Thrombosis and Hemostasis*, **25**(2), 183–97.

Cehaan, J. & Van Oeveren, W. (1998). Platelets and soluble fibrin promote plasminogen activation causing down regulation of platelet glycoprotein 1b/IX complexes: protection by a protein. *Thrombosis Research*, **92**, 171–9.

84   R.J. Schwartzman

Chomette, G., Auriol, M., Boubion, D. et al. (1980). Non-bacterial thrombotic endocarditis. Autopsy study, clinico-pathological correlations. *Annales Medecin Interne* (Paris), **131**, 443–7.

Cohendy, R., Lefrant, J.Y. & delaCoussaye, J.E. (1998). The use of antithrombin III CAT IV for disseminated intravascular coagulation (DIC) during septic shock. *Intensive Care Medicine*, **12**, 1344.

DeJonge, E., Levi, M., Stoutenbeek, C.P. et al. (1998). Current drug treatment strategies for disseminated intravascular coagulation. *Drugs*, **55**, 767–77.

Fareed, J., Bick, R.L., Squillaci, G. et al. (1983). Clinical and experimental utilization of a modified radioimmunoassay for B-beta 15–42 related peptides. *Clinical Chemistry*, **29**, 1161.

Felcher, A., Commichou, C., Cao, Q. et al. (1998). Disseminated intravascular coagulation and status epilepticus. *Neurology*, **51**, 629–31.

Fourrier, F. (1998). Therapeutic applications of antithrombin concentrates in systemic inflammatory disorders. *Blood Coagulation and Thrombolysis*, (Suppl. 2), S39–S45.

Fourrier, F., Jourdain, M. & Tournoys, A. (1998). Effect of a combined antithrombin III and protein C supplementation in porcine acute endotoxic shock. *Shock*, **10**, 364–70.

Francis, J.L. & Biggerstaff, J. et al. (1998). Hemostasis and malignancy. *Seminars in Thrombosis and Hemostasis*, **24**, 93–109.

Fulham, M.J., Gatenby, P. & Tuck, R.R. (1994). Focal cerebral ischemia and antiphospholipid antibodies: a case for cardiac embolism. *Acta Neurologica Scandinavica*, **90**, 417–23.

Gando, S., Nanzaki, S., Sasaki, S. et al. (1998a). Significant correlations between tissue factor and thrombin markers in trauma and septic patients with disseminated intravascular coagulation. *Thrombosis and Haemostasis*, **79**(6), 1111–15.

Gando, S., Nanzaki, S., Sasaki, S. et al. (1998b). Activation of the extrinsic coagulation pathway in patients with severe sepsis and septic shock. *Critical Care Medicine*, **26**, 2005–9.

Gando, S., Nanzaki, S. & Kemmotsu, O. (1999). Disseminated intravascular coagulation and sustained systemic inflammatory response syndrome predict organ dysfunctions after trauma: application of clinical decision analysis. *Annals of Surgery*, **229**(1), 121–7.

Garcia-Avello, A., Lorente, J.A., Cesar-Perez, J. et al. (1998). Degree of hypercoagulability and hyperfibrinolysis is related to organ failure and prognosis after burn trauma. *Thrombosis Research*, **89**(2), 59–64.

George, J.N., Gilcher, R.O., Smith, J.W. et al. (1998). Thrombotic thrombocytopenic purpura hemolytic uremic syndrome: diagnosis and management. *Journal of Clinical Apheresis*, **13**, 120–5.

Hjorth-Hansen, H., Seidel, C., Lamvid, J. et al. (1999). Elevated serum concentrations of hepatocyte growth factor in acute myelocytic leukemia. *European Journal of Haematology*, **62**, 129–34.

Hori, Y., Wada, H., Mori, Y. et al. (1999). Plasma sFas and rFas ligand levels in patients with thrombotic thrombocytopenic purpura and in those with disseminated intravascular coagulation. *American Journal of Hematology*, **61**, 21–5.

Inceman, S. & Tangun, Y. (1969). Chronic defibrination syndrome due to a giant hemangioma associated with microangiopathic hemolytic anemia. *American Journal of Medicine*, **46**, 997.

Jichici, D.F. & Frank, J.I. (1997). Thrombolytic therapy in neurointensive care. *Critical Care Clinics*, **13**, 201–27.

Johnson, R.T. & Richardson, E.P. (1968). The neurological manifestations of systemic lupus erythematosus. *Medicine*, **47**, 337–69.

Johnson, K., Choi, Y., DeGroot, E. et al. (1998). Potential mechanisms for a proinflammatory vascular cytokine response to coagulation activation. *Journal of Immunology*, **160**, 5130–5.

Kagawa, H., Komiyama, Y., Nakamura, S. et al. (1998). Expression of functional tissue factor on small vesicles of lipopolysaccharide-stimulated human endothelial cells. *Thrombosis Research*, **91**, 297–304.

Katsaros, D. & Grundfest-Broniatowski, S. (1998). Successful management of visceral Klippel–Trenaunay–Weber syndrome with the antifibrinolytic agent tranexamic acid (cyclocapron: a case report). *Annals of Surgery*, **64**(4), 302–4.

Kearsley, J.H. & Tattersall, M.H. (1982). Cerebral embolism in cancer patients. *Quarterly Journal of Medicine*, **81**, 279–91.

Kravans, J.R., Jackson, D.P., Conley, C.L. et al. (1957). The nature of the hemorrhagic disorder accompanying hemolytic transfusion reactions in man. *Blood*, **12**, 834–43.

Lopez, Y., Paloma, M.J., Rifon, et al. (1999). Measurement of prethrombotic markers in the assessment of acquired hypercoagulable states. *Thrombosis Research*, **93**, 71–8.

McKay, D.G. & Margaretten, W. (1967). Disseminated intravascular coagulation in virus diseases. *Archives of Internal Medicine*, **120**, 129.

Malhotra, R., Priest, R., Foster, M.R. et al. (1998). P-selectin binds to bacterial lipopolysaccharide. *European Journal of Immunology*, **28**, 983–8.

Maruyama, I. (1998). Biology of endothelium. *Lupus*, (Suppl. 2), S541–3.

Maulight, G.M., Binder, P.A. & Crosby, W.A. (1972). Disseminated intravascular coagulation in miliary tuberculosis. *Archives of Internal Medicine*, **30**, 388–9.

Meijer, K., Smid, W.M., Geerards, S. et al. (1998). Hyperfibrinogenolysis in desseminated adenocarcinoma. *Blood Coagulation Fibrinolysis*, **3**, 279–83.

Muller-Berghous, G. (1989). Pathophysiologic and biochemical events in disseminated intracoagulation: dysregulation of procoagulant and anticoagulant pathways. *Seminars in Thrombosis and Hemastasis*, **15**, 58.

Musio, F., Bohen, E.M., Yuan, C.M. et al. (1998). Review of thrombotic thrombocytopenic purpura in the setting of systemic lupus erythematosus. *Seminars in Arthritis and Rheumatism*, **28**, 1–19.

Niewiarowski, S., Regoeczi, E. & Stewart, G.J. (1972). Platelet interaction with polymerizing fibrin. *Journal of Clinical Investigations*, **51**, 685–99.

Oeth, P., Yao, J., Fan, S.T. et al. (1998). Retinoic acid selectively inhibits lipopolysaccharide induction of tissue factor gene expression in human monocytes. *Blood*, **91**, 2857–65.

Ojeda, V.J., Frost, F. & Mastaglia, F.L. (1985). Non-bacterial thrombotic endocarditis. *Medical Journal of Australia*, **142**, 629–31.

Ozier, Y. (1998). The paradox of disseminated intravascular coagulation. *Annales Francaises Anesthesie et de Reanimation*, (Suppl. 17), S18–S22.

Perouansky, M., Oppenheim, A., Sprung, C.L. et al. (1999). Effect of haemofiltration on pathological fibrinolysis due to severe sepsis in case report. *Resuscitation*, **40**, 53–6.

Persoons, M.C., Stals, F.S., van dam Mieras, M.C. et al. (1998). Multiple organ involvement during experimental cytomegalovirus infection is associated with disseminated vascular pathology. *Journal of Pathology*, **184**(1), 103–9.

Rocha, E., Paramo, J.A., Montes, R. et al. (1998). Acute generalized, wide spread bleeding. Diagnosis and management. *Haematologica*, **83**(11), 1024–37.

Rosen, P. & Armstrong, D. (1973). Non-bacterial thrombotic endocarditis in patients with malignant neoplastic disease. *American Journal of Medicine*, **54**, 23.

Schwartzman, R.J. & Hill, J.B. (1982). Neurologic complications of disseminated intravascular coagulation. *Neurology*, **32**, 791–7.

Shimura, M., Wada, H., Nakasaki, T. et al. (1999). Increased truncated form of plasma tissue factor pathway inhibitor levels in patients with disseminated intravascular coagulation. *American Journal of Hematology*, **60**(2), 94–8

Shoj, N., Nakada, T., Sugano, O. et al. (1998). Acute onset of coagulopathy in a patient with Kasabach–Merritt Syndrome following transurethral resection of bladder tumor. *Urology International*, **61**(2), 115–18.

Silverstein, A. (1968). Thrombotic thrombocytopenic purpura: the initial neurologic manifestations. *Archives of Neurology*, **18**, 358–62.

Sterchele, D.F. (1969). Consumptive coagulopathy in obstetrics and gynecology. Thrombosis it diathesis. *Hemorrhagica*, (Suppl.) **36**, 177.

Timperley, W.R., Preston, F.E. & Ward, J.D. (1974). Cerebral intravascular coagulation in diabetic ketoacidosis. *Lancet*, **1**, 952–6.

Verstraete, M., Vermylen, J. & Collen, D. (1974). Intravascular coagulation in liver disease. *Annual Review of Medicine*, **25**, 447–55.

Wada, H., Sakuragawa, N. & Shibu, H. (1998). Hemostatic molecular markers before onset of disseminated intravascular coagulation in leukemia patients. *Seminars in Thrombosis and Hemostasis*, **24**, 293–7.

Weiss, D.J. & Rashid, J. (1998). The sepsis coagulant axis: a review. *Journal of Veterinary Internal Medicine*, **12**, 317–24.

Weltermann, A., Mitterbaur, G.J., Mitterbaur, M. et al. (1998). Disseminated intravascular coagulation (DIC) with massive hyperfibrinolysis in metastatic uterine cancer. Observations on the effects on the coagulopathy of various treatments. *Wiener Klinische Wochenschrift*, **11**, 53–7.

Wijdicks, E.F. & Scott, J.P. (1998). Stroke in the medical intensive-care unit. *Mayo Clinic Proceedings*, **73**(7), 642–6.

Wurthner, J.V., Kohler, G., Behringer, D. et al. (1999). Leukostasis followed by hemorrhage complicating the initiation of chemotherapy in patients with acute myeloid leukemia and hyperleukocytosis: a clinicopathologic report of four cases. *Cancer*, **85**, 368–74.

Yamamuro, M., Wada, H., Kumeda, K. et al. (1998). Changes in plasma tissue factor pathway inhibitor levels during the clinical course of disseminated intravascular coagulation. *Blood Coagulation and Fibrinolysis*, **9**, 491–7.

11

Disorders of coagulation

Bruce M. Coull[1] and Peter T. Skaff[2]

[1]Department of Neurology, Arizona Health Sciences Center and
[2]Department of Neurology, University of Arizona College of Medicine, Tucson, AZ, USA

Introduction

Despite a careful and thorough evaluation for the underlying cause, stroke etiology remains cryptogenic in about one-third of cases in elderly adults, with even a higher proportion of unexplained causes of stroke in young individuals. It is likely that a significant number of unexplained strokes result from hemostatic abnormalities but, excluding antiphospholipid antibody related causes, currently definable intrinsic abnormalities in hemostasis probably account for less than 10% of ischemic strokes. One important exception, where hemostatic abnormalities play an important role, is cerebral vein or sinus occlusion. In the pathogenesis of most ischemic strokes, the pathological thrombus forms when normal coagulation pathways are activated in a focal region of the vasculature such as in complicated atheromatous plaque, or after mechanical, immunological or other related injury to the vascular endothelium or within a damaged cardiac chamber. In these instances, the coagulation system is responding 'normally' in a pathological environment. On the other hand, it has been estimated that up to 30% of individuals with Stroke or TIA harbour a platelet disorder or coagulation abnormality that predisposes to thrombosis (Bick & Kaplan, 1998). With completion of the human genome project, many new mutations within the coagulation system that are associated with an increased risk of stroke are likely to be identified.

Most individuals with stroke do not require an extensive evaluation for an obscure clotting disorder. However, although accounting for a small percentage of causes of strokes overall, in some specific clinical instances, a careful evaluation should be conducted to identify abnormalities of hemostasis. A predisposition to thrombotic events is termed a prethrombotic state. Recent advances in molecular genetics have greatly increased the recognition of potential causes of the prethrombotic state.

Abnormalities in coagulation that increase risk of CNS hemorrhage

Alterations in hemostasis that cause intracerebral hemorrhage (ICH) are most often the result of excessive anticoagulation with warfarin. They may result as an untoward complication of thrombolytic therapy or less often as a complication of therapies that utilize antiaggregate drugs. Iatrogenic causes, along with other abnormalities in clotting, account for fewer than 10% of all cases of ICH. Intracerebral hemorrhage sometimes occurs as a result of severe deficiencies in coagulation factors VIII, IX and with certain mutations in factor XIII. Other very uncommon causes include severe thrombocytopenia and certain other impairments of platelet and coagulation function. CNS bleeds are an uncommon complication of hereditary disorders of hemostasis such as von Willebrand's disease (1 to 2% prevalence), afibrinogenemia, and Glanzmann's thrombasthenia, characterized by dysfunction of the platelet GPIIb/IIa receptor, but ICH has been reported in infants and children with these disorders. Several gene polymorphisms are associated with an increased frequency of ICH including polymorphisms in factor XIII, α1-antichymotrypsin, and apolipoprotein E (α2 and α4) although the apo E alleles affect amyloid angiography and not clotting (Vila et al., 2000; Catto et al., 1998; O'Donnell et al., 2000). Mucocutaneous bleeds are much more common than CNS hemorrhage in most of the inherited bleeding disorders, whereas intracranial bleeds rarely occur spontaneously, but more often happen as a consequence of minor head trauma or by the concurrent use of medicines that affect coagulation.

Systemic diseases including hepatic and renal failure, leukemia, bone marrow failure, certain immune diseases and cancer chemotherapy are all associated with CNS bleeding complications. With the increasing use of drugs that affect hemostasis, the prevalence of ICH as a complication of such therapy is likely to increase. The major acquired abnormality of hemostasis associated with ICH is due to excessive anticoagulation with warfarin. The risk of intracranial hemorrhage is increased by the regular use of aspirin for either primary or secondary prevention of stroke (RR 1.35) (Hart et al., 2000). When aspirin is combined with warfarin for stroke prophylaxis the risk of intracranial hemorrhage more than doubles (RR 2.4; 95% CI = 1.2–4.8) (Hart et al., 1999).

When platelet count falls below $10\,000/mm^3$, the risk of CNS bleeds increases, but ICH can happen with higher platelet counts if platelet function is impaired because of hepatic or renal failure, with the concurrent use of platelet active drugs or in the presence of antibodies that bind to the platelet membrane such as may occur with idiopathic thrombocytopenic purpura (ITP). In certain prothrombotic states such as disseminated intravascular coagulation (DIC) and thrombotic thrombocytopenic purpura (TTP), discussed in detail elsewhere in this text, thrombocytopenia may be induced in the presence of ongoing intravascular thrombosis. Although DIC and TTP more often produce ischemic events, parenchymal hemorrhage also occurs. A particularly malignant condition in pregnancy in which brain bleeds occur is the HELLP syndrome characterized by hemolysis, elevated liver enzymes and low platelets due to DIC (Isler et al., 1999). With TTP, ischemic lesions combined with intracerebral hematomas in the same individual are described (Guzzini et al., 1998). In contradistinction to platelet consumption syndromes, very high platelet counts that occur with essential thrombocythemia are sometimes associated with a predilection for bleeding rather than thrombosis.

Every patient who presents with intracranial hemorrhage should receive a careful evaluation of the clotting system. Screening tests include a CBC with differential and platelet count, a prothrombin time and activated partial thromboplastin time (aPTT). A bleeding time, factor VIII clotting activity and plasma fibrinogen level may help to identify any bleeding diathesis. If the screening coagulation panel is abnormal, more sophisticated tests to identify a specific abnormality are often needed. A detailed discussion of these is beyond the scope of this chapter. Treatment for patients with a bleeding disorder can be complex but simple measures often include plasma exchange, administration of vitamin K and the use of cryoprecipitate and platelet transfusions. Recombinant factor VIIa administra-

tion could represent an emerging new treatment for acute hemorrhage (Hedner, 1998).

Abnormalities of coagulation that increase the risk of thrombosis

A concept that remains important today but dates back over a hundred years to insights of Virchow is the pivotal role played by chronic inflammation in atherothrombosis. An understanding of the role of inflammation in thrombotic disease such as stroke remains an important focus of investigation that could lead to better diagnosis and preventive treatments of stroke. A large number of population studies from throughout the world, including case control, cross-sectional and prospective epidemiological studies, provide strong evidence of the link between chronic inflammation and risk factors for stroke and cardiovascular disease such as hypertension, diabetes mellitus, tobacco smoking, elevated lipids and atrial fibrillation (Lee et al., 1993; Mendall et al., 1996; Tracy, 1999; Feinberg et al., 1999). This relationship is mediated largely by atherosclerosis and by the occurrence of complicated thrombotic events. In patients with cerebrovascular disease, various hematological markers of inflammation including elevations in C reactive protein (CRP), and plasma fibrinogen are associated with increased activation of coagulation as evidenced by increases in prothrombin fragment F1.2, thrombin–antithrombin, D-dimer and the platelet protein beta-thromboglobulin (Feinberg et al., 1996; Ridker, 1998; Ellis et al., 2000). Other studies indicate acute phase protein activation including fibrinogen and CRP is present in both an acute stroke and in subjects with risk factors for stroke lending credence to the notion that an inflammatory response promotes longstanding vascular damage and may have a role in 'triggering' the thrombotic event (Beamer et al., 1998; Gussekloo et al., 2000; Canova et al., 1999). It is possible that the relationship between inflammation and atherogenesis may, in part, be explained by the presence of infectious organisms such as chlamydiae pneumonae within atheromatous plaques (Grau, 1997; Ridker, 1998). While the measurement of markers of inflammation and coagulation activation has provided important insights into the pathobiology of cerebrovascular disease, the clinical utility of obtaining such measurements in the individual patient for purposes of diagnosis or treatment remains unproven (Matsuo et al., 2000).

Fibrinogen

Elevated plasma levels of fibrinogen are associated with an increased risk for venous thromboses and arterial vascular occlusive events including myocardial infarction and stroke. Although the association with cerebrovascular disease is observed in many of the large epidemiological studies, the utility of measuring fibrinogen levels in a given subject remains undefined. Almost 300 mutations in the genes that code for fibrinogen proteins have been described. Roughly half of these have not been associated with any clinical abnormality, whereas 25% of mutations have a hemorrhagic tendency and 20% predispose to thrombotic events (Martinez, 1997). Larger clinical studies are needed to determine if testing for specific mutations in the fibrinogen genes will prove to be of clinical utility.

When fibrinogen levels fall below 50 mg/dl the risk of bleeding, including ICH, is increased. An example is congenital hypofibrinogenemia, which has been associated with cases of ICH (Goodwin, 1989; Haverkate & Samama, 1995). However, since the von Willebrand factor can also bind to the fibrinogen receptor on platelets, the bleeding tendency with severe decreases in plasma fibrinogen levels is blunted. Afibrinogenemia is an autosomal recessive disorder with an estimated incidence of 2 per million live births (Al-Mondhiry & Ehmann, 1994). Spontaneous and recurrent episodes of ICH are reported with afibrinogenemia (Menart et al., 1998; Henselmans et al., 1999). Henselmans and colleagues (1999) recently called attention to the difficulty of standard imaging techniques with CT and MRI to identify the intracerebral hematoma in such cases since clot formation is incomplete without fibrin.

Antithrombin, heparin cofactor II, protein C and protein S

Thrombus formation results from a complex but exquisite interaction of molecules that induces platelet adhesion and aggregation in concert with thrombin activation and fibrin formation by convergence of the prothrombinase complex. In order to confine thrombosis to a local region of vascular injury, this process is carefully regulated by the intricate and complex interactions of antithrombin, heparin cofactor II (HCII), protein C and protein S. These hemostatic regulatory proteins serve to confine and focus the thrombotic process. In the presence of heparin, antithrombin inhibits thrombin and factor Xa, whereas HCII only inhibits thrombin activity. Protein C, when complexed with protein S, inactivates factor Va and VIII:C thereby effectively turning off the prothrombinase complex. Both the genetic and acquired abnormalities in these regulatory proteins are associated with a prethrombotic state. Various mutations in the genes that code for these regulatory proteins may result in a decreased biological function or decreased amount of protein. Disseminated intravascular coagulation (DIC),

nephrotic syndrome, severe liver disease, postoperative state, infection and massive thromboses, are among the clinical events that can produce an acquired deficiency in some or all of these proteins. Oral contraceptive use and other treatments with high doses of estrogen in women lower levels of protein S. Most of the thrombotic events associated with an abnormality in these regulatory proteins are venous rather than arterial. However, some cases of arterial strokes are reported in children and younger adults who have deficiencies in these proteins (Vomberg & Breederveld, 1987). Gaustadnes and colleagues (1999) in a study of 403 Danish subjects with thrombotic events found a cumulative prevalence of deficiency in the regulatory proteins in 2.4% of patients with stroke and 11.1% of individuals with venous thrombosis. The predilection to venous rather than arterial events is currently incompletely understood, but one serious complication resulting from deficiency or dysfunction of the regulatory clotting proteins is saggital sinus and cerebral vein occlusion. Although cerebral venous thrombosis has an estimated annual incidence of one case per 100 000 persons per year, compared with approximately 63 arterial strokes occurring for each case of CVT, subjects should receive a careful evaluation for abnormalities in the hemostatic regulatory proteins (Daif et al., 1995).

A single point mutation in the factor V gene (factor V Leiden) causes resistance to inactivation of factor Va by activated protein C (APC). Although the prevalence in some Caucasian populations may be as high as 15%, the factor V Leiden mutation does not seem to predispose to ischemic stroke in elderly individuals (Ridker et al., 1995; Press et al., 1996). However, especially when associated with other risk factors for thrombotic events, the mutation may contribute to stroke in younger individuals (Catto et al., 1995). Acquired APC resistance may occur when factor VIII:C levels are elevated such as with the use of oral contraceptives.

Fibrinolytic system

Hypoactivity of the fibrinolytic system can predispose to thrombic events including venous and arterial strokes. In general, when fibrinolysis is impaired, venous occlusions predominate over arterial events. An important exception may be chronic atrial fibrillation in which hypofibrinolysis in addition to other components of a prethrombotic state predisposes to systemic embolism (Roldan et al., 1998). Diminished fibrinolytic activity may result from increased amounts of plasminogen activator inhibitor type 1(PAI-1) or from diminished plasminogen levels or decreased amounts of tissue plasminogen activator (t-PA).

Impairments in fibrinolytic activity have been observed in individuals with generalized atherosclerosis and especially in individuals with diabetes mellitus. Catto and colleagues (1997) studied a common single nucleotide insertion/deletion (4G/5G) polymorphism in the PAI-1 gene that is associated with increased circulating levels of PAI-1. They found no difference in genotype frequency between all cases or among subtypes of stroke when compared with controls, but PAI-1 activity was significantly higher in patients with stroke than in controls both at stroke onset and three months after stroke. A recent nested case control study from Sweden (MONICA) found a significantly increased risk for first-ever stroke, especially of hemorrhagic type, among subjects with high plasma levels of the tPA/PAI-1 complex but increased stroke risk was not found with increased PAI-1 levels alone (Johansson et al., 2000).

Polycythemia vera and essential thrombocythemia

Polycythemia vera (PV) and essential thrombocythemia (ET) usually affect individuals older than age 50 and occur with the frequency of 1 to 3 per 100000. Since the prognosis differs, PV must be distinguished from hemoconcentration and secondary erythrocytosis. Both PV and ET are associated with transient ischemic attacks, migraine-like headache, seizures and stroke. Major thrombotic complications such as these may occur in up to 20% of individuals with PV and 10% of affected individuals with ET. In PV, the thrombotic episode often precedes, and leads to establishment of, the diagnosis. In a retrospective cohort study of 1213 patients with PV, thrombotic events occurred at the rate of 3.4/100 pts/yr (Gruppo Italiano Studio Policitemia, 1995). Stroke comprised approximately 10% and TIA 20% of the thrombotic events. Individuals over the age of 70, and those with previous occlusive events or untreated PV are at greatest risk of thromboses. In ET, the platelet count is not predictive of vascular occlusive events and, in fact, hemorrhage is associated with higher rather than lower platelet counts. Although low dose aspirin may increase the risk of bleeding in ET, on balance such therapy reduces the risk of stroke and related thrombotic events (Murphy, 1999).

Sickle cell disease

Stroke including venous, arterial and hemorrhagic is unfortunately a common and potentially devastating consequence of sickle cell disease (SCD). As the result of a point mutation in the α-chain of hemoglobin, approximately 8.5% of American Blacks have sickle trait (HbSA), while SCD (HbSS) occurs in approximately 0.16%. Individuals who are homozygous for the sickle cell gene are at much greater risk than those with other genotypes and have a stroke rate of approximately 0.61 per 100 patient–years. Incidence varies with age and is highest during the first decade of life (Ohene-Frempong et al., 1998; Gill et al., 1995).

Most cerebrovascular events associated with SCD are ischemic, though 22 to 34% are hemorrhagic (Ohene-Frempong et al., 1998; Earley et al., 1998). Clinically evident ischemic stroke occurs in approximately 7% of SCD patients by age 12, while clinically silent strokes demonstrated by magnetic resonance imaging (MRI) occur in 17 to 22% (Earley et al., 1998; Armstrong et al., 1996). SCD may be the most common cause of ischemic stroke in children. Among the mixed ethnicity population of children under 15 years old studied in the Baltimore–Washington Cooperative Young Stroke Study, SCD accounted for 39% of all ischemic strokes (12% of hemorrhagic strokes) and 58% of ischemic strokes among Blacks (Earley et al., 1998). The risk of stroke recurrence in untreated patients is at least 50% (Wang et al., 1991; Pegelow et al., 1995). Chronic transfusion therapy to maintain the HbS concentration below 30% significantly reduces the rate of recurrence, but does not completely eliminate the risk (Pegelow et al., 1995). Bone marrow transplantation offers the possibility of a cure for SCD (Walters et al., 1996, 2000), but frequent neurologic complications in patients with a history of stroke have also been reported (Walters et al., 1995).

Although the mechanism by which vascular disease develops in SCD has not been completely elucidated, it is clear that large vessel intracerebral arteriopathy is present in SCD patients who have had cerebrovascular events (Moran et al., 1998). Intracerebral arterial disease can be reliably demonstrated by various means including arteriography, magnetic resonance arteriography (MRA) and transcranial Doppler (TCD) (Moran et al., 1998; Seibert et al., 1998; Siegel et al., 1995). Moreover, cerebrovascular disease demonstrated by MRA and TCD may be predictive of future stroke (Seibert et al., 1998). A recent primary prevention of stroke trial in patients with demonstrable intracranial stenosis by TCD was terminated prematurely because of a 92% reduction in the risk of stroke among subjects receiving prophylactic transfusion (Adams et al., 1998).

Homocysteinemia

Unlike some prethrombotic states that predispose to venous thromboses, elevated plasma levels of homocysteine, a sulfur-containing amino acid, are associated with both arterial and venous strokes. Arguably, hyperhomocysteinemia may not be a truly prethrombotic state since experimental evidence suggests that elevated plasma homocysteine activates coagulation via endothelial injury. In normal individuals, total plasma homocysteine (tHcy) levels that include a variety of mixed disulfide-bound forms are maintained at less than 15 μmol/ l of which only a small fraction is the injurious free thiol (<1%) (Hankey & Eikelboom, 1999). Although experimental studies indicate that homocysteine injures the vascular endothelium, causing a vasculopathy that predisposes to occlusive events, the exact mechanism by which this happens is currently unknown. Homocystinuria, an inherited metabolic disorder characterized by a 20–fold or more increase in plasma homocysteine, occurs with an estimated incidence of approximately 1 in 332 000 live births (Mudd et al., 1985). Homocystinuria is usually caused by a defect in the cystathionine beta synthase (CBS) gene and subjects, if untreated, have a 50% chance of experiencing a vascular occlusive event by age 30. In a longitudinal follow-up of 629 subjects with homocystinuria reported by Mudd et al. (1985) about one-third of the vascular events were either venous or arterial strokes. Recent evidence suggests that effective treatment of homocystinuria significantly reduces the incidence of vascular events (Yap et al., 2000). Some individuals with homocystinuria have a Marfanoid appearance, lenticular dislocation, seizures and cognitive impairment, but this characteristic phenotype is not invariant and individuals may appear entirely normal.

Case control studies have shown that a modest (two to five times) increase in plasma homocysteine is also a potential significant independent risk factor for stroke (Perry, 1999; Boushey et al., 1995). One large meta-analysis of approximately 4000 cases estimated that an elevated tHcy increased the odds ratio for stroke by about 2.5 (95% CI; 2.0 to 3.0) (Perry, 1999). A recently completed case control study of 1550 subjects, of whom 750 had atherosclerosis, recruited from 19 centres in Europe found a twofold increase risk of atherosclerosis among subjects with the highest tHCY compared to subjects with lower levels of homocysteine (Graham et al., 1997). This relationship was independent of other typical epidemiological risk factors for stroke, but had a multiplicative effect on smoking and hypertension on the risk of atherosclerosis. The association with cerebrovascular disease is strongest for carotid atherosclerosis and related large artery, non-cardioembolic stroke (Eikelboom et al., 2000; Malinow et al., 1993). Some prospective studies provide less convincing data on the relationship between homocysteinemia and risk of stroke (Perry et al., 1995; Verhoef et al., 1994). Factors that accompany elevated tHcy include increasing age, male gender, tobacco smoking, renal impairment and an atherogenic diet that is deficient in folate and vitamin B12. A common genetic polymorphism in the methylene tetrahydrofolate reductase gene (MTHFR)677CαT when homozygous is associated with modest elevation in levels of tHcy in individuals with low dietary folate whereas several mutations in the CBS gene are associated with severe hyperhomocysteinemia (Gaustadnes et al., 2000). Paradoxically, a relationship between the homozygous (MTHFR)677CαT mutation and risk of vascular events including stroke in adults is not established but the co-existence of the (MTHFR)T/T mutation with CBS variants does appear to convey increased risk of thromboses (Gaustadnes et al., 2000). Prospective studies are currently ongoing to determine if dietary supplementation with folic acid and vitamins B12 and B6 to reduce levels of tHcy will likewise have a beneficial effect by decreasing recurrent stroke and related vascular events (Hankey & Eikelboom, 1999).

Platelet abnormalities and stroke

Essential thrombocythemia is a myeloproliferative disorder characterized by isolated clonal-mediated thrombocytosis with peripheral blood platelet counts greater than 600 000/mm^3. The platelets are morphologically and functionally normal. Many individuals with essential thrombocythemia are asymptomatic but cerebrovascular manifestations include TIA and stroke as well as migraine-like headaches. Brain infarction as a result of essential thrombocythemia is infrequent but Casto and colleagues report 6 cases of large artery occlusive stroke in subjects with ET (1994). Individuals older than age 60 and those having already experienced a vascular event or with platelet counts greater than 1.5×10^6 are at increased risk of stroke and related vascular thromboses. Cigarette smoking also increases the risk of stroke in ET. In a prospective study of 114 subjects with ET, Cortelazzo et al. (1995) observed a 14% occurrence of thrombotic events including two ischemic strokes and 5 TIAs. Risk of cerebrovascular events was reduced in the group of patients treated with hydroxyurea. Although not well studied, low dose aspirin therapy may reduce the risk of thrombotic events.

A reportedly common but often overlooked autosomal dominant platelet disorder that is associated with unexplained arterial and venous stroke is the 'sticky platelet syndrome'. First described by Mammen, the SPS is diagnosed by the hyperaggregatable responsiveness of platelets to epinephrine and ADP in ex vivo testing (Mammen, 1999). The molecular basis of the increased platelet responsiveness is unknown. In a small series of patients with arterial occlusions evaluated in a coagulation clinic,

Bick identified the SPS in 26% of patients with stroke and in 33% of subjects with TIA (Bick & Kaplan, 1998; Bick, 1998). It is possible that the SPS is in some way related to genetic variants in platelet glycoprotein receptors reported by Reiner and colleagues (2000) that increase the risk of stroke in young women. Since testing for platelet functional abnormalities is prone to artifactual interference and is technically demanding, testing to identify individuals with the SPS remains problematic.

Genetic polymorphisms and stroke

With the ongoing explosive growth of molecular genetics and near completion of the human genome project, genetic mutations that impart increased and sometimes-decreased risk of stroke are being increasingly identified in a variety of diverse populations. Virtually hundreds of polymorphisms that may affect clotting and platelet-related proteins have been described and this number is likely to increase greatly in the near future as more cohort studies of subjects with risk of stroke are studied (Lane & Grant, 2000). From an epidemiological standpoint, the potential importance of a genetic polymorphism will depend in part upon its prevalence in a given population as well as on the relative risk imparted by the variant allele in either the hetero- or homozygous state. Genetic insights into the hematological risk factors for stroke may also eventually lead to a more fundamental understanding of stroke mechanisms and possibly to novel therapies for stroke prevention. One such example is the Val34Leu mutation in the Factor XIII gene that may impart a protective role in ischemic stroke. Factor XIII stabilizes fibrin clots via a mechanism that causes tight covalent bonds between fibrin monomers (Kohler & Grant, 1999). In a case control study, Elbaz and colleagues (2000) found that carrying the Val34Leu allele was associated with an OR for ischemic stroke of 0.58 (95% CI = 0.44–0.75). It is possible that the Val34Leu mutation causes the fibrin clot to be more susceptible to thrombolysis by tPA. Larger trials will be needed to confirm this observation but, if substantiated, it may be possible to develop drugs that similarly interfere with fibrin clot stabilization in a beneficial way for stroke prevention.

Genetic polymorphisms that confer a prethrombotic state are often associated with saggital sinus and cerebral vein occlusion (Martinelli et al., 1996; Norland et al., 1997). One recently identified and relatively common polymorphism that in small case control studies appears to impart an increased risk of both arterial and venous strokes is the prothrombin 20210 A variant (G 20210 A) (De Stefano et al.,

1998). In one study, 20% of subjects with cerebral vein thrombosis possessed the G 20210 A allele compared with only 3% of controls. The odds ratio for the G 20210 A variant in these subjects with cerebral vein thrombosis when compared to healthy controls was 10.2 (Martinelli et al., 1998). The mechanism by which the G 20210 A variant increases risk of stroke is currently unknown (Neufeld, 1998). The coincidence of the factor V Leiden mutation and the G 20210 A variant in a subject with puerperal cerebral vein thrombosis is reported (Weih et al., 1998). The occurrence of combinations of two or more polymorphisms that favour thrombosis may be one import way that such mutations confer risk of stroke (Chaturvedi & Dzieczkowski 1999; Gemmati et al., 1998). Prothrombotic mutations also appear to have a potential interaction with conventional risk factors for stroke.

Evaluation and treatment

Standard hematological indices are usually obtained as part of the routine evaluation of almost every patient with stroke and TIA. For the majority of patients with stroke, such measures suffice to exclude many of the hematological conditions that could contribute to the cause or outcome of stroke. Additional testing that can be useful in many stroke patients includes measurement of plasma fibrinogen and homocysteine levels. In only a relatively few cases are extensive studies of hemostasis indicated in order to identify an underlying prothrombotic state. Before proceeding with a potentially expensive and often 'low yield' investigation to identify a coagulation abnormality, the clinician should carefully consider how such information would influence eventual treatment. In particular, the prothrombotic state may be a transient phenomenon caused by an acute phase response after surgery, infection or related to other clinical situations such as parturition. Abnormalities in hemostasis that are identified in such settings may be difficult to interpret from the perspective of both long-term thrombotic risk and the necessity of prolonged anticoagulation.

A detailed investigation to identify a prothrombotic state should be considered in most patients with saggital sinus and cerebral vein thrombosis and in children and young adults with moya-moya and other unexplained episodes of stroke and TIA and in subjects with a strong family history of stroke or other recurrent thrombotic events. Elderly patients with cryptogenic stroke are also candidates for a thorough hematological evaluation as, theoretically, are individuals with patent foramen ovale who experience cerebrovascular symptoms although

Table 11.1. *Prothrombotic states commonly associated with cerebrovascular disease*

Prothrombotic state	Screening test	Specific test
Hyperhomocysteinemia	Fasting and PML homocysteine	Genetic polymorphisms
Antiphospholipid antibody	aPTT, platelet count, mixing study	
– Lupus anticoagulant		ELISA
– Anticardiolipin antibody		ELISA
Activated protein C resistance	APCR assay	Various assays[a]
Protein C deficiency	DRVVT	Various assays[a]
Protein S deficiency	APCR assay	Various assays[a]
Factor V leiden	DRVVT, APCR assay	Factor V test, DNA
Antithrombin deficiency		Various assays[a]
Prothrombin G 20210A		PCR
DIC	CBC, fibrin split products	
TTP	CBC, BUN, bilirubin,	Bone marrow biopsy
Polycythemia vera	Hemoglobin, hematocrit	Erythropoetin
Essential thrombocythemia	Platelet count	Bone marrow biopsy
Sickle cell disease	CBC with manual differential	Hemoglobin genotype
Dysfibrinogenemia	Fibrinogen level, clotting time	Various assays[a]

Notes:

APCR = activated protein C resistance, DIC = disseminated intravascular coagulation, DRVVT = dilute Russell viper venom time, PML = post-methionine load, TTP = thrombotic thrombocytopenia purpura.

[a] Tests for both protein function and quantity are available for protein C, S, and antithrombin.

there are no prospective studies that define benefit to such an approach.

Table 11.1 lists the prothrombotic states most commonly evaluated in subjects with stroke and TIA. When testing for prothrombotic state, it is useful to employ functional tests of hemostasis in addition to specific measures of clotting factors, regulatory proteins and genetic polymorphisms. For example, functional testing for APC resistance will help to identify conditions other than factor V Leiden that impair inactivation of Va. Unfortunately, many of the sophisticated functional tests for various coagulation pathways are not widely available. In addition, many functional and quantitative measures of hemostasis are affected by concurrent treatment with anticoagulants including heparin and warfarin. Testing for the common genetic polymorphisms such as factor V Leiden and the prothrombin G 20210 A is commercially available, but many other genetic polymorphisms remain investigational. The factor V Leiden and the prothrombin G 20210 A mutations are more prevalent than abnormalities in protein C, S and antithrombin. Testing for platelet function abnormalities includes performing a bleeding time, ex vivo aggregometry or possibly by employing shear induced platelet aggregation with systems such as the PFA-100analyser (Mammen et al., 1998). It is important to pursue a complete testing profile when defining a prethrombotic state, since some

patients at increased risk for thrombotic events have more than one factor contributing to the presence of thrombophilia. Once identified, many patients with a defined prethrombotic state are placed on long-term anticoagulation. Unfortunately, the benefits to this approach remain unknown since there is a dearth of data about treatment outcomes with respect to stroke for most individuals with prothrombotic states.

References

Adams, R.J., McKie, V.C., Hsu, L. et al. (1998). Prevention of a first stroke by transfusions in children with sickle cell anemia and abnormal results on transcranial Doppler ultrasonography. *New England Journal of Medicine*, **339**(1), 5–11.

Al-Mondhiry, K. & Ehmann, W.C. (1994). Congenital afibrinogenemia. *American Journal of Hematology*, **46**, 343–7.

Armstrong, F.D., Thompson, R.J., Wang, W. et al. (1996). Cognitive function and brain resonance imaging in children with sickle cell disease. *Pediatrics*, **97**, 864–70.

Beamer, N.B., Coull, B.M., Clark, W.M., Briley, D.P., Wynn, M. & Sexton, G. (1998). Persistent inflammatory response in stroke survivors. *Neurology*, **50**, 1722–8.

Bick, R.L. (1998). Sticky platelet syndrome: A common cause of unexplained venous and arterial thrombosis – results of prevalence and treatment outcome. *Clinical and Applied Thrombosis and Hemostasis*, **4**, 1–5.

Bick, R.L. & Kaplan, H. (1998). Current concepts of thrombosis: prevalent trends for diagnosis and management. *Medical Clinics of North America*, **82**, 409–58.

Boushey, C.J. & Beresford, S.A.A., Omenn, G.S. & Motutsky, A.G. (1995). A quantitative assessment of plasma homocysteine as a risk factor for vascular disease: probable benefits of increasing folic acid intake. *Journal of the American Medical Association*, **274**, 1049–57.

Canova, C.R., Courtin, C. & Reinhart, W.H. (1999). C-reactive protein (CRP) in cerebro-vascular events. *Atherosclerosis*, **147**, 49–53.

Casto, L., Camerlingo, M., Finazzi, G., Censori, B., Barbui, T. & Mamoli, A. (1994). Essential thrombocytemia and ischemic stroke: report of six cases. *Italian Journal of Neurological Sciences*, **15**, 359–62.

Catto, A., Carter, A., Ireland, H. et al. (1995). Factor V Leiden mutation and thrombin generation in relation to the development of acute stroke. *Arteriosclerosis, Thrombosis and Vascular Biology*, **15**, 783–785.

Catto, A.J., Carter, A.M., Stickland, M.H., Bamford, J.M., Davies, J.A. & Grant, P.J. (1997). Plasminogen activator inhibitor -1 4G/5G promoter polymorphism and levels in subjects with cerebrovascular disease. *Thrombosis and Haemostasis*, **77**, 730.

Catto, A.J., Kohler., H.P., Bannan, S., Stickland, M., Carter, A. & Grant, P.J. (1998). Factor XIII Val 34 Leu: a novel association with primary intracerebral hemorrhage. *Stroke*, **29**, 813–16.

Chaturvedi, S. & Dzieczkowski, J.S. (1999). Protein S deficiency, activated protein C resistance and sticky platelet syndrome in a young woman with bilateral strokes. *Cerebrovascular Diseases*, **9**, 127–30.

Cortelazzo, S., Finazzi, G., Ruggeri, M. et al. (1995). Hydroxyurea for patients with essential thrombocythemia and a high risk of thrombosis. *New England Journal of Medicine*, **332**, 1132–6.

Daif, A. et al. (1995). Cerebral venous thrombosis in adults: a study of 40 cases from Saudi Arabia. *Stroke*, **26**, 1193–5.

De Stefano, V., Chiusolo, P., Paciaroni, K. et al. (1998). Prothrombin G20210A mutant genotype is a risk factor for cerebrovascular ischemic disease in young patients. *Blood*, **91**, 3562–5.

Earley, C.J., Kittner, S.J., Feeser, B.R. et al. (1998). Stroke in children and sickle-cell disease: Baltimore-Washington Cooperative Young Stroke Study. *Neurology*, **51**(1), 169–76.

Eikelboom, J.W., Hankey, G.J., Anand, S.S., Lofthouse, E., Staples, N. & Baker, R.I. (2000). Association between high homocyst(e)ine and ischemic stroke due to large- and small-artery disease but not other etiologic subtypes of ischemic stroke, *Stroke*, **31**, 1069–75.

Elbaz, A., Poirier, O., Canaple, S., Chedru, F., Cambien, F. & Amarenco, P. (2000). The association between the Val34Leu polymorphism in the factor XIII gene and brain infarction. *Blood*, **95**, 586–91.

Ellis, M.H., Kesler, A., Friedman, Z., Drucker, I., Radnai, Y. & Kott, E. (2000). Value of prothrombin fragment 1.2 (F 1.2) in the diagnosis of stroke in young patients with antiphospholipid antibodies. *Clinical and Applied Thrombosis–Hemostasis*, **6**, 61–4.

Feinberg, W.M., Erickson, L.P., Bruck, D. & Kittleson, J. (1996). Hemostatic markers in acute ischemic stroke. *Stroke*, **27**, 1296–300.

Feinberg, W.M., Pearce, L.A., Hart, R.G. et al. (1999). Markers of thrombin and platelet activity in patients with atrial fibrillation: correlation with stroke among 1531 participants in the stroke prevention in atrial fibrillation III study. *Stroke*, **30**, 2547–53.

Gaustadnes, M., Rudiger, N., Moller, J. et al. (1999). Thrombophilic predisposition in stroke and venous thromboembolism in Danish patients. *Blood Coagulation and Fibrinolysis*, **10**, 251–9.

Gaustadnes, M., Rudiger, N., Rasmussen, K. & Ingerslev, J. (2000). Intermediate and severe hyperhomocysteinemia with thromboses: a study of genetic determinates. *Thrombosis and Haemostasis*, **83**, 554–8.

Gemmati, D., Serino, M.L., Moratelli, S. et al. (1998). Coexistence of antithrombin deficiency, factor V Leiden and hyperhomocysteinemia in a thrombotic family. *Blood Coagulation and Fibrinolysis*, **9**, 173–6.

Gill, F.M., Sleeper, L.A., Weiner, S.J. et al. (1995). Clinical events in the first decade in a cohort of infants with sickle cell disease. *Blood*, **86**(2), 776–83.

Goodwin, T.M. (1989). Congenital hypofibrinogenemia in pregnancy, *Obstetric and Gynecology Survey*, **44**, 157–61.

Graham, I.M., Daly, L.E., Refsum, H.M. et al. (1997). Plasma homocysteine as a risk factor for vascular disease: the European Concerted Action Project. *Journal of the American Medical Association*, **277**, 1775–82.

Grau, A.J. (1997). Infection, inflammation, and cerebrovascular ischemia. *Neurology*, **49**(5 Suppl. 4), S47–51.

Gruppo Italiano Studio Policitemia. (1995). Polycythemia vera: the natural history of 1213 patients followed for 20 years. *Annals of Internal Medicine*, **123**, 656–64.

Gussekloo, J., Schaap, M.C., Frolich, M., Blauw, G.J. & Westendorp, R.G. (2000). C-reactive protein is a strong but nonspecific risk factor of fatal stroke in elderly persons, *Arteriosclerosis, Thrombosis and Vascular Biology*, **20**, 1047–51.

Guzzini, F., Conti, A. & Esposito, F. (1998). Simultaneous ischemic and hemorrhagic lesions of the brain detected by CT scan in a patient with thrombotic thrombocytopenic purpura. *Haematologica*, **83**, 280.

Hankey, G.J. & Eikelboom, J.W. (1999). Homocysteine and vascular disease. *Lancet*, **354**, 407–13.

Hart, R.G., Benavente, O. & Pearce, L.A. (1999). Increased risk of intracranial hemorrhage when aspirin is combined with warfarin: a meta-analysis and hypothesis. *Cerebrovascular Diseases*, **9**, 215–19.

Hart, R.G., Halperin, J.L., McBride, R., Benavente, O., Man-Son-Hing, M. & Kronmal, R.A. (2000). Aspirin for the primary prevention of stroke and other major vascular events: meta-analysis and hypothesis. *Archives of Neurology*, **57**, 326–32.

Haverkate, F. & Samama, M.M. (1995). Familial dysfibrinogenemia and thrombophilia. Report on a study of SSC Subcommittee on fibrinogen. *Thrombosis Haemostasis*, **73**, 151–61.

Hedner, U. (1998). Recombinant activated factor VII as a universal hemostatic agent. *Blood Coagulation and Fibrinolysis*, **9**(Suppl. 1) S147–52.

Henselmans, J.M.L., Jeije, K., Haaxma, R. et al. (1999). Recurrent spontaneous intracerebral hemorrhage in a congenitally afibrinogenemic patient: Diagnostic pitfalls and therapeutic options. *Stroke*, **30**, 2479–82.

Isler, C.M., Rinehart, B.K., Terrone, D.A., Martin, R.W., Magann, E.F. & Martin, J.N. Jr. (1999). Maternal mortality associated with HELLP (hemolysis, elevated liver enzymes, and low platelets) syndrome. *American Journal of Obstetrics and Gynecology*, **18**, 924.

Johansson, L., Jansson, J.H., Boman, K., Nilsson, T.K., Stegmayr, B. & Hallmans, G. (2000). Tissue plasminogen activator, plasminogen activator inhibitor-1, and tissue plasminogen activator/plasminogen activator inhibitor-1 complex as risk factors for the development of a first stroke. *Stroke*, **31**, 26–32.

Kohler, H.P. & Grant, P.J. (1999). The role of factor XIII Val34Leu in cardiovascular disease. *Quarterly Journal of Medicine*, **92**, 67–72.

Lane, D.A. & Grant, P.J. (2000). Role of hemostatic gene polymorphisms in venous and arterial thrombotic disease. *Blood*, **95**, 1517–32.

Lee, A.J., Lowe, G.D.O., Woodward, M. & Tunstall-Pedoe, H. (1993). Fibrinogen in relation to personal history of prevalent hypertension, diabetes, stroke, intermittent claudication, coronary heart disease, and family history: the Scottish Heart Health Study. *British Heart Journal*, **69**, 338–42.

Malinow, R.M., Nieto, J., Szklo, M., Chambles, L.E. & Bond, G. (1993). Carotid artery intimal-medial wall thickening and plasma homocyst(e)ine in asymptomatic adults: the Atherosclerosis Risk in Communities study. *Circulation*, **87**, 1107–13.

Mammen, E.F. (1999). Sticky platelet syndrome. *Seminars in Thrombosis and Hemostasis*, **25**, 361–5.

Mammen, E.F., Comp, P.C., Gosselin, R. et al. (1998). PFA-100 system: a new method for assessment of platelet function. *Seminars in Thrombosis and Hemostasis*, **24**, 195–202.

Martinelli, I., Landi, G., Merati, G., Cella, R., Tosetta, A. & Mannucci, P.M. (1996). Factor V gene mutation is a risk factor for cerebral venous thrombosis. *Thrombosis Haemostasis*, **75**, 393.

Martinelli, I., Sacchi, E., Landi, G. et al. (1998). High risk of cerebral vein thrombosis in carriers of a prothrombin-gene mutation and in users of oral contraceptives. *New England Journal of Medicine*, **338**, 1793–7.

Martinez, J. (1997). Congenital dysfibrinogenemia. *Current Opinion in Hematology*, **4**, 357–65.

Matsuo, T., Kobayashi, H., Kario, K. & Suzuki, S. (2000). Fibrin D-dimer in thrombogenic disorders. *Seminars in Thrombosis and Hemostasis*, **26**, 101–7.

Menart, C., Sprunck, N., Duhaut, P. et al. (1998). Recurrent spontaneous intracerebral hematoma in a patient with afibrinogenemia. *Thrombosis Haemostasis*, **79**, 241–2.

Mendall, M.A., Patel, P., Ballam, L., Strachan, D. & Northfield, T.C. (1996). C-reactive protein and its relation to cardiovascular risk factors: a population based cross sectional study. *British Medical Journal*, **312**, 1061–5.

Moran, C.J. et al. (1998). Sickle cell disease: imaging of cerebrovascular complications. *Radiology*, **206**(2), 311–21.

Mudd, S., H., Skovby, F., Levy, H.L. et al. (1985). The natural history of homocystinuria due to cystathionine beta-synthase deficiency. *American Journal of Human Genetics*, **37**, 1–31.

Murphy, S. (1999). Diagnostic criteria and prognosis in polycythemia vera and essential thrombocythemia. *Seminars in Hematology*, **36**(Suppl. 2), 9–13.

Neufeld, E.J. (1998). Coagulation disorders and treatment strategies: update on genetic risk factors for thrombosis and atherosclerotic vascular disease. *Hematology/Oncology Clinics of North America*, **12**, 1194–209.

Norland, L., Zoller, B. & Ohlin, A.K. (1997). A novel thrombomodulin gene mutation in a patient suffering from saggital sinus thrombosis. *Thrombosis and Haemostasis*, **78**, 1164.

O'Donnell, H.C., Rosand, J., Knudsen, K.A. et al. (2000). Apolipoprotein E genotype and the risk of recurrent lobar intracerebral hemorrhage. *New England Journal of Medicine*, **342**(4), 240–5.

Ohene-Frempong, K., Weiner, S.J., Sleeper, L.A. et al. (1998). Cerebrovascular accidents in Sickle Cell disease: rates and risk factors. *Blood*, **91**(1), 288–94.

Pegelow, C.H., Adams, R.J., McKie, V. et al. (1995). Risk of recurrent stroke in patients with sickle cell disease treated with erythrocyte infusions. *Journal of Pediatrics*, **126**, 896.

Perry, I.J. (1999). Homocysteine and risk of stroke. *Journal of Cardiovascular Risk*, **6**, 235–40.

Perry, I.J., Refsum, H., Morris, R.W., Ebrahim, S.B., Ueland, P.M. & Shaper, A.G. (1995). Prospective study of serum total homocysteine concentration and risk of stroke in middle-aged British men. *Lancet*, **346**, 1395–8.

Press, R.D., Liu, X.Y., Beamer, N. & Coull, B.M. (1996). Ischemic Stroke in the Elderly: role of the Common Factor V Mutation Causing Resistance to Activated Protein C. *Stroke*, **27**, 44–8.

Reiner, A.P. & Kumar, P.N., Schwartz, S.M. et al. (2000). Genetic variants of platelet glycoprotein receptors and risk of stroke in young women. *Stroke*, **31**, 1628–33.

Ridker, P.M. (1994). C-reactive protein and risks of future myocardial infarction and thrombotic stroke. *European Heart Journal*, **19**, 1–3.

Ridker, P.M. (1998). Inflammation, infection, and cardiovascular risk: how good is the clinical evidence? *Circulation*, **97**, 1671–4.

Ridker, P.M., Hennekens, C.H., Lindpaintner, K. et al. (1995). Mutation in the gene coding for coagulation factor V and the risk of myocardial infarction, stroke, and venous thrombosis in apparently healthy men. *New England Journal of Medicine*, **332**, 912–17.

Roldan, V., Marin, F., Marco, P., Martibez, J.G., Calatayud, R. & Sgort, F. (1998). Hypofibrinolysis in atrial fibrillation. *American Heart Journal*, **136**, 956–60.

Seibert, J.J. et al. (1998). Transcranial doppler, MRA and MRI as a screening examination for cerebrovascular disease in patients with sickle cell anemia: an 8-year study. *Pediatric Radiology*, **28**(3), 138–42.

Siegel, M.J. et al. (1995). Cerebral infarction in sickle cell disease:

transcranial doppler US versus neurologic examination. *Radiology*, **197**(1), 191–4.

Tracy, R.P. (1999). Epidemiological evidence for inflammation in cardiovascular disease. *Thrombosis Haemostasis*, **82**, 826.

Verhoef, P., Hennekens, C.H., Malinow, M.R., Kok, F.J., Willett, W.C. & Stampfer, M.J. (1994). A prospective study of plasma homocyst(e)ine and risk of ischemic stroke. *Stroke*, **25**, 1924–30.

Vila, N., Obach, V., Revilla, M., Oliva, R. & Chamorro, A. (2000). a1-antichymotrypsin gene polymorphism in patients with stroke, *Stroke*, **31**, 2103–5.

Vomberg, P.P. & Breederveld, C. (1987). Cerebral thromboembolism due to antithrombin III deficiency in two children, *Neuropediatrics*, **18**, 42–4.

Walters, M.C. et al. (1995). Neurologic complications after allogenic marrow transplantation for sickle cell anemia. *Blood*, **85**(4), 879–84.

Walters, M.C. et al. (1996). Bone marrow transplantation for sickle cell disease. *New England Journal of Medicine*, **335**(6), 369–76.

Walters, M.C. et al. (2000). Impact of bone marrow transplantation for symptomatic sickle cell disease: an interim report. *Blood*, **95**, 1918–24.

Wang, W.C. et al. (1991). High risk of recurrent stroke after discontinuance of five to twelve years of transfusion therapy in patients with sickle cell disease. *Journal of Pediatrics*, **118**, 377–82.

Weih, M., Mehracin, S., Valdueza, J.M. et al. (1998). Coincidence of factor V Leiden mutation and a mutation in the prothrombin gene at position 20210 in a patient with puerperal cerebral venous thrombosis, *Stroke*, **29**, 1739–40.

Yap, S., Naughten, E.R., Wilcken, B., Wilcken, D.E. & Boers, G.H.J. (2000). Vascular complications of severe hyperhomocysteinemia due to cystathionine β-synthase deficiency: effects of homocysteine-lowering therapy. *Seminars in Thrombosis and Hemostasis*, **26**, 335–340.

12

Moschcowitz syndrome (thrombotic thrombocytopenic purpura)

John Wade

West London Neurosciences Centre, Charing Cross Hospital, London, UK

Introduction

In 1929, Moschcowitz described the syndrome that is now referred to as thrombotic thrombocytopenic purpura (TTP). It is a severe multisystem disorder characterized by a heterogeneous array of fever, thrombocytopenia, microangiopathic hemolytic anemia, neurological symptoms, and renal involvement (Amorosi & Ultmann, 1966). It is more common in women than in men (ratio 3:2), and its peak frequency is in the third and fourth decades, but it has also been described in children and in the elderly (Ridolfi & Bell, 1981; Kwaan, 1987). TTP is a rare disorder; one case per year was diagnosed at the Johns Hopkins Hospital during 1960–80, at which time annual admissions ranged from 45625 to 51718 (Ridolfi & Bell, 1981). The mortality rate, which used to be extremely high (in excess of 90%) (Cahalane & Horn, 1959), has decreased with the introduction of plasma infusions and exchange, and now 85% of cases can be expected to go into remission. Approximately 40% of survivors, however, will suffer relapses (Rose & Eldor, 1987).

Pathology

The clinical manifestations are the results of widespread thrombosis of capillaries and arterioles, without much in the way of surrounding inflammatory reaction. The thrombus is composed primarily of platelets, with some fibrin in varying stages of organization, usually evident at the arteriolar-capillary junction. What characterizes TTP is the florid disseminated nature of the thrombotic process; in order of frequency, the most severely involved organs are the pancreas, adrenals, heart, brain, and kidney. With the exception of the lungs and liver, virtually all organs will be found to be affected if the histological examination is com-

prehensive enough (Ridolfi & Bell, 1981). The parenchymal changes in visceral organs are relatively mild with patchy focal necrosis and hemorrhage (Case Records of the Massachusetts General Hospital, 1968; Tapp et al., 1969).

Etiology

More than 90% of cases of TTP occur without an identifiable underlying cause, but in some cases the disorder appears to be triggered by infection, connective-tissue disease, immune-complex disease, drug reaction, neoplasia, or pregnancy (Ridolfi & Bell, 1981; Kwaan, 1987). Drugs that have been implicated include penicillamine and penicillin, but sometimes the association may be incidental rather than causal. Nonspecific prodromal symptoms precede the onset of TTP in 20% of cases, suggesting that viral illness can sometimes act as a trigger. Fifteen cases of TTP with coexistent HIV infection have been reported (Rarick et al., 1992). The third trimester of pregnancy and the postpartum period appear to predispose women to TTP, and unexpectedly large numbers of cases have been described in the obstetric literature (Ridolfi & Bell, 1981).

Clinical manifestations

Headache, confusion, disorientation, epilepsy and fluctuating focal neurological signs are common early presentations (Amorosi & Ultmann, 1966; Ridolfi & Bell, 1981). The onset is usually subacute, with symptoms of malaise, fatigue, and fever often preceding any neurological involvement by several weeks. Other prominent symptoms include hemorrhagic cutaneous lesions (petechiae, purpura and ecchymosis), abdominal pain, arthralgia, and myalgia. Although we emphasize that the presentation is usually subacute, TTP has recently been identified as a cause of sudden death, presumably due to involvement of the cardiac conduction system (Bell et al., 1990).

The most frequently observed neurological symptoms include confusion ($\cong$80%), headaches ($\cong$30%), pareses ($\cong$30%), and transient dysphasia or aphasia ($\cong$30%). Around 20% of these patients suffer one or more seizures, and approximately 10% progress to coma. Patients with severe neurological disease (aphasia, pareses, seizures, and coma) can recover completely with treatment, but some are left with residual deficits, despite prompt improvement in platelet count (Ben-Yehuda et al., 1988).

Laboratory findings

The blood picture reveals microangiopathic hemolytic anemia that is often severe, with hemoglobin values around 6.5 g dl^{-1} in about 40% of cases (Ridolfi & Bell, 1981). The red blood cell indices usually are normocytic and normochromic, but the peripheral blood invariably shows numerous fragmented and misshapen red blood cells. The reticulocyte count is variably elevated. The thrombocytopenia is usually severe, with platelet counts averaging in the vicinity of 20 000 mm^{-3}. The white cell count can be normal or modestly increased.

The hemolytic anemia characteristically is Coombs-negative, and there is no evidence that the anemia is autoimmune (Naeme, 1980). The red-cell hemolysis gives rise to an unconjugated bilirubinemia.

The majority of patients with TTP have normal or only mildly abnormal findings on coagulation studies (Jaffe et al., 1973; Ridolfi & Bell, 1981). Prothrombin times and partial thromboplastin times are normal in about 90% of patients and plasma fibrinogen concentrations are normal in about 80% (Ridolfi & Bell, 1981). It is very unusual to see fibrinogen concentrations fall below 100 mg.dl^{-1}. Fibrinogen–fibrin degradation products are usually normal, but occasionally weakly positive. There is an absence of fibrinolytic activity in the micro-vascular lesions of TTP, which serves to distinguish this condition from disseminated intravascular coagulation. Although the exact cause of TTP is unknown, the presence of von Willebrand factor (VWF) multimers has been implicated in the disease (Rock et al., 1996).

Biopsy of gingival tissue, bone marrow, spleen, and skin will reveal the characteristic microvascular hyaline thrombi in 30–50% of cases (Kennedy et al., 1980; Kwaan, 1987).

CT findings in the brain may be normal, even in patients with established focal neurological deficits, and normal findings usually portend complete recovery, without neurological deficit (Kay et al., 1991). In other cases, the CT findings may be abnormal, with acute infarcts, hemorrhages, or diffuse decreased attenuation in the white matter (Kay et al., 1991). Patients with brain-scan abnormalities tend to fare poorly; in the Mayo Clinic series, five of ten died, and four had permanent neurological deficits, whereas seven of ten patients with normal findings on brain scans recovered completely. The MRI experience has been limited, but punctate abnormalities deep in the white matter can be detected with MRI in patients who have normal CT findings (Tardy et al., 1993).

Treatment and outcome

Among the first 116 cases of TTP described, only four patients survived (Cahalane & Horn, 1959), and in 1966, a review of 271 cases reported mortality of 90% (Amorosi & Ultmann, 1966). Survival rates had risen to 46% by the time of the next major review (Ridolfi & Bell, 1981), and they are almost certainly better than that now. Increased awareness and earlier diagnosis of TTP are probably leading to detection of milder forms of the syndrome, in which the patients might be expected to fare better, but new forms of treatment, particularly plasmapheresis, have almost certainly contributed to the increased survival rate.

Both the rarity and severity of TTP have prevented the use of controlled clinical trials to develop treatment protocols. Survival rates for each new modality have been compared with those from the historical literature. In 1968, most survivors had been treated with corticosteroids and splenectomy, and that led to their continued use for two decades or so (Bukowski et al., 1981). During that time, a number of platelet-function inhibitors were also used, in combination with established treatments. The results were equivocal (Birgins et al., 1979; Bukowski et al., 1981; Rasone et al., 1982). The first report of plasma exchange leading to improvement was published in 1959 when a single case of TTP went into remission following exchange transfusion of fresh blood (Rubinstein et al., 1959). Subsequent studies have suggested complete remission in two thirds of patients following plasma-exchange transfusion (Byrnes, 1981; Gottschall et al., 1981; Myers, 1981). The rate of response is rapid: An initial rise in platelet count occurs after four exchanges, and the platelet count can be expected to exceed 150 000 mm^{-3} after an average of nine exchanges (Blitzer et al., 1987). Concomitant use of steroids (60–120 mg prednisolone per day) is recommended, because plasma exchange has not been evaluated as sole therapy. Plasma exchange with fresh frozen plasma produces a 50% response after seven exchanges and an 80% survival at one month, and it is more effective than plasma infusion (Rock et al., 1991) and cryosupernatant (plasma from which cryoprecipitate has been removed), which is relatively deficient in VWF multimers, is probably a more effective replacement fluid during plasma exchange (Rock et al., 1996; Perotti et al., 1996).

In patients with life-threatening findings at the time of diagnosis, the response rate to plasma exchange probably can be improved if vincristine sulfate (2 mg i.v.) is infused following the first plasma exchange (Abramson, 1978; Gutterman & Stevenson, 1982; Sennett & Conrad, 1986). Other modalities that should be considered in patients refractory to steroids/plasma exchange include high-dosage intravenous prostacyclin (Tardy et al., 1991), high dose cyclosporin (Hand et al., 1998), and high-dosage intravenous immunoglobulin (Kolodziej, 1993; Centurioni et al., 1995; Nosari et al., 1996). If all else fails, splenectomy should be considered (Hoffkes et al., 1995; Veltman et al., 1995). Antiplatelet agents are often used in conjunction with plasma exchange regimes, and there is now randomized trial data to validate usefulness in the acute phase. Moreover, at 1 year triclopidine (perhaps clopidogrel would work as well) reduces TTP relapses from 20%/year to 6%/year (Bobbio-Pallavicini et al., 1997).

An early review cited a relapse rate of around 7.5% (Ridolfi & Bell, 1981), but close observation of the steadily increasing numbers of patients surviving their first attacks suggests that the rate is much higher. In a study describing relapse rates for TTP survivors since 1977 (i.e. following plasma therapy), 12 of 38 suffered recurrent episodes (37%), with six patients suffering second relapses and two, further recurrent attacks (Rose & Eldor, 1987). Infections, pregnancy, and surgery were frequently associated with the initial episodes and the relapses. Relapse rates were surprisingly low in the Italian co-operative group study, where only 15% (9 out of 60) relapsed during a follow-up period of 10 years, and the difference in relapse rates between studies remains a mystery (Porta et al., 1996). Relapses can be managed successfully with additional plasma exchange or with splenectomy, which often induces long-term remission (Onundarson et al., 1992).

References

Abramson, N. (1978). Treatments for thrombotic thrombocytopenic purpura: plasma, vincristine, hemodialysis and exchange transfusions. *New England Journal of Medicine*, 298, 971–2.

Amorosi, E.L. & Ultmann, III E. (1966). Thrombotic thrombocytopenic purpura: report of 16 cases and review of the literature. *Medicine*, 45, 139–59.

Bell, M.D., Barnhart, & Martin, J.M. (1990). Thrombotic thrombocytopenic purpura causing sudden unexpected death – a series of eight patients. *Journal of Forensic Sciences*, 35, 601–13.

Ben-Yehuda, D., Rose, M., Michaeli, Y. & Eldor, A. (1988). Permanent neurological complications in patients with thrombotic thrombocytopenic purpura. *American Journal of Hematology*, 29, 7–8.

Birgins, H., Ernst, P. & Hansen, M. (1979). Thrombotic thrombocytopenic purpura: treatment with a combination of antiplatelet drugs. *Acta Medica Scandinavica*, 205, 437–9.

Blitzer, J.B., Granfortuna, J.M., Gottlieb, A.J. et al. (1987). Thrombotic thrombocytopenic purpura: treatment with plasmapheresis. *American Journal of Hematology*, 24, 329–39.

Bobbio-Pallavicini, E., Gugliotta, L., Centurioni, R. et al. (1997). Antiplatelet agents in thrombotic thrombocytopenic purpura (TTP). Results of a randomized multicenter trial by the Italian Cooperative Group for TTP. *Haematologica*, 82(4), 429–35

Bukowski, R.M., Hewlett, S. & Reimer, R.R. et al. (1981). Therapy of thrombotic thrombocytopenic purpura: an overview. *Seminars in Thrombosis and Hemostasis*, 7, 1–8.

Byrnes, J.J. (1981). Plasma infusion in the treatment of thrombotic thrombocytopenic purpura. *Seminars in Thrombosis and Hemostasis*, 7, 9–14.

Cahalane, S.F. & Horn, R.C. (1959). Thrombotic thrombocytopenic purpura of long duration. *American Journal of Medicine*, 27, 333.

Case Records of the Massachusetts General Hospital (1968). *New England Journal of Medicine*, 278, 1366.

Centurioni, R., Bobbio-Pallavicini, E., Porta, C. et al. (1995). Treatment of thrombotic thrombocytopenic purpura with high-dose immunoglobulins. Results in 17 patients. Italian Co-operative Group for TTP. *Haematologica*, Jul–Aug, 80(4), 325–31.

Gottschall, J.L., Pisciotta, A.V., Darin, J. et al. (1981). Thrombotic thrombocytopenic purpura: experience with whole blood exchange transfusion. *Seminars in Thrombosis and Hemostasis*, 7, 25–31.

Gutterman, L.A. & Stevenson, T.D. (1982). Treatment of thrombotic thrombocytopenic purpura with vincristine. *Journal of the American Medical Association*, 247, 1433–6.

Hand, J.P., Lawlor, E.R., Yong, C.K. & Davis, J.H., (1998). Successful use of cyclosporine A in the treatment of refractory thrombotic thrombocytopenic purpura. *British Journal of Haematology*, 100(3), 597–9.

Hoffkes, H.G., Weber, F., Uppenkamp, M. et al. (1995). Recovery by splenectomy in patients with relapsed thrombotic thrombocytopenic purpura and treatment failure to plasma exchange. *Seminars in Thrombosis and Hemostasis*, 21(2), 161–5.

Jaffe, E.A., Nachman, R.L. & Merskey, C. (1973). Thrombotic thrombocytopenic purpura – coagulation parameters in 12 patients. *Blood*, 42, 499.

Kay, A.C., Solberg, L.A., Nichols, D.A. & Pettit, R.M. (1991). Prognostic significance of computerised tomography of the brain in thrombotic thrombocytopenic purpura. *Mayo Clinic Proceedings*, 66, 602–6.

Kennedy, S.S., Zacharski, L.R. & Beck, L.R. (1980). Thrombotic thrombocytopenic purpura: analysis of 48 unselected cases. *Seminars in Thrombosis and Hemostasis*, **6**, 341–9.

Kolodziej, M. (1993). High-dose intravenous immunoglobulin as therapy for thrombotic thrombocytopenic purpura. *American Journal of Medical Science*, **305**, 101–2.

Kwaan, H.C. (1987). Clinicopathological features of thrombotic thrombocytopenic purpura. *Seminars in Hematology*, **24**, 71–81.

Moschcowitz, E. (1929). Hyaline thrombosis of the terminal arterioles and capillaries: a hitherto undescribed disease. *Proceedings of the New York Pathological Society*, **24**, 21–4.

Myers, T. I. (1981). Treatment of thrombotic thrombocytopenic purpura with combined exchange plasmapheresis and antiplatelet drugs. *Seminars in Thrombosis and Hemostasis*, **7**, 37–42.

Naeme, P.B. (1980). Immunologic and other factors in thrombotic thrombocytopenic purpura (TTP). *Seminars in Thrombosis and Hemostasis*, **6**, 416.

Nosari, A., Muti, G., Busnach, G., Cantoni, S., Strinchini, A. & Morra, E. (1996). Intravenous gamma globulin in refractory thrombotic thrombocytopenic purpura. *Acta Haematologica*, **96**(4), 255–7.

Onundarson, P.T., Rowe, J.M., Heal, J.M. & Francis, C.W. (1992). Response to plasma exchange and splenectomy in thrombotic thrombocytopenic purpura. *Archives of Internal Medicine*, **152**, 791–6.

Perotti, C., Torretta, L., Molinari, E. & Salvaneschi, L. (1996). Cryoprecipitate-poor plasma fraction (cryosupernatant) in the treatment of thrombotic thrombocytopenic purpura at onset. A report of four cases. *Haematologica*, **81**(2), 175–7.

Porta, C., Centurioni, R., Vianelli, N., Bobbio-Pallavicini, E., Gugliotta, L. & Billio, A., (1996). Thrombotic thrombocytopenic purpura and relapses: why do case series differ? *American Journal of Hematology*, **52**(3), 215–16.

Rarick, M.U., Espina, B., Mocharnuk, R., Trilling, Y. & Levine, A.M. (1992). Thrombotic thrombocytopenic purpura in patients with HIV infection; a report of three cases and review of the literature. *American Journal of Hematology*, **40**, 103–9.

Rasone, M.H., Ho, W.G. & Goldfinger, D. (1982). Ineffectiveness of aspirin and dipyridamine in the treatment of thrombotic thrombocytopenic purpura. *Seminars in Thrombosis and Hemostasis*, **7**, 25–31.

Ridolfi, R.L. & Bell, W.R. (1981). Thrombotic thrombocytopenic purpura: report of 25 cases and review of the literature. *Medicine*, **60**, 413–27.

Rock, G., Shumak, K.H., Buskard, N.A. et al. (1991). Comparison of plasma exchange with plasma infusion in the treatment of thrombotic thrombocytopenic purpura. *New England Journal of Medicine*, **325**(6), 393–7.

Rock, G., Shumak, K.H., Sutton, D.M., Buskard, N.A. & Nair, R.C. (1996). Cryosupernatant as replacement fluid for plasma exchange in thrombotic thrombocytopenic purpura. *British Journal of Haematology*, **94**(2), 383–6.

Rose, M. & Eldor, A. (1987). High incidence of relapses in thromhotic thrombocytopenic purpura: clinical study of 38 patients. *American Journal of Medicine*, **83**, 437–44.

Rubinstein, M.A., Kegan, E.M., Macgilvary, M.H. et al. (1959). Unusual remission in a case of thrombocytopenic purpura syndrome following fresh blood exchange transfusion. *Archives of Internal Medicine*, **51**, 1409–19.

Sennett, M.L. & Conrad, M.E. (1986). Treatment of thrombotic thrombocytopenic purpura: plasmapheresis, plasma transfusions and vincristine. *Archives of Internal Medicine*, **146**, 266–7.

Tapp, E., Geary, C.G. & Dawson, D.W. (1969). Thrombotic microangiopathy with macroscopic infarction. *Journal of Pathology*, **97**, 711.

Tardy, B., Page, Y., Contet, C. et al. (1991). Intravenous prostacyclin in thrombotic thrombocytopenic purpura: case report and review of the literature. *Journal of Internal Medicine*, **230**, 279–82.

Tardy, B., Page, Y., Convers, P., Mismetti, P., Barral, F. & Bertrand, I. C. (1993). Thrombotic thrombocytopenic purpura: MR findings. *American Journal of Neuroradiology*, **14**, 489–90.

Veltman, G.A., Brand, A., Leeksma, O. C. et al. (1995). The role of splenectomy in the treatment of relapsing thrombotic thrombocytopenic purpura. *Annals of Hematology*, **70**(5), 231–6.

13

Hyperviscosity and stroke

John F. Dashe

Tufts New England Medical Center, Boston, MA, USA

Introduction

There is a strong association of increased stroke risk with elevated hematocrit and fibrinogen levels. These facts have led to increasing interest in hemorheological factors and their role in the development of vascular disease and acute stroke. The neurological complications of the hyperviscosity syndromes are well described, but the relative importance of viscosity in the more common ischemic stroke subtypes is still uncertain.

Basic principles of blood viscosity

Viscosity is the resistance to flow that arises from the friction between adjacent layers of a fluid in motion, and is defined as the ratio of shear stress to shear rate. Shear stress is the tangential force between flowing layers of fluid, and shear rate is the velocity gradient between the layers of flow (Wood and Kee, 1985). For Newtonian fluids such as water or plasma, viscosity is a fixed property, and is independent of flow rate. Whole blood is a non-Newtonian fluid, and has an apparent viscosity that varies as a function of its shear rate. Blood viscosity increases at low shear rates (low velocity) and decreases at high shear rates (high velocity). At very low flow velocities, blood viscosity may be from 100 to 10 000 times that of water; at high flow velocities, it may be of the order of two to ten times that of water (Dintenfass, 1968).

Because of its non-Newtonian properties, blood viscosity is continuously changing in vivo as blood flows through vessels of different sizes and pressure gradients. In addition, shear rates cannot be measured directly, and their values are approximations for different parts of the circulation. For these reasons, a single in vitro measurement of blood viscosity has limited practical value (Thomas, 1982).

Blood viscosity is influenced by many factors including hematocrit, plasma protein and fibrinogen concentrations, cellular aggregation, red cell deformability and axial migration, vessel diameter and flow rate. Leukocytes and platelets make a relatively minor contribution to whole blood viscosity under normal conditions, but may be important in certain pathological conditions.

Effects of hyperviscosity in large and small vessels

Blood flow in the microcirculation (vessels with an internal diameter of 100 microns or less) is governed mainly by red cell deformability and plasma viscosity. Normal deformability allows erythrocytes with a diameter of 8 microns to squeeze through capillaries with diameters of 4 to 6 microns (Wood & Kee, 1985). Red cell deformability is determined by surface to volume area, cell morphology, mechanical properties of the membrane, and the viscosity of the cell contents (Koenig & Ernst, 1992). Normal deformability requires sufficient adenosine triphosphate (ATP) levels to maintain cell shape and actively extrude calcium. Excess intracellular calcium can cause gelation of hemoglobin and contraction of the cell membrane (Grotta et al., 1986). If intracellular ATP is depleted, as might occur in ischemic tissue, the red cell becomes more rigid, contributing to increased viscosity. Likewise, rigid erythrocytes in sickle cell blood cannot easily pass through the smaller vessels.

Because of the Fahraeus–Lindqvist effect (Fahraeus & Lindqvist, 1931), blood viscosity decreases as tube diameter decreases below 1 mm due to reduced contribution of normal red cells to viscous resistance (*Lancet* editorial, 1975). In these small vessels, blood viscosity approximates plasma viscosity, which becomes a direct determinant of

Table 13.1. *Hematological hyperviscosity syndromes*

Plasma abnormality	Increased cellularity	Decreased red cell deformability
Waldenstrom's macroglobulinemia	Polycythemia vera	Sickle cell anemia
Paraproteinemias	Erythrocytosis (Secondary polycythemia)	Spherocytosis
Congenital hyperfibrinogenemia	Stress polycythemia (Gaisbock's syndrome)	Hemoglobinopathies
	Hyperleukocytic leukemias	

Source: Modified from Dormandy et al. (1981).

capillary blood flow (Gaehtgens & Marx, 1987). Leukocytes may also play an important role at this level.

Red cell aggregation is a reversible process that causes most of the non-Newtonian flow behavior of whole blood. Large electrically positive macromolecules in plasma, mainly fibrinogen and globulins, facilitate bridging and reduce the electronic repulsion between red blood cells. In large vessels, migration of red cells to the vessel axis increases blood fluidity and oxygen transport, and the higher velocities and shear rates tend to break up aggregations of red cells. Under low flow conditions, and accompanying lower shear rates, the process tilts toward formation of red cell aggregates (rouleau), which increase blood viscosity and may result in diminished perfusion (Koenig & Ernst, 1992). The width of capillaries precludes the passage of red cell aggregates unless a rouleau formation enters end on (Wells, 1964). Elevated fibrinogen and paraprotein levels cause an increase in erythrocyte aggregation. Increased red cell aggregation also occurs with trauma, shock, burns, infection, complicated diabetes mellitus, malignancy, and rheumatic diseases. Red cell aggregation is increased in most conditions that are accompanied by an increased erythrocyte sedimentation rate (Somer & Meiselman, 1993).

Viscosity increases logarithmically at the lowest shear rates (Somer & Meiselman, 1993), and this effect is magnified at higher hematocrit levels. Conditions that cause low flow, such as a high-grade arterial stenosis or systemic hypotension and hypovolemia, increase blood viscosity based on the associated low shear rates. The end result is a further reduction in flow, potentially leading to a 'viscous, vicious circle' (Dintenfass, 1966; Thomas, 1982) consisting of reduced blood flow, aggregation of blood cells, and finally complete stasis favouring thrombus formation. Acute ischemia also induces an acute-phase reaction and a further deterioration of blood fluidity, mainly by increasing fibrinogen. With stasis or zero shear rate, cell aggregation causes an increased structural viscosity, which must be overcome for flow to be reestablished. The minimum force required to initiate flow in static blood is called the yield stress, and fibrinogen is the principle determinant of this property of blood (Wells, 1964).

Epidemiological evidence

Patients with acute and chronic cerebrovascular disease show abnormalities involving blood viscosity, plasma viscosity, hematocrit, red cell deformability and fibrinogen (Coull et al., 1991; Fisher & Meiselman, 1991; Ott et al., 1974; Sakuta, 1981; Thomas, 1982). The Framingham study suggested an epidemiological link between elevated hematocrit and risk of stroke (Kannel et al., 1972). A later report found that the risk of stroke increases progressively with fibrinogen level in men but not in women (Kannel et al., 1987). Average fibrinogen levels are higher in women and in populations with other cardiovascular risk factors, including elevated hematocrit, hypertension, diabetes, cigarette smoking, obesity, and hyperlipidemia (Kannel, 1997). Although fibrinogen is an acute-phase reactant, prospective epidemiological studies have shown that hematocrit, fibrinogen, blood viscosity and plasma viscosity are increased years before the onset of acute ischemic events and are positively associated with risk of stroke (Lowe et al., 1997). Plasma viscosity increases with age regardless of gender; is positively associated with untreated hypertension, hypercholesterolemia and smoking in men; and is raised in hypertension and severe obesity in women (Koenig & Ernst, 1992). In patients with a history of stroke and patients with risk factors for stroke, a low albumin–globulin ratio predicts a significantly increased risk for recurrent stroke (Beamer et al., 1993).

Hematological hyperviscosity syndromes

Diseases that cause hyperviscosity fall into three main categories: plasma abnormalities, increased cellularity, and decreased deformability (Table 13.1). Each has a different rheological mechanism that leads to a hyperviscous state.

Table 13.2. *Covert hyperviscosity states*

Diabetes
Inflammation
Atherosclerosis
Systemic low flow states/hemoconcentration in:
Burn injury
Inappropriate red cell transfusion
Dehydration
Circulatory shock

A fourth category of 'covert' hyperviscosity states is increasingly recognized (Table 13.2).

Plasma abnormalities

Plasma viscosity is determined mainly by the concentration of electrically neutral or slightly positively charged, non-spherical, high molecular weight proteins. These proteins, including fibrinogen, alpha-2 macroglobulins, and immunoglobulins, contribute to viscosity because of their physical characteristics as well as by their interactions with red cells. Fibrinogen is the principal determinant of plasma viscosity under normal conditions (Dormandy et al., 1981; Wells, 1970). Although it makes up about 4% of normal plasma proteins by weight, fibrinogen is responsible for more than one-fifth of the total plasma viscosity (Somer & Meiselman, 1993).

Increased production of high molecular weight globulins or macroglobulins is frequently found in patients with monoclonal and polyclonal immunoglobulinemias including lymphoma, Waldenstrom's macroglobulinemia, and less commonly in multiple myeloma (Fahey et al., 1965). The plasma hyperviscosity syndrome is a clinical entity characterized by mucous membrane bleeding, blurred vision, visual loss, lethargy, headache, dizziness, vertigo, tinnitus, paresthesias, and occasionally seizures (Dintenfass, 1966; Fahey et al., 1965; Pavy et al., 1980; Wells, 1970). Funduscopic examination may show retinal hemorrhages and papilledema. Pathologically, this syndrome is explained by extremely elevated plasma viscosity and hypervolemia; intense red cell aggregation results from the elevated paraproteins (Somer & Meiselman, 1993).

Increased cellularity

Polycythemia vera is the most common cause of increased cellularity, and is characterized by overproduction of erythroid, myeloid, and megakaryocytic cell lines, leading to elevated peripheral blood cell counts and an increased red cell mass. Cerebral blood flow (CBF) is diminished with the high hematocrits found in polycythemia (Thomas et al., 1977a). The most common neurological symptoms related to polycythemia include headache, dizziness or vertigo, paresthesias, scotomata, blurred vision and tinnitus (Silverstein et al., 1962), similar to the symptoms reported in the plasma hyperviscosity syndrome.

The frequency of brain infarction due to hyperviscosity in polycythemia vera is unclear. Prospective controlled studies addressing this issue are lacking. Grotta et al. (1986) concluded that polycythemia rarely, if ever, plays a role in focal cerebral infarction, but many other reports have noted an increased incidence of brain ischemia and thrombosis (Barabas et al., 1973; Chievitz & Thiede, 1962; Millikan et al., 1960; Silverstein et al., 1962). The nature of the brain events themselves (whether focal or diffuse) is often difficult to ascertain from these studies, as they generally do not provide detailed clinical–pathological correlation or precise definitions of the cerebral thrombotic events.

It is plausible that the increased hematocrit in polycythemia may impede flow and increase coagulability in the presence of large artery occlusive disease, and contribute to decreased microvascular flow in patients with hypertensive small vessel disease. Stroke could also be caused by the increased platelet counts and increased platelet reactivity found in myeloproliferative disorders such as polycythemia vera (Schafer, 1984). Pearson and Wetherley-Mein (1978) found that the incidence of vascular occlusive episodes correlated directly with the red cell mass; the same study showed an association between the frequency of thrombosis and thrombocytosis, but this association did not achieve statistical significance. Lacunar infarction (Pearce et al., 1983), Binswanger's disease (Caplan, 1995), cerebral venous thrombosis (Melamed et al., 1976), intracerebral hemorrhage, cerebral large artery thrombosis, large artery territorial infarction, and watershed infarction (Yazdi & Cote, 1986) have all been attributed to polycythemia (Barabas et al., 1973).

Erythrocytosis from increased erythropoietin (so-called secondary polycythemia) causes elevated hematocrit and hyperviscosity. Increased erythropoietin production can be triggered by a physiologic response to chronic hypoxia in a number of conditions including cyanotic congenital heart disease, hypoxic lung disease, hypoventilation due to the Pickwickian syndrome, and high altitude. Non-physiologically increased erythropoietin is associated with renal cysts, hydronephrosis, and a number of neoplasms (Grotta et al., 1986). Stress polycythemia, or Gaisbock's syndrome, also causes elevated hematocrit. High altitude induces a physiologic erythrocytosis, but the limited epidemiological data in the United States shows that stroke mortality actually declines with increasing altitude (Gordon et al., 1977). In a study of 122 adults with cyanotic congenital heart disease followed for 1 to 12 years and a total of 748 patient–years, Perloff et al., (1988) found no evidence of cerebral arterial thrombosis with brain infarct in any patients, irrespective of the severity of hyperviscosity symptoms or duration of follow-up. Symptoms of transient ischemic attack likewise did not occur, with the exception of one patient who had amaurosis fugax.

Children with congenital cyanotic heart disease have an increased incidence of stroke, most frequently due to cerebral venous thrombosis (Cottrill & Kaplan, 1973; Phornphutkul et al., 1973). Unlike adults, these children are likely to have a microcytic hypochromic red cell morphology consistent with iron deficiency, which has been shown to decrease red cell deformability (Cottrill & Kaplan, 1973; Phornphutkul et al., 1973). Thus, hyperviscosity in these children may be more related to decreased red cell deformability than to the level of hemoglobin or hematocrit.

Hyperleukocytic leukemias are associated with hyperviscosity. Normal white cells are by some estimates 1000 fold less deformable (and leukemic blast cells may be less deformable still) than normal red cells. The increased numbers of rigid leukemic cells tend to occlude small vessels and lead to global neurological dysfunction (Somer & Meiselman, 1993). Microinfarcts and petechial hemorrhages result. No strong evidence has emerged linking leukemic hyperviscosity to large artery brain infarction.

Decreased red cell deformability

In sickle cell disease, the hemoglobin HbS structure is less soluble than normal hemoglobin, and has a tendency toward polymerization when exposed to hypoxia or low pH. This causes the cell membrane to conform to a highly rigid sickle shape, and results in tremendously increased viscosity with abnormal flow and red blood cell sludging in the microcirculation and cerebral veins. Even oxygenated sickle blood from asymptomatic sickle patients has an elevated viscosity when compared to normal blood at the same hematocrit (Chien et al., 1970). Although the tissue damage is thought to occur in the microcirculation, large artery occlusive disease involving the distal internal carotid artery and Circle of Willis is a characteristic feature, occasionally developing into a Moya–Moya radiographic pattern (Stockman et al., 1972). The mechanism may be stasis and occlusion of the small vessels of the vaso vasorum that nourish the large arteries, leading to ischemia of the large artery walls, intimal proliferation, and gradual occlusion (Stockman et al., 1972). Sickle red cells may stimulate proliferation of the smooth muscle and fibrous components of arterial walls, leading to arterial stenoses.

The incidence of stroke in sickle cell disease is 8 to 17% for homozygotes (HbSS) (Grotta et al., 1986). Sickle patients are at risk for both cerebral infarction and intracerebral hemorrhage; the latter may develop from medial wall necrosis and rupture of cerebral arterioles (Stockman et al., 1972). Cerebral infarctions occur in both deep and subcortical structures. Both neuropathologic (Rothman et al., 1986) and neuroradiologic (Pavlakis et al., 1988) evidence indicates that the majority of brain infarcts in patients with sickle cell disease involve the high cortical convexity borderzone regions between the major arterial territories. Brainstem, spinal cord and retinal infarctions also occur (Grotta et al., 1986).

Other examples of decreased red cell deformability include hereditary spherocytosis, pyruvate kinase deficiency, and certain hemoglobinopathies; usually these disorders do not lead to major clinical symptoms or cerebrovascular involvement (Somer & Meiselman, 1993), although patients with brain infarction have been reported (van Hilten et al., 1989).

Other conditions associated with hyperviscosity

Diabetes, inflammation, and atherosclerosis have been termed 'covert' hyperviscosity syndromes (Somer & Meiselman, 1993), since their rheological manifestations are typically less pronounced than in the better known hematological hyperviscosity syndromes (Table 13.2). Diabetes is associated with a number of rheological abnormalities (McMillan, 1985, 1989); the arteriolar hyalinization found in this disease may be mediated by a diabetes-specific impairment in red cell deformability, causing an increase in peak tangential arteriolar wall force (Juhan et al., 1982; McMillan, 1997). The hematological stress syndrome, described in patients with cancer and other acute and chronic inflammatory diseases (Reizenstein, 1979), consists of increases in platelet numbers and adhesiveness, blood viscosity, plasma viscosity, erythrocyte sedimentation rate, and certain plasma proteins including fibrinogen and other coagulation factors, along with a decrease in fibrinolytic activity. This response is similar to the acute phase response to tissue injury and infection. Increased viscosity may occur in low-flow states that arise systemically from hemoconcentration in severe burns, inappropriate red cell transfusion, dehydration due to illness, and circulatory shock (Lowe, 1987).

The most important aspect of hyperviscosity could turn out to be its role in the pathogenesis of atherosclerosis. Evidence is accumulating that the atherosclerotic and thrombotic arterial lesions are promoted by altered rheological factors including fibrinogen, lipoproteins, plasma viscosity, hematocrit, red blood cell aggregation, and leukocyte activation (Koenig & Ernst, 1992). By this hypothesis, increased viscosity creates larger areas of decreased blood flow, thereby perpetuating the interaction of atherogenic elements with the endothelium (Sloop, 1996). In arterial hypertension, whole blood viscosity, plasma viscosity, hematocrit, fibrinogen, red cell aggregation and deformability are all increased (Hossmann et al., 1985; Letcher et al., 1981; Zannad et al., 1988). However, some have questioned whether the elevated viscosity found in acute and chronic vascular disease is a primary cause or a secondary consequence of atherosclerosis (Stuart et al., 1981).

Lipoproteins have direct effects on blood rheology. Increases in triglycerides, chylomicrons (Seplowitz et al., 1981), low density lipoprotein (LDL) and very low density lipoprotein (VLDL) cholesterol fractions lead to a concentration-dependent increase in plasma viscosity (Leonhardt et al., 1977; Rosenson & Lowe, 1998). Patients with hyperlipoproteinemia type II have elevated fibrinogen levels and increased blood viscosity, plasma viscosity and hematocrit, as well as elevated levels of alpha-2 antiplasmin (Lowe et al., 1982), an inhibitor of fibrinolysis. Elevated LDL causes increased viscosity by fostering red cell aggregation (Sloop, 1996), whereas high density lipoprotein (HDL) has anti-atherothrombotic properties that result in part from inhibition of platelet and erythrocyte aggregation and reduced blood viscosity (Rosenson & Lowe, 1998).

Cigarette smoking is associated with increased hemoglobin, fibrinogen levels, plasma viscosity, red cell aggregation, platelet aggregation, and leukocyte counts, resulting in a steep increase in whole blood viscosity in smokers (Ernst, 1995). The effect of smoking is dose dependent and largely reversible (Lowe, 1998).

Abnormal body temperature may have deleterious effects on viscosity. Increases in platelets, red cells, and viscosity in response to mild surface cooling provide a possible explanation for rise in cerebral thrombosis found in cold weather (Keatinge et al., 1984), and temperatures below 37 °C may produce abnormal rheologic changes in either the cellular or the protein components of blood (Kwaan & Bongu, 1999). Significant elevations in fibrinogen, plasma viscosity, and HDL cholesterol in the coldest six months compared with summer months correlate with the excess winter frequency of cardiovascular disease in the elderly (Stout & Crawford, 1991). Heat stress has been linked to increased platelet counts, red cell counts, blood viscosity, and plasma cholesterol levels, and these changes may explain the marked rise in recorded deaths from coronary and cerebral thrombosis during heat waves (Keatinge et al., 1986). Blood viscosity and hematocrit also follow a circadian variation with a morning peak (Kubota et al., 1987), which correlates with the peak time of ischemic stroke onset (Marsh et al., 1990).

Role of hyperviscosity in ischemic stroke subtypes

Outside of the overt hematological hyperviscosity syndromes, few studies have directly examined the role of rheological factors pertaining to ischemic strokes subtypes or vascular lesions. Tohgi et al., (1978) studied 432 consecutive patients with 'cerebral infarction' at autopsy and found that the risk of ischemic stroke rose dramatically for hematocrit values above 46%; the increase occurred predominantly in deeper regions rather than in cortex, but this trend did not reach statistical significance. The proportion of large versus small vessel infarcts is not clear from their data.

The majority of studies have focused on the microcirculation. In a study of 40 patients with lacunar strokes confirmed by clinical and radiological criteria, Schneider et al., (1985) found that erythrocyte aggregation, erythrocyte deformability, plasma viscosity, fibrinogen concentration and yield shear stress were pathological when compared to normal control patients, but hematocrit was not significantly different. A later study (Schneider et al., 1987) found that fibrinogen levels were significantly higher in 40 patients with lacunar infarcts and 21 patients with Binswanger's disease compared to 275 healthy control subjects without vascular risk factors. The Binswanger patients alone had consistently elevated plasma viscosity. Although most strongly associated with hypertension, Binswanger's disease may be associated with other conditions linked to hyperviscosity such as polycythemia, hyperglobulinemia, hyperlipidemia, and diabetes (Caplan, 1995). Kawamoto et al., (1991) found that asymptomatic patients with multiple lacunar infarcts by magnetic resonance imaging criteria showed a higher predicted whole blood viscosity and a lower high density lipoprotein (HDL) cholesterol than hypertensive and normotensive controls. Taken together, these studies suggest that hyperviscosity and altered rheological factors may be involved in the pathophysiology of small vessel ischemic disease.

Scant data exist regarding rheological factors and large vessel occlusive disease. In patients with angiographically confirmed carotid artery occlusion found after evaluation for TIA and minor stroke, infarct size on CT scans correlated significantly with increased hematocrit (Harrison et al., 1981). Oder et al., (1998) reported significantly higher blood viscosity in patients with sonographic abnormalities of one vertebral artery compared to controls.

Spontaneous echo contrast (SEC) seen in the left atrial cavity or appendage on echocardiographic examination has generated interest as a risk factor for cardioembolic stroke (Ansari & Maron, 1997; Daniel et al., 1988). In vitro, static erythrocytes are highly echogenic. The swirling smoke-like appearance of SEC is present at low shear rates but disappears at high shear rates. SEC is associated with cardiac abnormalities that produce low-flow states within the left atrium, including atrial fibrillation, mitral stenosis, and left atrial enlargement (Black & Stewart, 1993). Most left atrial thrombi are accompanied by SEC (Black & Stewart, 1993).

SEC is likely a consequence of protein-mediated red blood cell aggregation in the setting of low shear forces (Merino et al., 1992). Fatkin et al., (1997) showed that SEC can be reduced by inhibition of red cell aggregation using dextran 40 and poloxamer 188, but is unaltered by heparin and warfarin. SEC in patients with non-valvular atrial fibrillation is independently related to hematocrit, fibrinogen concentration and left atrial dimension (Black et al., 1993). In a study of 185 patients with atrial fibrillation, 46% of patients demonstrated SEC, and the severity of SEC was positively correlated with erythrocyte sedimentation rate, low-shear blood viscosity and anticardiolipin antibody (Fatkin et al., 1994). In 50 patients with acute or chronic cerebrovascular disease, Briley et al., (1994) found that the severity of SEC was related to elevated fibrinogen levels and concomitant increases in both plasma and serum viscosity; patients with severe SEC had double the prevalence of cardioembolic stroke compared to those with other causes of stroke.

Cerebral blood flow and oxygen delivery

Blood flow to an organ system is determined by the blood vessel size, the blood pressure, and the hemorheologic or flow properties of blood. In patients with polycythemia vera, CBF is low at high hematocrit levels, and reducing hematocrit dramatically increases the CBF (Thomas et al., 1977a, b). Other studies have confirmed an inverse relationship between hematocrit and viscosity on the one hand, and CBF on the other (Grotta et al., 1982; Thomas, 1982). These observations have been interpreted as evidence that hyperviscosity causes a reduction in CBF, since hematocrit is the primary factor influencing blood viscosity. A similar inverse relationship between fibrinogen levels and viscosity, and between fibrinogen levels and CBF, has been demonstrated (Grotta et al., 1982, 1985). However, other studies have found that the oxygen carrying capacity of the blood is the critical factor in determining CBF, reflecting a homeostatic and physiological mechanism designed to maintain transport and delivery of oxygen to the brain despite falling hematocrit and arterial oxygen content (Harrison, 1989; Wade, 1983).

The rationale behind hemodilution and phlebotomy is that reducing the hematocrit lowers whole blood viscosity, which in turn increases CBF to ischemic regions. To be useful, this increase in CBF must be sufficiently robust to overcome the diminished oxygen carrying capacity of the blood that results from lowering the hematocrit. The optimal hematocrit for oxygen delivery to most tissues has been estimated at 30 to 35% (Messmer et al., 1973; Wood & Kee, 1985). It is unclear if this relationship is true for brain (Asplund, 1989); Gaehtgens and Marx (1987) place the optimum hematocrit for cerebral oxygen delivery at 42%. Lowering viscosity by reducing hematocrit runs the risk of worsening ischemia if the CBF is in fact regulated by homeostatic mechanisms designed to maintain oxygen carrying capacity or oxygen delivery irrespective of viscosity. However, homeostatic regulation of CBF may be deranged in ischemic regions (Asplund, 1989), and the effect of hyperviscosity may take on greater importance as the physiological response to diminished oxygen delivery is blunted, or even exhausted as when vasodilation is maximal in an ischemic vascular bed (Grotta, 1987a).

The studies examining oxygen delivery after hematocrit reduction are conflicting. Wade (1983) reported a small but significant increase in oxygen transport to the brain following phlebotomy to reduce hematocrit in 20 patients with polycythemia vera, and Yamauchi et al., (1993) found that CBF and oxygen transport were increased in the hemisphere ipsilateral to carotid occlusion in five patients after hemodilution. Henriksen et al., (1981) reported that oxygen delivery capacity did not change significantly from baseline following hemodilution in six patients with slightly elevated hematocrit.

Treatment

Plasma hyperviscosity syndromes are treated by plasmapheresis or plasma exchange to remove the paraproteins and thereby reduce hyperviscosity and hypervolemia. Newer techniques of cell centrifugation, plasma separation and filtration may also be useful.

For many years, phlebotomy has been the mainstay for treatment of polycythemia, with the goal of keeping the hematocrit in the range of 45% or less. However, phlebotomy increases the risk of thrombosis, which is also associated with a history of prior thrombosis and advanced age (Berk et al., 1986). Supplemental phlebotomy is still useful for patients with severe hyperviscosity symptoms, and for those unable to tolerate myelosuppression. For leukocytic leukemias, leukapheresis is the treatment of choice to decrease levels of leukemic cells and blood viscosity (Somer & Meiselman, 1993).

Treatment of sickle cell anemia is aimed at maintaining the HbS concentration below 30% by repeated exchange transfusion, which reduces the risk of stroke in sickle cell disease (Pegelow et al., 1995). During acute crises, oxygen and intravenous fluids are used in an attempt to improve systemic and cerebral blood flow.

Despite some promising results in a few human stroke trials (Strand et al., 1984; Wood & Fleischer, 1982), the majority of hemodilution studies failed to show significant benefit (Asplund, 1989; Grotta, 1987b; Harrison, 1989). Many of these trials may have been flawed by late initiation of therapy beyond the therapeutic time window to salvage brain cells within the ischemic penumbra.

Other methods of lowering viscosity in acute stroke or chronic cerebrovascular disease could be useful to improve blood flow and ameliorate ischemia. Pentoxifylline increases erythrocyte (Schneider et al., 1983) and leukocyte deformability, and decreases viscosity (Muller, 1979). Omega-3 fatty acids available in the form of fish oils decrease fibrinogen levels (Radack et al., 1989) and blood viscosity, and may increase erythrocyte deformability (Simopoulos, 1991). They also have lipid lowering effects on triglycerides and total cholesterol (Haglund et al., 1990). However, the fibrinogen lowering effects of omega-3 fish oil consumption may not be evident at typical intake levels consumed by the US population (Archer et al., 1998).

Derivatives of fibric acid (fibrates), including clofibrate, gemfibrozil, fenofibrate, bezafibrate, and ciprofibrate, are most commonly used to treat elevations of VLDL cholesterol and plasma triglycerides (Miller & Spence, 1998). They also reduce plasma fibrinogen (Simpson et al., 1985). Heparin-induced extracorporeal LDL precipitation (HELP) is a method of rapidly reducing fibrinogen and lipoprotein levels in order to reduce viscosity (Walzl et al., 1994). Lipid-lowering therapy alone can improve whole blood viscosity. Koenig et al., (1992) found that the HMG-CoA reductase inhibitor lovastatin decreased plasma viscosity to the same extent as bezafibrate, but did not reduce fibrinogen.

Three fibrinolytic snake venoms – ancrod, batroxobin, and crotalase – act primarily by a proteolytic effect on circulating fibrinogen (Bell, 1997). Treatment with batroxobin or ancrod increases CBF and reduces blood viscosity (Grotta, 1987a; Izumi et al., 1996). Ticlopidine directly reduced the mean fibrinogen level in a study of patients with polycythemia vera (Finelli et al., 1991); in another study ticlopidine reduced fibrinogen levels of both healthy volunteers and patients with stable angina (de Maat et al., 1996). The mechanism of fibrinogen reduction by ticlopidine has not yet been elucidated. Ticlopidine and clopidogrel, by binding with ADP receptors, inhibit activation of the GpIIb/IIIa receptors and thereby reduce platelet binding with fibrinogen. Whether clopidogrel has direct effects on fibrinogen levels is unclear.

The thrombolytic agents including streptokinase (Jan et al., 1990) and urokinase decrease fibrinogen, plasma viscosity, and red cell aggregation (Koenig & Ernst, 1992). Tissue plasminogen activator (tPA) reduces fibrinogen and blood viscosity to a lesser degree than streptokinase (Jan et al., 1990). Improved blood fluidity may be an additional beneficial effect of these agents beyond their primary role in thrombolysis (Moriarty et al., 1988).

Conclusions

Hyperviscosity is an intriguing problem in stroke. The neurological symptoms described in the hematological hyperviscosity syndromes are global, non-specific for localization, and are generally reversible with treatment. Focal brain infarction and cerebral venous thrombosis are increased in sickle cell disease, and probably as well in polycythemia. Hyperviscosity, hyperfibrinoginemia, and altered rheological factors may increase the risk of acute stroke in certain conditions, including large vessel stenosis, low flow, and hypertensive small vessel disease. Hyperviscosity may also be important in the promotion of atherosclerosis and chronic cerebrovascular disease. Many treatment options are available to decrease viscosity and potentially improve flow, but outside of the hematological hyperviscosity syndromes our knowledge is limited regarding the usefulness of these treatments. Further study is needed to determine the role of hemorheology in the pathogenesis of cerebrovascular disease and ischemic stroke subtypes, keeping in mind the goal of effective prevention and treatment of these disorders.

References

Ansari, A. & Maron, B.J. (1997). Spontaneous echo contrast and thromboembolism. *Hospital Practice*, **32**, 109–11, 115–16.
Archer, S.L., Green, D., Chamberlain, M., Dyer, A.R. & Liu, K. (1998).

Association of dietary fish and n-3 fatty acid intake with hemostatic factors in the coronary artery risk development in young adults (CARDIA) study. *Arteriosclerosis, Thrombosis and Vascular Biology*, **18**, 1119–23.

Asplund, K. (1989). Randomized clinical trials of hemodilution in acute ischemic stroke. *Acta Neurologica Scandinavica* (Suppl.), **127**, 22–30.

Barabas, A.P., Offen, D.N. & Meinhard, E.A. (1973). The arterial complications of polycythaemia vera. *British Journal of Surgery*, **60**, 183–7.

Beamer, N., Coull, B.M., Sexton, G., de Garmo, P., Knox, R. & Seaman, G. (1993). Fibrinogen and the albumin–globulin ratio in recurrent stroke. *Stroke*, **24**, 1133–9.

Bell, W.R., Jr. (1997). Defibrinogenating enzymes. *Drugs*, **54** Suppl 3, 18–30; discussion 30–1.

Berk, P.D., Goldberg, J.D., Donovan, P.B., Fruchtman, S.M., Berlin, N.I. & Wasserman, L.R. (1986). Therapeutic recommendations in polycythemia vera based on Polycythemia Vera Study Group protocols. *Seminars in Hematology*, **23**, 132–43.

Black, I.W. & Stewart, W.J. (1993). The role of echocardiography in the evaluation of cardiac source of embolism: left atrial spontaneous echo contrast. *Echocardiography*, **10**, 429–39.

Black, I.W., Chesterman, C.N., Hopkins, A.P., Lee, L.C., Chong, B.H. & Walsh, W.F. (1993). Hematologic correlates of left atrial spontaneous echo contrast and thromboembolism in nonvalvular atrial fibrillation. *Journal of the American College of Cardiology*, **21**, 451–7.

Briley, D.P., Giraud, G.D., Beamer, N.B. et al. (1994). Spontaneous echo contrast and hemorheologic abnormalities in cerebrovascular disease. *Stroke*, **25**, 1564–9.

Caplan, L.R. (1995). Binswanger's disease – revisited. *Neurology*, **45**, 626–33.

Chien, S., Usami, S. & Bertles, J.F. (1970). Abnormal rheology of oxygenated blood in sickle cell anemia. *Journal of Clinical Investigation*, **49**, 623–34.

Chievitz, E. & Thiede, T. (1962). Complications and causes of death in polycythaemia vera. *Acta Medica Scandinavica*, **172**, 513–23.

Cottrill, C.M. & Kaplan, S. (1973). Cerebral vascular accidents in cyanotic congenital heart disease. *American Journal of Diseases of Children*, **125**, 484–7.

Coull, B.M., Beamer, N., de Garmo, P. et al. (1991). Chronic blood hyperviscosity in subjects with acute stroke, transient ischemic attack, and risk factors for stroke. *Stroke*, **22**, 162–8.

Daniel, W.G., Nellessen, U., Schroder, E. et al. (1988). Left atrial spontaneous echo contrast in mitral valve disease: an indicator for an increased thromboembolic risk. *Journal of the American College of Cardiololgy*, **11**, 1204–11.

de Maat, M.P., Arnold, A.E., van Buuren, S., Wilson, J.H. & Kluft, C. (1996). Modulation of plasma fibrinogen levels by ticlopidine in healthy volunteers and patients with stable angina pectoris. *Thrombosis and Haemostasis*, **76**, 166–70.

Dintenfass, L. (1966). A preliminary outline of the blood high viscosity syndromes. *Archives of Internal Medicine*, **118**, 427–35.

Dintenfass, L. (1968). Internal viscosity of the red cell and a blood viscosity equation. *Nature*, **219**, 956–8.

Dormandy, J.A., Yates, C.J. & Berent, G.A. (1981). Clinical relevance of blood viscosity and red cell deformability including newer therapeutic aspects. *Angiology*, **32**, 236–42.

Ernst, E. (1995). Haemorheological consequences of chronic cigarette smoking. *Journal of Cardiovascular Risk*, **2**, 435–9.

Fahey, J.L., Barth, W.F. & Solomon, A. (1965). Serum hyperviscosity syndrome. *Journal of the American Medical Association*, **192**, 464–7.

Fahraeus, R. & Lindqvist, T. (1931). Viscosity of blood in narrow capillary tubes. *American Journal of Physiology*, **96**, 562–68.

Fatkin, D., Herbert, E. & Feneley, M.P. (1994). Hematologic correlates of spontaneous echo contrast in patients with atrial fibrillation and implications for thromboembolic risk. *Amercian Journal of Cardiology*, **73**, 672–6.

Fatkin, D., Loupas, T., Low, J. & Feneley, M. (1997). Inhibition of red cell aggregation prevents spontaneous echocardiographic contrast formation in human blood. *Circulation*, **96**, 889–96.

Finelli, C., Palareti, G., Poggi, M. et al. (1991). Ticlopidine lowers plasma fibrinogen in patients with polycythaemia rubra vera and additional thrombotic risk factors. A double-blind controlled study. *Acta Haematologica*, **85**, 113–18.

Fisher, M. & Meiselman, H.J. (1991). Hemorheological factors in cerebral ischemia. *Stroke*, **22**, 1164–9.

Gaehtgens, P. & Marx, P. (1987). Hemorheological aspects of the pathophysiology of cerebral ischemia. *Journal of Cerebral Blood Flow and Metabolism*, **7**, 259–65.

Gordon, R.S., Jr., Kahn, H.A. & Forman, S. (1977). Altitude and CBVD death rates show apparent relationship. *Stroke*, **8**, 274.

Grotta, J.C. (1987a). Can raising cerebral blood flow improve outcome after acute cerebral infarction? *Stroke*, **18**, 264–7.

Grotta, J.C. (1987b). Current status of hemodilution in acute cerebral ischemia. *Stroke*, **18**, 689–90.

Grotta, J., Ackerman, R., Correia, J., Fallick, G. & Chang, J. (1982). Whole blood viscosity parameters and cerebral blood flow. *Stroke*, **13**, 296–301.

Grotta, J., Ostrow, P., Fraifeld, E., Hartman, D. & Gary, H. (1985). Fibrinogen, blood viscosity, and cerebral ischemia. *Stroke*, **16**, 192–8.

Grotta, J.C., Manner, C., Pettigrew, L.C. & Yatsu, F.M. (1986). Red blood cell disorders and stroke. *Stroke*, **17**, 811–17.

Haglund, O., Wallin, R., Luostarinen, R. & Saldeen, T. (1990). Effects of a new fluid fish oil concentrate, ESKIMO-3, on triglycerides, cholesterol, fibrinogen and blood pressure. *Journal of Internal Medicine*, **227**, 347–53.

Harrison, M.J. (1989). Influence of haematocrit in the cerebral circulation. *Cerebrovascular and Brain Metabolism Reviews*, **1**, 55–67.

Harrison, M.J., Pollock, S., Kendall, B.E. & Marshall, J. (1981). Effect of haematocrit on carotid stenosis and cerebral infarction. *Lancet*, **ii**, 114–15.

Henriksen, L., Paulson, O.B. & Smith, R.J. (1981). Cerebral blood flow following normovolemic hemodilution in patients with high hematocrit. *Annals of Neurology*, **9**, 454–7.

Hossmann, V., Auel, H., Bonner, G. et al. (1985). Haemorheology in adolescent hypertensives. *Journal of Hypertension. Supplement*, (Suppl. 3), S331–3.

Izumi, Y., Tsuda, Y., Ichihara, S., Takahashi, T. & Matsuo, H. (1996). Effects of defibrination on hemorheology, cerebral blood flow velocity, and CO_2 reactivity during hypocapnia in normal subjects. *Stroke*, **27**, 1328–32.

Jan, K.M., Powers, E., Reinhart, W. et al. (1990). Altered rheological properties of blood following administrations of tissue plasminogen activator and streptokinase in patients with acute myocardial infarction. *Advances in Experimental Medicine and Biology*, **281**, 409–17.

Juhan, I., Vague, P., Buonocore, M., Moulin, J.P., Jouve, R. & Vialettes, B. (1982). Abnormalities of erythrocyte deformability and platelet aggregation in insulin-dependent diabetics corrected by insulin in vivo and in vitro. *Lancet*, **i**, 535–7.

Kannel, W.B. (1997). Influence of fibrinogen on cardiovascular disease. *Drugs*, **54**(Suppl. 3), 32–40.

Kannel, W.B., Gordon, T., Wolf, P.A. & McNamara, P. (1972). Hemoglobin and the risk of cerebral infarction: the Framingham Study. *Stroke*, **3**, 409–20.

Kannel, W.B., Wolf, P.A., Castelli, W.P. & D'Agostino, R.B. (1987). Fibrinogen and risk of cardiovascular disease. The Framingham Study. *Journal of the American Medical Association*, **258**, 1183–6.

Kawamoto, A., Shimada, K., Matsubayashi, K., Nishinaga, M., Kimura, S. & Ozawa, T. (1991). Factors associated with silent multiple lacunar lesions on magnetic resonance imaging in asymptomatic elderly hypertensive patients. *Clinical and Experimental Pharmacology and Physiology*, **18**, 605–10.

Keatinge, W.R., Coleshaw, S.R., Cotter, F., Mattock, M., Murphy, M. & Chelliah, R. (1984). Increases in platelet and red cell counts, blood viscosity, and arterial pressure during mild surface cooling: factors in mortality from coronary and cerebral thrombosis in winter. *British Medical Journal*, **289**, 1405–8.

Keatinge, W.R., Coleshaw, S.R., Easton, J.C., Cotter, F., Mattock, M. B. & Chelliah, R. (1986). Increased platelet and red cell counts, blood viscosity, and plasma cholesterol levels during heat stress, and mortality from coronary and cerebral thrombosis. *American Journal of Medicine*, **81**, 795–800.

Koenig, W. & Ernst, E. (1992). The possible role of hemorheology in atherothrombogenesis. *Atherosclerosis*, **94**, 93–107.

Koenig, W., Hehr, R., Ditschuneit, H.H. et al. (1992). Lovastatin alters blood rheology in primary hyperlipoproteinemia: dependence on lipoprotein(a)? *Journal of Clinical Pharmacology*, **32**, 539–45.

Kubota, K., Sakurai, T., Tamura, J. & Shirakura, T. (1987). Is the circadian change in hematocrit and blood viscosity a factor triggering cerebral and myocardial infarction? *Stroke*, **18**, 812–13.

Kwaan, H.C. & Bongu, A. (1999). The hyperviscosity syndromes. *Seminars in Thrombosis and Hemostasis*, **25**, 199–208.

Lancet (1975). Editorial: Haemorheology, blood-flow and venous thrombosis. *Lancet*, **ii**, 113–14.

Leonhardt, H., Arntz, H.R. & Klemens, U.H. (1977). Studies of plasma viscosity in primary hyperlipoproteinaemia. *Atherosclerosis*, **28**, 29–40.

Letcher, R.L., Chien, S., Pickering, T.G., Sealey, J.E. & Laragh, J.H. (1981). Direct relationship between blood pressure and blood viscosity in normal and hypertensive subjects. Role of fibrinogen and concentration. *American Journal of Medicine*, **70**, 1195–202.

Lowe, G.D. (1987). Blood rheology in general medicine and surgery. *Bailliere S Clinical Haematology*, **1**, 827–61.

Lowe, G.D. (1998). Etiopathogenesis of cardiovascular disease: hemostasis, thrombosis, and vascular medicine. *Annals of Periodontology*, **3**, 121–6.

Lowe, G.D., McArdle, B.M., Stromberg, P., Lorimer, A.R., Forbes, C.D. & Prentice, C.R. (1982). Increased blood viscosity and fibrinolytic inhibitor in type II hyperlipoproteinaemia. *Lancet*, **i**, 472–5.

Lowe, G.D., Lee, A.J., Rumley, A., Price, J.F. & Fowkes, F.G. (1997). Blood viscosity and risk of cardiovascular events: the Edinburgh Artery Study. *British Journal of Haematology*, **96**, 168–73.

McMillan, D.E. (1985). Hemorheologic changes in diabetes and their role in increased atherogenesis. *Hormone and Metabolic Research. Supplement Series*, **15**, 73–9.

McMillan, D.E. (1989). Increased levels of acute-phase serum proteins in diabetes. *Metabolism*, **38**, 1042–6.

McMillan, D.E. (1997). Development of vascular complications in diabetes. *Vascular Medicine*, **2**, 132–42.

Marsh, E.E.D., Biller, J., Adams, H.P., Jr. et al. (1990). Circadian variation in onset of acute ischemic stroke. *Archives of Neurology*, **47**, 1178–80.

Melamed, E., Rachmilewitz, E.A., Reches, A. & Lavy, S. (1976). Aseptic cavernous sinus thrombosis after internal carotid arterial occlusion in polycythaemia vera. *Journal of Neurology, Neurosurgery and Psychiatry*, **39**, 320–4.

Merino, A., Hauptman, P., Badimon, L. et al. (1992). Echocardiographic 'smoke' is produced by an interaction of erythrocytes and plasma proteins modulated by shear forces. *Journal of the American College of Cardiology*, **20**, 1661–8.

Messmer, K., Gornandt, L., Jesch, F., Sinagowitz, E., Sunder-Plassmann, L. & Kessler, M. (1973). Oxygen transport and tissue oxygenation during hemodilution with dextran. *Advances in Experimental Medicine and Biology*, **37**, 669–80.

Miller, D.B. & Spence, J.D. (1998). Clinical pharmacokinetics of fibric acid derivatives (fibrates). *Clinical Pharmacokinetics*, **34**, 155–62.

Millikan, C.H., Siekert, R.G. & Whisnant, J.P. (1960). Intermittent carotid and vertebral-basilar insufficiency associated with polycythemia. *Neurology*, **10**, 188–96.

Moriarty, A.J., Hughes, R., Nelson, S.D. & Balnave, K. (1988). Streptokinase and reduced plasma viscosity: a second benefit. *European Journal of Haematology*, **41**, 25–36.

Muller, R. (1979). Pentoxifylline – a biomedical profile. *Journal of Medicine*, **10**, 307–29.

Oder, B., Oder, W., Lang, W., Marschnigg, E. & Deecke, L. (1998). Hypoplasia, stenosis and other alterations of the vertebral artery: does impaired blood rheology manifest a hidden disease? *Acta Neurologica Scandinavica*, **97**, 398–403.

Ott, E.O., Lechner, H. & Aranibar, A. (1974). High blood viscosity syndrome in cerebral infarction. *Stroke*, **5**, 330–3.

Pavlakis, S.G., Bello, J., Prohovnik, I. et al. (1988). Brain infarction in sickle cell anemia: magnetic resonance imaging correlates. *Annals of Neurology*, **23**, 125–30.

Pavy, M.D., Murphy, P.L. & Virella, G. (1980). Paraprotein-induced hyperviscosity. A reversible cause of stroke. *Postgraduate Medicine*, **68**, 109–12.

Pearce, J.M., Chandrasekera, C.P. & Ladusans, E.J. (1983). Lacunar infarcts in polycythaemia with raised packed cell volumes. *British Medical Journal*, **287**, 935–6.

Pearson, T.C. & Wetherley-Mein, G. (1978). Vascular occlusive episodes and venous haematocrit in primary proliferative polycythaemia. *Lancet*, **2**, 1219–22.

Pegelow, C.H., Adams, R.J., McKie, V. et al. (1995). Risk of recurrent stroke in patients with sickle cell disease treated with erythrocyte transfusions. *Journal of Pediatrics*, **126**, 896–9.

Perloff, J.K., Rosove, M.H., Child, J.S. & Wright, G.B. (1988). Adults with cyanotic congenital heart disease: hematologic management. *Annals of Internal Medicine*, **109**, 406–13.

Phornphutkul, C., Rosenthal, A., Nadas, A.S. & Berenberg, W. (1973). Cerebrovascular accidents in infants and children with cyanotic congenital heart disease. *American Journal of Cardiology*, **32**, 329–34.

Radack, K., Deck, C. & Huster, G. (1989). Dietary supplementation with low-dose fish oils lowers fibrinogen levels: a randomized, double-blind controlled study. *Annals of Internal Medicine*, **111**, 757–8.

Reizenstein, P. (1979). The haematological stress syndrome. *British Journal of Haematology*, **43**, 329–34.

Rosenson, R.S. & Lowe, G.D. (1998). Effects of lipids and lipoproteins on thrombosis and rheology. *Atherosclerosis*, **140**, 271–80.

Rothman, S.M., Fulling, K.H. & Nelson, J.S. (1986). Sickle cell anemia and central nervous system infarction: a neuropathological study. *Annals of Neurology*, **20**, 684–90.

Sakuta, S. (1981). Blood filterability in cerebrovascular disorders, with special reference to erythrocyte deformability and ATP content. *Stroke*, **12**, 824–8.

Schafer, A.I. (1984). Bleeding and thrombosis in the myeloproliferative disorders. *Blood*, **64**, 1–12.

Schneider, R., Schmid-Schonbein, H. & Kiesewetter, H. (1983). The rheological efficiency of parenteral pentoxifylline (Trental) in patients with ischemic brain lesions. Preliminary results. *European Neurology*, **22**(Suppl. 1), 98–104.

Schneider, R., Korber, N., Zeumer, H., Kiesewetter, H., Ringelstein, E.B. & Brockmann, M. (1985). The haemorheological features of lacunar strokes. *Journal of Neurology*, **232**, 357–62.

Schneider, R., Ringelstein, E.B., Zeumer, H., Kiesewetter, H. & Jung, F. (1987). The role of plasma hyperviscosity in subcortical arteriosclerotic encephalopathy (Binswanger's disease). *Journal of Neurology*, **234**, 67–73.

Seplowitz, A.H., Chien, S. & Smith, F.R. (1981). Effects of lipoproteins on plasma viscosity. *Atherosclerosis*, **38**, 89–95.

Silverstein, A., Gilbert, H. & Wasserman, L.R. (1962). Neurologic complications of polycythemia. *Annals of Internal Medicine*, **57**, 909–16.

Simopoulos, A.P. (1991). Omega-3 fatty acids in health and disease and in growth and development. *American Journal of Clinical Nutrition*, **54**, 438–63.

Simpson, I.A., Lorimer, A.R., Walker, I.D. & Davidson, J.F. (1985).

Effect of Ciprofibrate on platelet aggregation and fibrinolysis in patients with hypercholesterolaemia. *Thrombosis and Haemostasis*, **54**, 442–4.

Sloop, G.D. (1996). A unifying theory of atherogenesis. *Medical Hypotheses*, **47**, 321–5.

Somer, T. & Meiselman, H.J. (1993). Disorders of blood viscosity. *Annals of Medicine*, **25**, 31–9.

Stockman, J.A., Nigro, M.A., Mishkin, M.M. & Oski, F.A. (1972). Occlusion of large cerebral vessels in sickle-cell anemia. *New England Journal of Medicine*, **287**, 846–9.

Stout, R.W. & Crawford, V. (1991). Seasonal variations in fibrinogen concentrations among elderly people. *Lancet*, **338**, 9–13.

Strand, T., Asplund, K., Eriksson, S., Hagg, E., Lithner, F. & Wester, P. O. (1984). A randomized controlled trial of hemodilution therapy in acute ischemic stroke. *Stroke*, **15**, 980–9.

Stuart, J., George, A.J., Davies, A.J., Aukland, A. & Hurlow, R.A. (1981). Haematological stress syndrome in atherosclerosis. *Journal of Clinical Pathology*, **34**, 464–7.

Thomas, D.J. (1982). Whole blood viscosity and cerebral blood flow. *Stroke*, **13**, 285–7.

Thomas, D.J., du Boulay, G.H., Marshall, J. et al. (1977a). Cerebral blood-flow in polycythaemia. *Lancet*, **ii**, 161–3.

Thomas, D.J., Marshall, J., Russell, R.W. et al. (1977b). Effect of haematocrit on cerebral blood-flow in man. *Lancet*, **ii**, 941–3.

Tohgi, H., Yamanouchi, H., Murakami, M. & Kameyama, M. (1978). Importance of the hematocrit as a risk factor in cerebral infarction. *Stroke*, **9**, 369–74.

van Hilten, J.J., Haan, J., Wintzen, A.R. et al. (1989). Cerebral infarction in hereditary spherocytosis. *Stroke*, **20**, 1755–6.

Wade, J.P. (1983). Transport of oxygen to the brain in patients with elevated haematocrit values before and after venesection. *Brain*, **106**, 513–23.

Walzl, B., Walzl, M. & Lechner, H. (1994). Extracorporeal fibrinogen and platelet precipitation as a new haemorheological treatment for acute stroke. *Journal of the Neurological Sciences*, **126**, 25–9.

Wells, R. (1970). Syndromes of hyperviscosity. *New England Journal of Medicine*, **283**, 183–6.

Wells, R.E.J. (1964). Rheology of blood in the microvasculature. *New England Journal of Medicine*, **270**, 832–9.

Wood, J.H. & Fleischer, A.S. (1982). Observations during hypervolemic hemodilution of patients with acute focal cerebral ischemia. *Journal of the American Medical Association*, **248**, 2999–3004.

Wood, J.H. & Kee, D. (1985). Hemorheology of the cerebral circulation in stroke. *Stroke*, **16**, 765–72.

Yamauchi, H., Fukuyama, H., Ogawa, M., Ouchi, Y. & Kimura, J. (1993). Hemodilution improves cerebral hemodynamics in internal carotid artery occlusion. *Stroke*, **24**, 1885–90.

Yazdi, R. & Cote, C. (1986). Watershed infarction in a case of polycythemia vera. *Clinical Nuclear Medicine*, **11**, 665–6.

Zannad, F., Voisin, P., Brunotte, F., Bruntz, J.F., Stoltz, J.F. & Gilgenkrantz, J.M. (1988). Haemorheological abnormalities in arterial hypertension and their relation to cardiac hypertrophy. *Journal of Hypertension*, **6**, 293–7.

14

Calcium, hypercalcemia, magnesium, and brain ischemia

Galen V. Henderson[1] and Louis R. Caplan[2]

[1]Department of Neurology, Brigham and Women's Hospital and
[2]Beth Israel Deaconess Medical Center, Boston, MA, USA

Introduction

Calcium is a very important constituent of many organs of the body especially bones and teeth. Normal calcium and magnesium ion concentrations are crucial for the maintenance of homeostatsis and are instrumental in many body functions. Calcium is an important mediator of striatal and smooth muscle contraction, and is integral in many coagulation and other blood reactions. The concentration of ionized calcium is normally much higher in the extracellular spaces than within cells. Excessive entry of calcium into cells promotes cell death (Siesjo & Bengtson, 1989; Siesjo, 1991; Choi, 1995; Orrenius et al., 1992). Hypercalcemia is a relatively common biochemical abnormality that is often caused by hyperparathyroidism but may also be related to a number of pathological entities that include cancer, bone metastases, sarcoidosis, and many other conditions.

Calcium has recently become recognized as a key mediator of cell death in cerebrovascular pathophysiology. Reviews of the neurological manifestations of hypercalcemia rarely discuss stroke, although such has been reported. Magnesium is another important metallic ion that sometimes functions in a reciprocal way to calcium. We herein review the role of calcium in causing and promoting brain ischemia.

Theoretical considerations

Three different effects of hypercalcemia are posited to contribute to the development and severity of brain ischemia: (i) hypercalcemia stimulates vascular smooth muscle causing vasoconstriction, (ii) increased calcium concentrations enhance platelet aggregation and activate the bodies intrinsic coagulation system, and (iii) calcium entry into cells, a process enhanced by an elevated extracellular to intracellular calcium ion gradient, causes cytotoxic effects which promote cell death and brain infarction.

Calcium is an essential mediator of smooth muscle contraction. Contraction of the smooth muscle of blood vessels is often initiated by stimulation of alpha adrenergic receptors which in turn leads to a release of membrane bound calcium. The increase in calcium ion concentration promotes entry of calcium ions through voltage controlled or receptor-operated channels into the cytosol of smooth muscle cells (Tymianski, 1996). Calcium ions bind with the protein calmodulin and activate myosin light chain kinase, which in turn phosphorylates myosin heads. This reaction activates ATPase, an enzyme that cleaves ATP causing conformational change in myosin, and stimulating smooth muscle contraction. When calcium is not present, ATPase activity in smooth muscle is extremely slight, ATP cannot be cleaved, and the contractile process does not take occur. This process is slow and other factors besides calcium ions can have large effects on the intensity of the contractile process (Guyton, 1986).

The role of calcium in smooth muscle contraction has been better understood since clarification of the relationship of calcium to magnesium. Altura et al. (1997) studied 98 patients admitted to hospitals with a diagnosis of either ischemic or hemorrhagic stroke. The stroke patients had early and significant deficits in serum ionized magnesium, but not in total magnesium. Twenty five per cent had >65% reductions in the mean serum ionized magnesium level compared to controls. The stroke patients had significant elevation in the serum ionized calcium/ionized magnesium ratio, a sign of increased vascular tone and vasoconstriction of intracranial arteries. In animals, low concentrations of ionized magnesium resulted in rapid and marked elevations in cytosolic free calcium ions.

Coincident with the rise in intracellular calcium, many of the cerebral vascular smooth muscle cells contracted causing vasospasm. Reintroduction of normal extracellular magnesium ion concentrations failed to either lower the intracellular calcium overload or reverse the rounding-up of the cerebral vascular cells (Altura et al., 1997). These results suggest that changes in magnesium metabolism play an important role in stroke syndromes and in the etiology of intracranial artery vasoconstriction associated with subarachnoid hemorrhage.

Calcium is essential for blood clotting. It is required at multiple levels within the intrinsic and extrinsic pathways of coagulation to form activated blood coagulation factors and convert prothrombin to thrombin. Calcium also plays a role in ADP-induced platelet aggregation and participates in platelet adhesion reactions to various surfaces. Various substances have been used to reduce the concentration of calcium ions in the blood. With potassium citrate, the citrate ion combines with calcium in the blood to cause an un-ionized calcium compound; the lack of ionic calcium prevents coagulation (Guyton, 1986). Severe hypercalcemia can trigger diffuse intravascular coagulation (Bauermeister et al., 1967).

Entry of calcium into cells is known to contribute to cell death. In neurons, the total intracellular calcium content is in the millimolar range, but its physiological intracellular concentration is very low, $<0.1\ \mu M$. To maintain such a large gradient across the cell membrane, the movement of calcium is subject to strict and sensitive control and multiple mechanisms are involved in it homeostasis (Blaustein, 1988; Siesjo & Bengtson, 1989; Miller, 1991). A rise in intracellular calcium can be brought about by one or more of three mechanisms: activation of influx, curtailment of efflux, and reduction in the intracellular calcium buffering capacity, which includes release from internal stores. In hypoxia and ischemia, ATP production fails. The sodium–potassium channels fail, resulting in membrane depolarization. Brain hypoxia leads to a cascade of metabolic changes. Lactate, potassium, free radicals that contain active oxygen species, prostaglandins, leukotrienes, and thromboxane A2 are all present in extracellular fluid in the hypoxic zone in much higher than normal levels. These biochemical changes alter cell membrane function and open voltage-dependent ion channels causing a rise in intracellular calcium (Siesjo & Bengtson, 1989). Other calcium-related damage includes: changes in protein phosphorylation, enhanced proteolysis and microtubular disassembly, production of free radicals, and mitochondrial calcium overload. The combinations of these processes trigger apoptosis and necrotic cell death (Siesjo, 1991; Siesjo & Bengtson, 1989).

Stroke and hypercalcemia – prior reports

The most extensive analysis of the relation between hypercalcemia and stroke was a report by Bostrom and Alveryd (1972) concerning their experience in Stockholm. Among 170 patients with hypercalcemia referred for parathyroid exploration, nine had well-defined strokes. The brain event consisted of a sudden or stepwise onset of severe focal deficits, usually hemiparesis or quadriparesis, without seizures. Although the patients were not evaluated with angiography or modern imaging technology, the events were most likely to be brain infarcts. Four of the nine stroke patients had necropsies that documented brain infarcts in three patients, occlusion of one vertebral and the basilar artery in one patient, and putaminal hemorrhage in one hypertensive patient. The average age of these nine patients was 71.6 years. Some patients also had hypertention; two had atrial fibrillation. Bostrom and Alveryd (1972) screened 2 268 consecutive internal medicine emergency patients for hypercalcemia and identified 12 with hyperparathyroidism, of whom three had had recent strokes. They also screened 86 consecutive stroke patients by repeated measurements of serum calcium and identified two patients with hyperparathyroidism among those patients with brain infarction. No patient with intracerebral hemorrhage was found to be hypercalcemic.

Gorelick and Caplan (1985) reviewed their experience with hypercalcemia and stroke at the Michael Reese Hospital in Chicago. During a 2-year period, among 502 patients seen by the stroke service, six stroke patients had hypercalcemia. The patients were all black and five of the six were women. All were hypertensive and elderly and all had hyperparathyroidism. A parathyroid adenoma and parathyroid hyperplasia were found in two patients; the others all had elevated parathyroid hormone levels. In four patients the hypercalcemia was found at the time of the strokes while the other two patients were known to have hypercalcemia for 5 and 7 years respectively. Three patients had single strokes with sudden onset of hemiplegia. The other patients had multiple instances of multiple focal neurological symptoms and signs that occurred during days, weeks, or months. Two patients had decreased consciousness and two had seizures (Gorelick & Caplan, 1985). Angiography in three patients showed distal branch artery occlusions (two patients) and the third had severe large artery and distal branch narrowing most likely caused by vasoconstriction. The patient with intracranial artery vasoconstriction was a psychotic woman with known longstanding hypercalcemia. She had refused treatment. She was lethargic, restless, confused, and she often hallucinated. She had seizures and multifocal findings on examination. After parathyroidectomy and normalization of serum calcium levels, the patients improved (Gorelick & Caplan, 1985).

Focal seizures have been noted in hypercalcemic patients (Bauermeister et al., 1967; Herishanu et al., 1970; Gorelick & Caplan, 1985). One patient with parathyroid adenoma and acute pancreatitis died after developing focal seizures that led to stupor. Necropsy revealed multiple cerebral microthrombi and scattered microinfarcts and small hemorrhages (Bauermeister et al., 1967).

Case reports have identified vasospasm as the probable mechanism for brain ischemia in some patients with hypercalcemia (Walker et al., 1980; Streeto, 1969; Yarnell & Caplan, 1986).

A 52-year-old woman with hypertension and severe hypercalcemia was evaluated for headache and polyuria (Walker et al., 1980). She developed a left hemiparesis, fluent aphasia, and bilateral Babinski signs. CT scan showed two separate right cerebral infarcts in the parasaggittal parietal lobe in the anterior cerebral artery territory and in the occipital lobe in the posterior cerebral artery territory. Angiography showed intense spasm of the distal right internal carotid and proximal left anterior cerebral and middle cerebral arteries. Localized areas of spasm were also identified in distal cortical branches, and transit of blood was slow through both cerebral hemispheres. After treatment of hypercalcemia, she improved clinically, and repeat angiography showed a marked decrease in cerebral vasospasm (Walker et al., 1980). The patient reported by Yarnell and Caplan (1986) was a 42-year-old hypertensive man who had a brainstem stroke that evolved during 1 week. Two angiograms (performed on days 8 and 20 of the stroke) showed an irregular constriction beginning at the midportion of the basilar artery extending from the anterior inferior cerebellar artery origins to the superior cerebellar artery origins. Serum calcium and parathyroid hormone levels were persistently high. He had a parathyroidectomy. Repeat angiography 18 months after the stroke showed complete normalization of the basilar artery narrowing, identifying vasoconstriction related to hypercalcemia as the explanation for the findings on the initial angiograms (Yarnell & Caplan, 1986).

In some patients, stroke was accompanied by sleepiness, restlessness, confusion, stupor, muscle weakness, hallucination, altered intellectual function and psychosis. In a single case report by Streeto (1969), a patient with hypercalcemia caused by vitamin D intoxication, had visual hallucinations, ataxia and hemianopia. The symptoms in this patient mimicked those often found in patients with vertebro-basilar arterial disease.

Hypercalcemia is most commonly found in older patients and is often accompanied by hypertension. It is often difficult to decide how much of the cerebrovascular pathology in patients with ischemic stroke is related to the elevated serum calcium level and how much is better explained by coexisting hypertension and atherosclerosis.

Investigators have also actively explored the role of calcium and calcium channel blocking agents in contributing to intracranial arterial vasoconstriction related to subarachnoid hemorrhage. The rationale for the use of calcium antagonists in the prevention or treatment of secondary brain ischemia was based on the assumption that these drugs reduce the frequency of vasospasm by counteracting the influx of calcium into vascular smooth-muscle cells. The antivasospastic effect of calcium antagonists was confirmed by many in vitro studies that used intracranial arteries and also by in vivo assessments of arterial lumen changes after experimental subarachnoid hemorrhage. Clinical trials have been undertaken with three calcium antagonists: nimodipine, AT877 (Asahi Chemical Industry Company, Japan), and nicardipine, of which nimodipine was the most extensively used and studied (Feigin et al., 1998). In a review of reported randomized controlled trials of calcium antagonists in patients with subarachnoid hemorrhage, pooled data from trials on all three calcium antagonists, totaling 2434 randomized patients, showed a significant reduction in the frequency of poor outcome, which resulted from a reduction in the frequency of secondary brain ischemia (Feigin et al., 1998). When analysed separately, the nimodipine trials showed a significant reduction in the frequency of a poor outcome, but the nicardipine and AT877 trials did not. Nicardipine and AT877 significantly reduced the frequency of vasospasm, whereas the nimodipine trials showed only a trend toward reduction of a vasospasm. These data suggest that the administration of nimodipine improves outcome in patients with subarachnoid hemorrhage, but it is uncertain whether nimodipine acts by reducing the frequency of vasospasm or through a neuroprotective mechanism, or both. Nicardipine and AT877 reduce the frequency of vasoconstriction, but the effect on overall outcome remains uncertain. Calcium channel blockers have also been used to prophylactically treat common migraine and patients with classic and basilar artery migraine. The rationale behind the use of calcium-channel blockers in migrane is to prevent vasoconstriction.

Dietary calcium and other electrolytes

Recently, there has been some interest in the role of dietary intake of calcium and its relationship to stroke. Iso et al.

(1999) prospectively studied calcium, potassium and magnesium intake and the risk of stroke among 85 746 women who filled out dietary questionnaires. After 1.6 million-years of follow-up, there were 690 strokes (129 subarachnoid hemorrhages, 74 intraparenchymal hemorrhages, 386 ischemic strokes, and 101 strokes of undetermined type). Women in the highest quintile of calcium intake had an adjusted relative risk of ischemic stroke 0.69 compared with those in the lowest quintile (Iso et al., 1999). These investigators concluded that low calcium intake and low potassium intake, might contribute to the increased risk of ischemic stroke in middle-aged women. Due to the design of the study, it remains possible that women in the lowest quintile of calcium had unknown characteristics that may have made them susceptible to ischemic stroke.

References

Altura, B.T., Memon, Z.I., Zang, A. et al. (1997). Low levels of serum ionized magnesium are found in patients early after stroke which result in rapid elevation in cytosolic free calcium and spasm in cerebral vascular muscle cells. *Neuroscience Letters*, **230**, 37–40.

Bauermeister, D.E., Jennings, E.R., Cruse, D.R. & Sedgwick, V.D. (1967). Hypercalcemia with seizures, a clinical paradox. *Journal of the American Medical Association*, **201**, 146–8.

Blaustein, M.P. (1988). Calcium transport and buffering in neurons. *Trends in Neuroscience*, **11**, 438–43.

Bostrom, H. & Alveryd, A. (1972). Stroke in hyperparathyroidism. *Acta Medica Scandinavica*, **192**, 299–308.

Choi, D. (1995). Calcium: still center-stage in hypoxic–ischemic neuronal death. *Trends in Neuroscience*, **18**, 58–60

Feigin, V.L., Rinkel, G.J.E., Algra, A. et al. (1998). Calcium antagonists in patients with subarachnoid hemorrhage: a systemic review. *Neurology*, **50**, 876–83.

Gorelick, P.B. & Caplan, L.R. (1985). Calcium, hypercalcemia, and stroke. Current concepts of cerebrovascular disease. *Stroke*, **20**, 13–17.

Guyton, A.C. (1986). *Textbook of Medical Physiology*, 7th edn. W.B. Saunders Company.

Herishanu, U., Abramsky, O. & Lavy, S. (1970). Focal neurological manifestation in hypercalcemia. *European Neurology*, **4**, 283–8.

Iso, H., Stampfer, M.J., Manson, J.E. et al. (1999). Prospective study of calcium, potassium and magnesium intake and the risk of stroke in women. *Stroke*, **30**, 1772–9.

Miller, R.J. (1991). The control of neuronal Ca^{2+} homeostasis. *Progress in Neurobiology*, **37**, 255–85.

Orrenius, S., Burkitt, M.J., Kass, G.E.N., Dypbukt, J.M. & Nicotera, P. (1992). Calcium ions and oxidative cell injury. *Annals of Neurology*, **32**, S33–42.

Siesjo, B. (1991). The role of calcium in cell death. In *Neurodegenerative Disorders: Mechanisms and Prospects for Therapy*, ed. D. Price, A. Aguayo & H. Thoenen, pp. 35–59. Chichester, UK: Wiley.

Siesjo, B.K. & Bengtson, F. (1989). Calcium fluxes, calcium antagonists, and calcium related pathology in brain ischemia, hypoglycemia and spreading depression: a unifying hypothesis. *Journal of Cerebral Blood Flow and Metabolism*, **9**, 127–40.

Streeto, J.M. (1969). Acute hypercalcemia simulating basilar artery insufficiency. *New England Journal of Medicine*, **280**, 427–9.

Tymianski, M. (1996). Cytosolic calcium concentrations and cell death in vitro. *Advances in Neurology*, **71**, 85–105.

Walker, G.L., Williamson, P.M., Ravich, R.M.B. & Roche, J. (1980). Hypercalcemia associated with cerebral vasospasm causing infarction. *Journal of Neurology, Neurosurgery and Psychiatry*, **43**, 464–7.

Yarnell, P. & Caplan, L.R. (1986). Basilar artery narrowing and hyperparathyroidism: illustrative case. *Stroke*, **17**, 1022–24.

15

Cerebral vasoconstriction syndromes

Aneesh B. Singhal[1], W. Koroshetz[2] and Louis R. Caplan[3]

[1]Department of Neurology and [2]Neurological Intensive Care Unit, Harvard Medical School and
[3]Beth Israel Deaconess Medical Center, Boston, MA, USA

Introduction

Segmental narrowing or 'beading' of intracranial arteries on contrast cerebral angiograms is commonly associated with atherosclerosis, infection, vasculitis and fibromuscular dysplasia. In these conditions the arteries are histologically abnormal and the luminal narrowing is progressive unless the underlying disorder can be treated. Several other conditions, however, are associated with reversible narrowing of segments of histologically normal arteries, demonstrable by serial angiography. This phenomenon of reversible segmental arterial vasoconstriction, sometimes called 'vasospasm', is poorly understood and affects cerebral as well as extracerebral vessels (see Table 15.1). Intracranial vasoconstriction can occasionally persist for days to weeks and can be severe enough to precipitate cerebral ischemia and stroke. Though much less common than cerebral embolism and carotid stenosis, reversible cerebral arterial vasoconstriction (RCV) is an important cause of stroke, particularly in young individuals. RCV can be spontaneous, but more often it is precipitated by drugs or associated with other conditions. In this chapter, the spontaneous form will be discussed in detail and other conditions with RCV outlined briefly.

'Spontaneous' RCV

Call–Fleming syndrome, postpartum angiopathy

History

Stroke and brain ischemia were associated with intracranial arterial 'spasm' for decades, but after the recognition of carotid artery stenosis, embolic stroke and lacunar disease in the 1960s, subarachnoid hemorrhage and migraine emerged as the only two conditions associated with stroke related to possible cerebral vasospasm. In the 1970s, several unusual cases were reported of women who, during pregnancy or early puerperium, developed sudden headaches, nausea, vomiting, seizures and focal neurological deficits, and recovered spontaneously within a few weeks (Fisher, 1971; Millikan, 1976). Cerebrospinal fluid was normal and known thromboembolic etiologies were ruled out. Cerebral angiograms showed slow arterial filling or arterial irregularities that were reversible on serial angiograms. At the Second Conference on Cerebrovascular Diseases, Rascol et al. (1980) presented four such cases, and the entity came to be recognized as 'postpartum angiopathy'.

Similar cases continued to be reported in association with pregnancy (Dupuy et al., 1979; Rousseaux & Guyot, 1981; Rousseaux et al., 1983; Henry et al., 1984), migraine (Henry et al., 1984; Serdaru et al., 1984; Geraud & Fabre, 1984; Laurent et al., 1984; Michel et al., 1985; Case Records of the Massachussetts General Hospital, 1985; Fisher, 1986a) and unruptured intracranial aneurysms (Day & Raskin, 1986; Clarke et al., 1988). Since the ergot derivatives were frequently used in pregnancy and migraine and were known to have vasoconstrictive effects, increased sympathomimetic tone was often implicated in the pathophysiology. Identical cases (Snyder & McCelland, 1978; Bettoni et al., 1984; Van Calanbergh, 1986; Cucciniello et al., 1987) were also posited to have 'isolated benign cerebral vasculitis' since the clinical and angiogram features were virtually indistinguishable and they appeared to respond completely to a short course of steroids, unlike other biopsy-proven cases of cerebral vasculitis. In 1987, Marie Fleming presented two cases with RCV at a Boston Society of Neurology and Psychiatry meeting. Dr C. Miller Fisher recognized the similarity between these and the other previously published cases of RCV (including postpartum

Table 15.1. *Conditions with reversible arterial vasoconstriction*

(*a*) Reversible cerebral vasoconstriction

Spontaneous –
  Call–Fleming syndrome (incl. 'postpartum angiopathy';
    postcarotid endarterectomy)

  Headache disorders –
    classic and common migraine, crash migraine, benign
    orgasmic headache, benign exertional headache,
    thunderclap headache

Associated with –
  Subarachnoid hemorrhage

  Mechanical trauma (head injury, vascular neurosurgery,
    tumours)

  Unruptured intracerebral aneurysms

  Drugs –
    ergot derivatives (bromocryptine, ergotamine, lisuride)
    nasal decongestants (ephedrine, phenylpropanolamine)
    drugs of abuse (cocaine, amphetamines, LSD, heroin,
      marihuana)
    serotonergic drugs (sumatriptan, serotonin reuptake
      inhibitors)
    Erythropoetin[a], intravenous immune globulin (IVIg)

  Tumours – Pheochromocytoma, Carcinoid tumour

  Hypercalcemia

  Eclampsia[a]

  Porphyria[a]

(*b*) Reversible vasoconstriction of systemic arteries

Extremities: Raynaud's phenomenon, digit ischemia from
  vasoconstrictive drugs

Coronary: Prinzmetal's angina, cocaine-induced coronary
  vasospasm

Renal: possible small-vessel vasoconstriction due to tacrolimus,
  cyclosporine

Mesenteric: associated with carcinoid tumour, sumatriptan

Uterine: eclampsia

Note:
[a] Conditions associated with Reversible Posterior
  Leukoencephalopathy Syndrome.

angiopathy). In a collaborative effort they reported 19 cases as 'Reversible Cerebral Arterial Segmental Vasoconstriction syndrome' (Call et al., 1988), which is now known as the Call–Fleming syndrome. In their report the vasoconstriction was either spontaneous or associated with vasoactive drugs (ergot derivatives), unruptured saccular aneurysms, carotid endarterectomy and Guillain–Barre syndrome. Although the precise pathophysiology was unknown, 'migrainous vasospasm' was considered likely.

Clinical features

The Call–Fleming syndrome predominantly affects women, usually of childbearing age (20–50 years). Many cases are associated with pregnancy and puerperium (Fisher, 1971; Millikan, 1976; Rascol et al., 1980; Dupuy et al., 1979; Rousseaux & Guyot, 1981; Rousseaux et al., 1983; Henry et al., 1984; Bogousslavsky et al., 1989; Kulig et al., 1991; Barinagarrementeria et al., 1992; Raroque et al., 1993; Janssens et al., 1995; Comabella et al., 1996; Lucas et al., 1996; Chartier et al., 1997; Roh & Park, 1998; Sugiyama et al., 1997), possibly due to the frequent use of vasoactive ergot derivatives. Symptoms may begin during delivery or during the first 1–2 weeks thereafter. Some women have developed the syndrome at the time of the menopause. Few cases have followed carotid endarterectomy (Call et al., 1988; Brick et al., 1990; Lopes-Valdes et al., 1997). There is often a history of migraine (Serdaru et al., 1984; Geraud & Fabre, 1984; Laurent et al., 1984; Michel et al., 1985; Case Records of the Massachusetts General Hospital, 1985; Fisher, 1986a; Breen et al., 1994; Martin-Araguz et al., 1997), and four cases have been associated with thunderclap headache (Day & Raskin, 1986; Clarke et al., 1988; Singhal et al., 1999). Emotional disturbances (e.g. sudden fear, orgasm, excitement) are sometimes reported at the onset (Call et al., 1988; Iglesias & Baron, 1994). We have encountered a young man whose syndrome was precipitated by an intense burning sensation of the palate after ingestion of a spicy red jalapeno pepper! Presentation is usually dramatic with abrupt onset of severe headaches, nausea, focal deficits and sometimes seizures. The catastrophic headaches often warrant an evaluation for subarachnoid hemorrhage that turns out to be negative. Blood pressure may be normal or elevated, though usually not elevated to the levels seen in hypertensive encephalopathy. The headaches may be generalized or localized to the occiput or vertex, may recur intermittently for a few weeks, and may be exacerbated by physical exertion, straining or coughing. Generalized motor seizures may initially occur and are attributed to brain ischemia from severe vasoconstriction. Neurological deficits, if present, occur in the first few days after onset of the headache and often localize to the occipital lobes and 'borderzone' arterial territories. Cortical blindness, Balint's syndrome, flashing lights and scotomas in the visual fields, confusion, apraxia, dysarthria, aphasia, numbness, hemiparesis and ataxia have been reported. The clinical deficits usually recover within days to weeks, and headaches usually improve within a few weeks or months, either spontaneously or after treatment with vasodilators or steroids. Some cases are associated with a devastating course and even death (Beuckle et al., 1964)

Differential diagnosis

Cases with RCV are difficult to diagnose, and on initial evaluation the two major considerations are subarachnoid hemorrhage and primary cerebral vasculitis. The former is ruled out by the absence of blood on brain imaging or cerebrospinal fluid. Vasculitis is suggested by the presence of 'beading' on cerebral angiograms. However, as opposed to patients with this inflammatory and often fatal condition, patients with RCV usually present with sudden onset of headache, have normal CSF, and recover without immunosuppressive treatment. Calabrese et al. (1993) have suggested the term 'benign angiopathy' to emphasize these important differences between the two conditions (Calabrese et al., 1993). Given the presence of sudden severe headaches and posterior-predominant neurological symptoms, hypertensive encephalopathy and vertebral artery dissection should be considered in the differential diagnoses.

Etiology

The etiology of the sudden, prolonged and spontaneously reversible vasoconstriction in the Call–Fleming syndrome is not understood. Most reports have implicated 'migrainous vasospasm' in view of the frequent prior history of migraine and the severe headache, nausea, vomiting and visual symptoms that characterize the onset. The association of cerebral vasoconstriction with conditions like subarachnoid hemorrhage, carotid endarterectomy, head injury, surgery, hypercalcemia, hypertension and use of sympathomimetic or serotonergic drugs, lead to speculation that chemical factors, e.g. circulating catecholamines, serotonin, endothelin-1, calcium as well as mechanical factors, e.g. shear stress, may be involved in the pathophysiology. The frequent occurrence in women, particularly

around the time of delivery and menopause, suggests a role for hormonal influences.

Investigations

Blood counts, sedimentation rate, electrolytes, liver and renal function tests are invariably normal. Cerebrospinal fluid (CSF) examination, performed to rule out subarachnoid hemorrhage and vasculitis, is usually normal although mild elevations of CSF protein have been reported. Toxicology screens, rheumatoid factor, ANA, and urine VMA, 5–HIAA and ALA may be useful to rule out other conditions listed in the table. In reports of RCV, brain and temporal artery biopsy have been normal (Serdaru et al., 1984; Call et al., 1988; Singhal et al., 1999). There appears to be no role for biopsy other than to exclude a possible diagnosis of cerebral vasculitis.

Neuroimaging

Computerized tomograms and magnetic resonance imaging scans of the brain may show multifocal areas of infarction usually in posterior or 'borderzone' locations, similar to migraine-associated strokes. The calcarine cortex and medial occipital lobes are usually spared and this helps differentiate from embolic posterior cerebral artery strokes. In a recently reported case (Singhal et al., 1999), initial diffusion-weighted MRI (DWI) showed small occipital strokes but perfusion weighted MRI showed large surrounding areas of hypoperfusion; a second DWI showed enlargement of strokes within the areas of hypoperfusion (Fig. 15.1). These findings suggest that the infarctions result from severe vasoconstriction and hypoperfusion. Areas of brain hemorrhage, possibly resulting from reperfusion injury, have been reported (Rousseaux et al., 1983; Comabella et al., 1996; Roh & Park, 1998; Sugiyama et al., 1997; Breen et al., 1994). Contrast cerebral angiograms are by definition abnormal, and the intracranial portions of Circle of Willis arteries seem to be selectively involved. Multifocal areas of segmental narrowing and dilatation are characteristic, mostly in large and medium-sized arteries like the posterior and middle cerebral arteries and their branches. These abnormalities resolve in weeks or months (Fig. 15.2). The four patients with thunderclap headache mentioned earlier (Day & Raskin, 1986; Clarke et al., 1988; Singhal et al., 1999) also had small, unruptured, intracranial carotid artery aneurysms. Thunderclap headache is an entity independently associated with vasoconstriction (Slivka & Philbrook, 1995; Dodick et al., 1999) and the prevailing view is that the aneurysms in these cases were probably incidental (Dodick et al., 1999; Wijdicks et al., 1988). Transcranial Doppler studies may show diffusely elevated blood flow velocities and as suggested by Bogousslavsky et al. (1989), can be used in follow-up to establish reversal of vasoconstriction (Fig. 15.3). CT- and MR- angiograms are other useful noninvasive follow-up tests.

Treatment

There is no specific or established treatment. Vasodilators (e.g. calcium channel blockers) and steroids have been administered but resolution is usually spontaneous and occurs within weeks to months. Serial angiograms invariably show complete resolution of vasoconstriction. Despite the severe migraine-like headaches, antimigraine drugs like sumatriptan and ergot derivatives are best avoided since they have vasoconstrictive effects that may precipitate further vasoconstriction and lead to stroke. As discussed below, acute headaches are sometimes associated with vasoconstriction and further study is required to see if these drugs are contraindicated in all patients with acute, severe headaches.

RCV in headache disorders

RCV has been seen on serial angiograms in several patients with migraine (Dukes & Veith, 1964; Jensen et al., 1981;

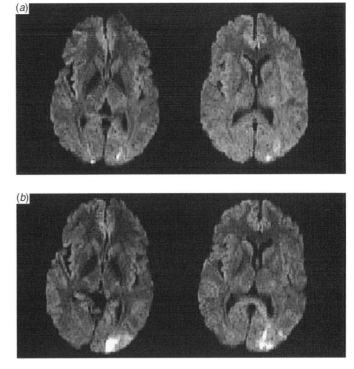

Fig. 15.1. Serial diffusion-weighted imaging (DWI) in a patient with Call–Fleming Syndrome. (*a*) Initial DWI showing small occipital infarctions. Surrounding areas of hypoperfusion, suggesting vasoconstriction, were present on perfusion MR imaging (not shown). (*b*) DWI after 1 week: enlargement of strokes within the hypoperfused areas.

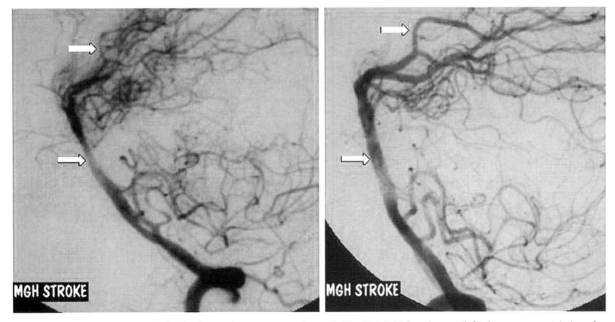

Fig. 15.2. Contrast angiogram in Call–Fleming syndrome, same patient as in Fig. 15.1. Initial angiogram (left) shows vasoconstriction of the basilar and posterior cerebral arteries (arrows). Repeat angiogram after 4 months (right) shows complete reversal of vasoconstriction.

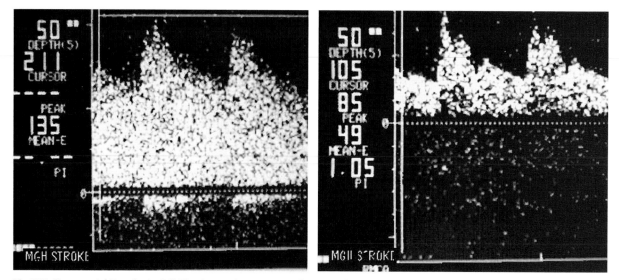

Fig. 15.3. Transcranial Doppler in Call–Fleming syndrome: severe elevation of right MCA blood velocity at time of presentation (left); marked reduction in right MCA blood velocity when test is repeated after 3 months (right).

Masuzawa et al., 1983; Garnic & Schellinger, 1983; Monteiro et al., 1985; Jensen, 1986; Fisher, 1986a; Schon & Harrison, 1987; Thie et al., 1988; Rothrock et al., 1988; Spierings, 1990; Solomon et al., 1990; Cole & Aube, 1990; Schulman & Hershey, 1991; Gomez et al., 1991; Caplan, 1991; Sanin & Mathew, 1993; Nighoghossian et al., 1998; Meschia et al., 1998) and is considered an important mechanism for the prolonged neurological deficits and strokes associated with migraine. Migraine-associated vasoconstriction may be spontaneous (Dukes & Veith, 1964; Jensen et al., 1981; Masuzawa et al., 1983; Garnic & Schellinger, 1983; Monteiro et al., 1985; Jensen, 1986; Fisher, 1986a; Schon & Harrison, 1987; Thie et al., 1988; Rothrock et al., 1988; Spierings, 1990; Solomon et al., 1990; Cole & Aube, 1990; Schulman & Hershey, 1991; Gomez et al., 1991; Caplan, 1991) or secondary to use of vasoactive drugs like ergot derivatives and sumatriptan (Sanin & Mathew, 1993; Nighoghossian et al., 1998; Meschia et al., 1998). RCV has been described with 'acute migraine variants' like thunderclap headache (Slivka & Philbrook, 1995; Dodick et al., 1999), crash migraine (Fisher, 1984), benign orgasmic headache and benign exertional headache (Silbert et al., 1989; Jackson et al., 1993; Kapoor et al., 1990). Since the Call–Fleming syndrome is frequently associated with migraine and thunderclap headache, the distinction between migraine-associated 'vasospasm' and Call–Fleming syndrome is not clear. The similarity between these two conditions has been noted in several reports (Martin-Araguz et al., 1997; Singhal et al., 1999; Iglesias & Baron, 1994; Jackson et al., 1993). In general, patients with Call–Fleming syndrome have a more acute onset of headache and prolonged arterial vasoconstriction.

'Secondary' RCV

Subarachnoid hemorrhage

Subarachnoid hemorrhage (SAH) is the best studied form of RCV and will be discussed only briefly in this chapter. Cerebral arterial 'vasospasm' is known to occur 5–15 days after SAH, usually in the segment of the artery that is surrounded by blood clot (Fisher et al., 1977; Kistler et al., 1983). Severity of vasoconstriction corresponds to the thickness of the clot and severe arterial narrowing may lead to delayed ischemic neurological deficits. In SAH, it is proposed that there is denervation of blood vessels resulting in functional supersensitivity to vasoactive compounds (catecholamines, histamine, serotonin, angiotensin, free radicals, heme degradation products, thromboxane A2, prostaglandins) found in the circulation or released by lysis of red blood cells. Initially the vasospasm is reversible, but severe and prolonged vasoconstriction may lead to endothelial damage and necrosis within the vessel wall, making it less distensible.

Unruptured saccular aneurysms

Cerebral vasoconstriction has been associated with unruptured saccular aneurysms, i.e. without the presence of subarachnoid blood, in a few case reports (Friedman et al.,

1983; Raynor & Messer, 1980; Bloomfield & Sonntag, 1985; Peerless, 1980; Fein, 1980). In most cases the aneurysms were located in the anterior circulation. Arterial narrowing was documented before surgery, immediately after application of the surgical clip, or as a delayed phenomenon. Vasoconstriction occurred in the region of the aneurysm, at a distant site, or as a diffuse phenomenon. Common presenting symptoms were insidious or intractable headache and cranial nerve palsies. The vasoconstriction was sometimes severe enough to cause stroke and was difficult to treat in most cases.

It has been speculated that sudden expansion of the aneurysm may lead to regional endothelial damage with impaired vasodilator production, but this cannot account for cases with distant or diffuse vasoconstriction. Another hypothesis is that surgical manipulation or sudden expansion of the aneurysm causes hypothalamic dysfunction that somehow contributes to vasoconstriction. Since some patients had intense headache, some authors have suggested that pain and stress may stimulate release of endorphins, which trigger release of vasoactive neurotransmitters from the hypothalamus.

Mechanical trauma and neurosurgical manipulation

Cerebral vasospasm has been described in cases of head injury (Suwanwela & Suwanwela, 1972), intracranial vascular procedures (Khodadad, 1973), and after resection of various intracranial tumors (Mawk et al., 1979; Camp et al., 1980; Wilkins, 1980; Ono et al., 1981; Mawk, 1983; Hyde-Rowan et al., 1983; LeRoux et al., 1991; Aoki et al., 1995; Cervoni et al., 1996; Bejjani et al., 1997; Chang et al., 1999). In most of these cases, vasospasm has been related to direct mechanical injury to the vessel wall or contamination of the subarachnoid space with blood. The common association of vasoconstriction with resection of pituitary adenomas and other seller region tumours possibly supports the role of the hypothalamus in causing vasospasm.

Drugs

Angiographic cerebral vasoconstriction has been reported with use of cocaine, amphetamines, heroin, LSD and nasal decongestants (Citron et al., 1970; Krendel et al., 1990; Glick et al., 1987; Margolis et al., 1971; Rumbaugh et al., 1971; Lignelli & Buchheit, 1971; Sobel et al., 1971; Leiberman et al., 1974; Cahill et al., 1981; Yu et al., 1983; Le Coz et al., 1988; Barinagarrementeria et al., 1990; Martin et al., 1995; Ryu & Lin, 1995). Some of these cases (Citron et al., 1970; Krendel et al., 1990; Glick et al., 1987) have had inflammatory CSF findings or pathologic evidence for

inflammation. In others there is no evidence for inflammation and vasoconstriction has been attributed to sympathomimetic drug effects. As mentioned above the ergot derivatives have also been implicated in postpartum angiopathy and migraine-associated vasoconstriction due to their sympathomimetic actions. Recently, vasoconstriction and Call–Fleming syndrome have been described in patients using serotonergic drugs like sumatriptan, selective serotonin reuptake inhibitors, trazodone and dextromethorphan (Singhal et al., 1999; Nighoghossian et al., 1998; Meschia et al., 1998; Conde Lopez et al., 1998).

Catecholamine-secreting tumours

RCV has been described in two patients with pheochromocytoma and one patient with an atypical carcinoid tumour, where the mechanism was related to high levels of circulating catecholamines (Armstrong & Hayes, 1961; Razavi et al., 1999; Nighoghossian et al., 1994).

Hypercalcemia

Hypercalcemia has been associated with headache, confusion, nausea, vomiting, seizures, hemiparesis, hemianopia and cortical blindness. Neurological deficits are usually transient, but permanent deficits from brain infarction have been reported (Anderson & Lindholm, 1967; Bostrom & Alveryd, 1972; Walker et al., 1980; Kaplan, 1998; Yamamoto et al., 1999). Angiograms and Single Photon Emission Computerized Tomogram (SPECT) studies have documented RCV in cases with hypercalcemia-related brain infarction (Bostrom & Alveryd, 1972; Walker et al., 1980; Kaplan, 1998; Yamamoto et al., 1999; Yarnell & Caplan, 1986). The mechanism has been related to hypercalcemia-induced actin-myosin coupling with activation of vascular smooth muscle. This is discussed in Chapter 14.

Miscellaneous

Eclampsia, severe hypertension and porphyria can cause the 'Reversible Posterior Leukoencephalopathy Syndrome' (RPLS) (Hinchey et al., 1996), a condition characterized by headache, altered mentation, visual symptoms, seizures and posterior-predominant white matter edema on brain imaging. The pathophysiology of RPLS is related to endothelial damage and disordered cerebral autoregulation. It is believed that the cerebral microcirculation is primarily affected; however, some patients with eclampsia, porphyria and RPLS have had vasoconstriction of large cerebral vessels on angiogram (Trommer et al., 1988; Will et al., 1987; Black et al., 1995; Ito et al., 1997). Similarly, intravenous immune globulin treatment has been associated with stroke and reversible, posterior-predominant encephalopathy from vasoconstriction affecting small as well as large vessels (Voltz et al., 1996; Sztajzel et al., 1999). Lastly, transient retinal and cerebral vasoconstriction has been associated with the systemic, small-vessel vasoconstriction of Raynaud's phenomenon, particularly in patients who also have migraine (Storimans et al., 1998; Detry-Morel et al., 1995; Levy et al., 1984; Ferracioli et al., 1999).

References

Andersson, L. & Lindholm, T. (1967). Less common manifestations of hyperparathyroidism. *Acta Medica Scandinavica*, **182**, 411–18.

Aoki, N., Origitano, T.C. & al-Mefty, O. (1995). Vasospasm after resection of skull base tumors. *Acta Neurochirurgica (Wien)*, **132**, 53–8.

Armstrong, F.S. & Hayes, G.J. (1961). Segmental cerebral arterial constriction associated with pheochromocytoma. Report of a case with arteriograms. *Journal of Neurosurgery*, **18**, 843–6.

Barinagarrementeria, F., Mendez, A. & Vega, F. (1990). Cerebral hemorrhage associated with the use of phenylpropanolamine (Spanish). *Neurologia*, **5**(8), 292–5.

Barinagarrementeria, F., Cantu, C. & Balderrama, J. (1992). Postpartum cerebral angiopathy with cerebral infarction due to ergonovine use. *Stroke*, **23**, 1364–6.

Bejjani, G.K., Duong, D.H., Kalamarides, M., Ziyal, I. & Sullivan, B.J. (1997). Cerebral vasospasm after tumor resection. *Neurochirurgie*, **43**(3), 164–8.

Bettoni, L., Juvarra, G., Bortone, E. & Lechi, A. (1984). Isolated benign cerebral vasculitis. Case report and review. *Acta Neurologica Belgica*, **84**(4), 161–73.

Beuckle, R.M., DuBoulay, G. & Smith, B. (1964). Death due to cerebral vasospasm. *Journal of Neurology, Neurosurgery and Psychiatry*, **27**, 440–4.

Black, K.S., Mirsky, P., Kalina, P. et al. (1995). Angiographic demonstration of reversible cerebral vasospasm in porphyric encephalopathy. *American Journal of Neuroradiology*, **16**(8), 1650–2.

Bloomfield, S.M. & Sonntag, V.K. (1985). Delayed cerebral vasospasm after uncomplicated operation on an unruptured aneurysm: case report. *Neurosurgery*, **17**(5), 792–6.

Bogousslavsky, J., Respland, P.A., Regli, F. & Dubuis, P.Y. (1989). Postpartum cerebral angiopathy: reversible vasoconstriction assessed by Transcranial Doppler Ultrasounds. *European Neurology*, **29**(2), 102–5.

Bostrom, H. & Alveryd, A. (1972). Stroke in hyperparathyroidism. *Acta Medica Scandinavica*, **192**, 299–308.

Breen, J.C., Caplan, L.R., Wityk, R.J. & Wu, J. (1994). Reversible vasoconstriction, brain hemorrhage, and edema associated with severe migraine. *Stroke*, **25**(1), 262.

Brick, F.J., Dunker, R.O. & Gutierrez, A.R. (1990). Cerebral vasoconstriction as a complication of carotid endarterectomy. *Journal of Neurosurgery*, **73**, 151–3.

Cahill, D.W., Knipp, H. & Mosser, J. (1981). Intracranial hemorrhage with amphetamine abuse. *Neurology*, **31**, 1058.

Calabrese, L.H., Gragg, L.A. & Furlan, A.J. (1993). Benign angiopathy: a distinct subset of angiographically defined primary angiitis of the central nervous system. *Journal of Rheumatology*, **20**, 2046–50.

Call, G.K., Fleming, M.L., Sealfon, S., Levine, H., Kistler, J.P. & Fisher, C.M. (1988). Reversible cerebral segmental vasoconstriction. *Stroke*, **19**(9), 1159–70.

Camp, P.E., Paxton, H.D., Buchan, G.C. & Gahbauer, H. (1980). Vasospasm after transsphenoidal hypophysectomy. *Neurosurgery*, **7**, 382–6.

Caplan, L. (1991). Migraine and vertebrobasilar ischemia. *Neurology*, **41**, 55–61.

Case records of the Massachusetts General Hospital (case 35–1985). (1985). *New England Journal of Medicine*, **313**, 566–75.

Cervoni, I., Salovati, M. & Santoro, A. (1996). Vasospasm following tumor removal: report of five cases. *Italian Journal of Neurological Science*, **17**(4), 291–4.

Chang, S.D., Yap, O.W.S. & Adler, J.R. (1999). Symptomatic vasospasm after resection of a suprasellar pilocytic astrocytoma: case report and possible pathogenesis. *Surgical Neurology*, **51**, 521–7.

Chartier, J.P., Bousigue, J.Y., Teisseyre, A., Morel, C. & Delpeuch-Formosa, F. (1997). Angiopathie cerebrale du post-partum d'origine iatrogenique. *Revue Neurologie (Paris)*, **153**, 212–14.

Citron, B.P., Halpern, M., McCarron, M. et al. (1970). Necrotizing angiitis associated with drug abuse. *New England Journal of Medicine*, **283**(19), 1003–11.

Clarke, C.E., Shepherd, D.I., Chishti, K. & Victoratos, G. (1988). Thunderclap headache. *Lancet*, **ii**, 625.

Cole, A. & Aube, M. (1990). Migraine with vasospasm and delayed intracerebral hemorrhage. *Archives of Neurology*, **47**, 53–6.

Comabella, M., Alvarez-Sabin, J., Rovira, A. & Codina, A. (1996). Bromocryptine and postpartum cerebral angiopathy: a causal relationship? *Neurology*, **46**, 1754–6.

Conde Lopez, V.J.M., Ballesteros Alcaled, M.C., Blanco Garrote, J.A. & Marco Llorente, J. (1998). Cerebral infarction in an adolescent girl following an overdose of paroxetine and caffedrine combined with theodrenaline. *Actas Luso España Neurologica Psiquiatric Cienc Afines*, **26**(5), 333–8. Spanish.

Cucciniello, B., Martellotta, N., Citro, E., Marchese, E., De Trana, L. & Lupo, F.A. (1987). A case of benign acute cerebral angiopathy. *Acta Neurologica (Napoli)*, **9**(4), 291–6.

Day, J.W. & Raskin, N.H. (1986). Thunderclap headache: symptom of unruptured cerebral aneurysm. *Lancet*, **ii**, 1247–8.

Detry-Morel, M., Boschi, A., Gehenot, M. & Geubel, A. (1995). Bilateral transient visual obscurations with headaches during alpha-II interferon therapy: a case report. *European Journal of Ophthalmology*, **5**(4), 271–4.

Dodick, D.W., Brown, R.D. Jr., Britton, J.W. & Huston, J. III. (1999). Nonaneurysmal thunderclap headache with diffuse, multifocal, segmental, and reversible vasospasm. *Cephalalgia*, **19**, 118–23.

Dukes, H.T. & Veith, R.G. (1964). Cerebral arteriography during migraine prodrome and headache. *Neurology*, **14**, 636–9.

Dupuy, B., Lechelavallier, B., Chevallier, D., Theron, J. & Dikstra, R.

(1979). Complications vasculaires cerebrales a rechute liees a la prise de Methergin en milieu obstetrical. *Reviews of Otoneuroophthalmology*, **51**, 293–9.

Fein, J.M. (1980). Unruptured aneurysms and cerebral vasospasm. In *Cerebral Arterial Spasm: Proceedings of the Second International Workshop on Cerebral Vasospasm*, ed. R.H. Wilkins, pp. 499–504. Baltimore: Williams and Wilkins.

Ferraccioli, G., Di Poi, E., Di Gregorio, F., Giazomuzzi, F. & UgoPaolo, G. (1999). Changes in regional cerebral blood flow after a cold hand test in systemic lupus erythematosus patients with Raynaud's syndrome. *Lancet*, **354**(9196), 2135–6.

Fisher, C.M. (1971). Cerebral ischemia – less familiar types. (Review). *Clinical Neurosurgery*, **18**, 267–336.

Fisher, C.M. (1984). Painful states: a neurologic commentary. *Clinical Neurosurgery*, **31**, 32–53.

Fisher, C.M. (1986a). Late life migraine accompaniments – further experience. *Stroke*, **17**(5), 1033–42.

Fisher, C.M. (1986b). Unusual vascular events in the territory of the posterior cerebral artery. *Canadian Journal of Neurological Science*, **13**, 1–7.

Fisher, C.M. Roberson, G.H. & Ojemann, R.G. (1977). Cerebral vasospasm with ruptured saccular aneurysm – the clinical manifestations. *Neurosurgery*, **1**, 243–8.

Friedman, P., Gass, H. & Magidson, M. (1983). Vasospasm with an unruptured and unoperated aneurysm. *Surgical Neurology*, **19**, 21–5.

Garnic, J.D. & Schellinger, D. (1983). Arterial spasm as a finding intimately associated with onset of vascular headache. *Neuroradiology*, **24**, 273–6.

Geraud, G. & Fabre, N. (1984). Angiopathie cerebrale aigne benigne. *Presse Medecin*, **13**, 1095.

Glick, R., Hoying, J., Cerullo, L. & Perlman, S. (1987). Phenylpropanolamine: an over-the-counter drug causing central nervous system vasculitis and intracerebral hemorrhage. *Neurosurgery*, **20**, 969–74.

Gomez, C.R., Gomez, S.M., Puricelli, M.S. & Malik, M.M. (1991). Transcranial Doppler in reversible migrainous vasospasm causing cerebellar infarction: report of a case. *Angiology*, **42**(2), 152–6.

Henry, P.Y., Larre, P., Aupy, M., Lafforgue, J.L. & Orgogozo, J.M. (1984). Reversible cerebral arteriopathy associated with the administration of ergot derivatives. *Cephalalgia*, **4**(3), 171–8.

Hinchey, J., Chaves, C., Appignani, B. et al. (1996). A reversible posterior leukoencephalopathy syndrome. *New England Journal of Medicine*, **334**, 494–500.

Hyde-Rowan, M.D., Roessmann, U. & Brodkey, J.S. (1983). Vasospasm following transsphenoidal tumor removal associated with the arterial changes of oral contraception. *Surgical Neurology*, **20**, 120–4.

Iglesias, S. & Baron, J.C. (1994). Unusual triggering circumstances of acute benign cerebral angiopathy. A link with exertional headache? *Reviews in Neurology*, **150**(3), 241–4.

Ito, Y., Niwa, H., Iida, T. et al. (1991). Post-transfusion reversible posterior leukoencephalopathy syndrome with cerebral vasoconstriction. *Neurology*, **49**(4), 1174–5.

Jackson, M., Lennox, G., Jaspen, T. & Jefferson, D. (1993). Migraine angiitis precipitated by sex headache and leading to watershed infarction. *Cephalalgia*, **13**(6), 427–30.

Janssens, E., Hommel, M., Mounier-Vehier, F. et al. (1995). Postpartum cerebral angiopathy possibly due to bromocryptine therapy. *Stroke*, **26**, 128–30.

Jensen, I. (1986). Unusual angiographic appearance during attack of hemiplegic migraine. *Headache*, **26**, 295–6.

Jensen, T., Olivarius, B., Kraft, M. & Hansen, H. (1981). Familial hemiplegic migraine – a reappraisal and a long-term follow-up study. *Cephalalgia*, **1**, 33–9.

Kaplan, P. (1998). Reversible hypercalcemic cerebral vasoconstriction with seizures and blindness: a paradigm for eclampsia? *Clinical Electroencephalography*, **29**(3), 120–3.

Kapoor, R., Kendall, B.E. & Harrison, M.J.G. (1990). Persistent segmental cerebral artery constrictions in coital cephalgia. *Journal of Neurology, Neurosurgery and Psychiatry*, **53**, 266–70.

Khodadad, G. (1973). Middle cerebral artery embolectomy and prolonged widespread vasospasm. *Stroke*, **4**, 446–50.

Kistler, J.P., Crowell, R.M., Davis, K.R. et al. (1983). The relation of cerebral vasospasm to the extent and location of subarachnoid blood visualized by CT scan: a prospective study. *Neurology*, **33**, 424–36.

Krendel, D.A., Ditter, S.M., Frankel, M.R. & Ross, W.K. (1990). Biopsy-proven cerebral vasculitis associated with cocaine abuse. *Neurology*, **40**, 1092–4.

Kulig, M., Moore, L., Kirk, M., Smith, D., Stallworth, J. & Rumack, B. (1991). Bromocryptine-associated headache: possible life-threatening sympathomimetic interaction. *Obstetrics and Gynecology*, **78**, 941.

Laurent, B., Michel, D., Antoine, J.C. & Montagnon, D. (1984). Migraine basilaire avec alexie sans agraphie: spasme arteriale a l'arteriographie et effet de la naloxone. *Revue Neurologie (Paris)*, **140**(11), 663–5.

Le Coz, P., Woimant, F., Rougemont, D. et al. (1988). Angiopathies cerebrales benignes et phenylpropanolamine. *Revue Neurologie (Paris)*, **144**(4), 295–300.

LeRoux, P.D., Haglund, M.M., Mayberg, M.R. & Winn, H.R. (1991). Symptomatic cerebral vasospasm following tumor resection: report of 2 cases. *Surgical Neurology*, **36**, 25–31.

Levy, A., Kuritzky, A., Salamon, F. et al. (1984). Raynaud's phenomenon complicated by recurrent brain infarction. *Headache*, **24**, 256–8.

Lieberman, A.N., Bloom, W., Kishore, P.S. & Lin, J.P. (1974). Carotid artery occlusion following ingestion of LSD. *Stroke*, **5**, 213.

Lignelli, G.J. & Buchheit, W.A. (1971). Angiitis in drug abusers. *New England Journal of Medicine*, **284**, 112.

Lopes-Valdes, E., Chang, H.M., Pessin, M.S. & Caplan, L.R. (1997). Cerebral vasoconstriction after carotid surgery. *Neurology*, **49**, 303–4.

Lucas, C., Deplanque, D., Salhi, A., Hachulla, E. & Doumith, S. (1996). Angiopathie benigne du post-partum: un cas clinicoradiologique associe a la prise de bromocryptine. *Revue Medécin Interne*, **17**(10), 839–41.

Margolis, M.T. & Newton, T.H. (1971). Methamphetamine ('speed') arteritis. *Neuroradiology*, 2, 179.

Martin, K., Rogers, T. & Kavanaugh, A. (1995). Central nervous system angiopathy associated with cocaine abuse. *Journal of Rheumatology*, 22, 780–2.

Martin-Araguz, A., Fernandez-Armayor, V., Moreno-Martinez, J.M. et al. (1997). Segmental arteriographic anomalies in migrainous cerebral infarct. *Reviews of Neurology*, 25(138), 225–9.

Masuzawa, T., Shinoda, S., Furuse, M., Nakahara, N., Abe, F. & Sato, F. (1983). Cerebral angiographic changes on serial examination of a patient with migraine. *Neuroradiology*, 24, 277–81.

Mawk, J.R. (1983). Vasospasm after pituitary surgery (letter). *Journal of Neurosurgery*, 58, 972.

Mawk, J.R., Ausman, J.I., Erikson, D.L. & Maxwell, R.E. (1979). Vasospasm following transcranial removal of large pituitary adenomas. *Journal of Neurosurgery*, 50, 229–32.

Meschia, J.F., Malkoff, M.D. & Biller, J. (1998). Reversible segmental cerebral arterial vasospasm and cerebral infarction: possible association with excessive use of Sumatriptan and Midrin. *Archives of Neurology*, 55, 712–14.

Michel, D., Vial, C., Antoine, J.C., Laurent, B., Portafaix, M. & Trillet, M. (1985). Acute benign cerebral angiopathy. A review of 4 cases. *Reviews of Neurology*, 141(12), 786–92.

Millikan, C.H. (1976) Discussion. Accidents vasculaires cerebraux chez les femmes agees de 15 a 45. In *Cerebrovascular Diseases, I Conference de le Salpetrière*, pp. 77–84. Paris: JB Baillière.

Monteiro, P., Carneiro, L., Lima, B. & Lopes, C. (1985). Migraine and cerebral infarction; three case studies. *Headache*, 25, 429–33.

Nighoghossian, N., Trouillas, P., Loire, R., Perrin, L., Trilet, V. & Gamondes, P. (1994). Catecholamine syndrome, carcinoid lung tumor and stroke. *European Neurology*, 34, 288–9.

Nighoghossian, N., Derex, L. & Trouillas, P. (1998). Multiple intra-cerebral hemorrhages and vasospasm following antimigrainous drug abuse. *Headache*, 38, 478–80.

Ono, M., Misumi, S. & Nukui, H. (1981). Vasospasm following removal of a large pituitary adenoma by the subfrontal approach. Report of a case and review of the literature. *Neurologica Medica Chirurgica (Tokyo)*, 21, 609–14.

Peerless, S. (1980). Postoperative cerebral vasospasm without sub-arachnoid hemorrhage. In *Cerebral Arterial Spasm: Proceedings of the Second International Workshop on Cerebral Vasospasm*, ed. R.H. Wilkins, pp. 496–8. Baltimore: Williams and Wilkins.

Raroque, H.G., Tesfa, G. & Purdy, P. (1993). Postpartum cerebral angiopathy. Is there a role for sympathomimetic drugs? *Stroke*, 24, 2108–10.

Rascol, A., Guiraud, B., Manelfe, C. & Clanet, M. (1980). Accidents vasculaires cerebraux de la grosesse et du post partum. In *Cerebrovascular Diseases, II Conference de le Salpetrière*, pp. 84–127. Paris: J.B. Baillière.

Raynor, R. & Messer, H. (1980). Severe vasospasm with an unrup-tured aneurysm: case report. *Neurosurgery*, 6, 92–5.

Razavi, M., Bendixen, B., Maley, J.E. et al. (1999). CNS pseudovas-culitis in a patient with pheochromocytoma. *Neurology*, 52(5), 1088–90.

Roh, J.K. & Park, K.S. (1998). Postpartum cerebral angiopathy with

intracerebral hemorrhage in a patient receiving lisuride. *Neurology*, 50, 1152–4.

Rothrock, J., Walicke, P., Swenson, M., Lyden, P. & Logan, W. (1988). Migrainous stroke. *Archives of Neurology*, 45, 63–7.

Rousseaux, P. & Guyot, J.F. (1981). Une nouvelle variete d'arteri-opathie cerebrale. A propos de 3 cas. *Neurochirurgie*, 27, 141.

Rousseaux, P., Scherpereel, B., Bernard, M.H. & Guyot, J.F. (1983). Acute benign cerebral angiopathy. 6 cases (French). *Presse Medecin*, 12(35), 2163–8.

Rumbaugh, C.L., Bergeron, R.T., Fang, H.C.H. & McCormick, R. (1971). Cerebral angiographic changes in the drug abuse patient. *Radiology*, 101, 335.

Ryu, S.J. & Lin, S.K. (1995). Cerebral arteritis associated with oral use of phenylpropanolamine: report of a case. *Journal of the Formos Medical Association*, 94(1–2), 53–5.

Sanin, L.C. & Mathew, N.T. (1993). Severe diffuse intracranial vasospasm as a cause of extensive migrainous cerebral infarc-tion. *Cephalalgia*, 13, 289–92.

Schon, F. & Harrison, M.J.H. (1987). Can migraine cause multiple segmental artery constrictions? *Journal of Neurology, Neurosurgery and Psychiatry*, 50, 492–4.

Schulman, E.A. & Hershey, B. (1991). An unusual angiographic picture in status migrainosus. *Headache*, 31, 396–8.

Serdaru, M., Chiras, J., Cujas, M. & Lhermitte, F. (1984). Isolated benign cerebral vasculitis or migrainous vasospasm? *Journal of Neurology, Neurosurgery and Psychiatry*, 47, 73–6.

Silbert, P.L., Hankey, G.J., Prentice, D.A. & Apsimon, H.T. (1989). Angiographically demonstrated arterial spasm in a case of benign sexual headache and benign exertional headache. *Australia and New Zealand Journal of Medicine*, 19, 466–8.

Singhal, A., Begleiter, A., Rordorf, G. & Koroshetz, W. (1999). Vasoconstriction and stroke related to the use of selective serot-onin reuptake inhibitors. *Neurology*, 52(6), A241, Abstract P03.129.

Slivka, A. & Philbrook, B. (1995). Clinical and angiographic features of thunderclap headache. *Headache*, 35, 1–6.

Snyder, B.D. & McCelland, R.R. (1978). Isolated benign cerebral vasculitis. *Archives of Neurology*, 35, 612–14.

Sobel, J., Espinas, O.E. & Friedman, S.A. (1971). Carotid artery obstruction following LSD capsule ingestion. *Archives of Internal Medicine*, 127, 290.

Solomon, S., Lipton, R.B. & Harris, P.Y. (1990). Arterial stenosis in migraine: spasm or arteriopathy? *Headache*, 30, 52–61.

Spierings, E.L.H. (1990). Angiographic changes suggestive of vasospasm in migraine complicated by stroke. *Headache*, 30, 727–8.

Storimans, C.W., Fekkes, D., van Dalen, A., Bleeker-Wagemakers, E.D. & Oosterhuis, J.A. (1998). Serotoninergic status in patients with hereditary vascular retinopathy syndrome. *British Journal of Ophthalmology*, 82(8), 897–900.

Sugiyama, Y., Muroi, A., Ishikawa, M., Tsukamoto, T. & Yamamoto, T. (1997). A benign form of isolated angiitis of the central nervous system in puerperium: an identical disorder to postpartum cere-bral angiopathy? *Internal Medicine*, 36(12), 931–4.

Suwanwela, C. & Suwanwela, N. (1972). Intracranial arterial narrowing and spasm in acute head injury. *Journal of Neurosurgery*, **36**, 314–23.

Sztajzel, R., Floch-Rohr, J. & Eggimann, P. (1999). High-dose intravenous immunoglobulin treatment and cerebral vasospasm: a possible mechanism of ischemic encephalopathy? *European Neurology*, **41**, 153–8.

Thie, A., Spitzer, K., Lachenmayer, L. & Kunze, K. (1988). Prolonged vasospasm in migraine detected by noninvasive transcranial Doppler ultrasound. *Headache*, **28**, 183–6.

Trommer, B.L., Homer, D. & Mikhael, M. (1988). Cerebral vasospasm and eclampsia. *Stroke*, **19**, 326–9.

Van Calanbergh, F., van den Bergh, V. & Wilms, G. (1986). Benign isolated arteritis of the central nervous system. *Clinical Neurological Neurosurgery*, **88**, 267–73.

Voltz, R., Rosen, F.V., Yousry, T., Beck, J. & Hohfeld, R. (1996). Reversible encephalopathy with cerebral vasospasm in a Guillain–Barré syndrome patient treated with intravenous immunoglobulin. *Neurology*, **46**(1), 250–1.

Walker, G., Williamson, P., Ravish, R. & Roche, J. (1980). Hypercalcemia associated with cerebral vasospasm causing infarction. *Journal of Neurology, Neurosurgery and Psychiatry*, **43**, 464–7.

Wijdicks, E.F.M., Kerkhoff, H. & Van Gijn, J. (1988). Cerebral vasospasm and unruptured aneurysm in thunderclap headache. *Lancet*, **ii**(8618), 1020.

Wilkins, R.H. (1980). Intracranial arterial spasms after procedures other than operations for intracranial aneurysms. In *Cerebral Arterial Spasm*, ed. R.H. Wilkins, pp. 505–9. Baltimore: Williams and Wilkins.

Will, A.D., Lewis, K.L., Hinshaw, D.B. et al. (1987). Cerebral vasoconstriction in toxemia. *Neurology*, **37**, 1555–7.

Yamamoto, Y., Georgiadis, A.L., Chang, H.M. & Caplan, L.R. (1999). Posterior cerebral artery territory infarcts in the New England Medical Center Posterior Circulation Registry. *Archives of Neurology*, **56**(7), 824–32.

Yarnell, P.R. & Caplan, L.R. (1986). Basilar artery narrowing and hyperparathyroidism: illustrative case. *Stroke*, **17**, 1022–4.

Yu, Y.J., Cooper, D.R., Wellenstein, D.E. & Block, B. (1983). Cerebral angiitis and intracerebral hemorrhage associated with methamphetamine abuse: case report. *Journal of Neurosurgery*, **58**, 109.

16

Eclampsia and stroke during pregnancy and the puerperium

Karla B. Kanis[1] and Louis R. Caplan[2]

[1]PAREXEL International, Waltham, MA, USA
[2]Beth Israel Deaconess Medical Center, Boston, MA, USA

Introduction

Toxemia of pregnancy (toxemia gravidarum) is an old term that included the wide spectrum of findings related to the acute or subacute development of hypertension during pregnancy. The term literally means a toxin in the blood reflecting the idea that some toxic substance released somehow from the uterus, placenta, or fetus was responsible for the disorder. The designations eclampsia and pre-eclampsia are now preferred.

Pre-eclampsia is characterized by hypertension, proteinuria, and edema. These findings usually develop during the second half of pregnancy usually after the 20th week of pregnancy. Pre-eclampsia may also develop during the early postpartum period. The blood pressure is usually around 140/90, or is elevated more than 30 mm Hg systolic or 15 mm Hg diastolic above the blood pressure in the first trimester. The hypertension may be quite labile because of sensitivity of the blood pressure to endogenous peptides and amines (Lindheimer & Katz, 1991). Proteinuria consists of more than 1+ proteinuria on dipstick testing, or greater than 300 mg protein in a 24-hour period. The edema of pre-eclampsia affects the hands and face in addition to the legs.

Pre-eclampsia may affect many organ systems and can lead to pulmonary edema, oliguria, renal failure, disseminated intravascular coagulopathy (DIC), and hepatic hemorrhages. Patients with pre-eclampsia may have neurologic symptoms including agitation, confusion, headache, difficulty concentrating, visual abnormalities including photophobia, hallucinations and blindness, that result from changes that affect the eye or the occipital lobe. Patients may become lethargic or comatose, and develop abnormally brisk reflexes. When seizures or coma occur in patients with pre-eclampsia, the condition is then designated as eclampsia. The diagnoses of pre-eclampsia and eclampsia are based on the clinical symptoms and signs, and laboratory abnormalities which may include elevated serum creatinine and uric acid, thrombocytopenia, decreased level of antithrombin lll, disseminated intravascular coagulation, and a syndrome characterized by hemolysis, elevated liver enzymes, and low platelets (HELLP syndrome).

The incidence of pre-eclampsia in the United States ranges between 6 and 10% of pregnancies (Chesley, 1978; Kaunitz et al., 1985; Schobel et al., 1996). Although the frequency of eclampsia has declined, pre-eclampsia and eclampsia are major causes of maternal and fetal mortality. The frequency of detection and treatment of pre-eclampsia depends on the availability and quality of prenatal care. Although classically considered as a disorder of pregnancy, puerperal eclampsia is also quite common. Many obstetricians will only use the term eclampsia when the findings occur during the first 48 hours after delivery, but identical findings can develop later during the first postpartum week. The clinical neurological symptoms and the imaging studies in patients presenting with these symptoms and signs greater than 2 days postpartum have been consistent with previously described patients with classic eclampsia (Raps et al., 1993; Stander et al., 1946).

Although pre-eclampsia is most often found in nulliparous, poorly nourished women, other high risk groups include multiparous women over the age of 35 who have extrauterine pregnancies, multiple pregnancies or hydatidiform moles (Sibai, 1989).

Strokes and encephalopathy associated with pre-eclampsia and eclampsia

In addition to the neurologic features of headache, confusion and seizures, some patients develop focal deficits of sudden onset, consistent with a clinical diagnosis of stroke. In two population-based studies, pre-eclampsia and eclampsia have accounted for 24–47% of ischemic strokes during pregnancy or the puerperium and have also accounted for 14–44% of intracerebral hemorrhages during this same time period (Kittner et al., 1996; Sharshar et al., 1995). Intraparenchymal hemorrhages are a common finding in fatal cases; they are found in >40% of patients studied at necropsy (Mas & Lamy, 1998a,b; Sheehan & Lynch, 1973; Richards et al., 1988).

Among the seven patients with hemorrhage in the 'Ile de France' study, eclampsia was associated with the HELLP syndrome (hemolysis, elevated liver enzymes, and low platelet count) in two patients, and with disseminated intravascular coagulopathy (DIC) in another two patients. The majority of intracerebral hemorrhages in the eclamptic patients (4/7) were lobar in location, with the brainstem (2/7) and lenticulostriate territory (1/7) accounting for the other locations.

The timing of ischemic strokes and intracerebral hemorrhages tends to cluster in the late third trimester and in the immediate postpartum period. Patients with intracerebral hemorrhage had a poorer outcome compared to the patients with ischemic stroke: three of the seven eclamptic women with hemorrhages died, and the remaining four patients had neurological sequelae, while there were no deaths among the seven women with ischemic strokes. At autopsy, intracerebral hemorrhages range from multiple scattered cortical and subcortical petechiae, to small hemorrhages most often located at cortical–subcortical junctions, to massive hematomas (Mas & Lamy, 1998a,b; Sheehan & Lynch, 1973; Richards et al., 1988).

More common than strokes is an encephalopathic disorder which is reversible if hypertension is effectively and rapidly controlled. The initial symptom is usually headache. Agitation, and reduced alertness follow. Visual aberrations are common and range from severe cortical blindness, to vivid visual hallucinations, to visual agnosias of the Balint type. Difficulty making new memories, impaired concentration, and loss of precision in language are often found when sought. Hemianopia can occur but is less common. Minor motor weakness and ataxia occur but frank paralysis is rare. If untreated, stupor and coma may intervene. The encephalopathy is identical to that found in patients with hypertensive encephalopathy, acute glomerulonephritis with uremia, and in some patients who are given immunosuppressant therapy after organ transplantation (Hinchey et al., 1996).

Brain and vascular imaging

Brain imaging has been used over the years to evaluate several possible central nervous system pathologic conditions that may account for acute neurologic changes in pregnant women. Imaging studies have assisted in the differential diagnosis of such processes as tumour, abscess, aneurysm, postpartum angiopathy, arteriovenous malformations, and dural venous sinus thrombosis, in patients with a clinical presentation similar to that of eclampsia. Computed tomography (CT) has also been used to separate hemorrhage from ischemia from encephalopathy in patients with typical eclampsia. CT scans in eclamptic women have most often shown white matter hypodensities that are usually symmetric, in the cerebral cortex, subcortical white matter, and the supratentorial deep grey matter. These abnormalities are predominantly located within the occipital and parietal areas, and are seen in women with severe pre-eclampsia and eclampsia who have an acute encephalopathy syndrome that usually includes acute development of cortical blindness and/or seizures (Dahmus et al., 1992; Duncan et al., 1989; Lau et al., 1987; Colosimo et al., 1985; Kirby & Jaindl, 1984).

Although CT scans have been abnormal in 33% of eclamptic patients (Dahmus et al., 1992), magnetic resonance imaging (MRI) scans are abnormal in 48–100% of patients with eclampsia (Digre et al., 1993; Raps et al., 1993; Dahmus et al., 1992; Sengar et al., 1997). The changes found on MRI include punctate or confluent areas of increased foci on T_2-weighted images in the centrum semiovale and the deep white matter, predominantly in the posterior parietal and occipital lobes (Dahmus et al., 1992; Hinchey et al., 1996), at the grey–white junction and in the external capsule, the basal ganglia, and occasionally in the cerebellum (Sengar et al., 1997). In pre-eclamptic patients, in one study, the abnormalities were present in the white matter only, and predominantly in the frontal and parietal areas, and not at the grey–white junction (Digre et al., 1993). In one study, these abnormalities were prevalent in the border-zone territory of the anterior, middle, and posterior cerebral arteries (Dahmus et al., 1992). Patients with eclampsia sometimes have a characteristic curvilinear abnormality at the grey–white matter junction, that was not seen in patients with pre-eclampsia, and this finding was used to help differentiate various causes of neurological symptoms in pregnant women (Digre, 1993; Sengar, 1997). Most often, there is no evidence of microhemorrhages or microinfarcts, but this may be secondary to the microscopic size of the lesions, and to the limits of the MR resolution. Figures 16.1 and 16.2 show MRIs from two different patients with eclampsia.

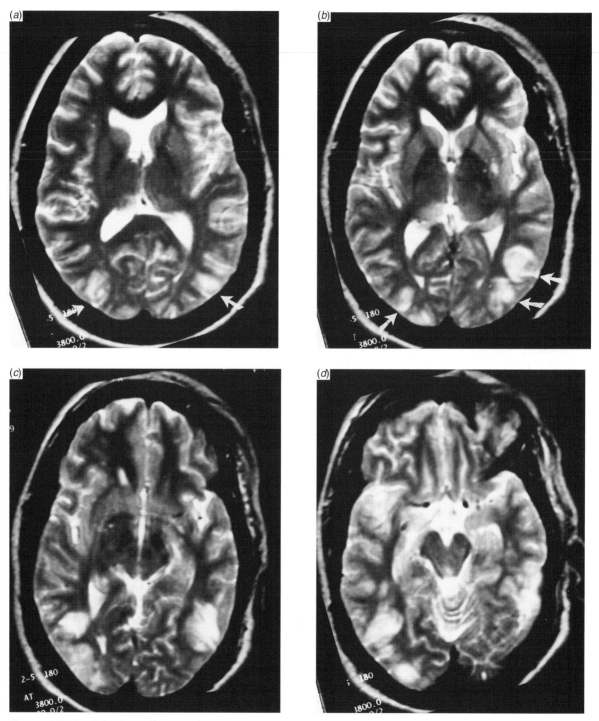

Fig. 16.1. MRI T$_2$-weighted scans from an eclamptic patient: a 28-week pregnant 33-year-old woman found unresponsive at home. BP 220/120. When aroused she had visual field defects and visual hallucinations. (*a*) and (*b*) are axial sections taken near the genu of the internal capsule showing hypersignals in the posterior portions of the temporal lobes (white arrows) and a signal abnormality shown in (*b*) in the posterior thalamus. (*c*) and (*d*) are axial sections taken through the midbrain showing larger regions of abnormal signal in the temporo-occipital lobes. (*e*) is a follow-up scan taken 6 weeks after the initial scans. The visual abnormalities had cleared but she still had difficulty with memory and concentration. The scan was taken in a plane close to (*b*); it shows clearing of the cortical/subcortical abnormalities with persistence of abnormal signals in the posterior thalamus.

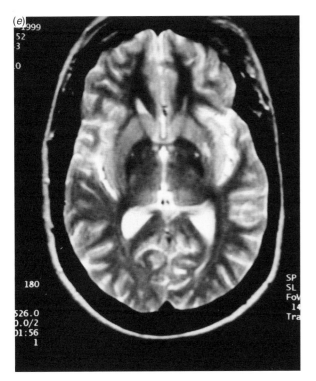

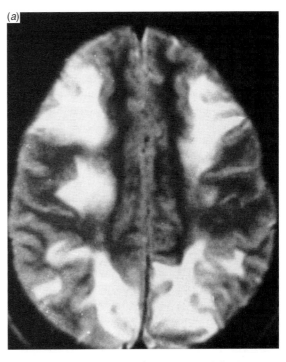

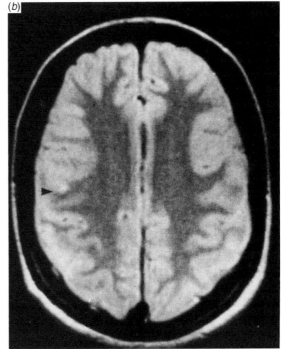

Fig. 16.1. (*cont.*)

The MRI abnormalities of hyperintense and hypointense signal on T_2-weighted and T_1-weighted images, respectively, located in the posterior parietal and occipital lobes have been shown to be reversible in most of the patients studied (Hinchey et al., 1996; Raps et al., 1993; Schwartz et al., 1992; Sanders et al., 1991; Raroque et al., 1990; Duncan et al., 1989; Sengar et al., 1997). Further analysis of the reversible abnormalities seen on T_2-weighted images, using diffusion-weighted imaging (DWI), has shown that these areas have an increased diffusion coefficient and are thus consistent with areas of vasogenic edema (Schaefer et al., 1997). CT and MRI showed similar areas of involvement in 30–80% of patients (Dahmus et al., 1992; Raroque et al., 1990). Hemorrhages are occasionally found but these are much less common than areas of vasogenic edema.

Vasoconstriction has been documented by angiography on several occasions in patients with eclampsia and focal neurologic signs such as lateral gaze paralysis or hemiparesis (Tommer et al., 1988; Call et al., 1988; Raps et al., 1993; Will et al, 1987). The vasoconstriction usually involves large arteries along the circle of Willis as well as small circumferential branch arteries. The constriction can be diffuse, but more often is multifocal with areas of vasoconstriction alternating with regions of vasodilatation, giving the vessels a sausage-shaped appearance. Magnetic resonance

Fig 16.2. Patient with postpartum eclampsia. She had left hemiparesis which cleared within 48 hours. MRI T_2-weighted sequences (TR 2000, TE 100) axial sections: (*a*) Right frontal and bilateral posterior parieto-occipital increased signals. (*b*) Disappearance of the hypersignals except for a small focal abnormality at the cortical–white matter junction (black arrowhead. (From Mas, J-L. & Lamy, C. 1998 with permission.)

angiography (MRA) has shown similar vascular abnormalities, (Sengar et al., 1997). The angiographic changes are
reversible when follow-up studies are performed. The
severity of the vasoconstriction does not correlate with the
severity of the hypertension (Easton et al., 1998).
Transcranial Doppler ultrasound (TCD) is a good non-
invasive way to monitor the vasoconstriction. Qureshi et
al. (1996) studied 11 women with eclampsia using TCD,
and found elevated blood flow velocities and lower average
pulsatility indexes compared to pre-eclamptic women and
those with normal pregnancies. TCD has also been used
effectively to study patients with postpartum cerebral
angiopathy (Bogousslavsky et al., 1989). Patients whose
angiography shows vasoconstriction have usually had
multifocal white matter abnormalities on brain imaging
scans.

Pathology

The kidneys usually show a very characteristic pathological change referred to as 'glomerular endotheliosis'.
(Lindheimer & Katz, 1991). The kidney glomeruli are
usually swollen as a result of swelling of endothelial cells
and mesangial cells. The swollen endothelial cells
encroach on the lumens of the capillaries (Lindheimer &
Katz, 1991). Thrombi and fibrin are often found within the
lumens of the kidney capillaries. Fibrinogen and fibrin are
often found between the basal lamina and endothelial cells
and within the cells (Cunningham et al., 1997). As a result
of the glomerular changes, the kidney often has decreased
ability to excrete sodium and the glomerular filtration rate
is reduced. Proteinuria results from the glomerular abnormalities.

The liver is also the seat of frequent pathological
changes. Periportal hemorrhagic necrosis develops in the
peripheral portion of liver lobules. (Cunningham et al.,
1997). Frank hemorrhages can occur and can lead to
enlargement of the liver and even rupture of the liver
capsule. Liver function tests are often abnormal.

As a result of the vascular damage at the precapillary and
capillary level, small ring hemorrhages and microinfarc-
tions may be found scattered in the cerebral cortex, usually
in an asymmetric distribution, and frequently in arterial
border-zone regions. These lesions are most commonly
seen in the occipital lobe, followed by the parietal lobe,
frontal lobe, and then the temporal lobe. These lesions are
rarely found in the cerebellum (Sheehan & Lynch, 1973).
The cortical lesions are only 0.3–1.0 mm in size, compared
to the subcortical hemorrhages that are 2 to 6 mm in size.
Small hemorrhages (3–5 mm) may also be located in the

deep white matter and in the caudate and brainstem. Large
intracerebral hemorrhages may occur in the basal ganglia,
pons or the cerebral hemispheres, and depending on the
location may extend to the ventricular system. In all the
hemorrhagic lesions, the pathology shows congested capillaries with surrounding hemorrhage.

The small cerebral blood vessels often show fibrinoid
necrosis of the vascular walls. Fibrin thrombi also occlude
some small arteries and arterioles. Perivascular small hemorrhages are also common (Easton et al., 1998).

Richards et al. (1988) correlated the neuroradiologic
findings and clinical status with neuropathologic findings
in seven patients, and have identified seven major neuropathological abnormalities including vasculopathy with
acute vessel wall damage, perivascular micro-hemor-
rhages/microinfarctions as listed above, and intracerebral
hemorrhages including subarachnoid and intraventricular
hemorrhage. They also described edema located throughout the brain and not limited to regions of microinfarc-
tions, hypoxic brain damage distributed diffusely and in
border-zone regions, and in one patient there was evidence of transtentorial herniation.

Differential diagnosis

The two most important differential diagnostic considerations are dural sinus thrombosis and a reversible cerebral
vasoconstriction syndrome. Cerebral dural sinus thrombosis is more common during the puerperium than during
pregnancy (Cantu & Baringarrementeria, 1993; Chopra &
Banarjee, 1989; Srinavasian 1983,1988). Headache and seizures are prominent features of both dural sinus occlusion
and eclampsia, but patients with dural sinus occlusions are
usually not hypertensive and the clinical and CT abnormalities in patients with dural sinus occlusions are usually
focal and not as multifocal as in eclampsia. The sagittal and
transverse dural sinuses are most often involved.

The reversible cerebral vasoconstriction syndrome is
another important consideration. This disorder is most
common in women and often develops in the postpartum
period (Call et al., 1988). The same condition has also been
called postpartum cerebral angiopathy when it develops in
the puerperium (Barinagarrementeria et al., 1992;
Bogousslavsky et al., 1989; Comabella et al., 1996; Raroque
et al., 1993; Roh & Park, 1998; Ursell et al., 1998) Headache,
seizures, and multifocal neurological symptoms and signs
may develop in postpartum cerebral angiopathy but the
white matter changes are usually not as extensive on brain
imaging as in eclampsia and most patients are not hypertensive. Hemorrhages can complicate the angiopathy (Roh

& Park, 1998; Ursell et al, 1998). This condition is discussed in Chapter 15. Some patients have taken pharmacological agents: bromocriptine (Comabella et al., 1996), ergonovine (Barinagarrementeria et al., 1992), and lisuride (Roh & Park, 1998) that might have promoted or caused the syndrome.

The differential diagnosis of the toxemias of pregnancy should also include other conditions that occur unrelated to pregnance, e.g. brain embolism from concurrent cardiac disease, bleeding diathesis, arterial dissection, etc.

Pathogenesis and pathophysiology of the pre-eclampsia–eclampsia syndromes

The cause of pre-eclampsia and eclampsia of pregnancy and the puerperum remains unknown. The most popular theory is that the syndrome is caused by some cytotoxic factor released from the placenta, uterus, or the products of conception.

The pathogenesis of neurologic involvement in eclampsia remains incompletely understood. Theories must explain the major features – occurrence during late pregnancy and the early postpartum period, hypertension, peripheral edema, cerebral vasoconstriction, reversible leukoencephalopathy related to vasogenic edema, and brain hemorrhages and infarcts.

The most popular explanation for the brain edema, and brain hemorrhages, is that the disorder represents a form of hypertensive encephalopathy that happens to occur during pregnancy and the early postpartum period. A review considers various investigators' opinions on this theory (Easton et al., 1998). The brain pathology in fatal cases of eclampsia is nearly identical to that found in patients with fatal hypertensive encephalopathy.

Cerebral perfusion is sensitive to changes in PCO_2 and hypoxia. When these factors are constant, the cerebral blood flow remains constant over a range of mean arterial blood pressures; thus the cerebral perfusion pressure is independent from the systemic arterial pressure. Elevations in blood pressure above the limits of autoregulation lead to increased cerebral blood flow and initial focal dilatation and then general vasodilatation which results in hypertensive encephalopathy (Auer, 1977; Strandgaard, 1973). Cerebral blood flow is increased in patients and experimental animals with acute hypertension (Dinsdale et al., 1974). Damage occurs at the precapillary and capillary levels with disruption of the vessel walls and the tight junctions resulting in extravasation of red cells and proteins into the perivascular space (Rodda & Denny-Brown, 1966; Ziylan, 1984) leading to ring hemorrhages and cerebral edema. The cortical microhemorrhages and microin-

farctions are located in the border-zone region as this is the area where there is the greatest change in arteriolar calibre and where the earliest consequence of advancing hypertension occurs (Johansson, 1974). The blood pressures usually recorded in patients with eclampsia are considerably lower than those found in patients with hypertensive encephalopathy.

The clinical, imaging, and pathological findings in eclampsia are identical to those found in patients with the reversible posterior leukoencephalopathy syndrome and, in fact, eclampsia is one cause of this syndrome (Hinchey et al., 1996). In other causes of the posterior leukoencephalopathy syndrome renal disease, often with azotemia, and pedal edema are frequent features. During pregnancy fluid retention is common. Many eclamptic patients have renal abnormalities. The fluid retention may contribute to increased blood volumes and to high-volume hypertension, and brain edema.

Mas and Lamy (Easton et al., 1998) posit that the toxemias of pregnancy and the puerperium represent an endotheliopathy. Glomerular endotheliosis, a characteristic kidney lesion in eclamptics, provides direct evidence of systemic endothelial injury. Additional evidence for systemic endothelial injury are the frequent biochemical abnormalities that are found in eclamptics. High circulating levels of von Willebrand factor, endothelin, and the cellular epitope of fibronectin have been reported (Easton et al., 1998). These substances are all known to be released by damaged endothelial cells. Endothelial changes in the brain lead to a breakdown in the normal blood/brain barrier and a capillary leak syndrome. The vasoconstriction and vasodilatation could also represent a vascular reaction to the endothelial abnormality that affects the brain blood vessels.

Schobel et al. (1996) showed that the rate of sympathetic nerve activity in patients with pre-eclampsia was more than three times higher than that found in normotensive pregnant women and more than twice as high as that found in hypertensive women who were not pregnant. The investigators showed conclusively that sympathetic overactivity was present in pre-eclamptic women. The heightened sympathetic nerve activity could cause or contribute to hypertension and vasoconstriction. The relationship between the sympathetic overactivity and the endotheliopathy is unclear.

Treatment

The treatment of patients with eclampsia and its resultant neurologic deficits is aimed at lowering the blood pressure, limiting and decreasing cerebral edema, and preventing seizures, with a goal of delivering a viable baby. Termination of pregnancy has long been recognized as an effective treatment. Delivery is associated with resolution of the eclamptic syndrome in most women (Donaldson, 1989). If possible, the fetus should be delivered immediately.

As the pathophysiology in most of the patients with eclampsia is thought to be a result of hypertensive encephalopathy, the treatment is to reduce the blood pressure to normal without resultant hypotension. As evidenced in most published cases, the neurological deficits and the abnormalities found on imaging studies are usually reversible when the blood pressure is effectively lowered. The antihypertensive drugs used in eclampsia prior to termination of the pregnancy should not interfere with fetal activity, metabolism or hemodynamics. Diazoxide, hydralazine, and nitroprusside have all been used over the years in woman with eclampsia. More recently newer agents such as intravenous labetolol and nifedipine have been introduced, studied, and have been found effective in the acute management of hypertensive emergencies of pregnancy (Vermillion et al., 1999; Scardo et al., 1999; Michael, 1986).

Obstetricians have, for a long time, used magnesium sulfate to treat eclamptic women. A recent randomized trial showed that magnesium sulfate was superior to phenytoin in preventing eclamptic seizures in hypertensive women admitted to the hospital for delivery (Lucas et al., 1995). Magnesium sulfate has also been shown to be superior to both phenytoin and diazepam in preventing recurrent seizures in women with eclampsia who have already had a seizure (Eclampsia Trial Collaborative Group, 1995). While the effectiveness of magnesium sulfate against seizures has been well shown, there is little data on blood pressure control when compared to antihypertensive drugs.

References

Auer, L. (1977). The role of cerebral perfusion pressure as origin of brain edema in acute arterial hypertension. *European Neurology*, **15**, 153–6.

Baringarrementeria, F., Cantu, C. & Balderrama, J. (1992). Postpartum cerebral angiopathy with cerebral infarction due to ergonovine use. *Stroke*, **23**, 1364–6.

Bogousslavsky, J., Despland, P.A., Regli, F. & Dubuis, P.Y. (1989). Postpartum cerebral angiopathy: reversible vasoconstriction assessed by transcranial Doppler ultrasound. *European Neurology*, **29**, 102–5.

Call, G.K., Fleming, M.C., Sealfon, S. et al. (1988). Reversible cerebral segmental vasoconstriction. *Stroke*, **19**, 1159–70.

Cantu, C. & Barinagarrementeria, F. (1993). Cerebral venous thrombosis associated with pregnancy and puerperium. Review of 67 cases. *Stroke*, **24**, 1880–4.

Chesley, L.C. (1978). *Hypertensive Disorders in Pregnancy*, p. 225. New York: Appelton-Century Crafts.

Chopra, J.S. & Banerjee, A.K. (1989). Primary intracranial sinovenous occlusions in youth and pregnancy. In *Handbook of Clinical Neurology*, Vol 10: *Vascular Diseases, part II*, ed. P.J. Vinken, G.W. Bruyn & H.L. Klawans, pp. 425–52. Amsterdam: Elsevier Science Publ.

Colosimo, C., Fileni, A., Moschini, M. & Guerrini, P. (1985). CT findings in eclampsia. *Neuroradiology*, **27**, 313–17.

Comabella, M., Alvarez-Sabin, J., Rovira, A. & Codina, A. (1996). Bromocriptine and postpartum cerebral angiopathy: a causal relationship? *Neurology*, **46**, 1754–6.

Cunningham, F.G., MacDonald, P.C., Gant, N.F. et al. (1997). Hypertensive disorders in pregnancy in *Williams' Obstetrics*, ed. F.G. Cunningham et al., pp. 693–744. 20th edn, Stamford, Connecticut: Appleton & Lange.

Dahmus, M.A., Barton, J.R. & Sibai, B.M. (1992). Cerebral imaging in eclampsia: magnetic resonance imaging versus computed tomography. *American Journal of Obstetrics and Gynecology*, **167**, 935–41.

Digre, K.B., Varner, M.W., Osborn, A.G. & Crawford, S. (1993). Cranial magnetic resonance imaging in severe preeclampsia vs. eclampsia. *Archives of Neurology*, **50**, 399–406.

Dinsdale, H.B., Robertson, D.M. & Haas, R.A. (1974). Cerebral blood flow in acute hypertension. *Archives of Neurology*, **31**, 80–7.

Donaldson, J.O. (1989). Eclampsia. In *Neurology of Pregnancy*, pp. 269–310. Philadelphia: WB Saunders.

Duncan, R., Hadley, D., Bone, I., Symonds, E.M., Worthington, B.S. & Rubin, P.C. (1989). Blindness in eclampsia: CT and MR imaging. *Journal of Neurology, Neurosurgery and Psychiatry*, **52**, 899–902.

Easton, J.D., Mas, J-L., Lamy, C. et al. (1998). Severe preeclampsia/eclampsia: hypertensive encephalopathy of pregnancy? *Cerebrovascular Disease*, **8**, 53–8.

Eclampsia Trial Collaborative Group. (1995). Which anticonvulsant for women with eclampsia? Evidence from the collaborative Eclampsia Trial. *Lancet*, **345**, 1455–63.

Hinchey, J., Chaves, C., Appignani, B. et al. (1996). A reversible posterior leukoencephalopathy syndrome. *New England Journal of Medicine*, **334**, 494–500.

Johansson, B. (1974). Regional changes of cerebral blood flow in acute hypertension in cats. *Acta Neurologica Scandinavica*, **50**, 366–72.

Kaunitz, A.M., Hughes, J.M., Grimes, D.A., Smith, J.C., Rochat, R.W., Kafrissen, M.E. (1985). Causes of maternal mortality in the United States. *Obstetrics and Gynecology*, **65**, 605–12.

Kirby, J.C., Jaindl, J.J. (1984). Cerebral CT findings in toxemia of pregnancy. *Radiology*, **151**, 114.

Kittner, S.J., Stern, B.J., Feeser, B.R. et al. (1996). Pregnancy and the risk of stroke. *New England Journal of Medicine*, **335**, 768–74.

Lau, S.P.C., Chan, F.L., Yu, Y.L. & Huang, C.Y. (1987). Cortical blindness in toxemia of pregnancy: findings on computed tomography. *British Journal Radiology*, **60**, 347–9.

Lindheimer, M.D. & Katz A.I. (1991). The kidney and hypertension in pregnancy. In *The Kidney*, 4th edn, ed. B.M. Brenner & F.C. Rector, pp. 1551–95. Philadelphia, W.B. Saunders.

Lucas, M.J., Leveno, K.J., Cunningham, F.G. (1995). A comparison of magnesium sulfate with phenytoin for the prevention of eclampsia. *New England Journal of Medicine*, **333**, 201–5.

Mas, J-L. & Lamy, C. (1998a). Stroke in pregnancy and the puerperium. *Journal of Neurology*, **245**, 305–13.

Mas, J-L. & Lamy, C. (1998b) Stroke in pregnancy and the postpartum period: in *Cerebrovascular Disease. Pathophysiology, Diagnosis, and Management*, M.D. Ginsberg & J. Bogousslavsky, pp. 1684–97. Malden, MA: Blackwell Science.

Michael, C.A. (1986). Intravenous labetolol and intravenous diazoxide in severe hypertension complicating pregnancy. *Australia and New Zealand Journal of Obstetrics and Gynecology*, **26**, 26–9.

Qureshi, A.I., Frankel, M.R., Ottenlips, J.R. & Stern, B.J. (1996). Cerebral hemodynamics in preeclampsia and eclampsia. *Archives of Neurology*, **53**, 1226–31.

Raps, E.C., Galetta, S.L., Broderick, M. & Atlas, S.W. (1993). Delayed peripartum vasculopathy: cerebral eclampsia revisited. *Annals of Neurology*, **33**, 222–5.

Raroque, H.G., Orrison, W.W. & Rosenberg, G.A. (1990). Neurologic involvement in toxemia of pregnancy: reversible MRI lesions. *Neurology*, **40**, 167–9.

Raroque, H.G., Tesfa, G. & Purdy, P. (1993). Postpartum cerebral angiopathy. Is there a role for sympathomimetic drugs? *Stroke*, **24**, 2108–10.

Richards, A., Graham, D. & Bullock, R. (1988). Clinicopathological study of neurological complications due to hypertensive disorders of pregnancy. *Journal of Neurology, Neurosurgery and Psychiatry*, **51**, 416–21.

Rodda, R. & Denny-Brown, D. (1966). The cerebral arterioles in experimental hypertension II. The development of arterionecrosis. *American Journal of Pathology*, **49**, 365–75.

Roh, J.K. & Park, K.S. (1998). Postpartum cerebral angiopathy with intracerebral hemorrhage in a patient receiving lisuride. *Neurology*, **50**, 1152–4.

Sanders, T.G., Clayman, D.A., Sanchez-Ramos, L., Vines, F.S., Russo, L. (1991). Brain in eclampsia: MR imaging with clinical correlation. *Radiology*, **180**, 475–8.

Scardo, J.A., Vermillion, S.T., Newman, R.B., Chauhan, S.P. & Hogg, B.B. (1999). A randomized, double-blind, hemodyanmic evaluation of nifedipine and labetolol in preeclamptic hypertensive emergencies. *American Journal of Obstetrics and Gynecology*, **181**, 862–6.

Schaefer, P.W., Buonanno, F.S., Gonzalez, R.G. & Schwamm, L.H. (1997). Diffusion-weighted imaging discriminates between cytotoxic and vasogenic edema in a patient with eclampsia. *Stroke*, **28**, 1082–5.

Schobel, H.P., Fischer, T., Heuszer, K., Geiger, H. & Schmieder, R.E. (1996). Preeclampsia – a state of sympathetic overactivity. *New England Journal of Medicine*, **335**, 1480–5.

Schwartz, R.B., Jones, K.M., Kalina, P. et al. (1992). Hypertensive encephalopathy: findings on CT, MR imaging, and SPECT imaging in 14 cases. *American Journal of Roentgenology*, **159**, 379–83.

Sengar, A.R., Gupta, R.K., Dhanuka, A.K., Roy, R. & Das, K. (1997). MR imaging, MR angiography, and MR spectroscopy of the brain in eclampsia. *American Journal of Neuroradiology*, **18**, 1485–90.

Sharshar, T., Lamy, C. & Mas, J.L. (1995). Incidence and causes of strokes associated with pregnancy and puerperium: a study in public hospitals of Ile de France. *Stroke*, **26**, 930–6.

Sheehan, H.L. & Lynch, J.B. (1973). Cerebral lesions. In *Pathology of Toxaemia of Pregnancy*, ed. H.L. Sheehan, & J.B. Lynch, pp. 525–54. London: Churchill Livingstone.

Sibai, B.M. (1989). Preeclampsia–eclampsia. In *Gynecology and Obstetrics*. Vol 2, ed. J.J. Sciarra, pp. 1–12. Philadelphia: J.B. Lippincott.

Srinivasan, K. (1983) Cerebral venous and arterial thrombosis in pregnancy and puerperium, a study of 135 patients. *Angiology*, **34**, 733–46.

Srinivasan, K. (1988). Puerperal cerebral venous and arterial thrombosis. *Seminars in Neurology*, **8**, 222–5.

Stander, H.J., Bonsners, R.W. & Stromme, W.B. (1946). Late postpartum eclampsia. *American Journal of Obstetrics and Gynecology*, **52**, 765–72.

Strandgaard, S. (1973). The lower and upper limit for autoregulation of cerebral blood flow. *Stroke*, **4**, 323.

Tommer, B.L., Homer, D. & Mikhael, M.A. (1988). Cerebral vasospasm and eclampsia. *Stroke*, **19**, 326–9.

Ursell, M.R., Marras, C.L., Farb, R., Rowed, D.W., Black, S.E. & Perry, J.R. (1998). Recurrent intracranial hemorrhage due to postpartum cerebral angiopathy. Implications for management. *Stroke*, **29**, 1995–8.

Vermillion, S.T., Scardo, J.A., Newman, R.B. & Chauhan, S.P. (1999). A randomized, double-blind trial of oral nifedipine and intravenous labetolol in hypertensive emergencies of pregnancy. *American Journal of Obstetrics and Gynecology*, **181**, 858–61.

Will, A.D., Lewis, K.L., Hinshaw, D.B. et al. (1987). Cerebral vasoconstriction in toxemia. *Neurology*, **37**, 1555–7.

Ziylan, Y.Z. (1984). Pathophysiology of opening of the blood–brain and blood–cerebrospinal fluid barriers in acute hypertension. *Experimental Neurology*, **84**, 18–28.

17

Stroke and substance abuse

John C.M. Brust

Harlem Hospital Center, New York, USA

The term 'substance abuse' refers to the non-medical use of an agent in a manner perceived as harmful. The use may or may not produce psychic dependence (addiction) or physical dependence (resulting in physical symptoms and signs upon withdrawal), and the agent may be either illicit or legally available. When alcohol and tobacco are included, countless people worldwide are substance abusers, and many of them are at increased risk for ischemic or hemorrhagic stroke (Brust, 1993, 1998; Kokkinos & Levine, 1993a).

Opiates

Opiate drugs include a large number of agonists, e.g. morphine, antagonists, e.g. naloxone, and mixed agonist/antagonists, e.g. pentazocine. The most widely abused opiate is the agonist heroin, and although the AIDS epidemic has led many users to adopt non-parenteral routes of administration, e.g. snorting or smoking, most heroin users inject the drug intravenously or subcutaneously. Infectious endocarditis is therefore a major risk, especially with *Staphylococcus aureus* and *Candida*. The aortic, mitral, and tricuspid valves are equally affected, and cerebral emboli are common. Strokes that result can be ischemic or hemorrhagic, the latter caused by rupture of either a septic 'mycotic' aneurysm or non-aneurysmal infectious vasculitis. Unlike saccular 'berry' aneurysms, septic aneurysmal rupture is often preceded by insidiously progressive neurological or systemic symptoms. Septic aneurysms may or may not disappear during appropriate antimicrobial therapy, and they can rupture during or following such treatment. It has been recommended, therefore, that septic aneurysms be angiographically sought in patients with endocarditis and suspicious neurological symptoms and that surgically accessible aneurysms be excised (Brust et al., 1990).

Hemorrhagic stroke in heroin users may be a consequence of hepatitis with liver failure and deranged clotting or of heroin nephropathy with uremia or malignant hypertension. Ischemic stroke may be a complication of meningitis or AIDS (Brust, 1997a).

A number of reports describe ischemic stroke in young heroin users without evidence of endocarditis, additional drug use, or other risk factors (Brust & Richter, 1976). In some patients, cerebral infarction was associated with loss of consciousness after intravenous injection of heroin. In others, ischemic stroke occurred in active users but did not follow overdose or a recent injection. Angiography in some suggested either large vessel or small vessel arteritis (unconfirmed pathologically). Suggestive of hypersensitivity were eosinophilia, hypergammaglobulinemia, a positive direct Coombs test, and a positive latex fixation test. In one patient hemiparesis was preceded by symptoms suggesting anaphylaxis (Woods & Strewler, 1972). Ischemic stroke has also followed heroin sniffing (Bartolomei et al., 1992). A young woman had an intracerebral hemorrhage within minutes of intravenous heroin (Knoblauch et al., 1983).

Stroke in heroin users could have a number of different mechanisms. Overdose causes hypoventilation and hypotension, and bilateral globus pallidus infarction is frequently found at autopsies of heroin users. Direct toxic injury from heroin or an adulterant is another possibility. Heroin is often mixed with quinine, and a variety of pharmacologically active and inactive ingredients find their way into the preparation (Caplan et al., 1982a).

Embolization of foreign material has not been documented in heroin users but is well recognized in users of other agents, including opiates. During the 1970s mixtures of pentazocine (Talwin) and tripelennamine (Pyribenzamine), 'Ts and Blues' became a popular form of drug abuse in the American Midwest. Oral tablets were crushed, suspended in water, and injected intravenously. Cerebral infarcts and hemorrhages were a frequent complication, and autopsies revealed talc and cellulose crystals in both pulmonary and brain arterioles. Cerebral angiography often showed arterial 'beading,' consistent with either multiple emboli or a vasoconstrictive or vasculitic reaction to the foreign material (Caplan et al., 1982b).

Foreign body embolism was also suspected in cases of ischemic stroke associated with parenteral use of paregoric, oral meperidine, and hydromorphone (Dilaudid) suppository (Brust, 1998).

Heroin myelopathy is probably ischemic in some cases. Several reports describe acute paraparesis, sensory loss, and urinary retention, occurring shortly after injection and often following a period of abstinence. Symptoms were sometimes present on awakening from coma, suggesting hypotension and border-zone infarction. In some patients, proprioception and vibratory sensation were spared, suggesting infarction in the territory of the anterior spinal artery (Pearson et al., 1972). In one case small vessel arteritis was found histologically (Judice et al., 1978).

Amphetamine and related agents

Amphetamine-like psychostimulants include dextroamphetamine, methamphetamine, methylphenidate (Ritalin), ephedrine, pseudoephedrine, phenylpropanolamine, and a large number of other agents marketed as decongestants or appetite suppressants. Ischemic or hemorrhagic stroke is a well-recognized complication of these drugs.

Dextroamphetamine and methamphetamine are often abused intravenously, and so strokes common to any parenteral drug use are encountered. Amphetamine overdose causes delirium, hypertension, malignant hyperthermia, vascular collapse, and death, and at autopsy there are cerebral edema and petechiae. Gross intracranial hemorrhage, however, has more often been associated with amphetamine use in the absence of other signs of overdose.

Over 30 such cases have been reported. Routes of administration were either intravenous, oral, or inhalation (Lloyd & Walker, 1995; Kokkinos & Levine, 1993a; Brust, 1998). Most cases involved dextroamphetamine or methamphetamine, but single cases involved pseudoephedrine or diethylpropion. Chronic use predominated. Severe headache usually occurred within minutes of drug use, and in most patients blood pressure was elevated. Computerized tomography (CT) showed either intracerebral or subarachnoid hemorrhage. In several cases cerebral angiographic 'beading' was present, and cerebral vasculitic changes were occasionally found at autopsy. Some of these strokes were therefore probably secondary to acute hypertension, some to acute vasculitis, and some to both.

Amphetamine-induced cerebral vasculitis has also caused ischemic stroke. In one report 14 polydrug abusers – all but two of whom used intravenous methamphetamine – developed a necrotizing arteritis that resembled polyarteritis nodosa, with systemic symptoms and signs and, in some, infarction or hemorrhage affecting the cerebrum, cerebellum, or brainstem (Citron et al., 1970). Such brain lesions have been found pathologically in other polydrug abusers (Brust, 1998; Bostwick, 1981; Kessler et al., 1978). In some reports, however, vasculitis has been presumed on the basis of angiographic 'beading,' which could have other causes, including multiple emboli, and subarachnoid hemorrhage (Rumbaugh et al., 1971; Rothrock et al., 1988). Experimental studies with monkeys and rats confirmed that cerebral vasculitis – often involving vessels smaller than those affected by polyarteritis nodosa – can follow either single or repeated intravenous administration of either methamphetamine or methylphenidate (Rumbaugh et al., 1976). It is unclear if such lesions are the result of direct toxicity or hypersensitivity.

Phenylpropanolamine (PPA) is an amphetamine-like drug sold over-the-counter in decongestants and diet preparations and also available by mail order as a 'legal stimulant.' Acute side effects include hypertension, severe headache, psychosis, seizures, and hemorrhagic stroke (Forman et al., 1989). Cases reported as 'cerebral arteritis' have been based on angiographic changes. PPA with caffeine, from a commercial diet preparation, caused subarachnoid hemorrhage in rats receiving it parenterally, but vasculitis was not described histologically (Mueller & Ertel, 1983)

Ephedrine and pseudoephedrine, also available over-the-counter, have caused hypertensive crisis and both ischemic and hemorrhagic stroke (Bruno et al., 1993; Loizou et al., 1982). In one case, cerebral angiography was initially normal but a week later showed 'beading,' and skin biopsy showed deposits of IgM and complement in dermal vessels, suggestive of circulating immune complexes (Wooten et al., 1983). Ischemic stroke has also been associated with the appetite suppressants phentermine and phendimetrazine (Kokkinos & Levine, 1993b).

3,4-methylenedioxymethamphetamine (MDMA, 'ecstasy'), a schedule I controlled substance in the United States, has both psychostimulant and hallucinogenic properties. MDMA became increasingly popular during the 1980s, especially on college campuses. Middle cerebral artery occlusion was reported in a young man 36 hours after use (Manchanda & Connolly, 1993).

Microembolization of talc to brain and retina was reported following intravenous (and inadvertent carotid artery) injection of crushed methylphenidate tablets (Chillar & Jackson, 1981; Mizutami et al., 1980).

Cocaine

Although cocaine's psychostimulatory effects are similar to those of amphetamine, its mode of action is different. Unlike amphetamine, cocaine blocks re-uptake of mono-amine neurotransmitters at synaptic nerve endings by binding to specific transporter proteins. Also unlike amphetamine, cocaine is a local anesthetic. Whether these different pharmacological properties confer different degrees of risk or different pathophysiological mechanisms for stroke is unclear.

The first report of stroke associated with cocaine use described cerebral infarction following intramuscular use (Brust & Richter, 1977). A handful of reports then described both ischemic and hemorrhagic stroke in intranasal users of cocaine hydrochloride. During the 1980s, cocaine production shifted to smokable alkaloidal 'crack,' which unlike cocaine hydrochloride can be administered in huge doses continuously over hours or even days. The resulting epidemic of use was accompanied by an upsurge in reports of cocaine-related stroke (Brust, 1993, 1998; Kaku & Lowenstein, 1990; Levine et al. 1990, 1991). By the mid-1990s over 300 cases had been described, about half ischemic and half hemorrhagic. (Although a case-control study failed to identify crack cocaine as a a risk factor for stroke (Qureshi et al. 1997), the number of reports involving young people without other risk factors, as well as cocaine's recognized actions on blood vessels, argues for causality. The negative findings in that study were perhaps related to a very high prevalence of cocaine use among controls.)

Ischemic strokes have included transient ischemic attacks and infarction of cerebrum, thalamus, brain stem, spinal cord, and retina. Infarction has occurred in pregnant women and in neonates whose mothers used cocaine shortly before delivery. As with amphetamine, cerebral vasculitis has sometimes been inferred on the basis of angiographic changes. In only five cases, however, was cerebral vasculitis confirmed pathologically, and in each case it was mild; most autopsies have shown histologically normal cerebral vessels, including cases with angiographic 'beading.'

Hemorrhagic strokes have been both intracerebral and subarachnoid, and of those patients receiving angiography, nearly half had vascular malformations or saccular aneurysms. Other hemorrhages include bleeding into embolic infarction or glioma. Intracerebral hemorrhages have occurred in post-partem women or their offspring.

Cocaine causes vasoconstriction by blocking re-uptake of norepinephrine at sympathetic nerve endings. Coronary artery constriction causes myocardial infarction and with it the risk of cardioembolic stroke. (Cocaine also causes a cardiomyopathy probably independent of coronary artery constriction.) Systemic artery constriction causes acute hypertension, predisposing to rupture of underlying vascular malformations or aneurysms. Cerebral artery constriction – a property verified angiographically in human volunteers (Kaufman et al., 1998) – causes cerebral ischemia. Infarcts are sometimes multiple and carry a high risk of hemorrhagic transformation if cerebral vasoconstriction clears while systemic hypertension is still present (Green et al., 1990). Animal studies, however, reveal greater complexity; cerebral vasodilatation as well as vasoconstriction occur, depending on species and whether the drug is administered intravenously or applied topically (Diaz-Tejedor et al., 1992).

In vitro studies have described both aggregation and deaggregation of platelets by cocaine (Jennings et al., 1993). Depletion of protein C and antithrombin III by cocaine has also been reported (Chokshi et al., 1989). Synergism between cocaine and ethanol is also recognized; in the presence of ethanol, cocaine is metabolized to cocaethylene, which binds more powerfully than cocaine itself to monoamine transporter proteins (Brust, 1993).

Relevant to cocaine and cerebrovascular disease are controversies over whether chronic cocaine use has long-term adverse effects on cognition and to what degree in utero exposure to cocaine affects psychomotor development. Human studies using controls demonstrate subtle cognitive impairment (Weinrieb & O'Brien, 1993), and CT studies show cerebral atrophy in chronic cocaine users (Pascual-Leone et al., 1991). Studies with positron emission tomography (PET) and single photon emission computerized tomography (SPECT) reveal irregularly decreased cerebral blood flow in chronic cocaine users, but the relationship of these changes to cognitive impairment or to cerebral ischemia is uncertain (Strickland & Stein, 1995).

Similarly, congenital anomalies and psychomotor retardation are difficult to blame on in utero cocaine exposure *per se*, for affected infants are likely to be victims of inadequate pre-natal care and exposure to other drugs, including ethanol and tobacco. Controlled studies suggest that in utero cocaine exposure causes hypertonic tetraparesis that tends to clear over the first two years of life as well as a small but lasting reduction in IQ (Chiriboga et al., 1999; Lester et al., 1998). Some investigators attribute such cocaine-related damage to fetal cerebral vasospasm (King et al., 1995).

Phencyclidine

Phencyclidine (PCP, 'angel dust') can be smoked, eaten, or injected. Low doses produce euphoria; higher doses produce psychosis. PCP's principal action is to block excitatory N-methyl-D-aspartate receptors. The basis of its circulatory effects is unclear but might involve specific receptors on blood vessels. Hypertension can appear either early or late during intoxication, and hemorrhagic stroke has either immediately followed use or occurred after a delay of a few days. Temporally related hypertensive encephalopathy is also described (Eastman & Cohen, 1975; Boyko et al., 1987).

LSD

The hallucinogenic drug D-lysergic acid diethylamide (LSD) is an ergot which in high doses causes severe hypertension and in vitro produces spasm of cerebral vessel strips. Ischemic stroke has occurred up to several days after LSD use, with cerebral angiography showing either progressive narrowing and occlusion of the internal carotid artery or more widespread intracranial arterial 'beading' (Sobel et al., 1971).

Marijuana

Reports of ischemic stroke in marijuana users are mostly unconvincing as to causality. Hypotension and cerebral vasospasm have been proposed as mechanisms, but neither has been documented in clinical reports. In humans, marijuana has unpredictable effects on cerebral blood flow (Mathew & Wilson, 1991).

Sedatives

Barbiturates, benzodiazepines, and other sedative drugs can cause cerebral infarction as a result of respiratory depression, hypotension, and decreased cerebral blood flow, but ischemic or hemorrhagic stroke has not otherwise been reported.

Inhalants

Inhaling the intoxicating vapors of household and industrial products is especially common among children. Death results from accidents, violence, suffocation, aspiration, and cardiac arrhythmia, but clinical stroke has not been reported.

Ethanol

The relationship between ethanol consumption and coronary artery disease follows a 'J-shaped curve' – that is, mild-to-moderate drinking decreases risk whereas heavy drinking increases risk (Ahlawat & Siwach, 1994). Heavy drinkers are therefore indirectly at increased risk for cardioembolic stroke as an aftermath of myocardial infarction. Ethanol also directly precipitates cardiac arrhythmia ('holiday heart'), and thromboembolism is a prominent feature of alcoholic cardiomyopathy.

Stroke independent of ethanol's cardiac effects has been extensively studied. Finnish investigators reported a temporal association of heavy drinking and both ischemic and hemorrhagic stroke, but those studies were retrospective and the findings could not be duplicated by others (Gorelick et al., 1989).

The relationship of chronic ethanol use and stroke has been addressed in many case-control and cohort studies. Contradictory findings are the result of differently selected endpoints, e.g. total stroke, ischemic stroke, hemorrhagic stroke, or stroke mortality, amount and duration of ethanol consumption, correction for other risk factors, e.g. hypertension and tobacco, ethnicity and socioeconomics of populations being studied, and selection of controls. A meta-analysis of 62 epidemiologic studies addressed the relationship of no drinking, 'moderate' drinking (less than two drinks or 1 oz of absolute alcohol daily), and heavier drinking to ischemic and hemorrhagic stroke. Among whites, a J-shaped curve similar to that found for coronary artery disease emerged for ischemic stroke; moderate drinking decreased risk and heavy drinking increased risk. Among Japanese, however, moderate drinking conferred no protection for ischemic stroke. In both populations both moderate and heavy drinking increased the risk of hemorrhagic stroke, both intracerebral and subarachnoid (Camargo, 1989).

More recently, the Northern Manhattan Stroke Study reported that drinking up to two drinks daily protected against ischemic stroke in whites, Hispanics, and African-Americans; higher doses increased risk. (A 'standard drink' was defined as 120 ml of wine, 360 ml of beer, or 45 ml of liquor.) There was no difference in the effect of wine, beer, or liquor (Sacco et al., 1999).

Studies with angiography and ultrasound parallel these clinical observations. Heavy ethanol consumption increases the risk of carotid artery atherosclerosis, whereas low ethanol consumption decreases it (Polomaki et al., 1993).

Multiple mechanisms probably explain the complex association of ethanol and stroke. Ethanol acutely and chronically raises blood pressure (Beilin, 1995). It lowers blood levels of low-density lipoproteins and raises the levels of high-density lipoproteins. Ethanol acutely decreases fibrinolytic activity, increases factor VII levels, and increases platelet reactivity to ADP. It also decreases plasma fibrinogen levels, increases levels of prostacyclin, decreases platelet function, and stimulates endothelial release of endothelin (Brust, 1998). Alcoholic liver disease impairs clotting. During withdrawal hemoconcentration and rebound platelet hyperaggregability occur. Acute ethanol intoxication causes cerebral vasodilatation, yet ethanol in vitro constricted cerebral artery segments, and in rats ethanol constricted cerebral arterioles (Gordon et al., 1995).

Tobacco

Smoking is a major risk factor for coronary artery and peripheral vascular disease. Case-control and cohort studies show that independent of these effects tobacco increases the risk for both ischemic and hemorrhagic stroke (Department of Health and Human Services, 1988; Shinton & Beevers, 1989). In women the risk of ischemic and hemorrhagic stroke is greater in those also taking oral contraceptives (Goldbaum et al., 1987). As with ethanol, multiple mechanisms probably contribute. Smoking aggravates atherosclerosis (Haapanen et al., 1989) and reduces the blood's oxygen carrying capacity (Benowitz, 1988). Nicotine damages endothelium, and acutely smoking raises blood pressure. Smoking also increases platelet reactivity, inhibits prostacyclin formation, and raises blood fibrinogen levels. Smoking-induced polycythemia increases blood viscosity.

References

Ahlawat, S.K. & Siwach, S.B. (1994). Alcohol and coronary artery disease. *International Journal of Cardiology*, **44**, 157.

Bartolomei, F., Nicoli, F., Swiader, L. & Gastaut, J.L. (1992). Accident vasculaire cerebral ischemique apres prise nasale d'heroine. Une nouvelle observation. *Presse Medécin*, **21**, 983.

Beilin, L.J. (1995). Alcohol and hypertension. *Clinical and Experimental Pharmacology and Physiology*, **22**, 185.

Benowitz, N.L. (1988). Pharmacologic aspects of cigarette smoking and nicotine addiction. *New England Journal of Medicine*, **319**, 1318.

Bostwick, D.G. (1981). Amphetamine induced cerebral vasculitis. *Human Pathology*, **12**, 1031.

Boyko, O.B., Burger, P.C. & Heinz, E.R. (1987). Pathological and radiological correlation of subarachnoid hemorrhage in phencyclidine abuse: case report. *Journal of Neurosurgery*, **67**, 446.

Bruno, A., Nolte, K.B. & Chapin, J. (1993). Stroke associated with ephedrine use. *Neurology*, **43**, 1313.

Brust, J.C.M. (1993). *Neurological Aspects of Substance Abuse*. London: Butterworth-Heinemann.

Brust, J.C.M. (1997a). AIDS and stroke. In *Cerebrovascular Disease. A Primer*, ed. K.M.A. Welch, L.R. Caplan, D.J. Reis, B.K. Siesjo & B. Weir, pp. 423–425. San Diego: Academic Press.

Brust, J.C.M. (1997b). Vasculitis owing to substance abuse. In *Vasculitis and the Nervous System*, ed. D. Younger, *Neurology Clinics*, vol. 15, pp. 945–957.

Brust, J.C.M. (1998). Stroke and substance abuse. In *Stroke: Pathophysiology, Diagnosis, and Treatment*, ed. H.J.M. Barnett, J.P. Mohr, F. Yatsu & B. Stein, pp. 979–1000. Edinburgh, London: Churchill-Livingstone.

Brust, J.C.M. & Richter, R.W. (1976). Stroke associated with addiction to heroin. *Journal of Neurology, Neurosurgery and Psychiatry*, **39**, 194.

Brust, J.C.M. & Richter, R.W. (1977). Stroke associated with cocaine abuse? *NY State Journal of Medicine*, **77**, 1473.

Brust, J.C.M., Dickinson, P.C.T., Hughes, J.E.O. & Holtzman, R.N.N. (1990). The diagnosis and treatment of cerebral mycotic aneurysms. *Annals of Neurology*, **27**, 238.

Camargo, C.A. (1989). Moderate alcohol consumption and stroke: the epidemiologic evidence. *Stroke*, **20**, 1611.

Caplan, L.R., Hier, D.B. & Banks, G. (1982a). Stroke and drug abuse. *Stroke*, **13**, 869.

Caplan, L.R., Thomas, C. & Banks, G. (1982b). Central nervous system complications of addition to 'Ts and Blues.' *Neurology*, **32**, 623.

Chillar, R.K. & Jackson, A.L. (1981). Reversible hemiplegia after presumed intracarotid injection of Ritalin. *New England Journal of Medicine*, **304**, 1305.

Chiriboga, C.A., Brust, J.C.M., Bateman, D. & Hauser, W.A. (1999). Dose–response effect of fetal cocaine exposure on newborn neurologic function. *Pediatrics*, **103**, 79.

Chokshi, S.K., Moore, R., Pandian, N.G. & Isner, J.M. (1989). Reversible cardiomyopathy associated with cocaine intoxication. *Annals of Internal Medicine*, **111**, 1039.

Citron, B.P., Halpern, M., McCarron, M. et al. (1970). Necrotizing angiitis associated with drug abuse. *New England Journal of Medicine*, **283**, 1003.

Department of Health and Human Services (1988). The Health Consequences of Smoking: Nicotine Addiction. A Report of the Surgeon General (DHHS Publ. No. [CDC] 88-8406). US Government Printing Office, Washington, DC.

Diaz-Tejedor, E., Tejada, J. & Munoz, J. (1992). Cerebral arterial changes following cocaine IV administration: an angiographic study in rabbits. *Journal of Neurology*, **239** (Suppl. 2), 538.

Eastman, J.W. & Cohen, S.N. (1975). Hypertensive crisis and death associated with phencyclidine poisoning. *Journal of the American Medical Association*, **231**, 1270.

Forman, H.P., Levin, S., Stewart, B., et al. (1989). Cerebral vasculitis and hemorrhage in an adolescent taking diet pills containing phenylpropanolamine: case report and review of the literature. *Pediatrics*, **83**, 737.

Goldbaum, G.M., Kendrick, J.S., Hogelin, G.C. & Gentry, E.M. (1987). The relative impact of smoking and oral contraceptive use on women in the United States. *Journal of the American Medical Association*, **258**, 1339.

Gordon, E.L., Nguyen, T.S., Ngai, A.C. & Winn, H.R. (1995). Differential effects of alcohols on intracerebral arterioles. Ethanol alone causes vasoconstriction. *Journal of Cerebral Blood Flow Metabolism*, **15**, 532.

Gorelick, P.B., Rodin, M.B., Langenberg, P. et al. (1989). Weekly alcohol consumption, cigarette smoking, and the risk of ischemic stroke: results of a case-control study at three urban medical centers in Chicago, Illinois. *Neurology*, **39**, 339.

Green, R., Kelly, K.M., Gabrielsen, T. et al. (1990). Multiple cerebral hemorrhages after smoking 'crack' cocaine. *Stroke*, **21**, 957.

Haapanen, A., Koskenvuo, M., Kaprio, J. et al. (1989). Carotid atherosclerosis in identical twins discordant for cigarette smoking. *Circulation*, **80**, 10.

Jennings, L.K., White, M.M., Saver, C.M., et al. (1993). Cocaine induced platelet defects. *Stroke*, **24**, 1352.

Judice, D.J., LeBlanc, H.J., McGarry, P.A. (1978). Spinal cord vasculitis presenting as spinal cord tumor in a heroin addict. *Journal of Neurosurgery*, **48**, 131.

Kaku, D.A. & Lowenstein, D.H. (1990). Emergence of recreational drug abuse as a major risk factor for stroke in young adults. *Annals of Internal Medicine*, **113**, 821.

Kaufman, M.J., Levin, J.M., Ross, M.H. et al. (1998). Cocaine-induced cerebral vasoconstriction detected in humans with magnetic resonance angiography. *Journal of the American Medical Association*, **279**, 376.

Kessler, J.T., Jorntner, B.S. & Adapon, B.D. (1978). Cerebral vasculitis in a drug abuser. *Journal of Clinical Psychiatry*, **39**, 559.

King, T.A., Perlman, J.M., Laptook, A.R. et al. (1995). Neurologic manifestations of *in utero* cocaine exposure in near term and term infants. *Pediatrics*, **96**, 259.

Knoblauch, A.L., Buchholz, M., Koller, M.G. & Kistler, H. (1983). Hemiplegie nach Injektion von Heroin. *Schweiz Medische Wochenschrift*, **113**, 402.

Kokkinos, J. & Levine, S.R. (1993a). Stroke. In *Neurologic Complications of Drug and Alcohol Abuse*, ed. J.C.M. Brust. *Neurologic Clinics*, vol. 11, 577–90.

Kokkinos, J. & Levine, S.R. (1993b). Possible association of ischemic stroke with phentermine. *Stroke*, **24**, 310.

Lester, B.M., LaGasse, L.L. & Seifer, R. (1998). Cocaine exposure and children: the meaning of subtle effects. *Science*, **282**, 63.

Levine, S.R., Brust, J.C.M., Futrell, N. et al. (1990). Cerebrovascular complications of the use of the 'crack' form of alkaloidal cocaine. *New England Journal of Medicine*, **323**, 699.

Levine, S.R., Brust, J.C.M., Futrell, N. et al. (1991). A comparative study of the cerebrovascular complications of cocaine: alkaloidal versus hydrochloride – a review. *Neurology*, **41**, 1173.

Lloyd, J.T.A. & Walker, D.R.H. (1995). Death after combined dexamphetamine and phenylzine. *British Medical Journal*, **2**, 168.

Loizou, L.A., Hamilton, J.G. & Tsementzis, S.A. (1982). Intracranial hemorrhage in association with pseudoephedrine overdose. *Journal of Neurology, Neurosurgery and Psychiatry*, **45**, 471.

Manchanda, S. & Connolly, M.J. (1993). Cerebral infarction in association with Ecstasy abuse. *Postgraduate Medical Journal*, **69**, 874.

Matthew, R.J. & Wilson, W.H. (1991). Substance abuse and cerebral blood flow. *American Journal of Psychiatry*, **148**, 292.

Mizutami, T., Lewis, R. & Gonatas, N. (1980). Medial medullary syndrome in a drug abuser. *Archives of Neurology*, **37**, 425.

Meuller, S.M. & Ertel, P.J. (1983). Subarachnoid hemorrhage associated with over-the-counter medications. *Stroke*, **14**, 16.

Palomaki, H., Kaste, M., Raininko, R. et al. (1993). Risk factors for cervical atherosclerosis in patients with transient ischemic attack or minor ischemic stroke. *Stroke*, **24**, 970.

Pascual-Leone, A., Dhuna, A. & Anderson, D.C. (1991). Cerebral atrophy in habitual cocaine abusers: a planimetric CT study. *Neurology*, **41**, 34.

Pearson, J., Richter, R.W., Baden, M.M. et al. (1972). Transverse myelopathy as an illustration of the neurologic and neuropathologic features of heroin addiction. *Human Pathology*, **3**, 109.

Qureshi, A.L., Akber, M.S., Czander, E. et al. (1997). Crack cocaine use and stroke in young patients. *Neurology*, **48**, 341.

Rothrock, J.F., Rubenstein, R. & Lyden, P.D. (1988). Ischemic stroke associated with methamphetamine inhalation. *Neurology*, **38**, 589.

Rumbaugh, C.L., Bergeron, R.T., Fang, H.C.H. & McCormick, R. (1971). Cerebral angiographic changes in the drug abuse patient. *Radiology*, **101**, 335.

Rumbaugh, C.L., Fang, H.C.H., Higgins, R.E. et al. (1976). Cerebral microvascular injury in experimental drug abuse. *Investigative Radiology*, **11**, 282.

Sacco, R.L., Elkind, M., Boden-Albala, B. et al. (1999). The protective effect of moderate alcohol consumption on ischemic stroke. *Journal of the American Medical Association*, **281**, 53.

Shinton, R. & Beevers, G. (1989). Meta-analysis of relation between cigarette smoking and stroke. *British Medical Journal*, **298**, 789.

Sobel, J., Espinas, O.E. & Friedman, S.A. (1971). Carotid artery obstruction following LSD capsule injection. *Archives of Internal Medicine*, **127**, 290.

Strickland, T.L. & Stein, R. (1995). Cocaine-induced cerebrovascular impairment: challenges to neuropsychological assessment. *Neuropsychology Review*, **5**, 69.

Weinrieb, R.M. & O'Brien, C.P. (1993). Persistent cognitive deficits attributed to substance abuse. In *Neurologic Complications of Drug and Alcohol Abuse*, ed. J.C.M. Brust. *Neurologic Clinics*, vol. 11, pp. 663–91.

Woods, B.T. & Strewler, G.J. (1972). Hemiparesis occurring six hours after intravenous heroin injection. *Neurology*, **22**, 863.

Wooten, M.R., Khangure, M.S. & Murphy, M.J. (1983). Intracerebral hemorrhage and vasculitis related to ephedrine abuse. *Annals of Neurology*, **13**, 337.

18

Paraneoplastic strokes

José Castillo[1] and Antoni Dávalos[2]

[1]Department of Neurology, Hospital Xeral de Galicia, Santiago de Compostela, Spain
[2]Department of Neurology, Hospital Universitari Doctor Josep, Trueta, Girona, Spain

Introduction

Paraneoplastic syndromes are a variety of disorders that accompany the clinical evolution of tumours, which are not produced directly by the primary neoplasm, nor by its metastasis, nor as a result of diagnostic or therapeutic procedures. These syndromes may evolve in parallel with the development of the tumour, but may also be independent of it and even precede the initial diagnosis of neoplasm.

It has been estimated that paraneoplastic syndromes are detected in 7–10% of patients at the time the tumour is diagnosed, although almost all patients with a malignant tumour present a paraneoplastic syndrome during the course of its evolution (Nathanson & Hall, 1997).

Paraneoplastic syndromes can affect any part of the nervous system. Occasionally, paraneoplastic syndromes arise from causal lesions in the central or peripheral nervous system, but neurological manifestations are more commonly due to lesions in non-neurological organs. The classic paraneoplastic neurological syndromes fall into the first group, while in the second group, the neurological manifestations are the result of blood vessel changes, blood-forming elements, hemostasia and coagulation disorders, metabolic changes and infections (Table 18.1). Cerebrovascular paraneoplastic manifestations are included in the second group of neurological paraneoplastic syndromes.

Frequency

Cerebrovascular disease is the second most common cause of central nervous system disease found at autopsy of patients with cancer, and must be considered in any patient who experiences cerebral symptoms. Fifteen per cent of patients with cancer present cerebrovascular disorders related to neoplastic disease and half of these patients have clinical symptoms before dying. In some patients, the cerebrovascular manifestations are due to the tumour itself, its metastases or to complications resulting from the diagnostic procedures or from treatment. However, in most cases, the paraneoplastic origin is the most common cause of strokes (Patchell & Posner, 1985; Graus et al., 1985).

Etiopathology

In all primary neurological paraneoplastic syndromes, the pathogenesis is autoimmune. Proteins normally expressed only in the nervous system are expressed ectopically by the tumour. However, the immune system does not recognize these proteins as its own and produces antibodies against the proteins that destroy antigenically vulnerable neurons (Dalmau & Posner, 1997).

In the secondary neurological paraneoplastic syndromes, that are responsible for most cerebrovascular diseases that appear in patients with cancer, the pathogenesis has been linked to autoimmunity or to the release of procoagulant substances by the tumor. Some of them are associated with intracerebral hemorrhages, others with cerebral infarcts and others with both (Table 18.2).

Microangiopathic hemolytic anemia, thrombocytopenia, von Willebrand's disease, antiphospholipid syndrome and vasculitis all fall within the first group of etiopathological mechanisms. Microangiopathic hemolytic anemia, usually accompanied by thrombocytopenia, is an autoimmune disease that is sometimes associated with mucinous adenocarcinomas, above all of the stomach, breast and lung (Staszewski, 1997). Thrombocytopenia of paraneoplastic origin may also be due to autoimmune thrombocytopenia, accompanying chronic lymphocytic leukemia,

Table 18.1. *Classification of neurological paraneoplastic syndromes*

Primary neurological paraneoplastic syndromes

Disorders of the brain and cranial nerves
Encephalomyelitis
Subacute cerebellar degeneration
Opsoclonus/myoclonus syndrome
Limbic encephalitis and other dementias
Brainstem encephalitis
Optic neuritis
Cancer-associated retinopathy

Disorders of the spinal cord
Necrotizing myelopathy
Subacute motor neuropathy
Stiff person (man) syndrome

Disorders of the peripheral nerve
Sensorimotor polyneuropathy
Subacute sensory neuronopathy
Guillain–Barré syndrome
Autonomic neuropathy

Disorders of the neuromuscular union
Lambert–Eaton myasthenic syndrome
Myasthenia gravis

Muscle disorders
Dermatomyositis, polymyositis
Carcinoid myopathies
Myotonia
Cachectic myopathy

Secondary neurological paraneoplastic syndromes

Disorder of the vessels
Vasculitis

Disorders of blood-forming elements
Thrombocytopenia
Thrombocytosis

Hemostasia and coagulation disorders
Disseminated intravascular coagulation
Non-bacterial thrombotic endocarditis
Acquired von Willebrand's disease
Hyperviscosity syndrome

Metabolic changes

Infections

Table 18.2. *Etiopathology of paraneoplastic strokes*

Intracerebral hemorrhage

Mediated by autoimmune mechanism
Autoimmune thrombocytopenia
Thrombotic thrombocytopenic purpura
Acquired von Willebrand's disease

Mediated by the release of procoagulant substances
Disseminated intravascular coagulation
Hyperviscosity due to myeloproliferative syndrome

Cerebral infarct

Mediated by autoimmune mechanism
Microangiopathic hemolytic anemia
Acquired von Willebrand's disease
Antiphospholipid syndrome
Vasculitis

Mediated by the release of procoagulant substances
States of hypercoagulability
Thrombocytosis
Bacterial thrombotic endocarditis
Disseminated intravascular coagulation
Hyperviscosity syndrome

B-cell lymphomas and, less commonly, in some solid tumours (lung and rectum), it may be due to thrombotic thrombocytopenic purpura (Steingart, 1988). In these cases, deposits of fibrin and platelet aggregates are found at the cerebral microcirculation. These give rise to micro-infarcts and subdural and intracerebral hemorrhaging. An acquired form of von Willebrand's disease has been reported as a paraneoplastic manifestation in patients with lymphoproliferative and myeloproliferative neoplasms and with systemic hemorrhages (Mohri et al., 1987).

The association of high levels of antiphospholipid antibodies with arterial and venous thrombosis is called antiphospholipid syndrome, which may be primary or associated with other diseases such as neoplasms (Harris et al., 1985; McNeil et al., 1991). Even though the link between the presence of antiphospholipid antibodies and thrombotic phenomena has clearly been established, we still do not know what the pathogenic mechanism is. One of the most widely accepted theories is based on the possible effects of the binding of antiphospholipid antibodies with phospholipids that make up the cellular membranes of the endothelium and platelets. The inhibiting effect of β_2–glycoprotein I on blood coagulation and platelet aggregation would be neutralized by antiphospholipid antibodies (Khamashta et al., 1990). Antiphospholipid syndrome might cause occlusion of the intracerebral arteries and of the large intracranial venous sinuses (Coull et al., 1992; Russell & Enevoldson, 1993).

Vasculitis is a heterogeneous group of multisystemic processes characterized by inflammation of the arterial wall. These inflammatory arteriopathies may lead to ischemia of the central nervous system by two different mechanisms, which are not mutually exclusive: firstly, arterial disease provides the right conditions for thrombosis to develop; and secondly, the change in the arterial wall can itself, though less commonly, cause stenosis of the vascular lumen to the point that it is destroyed.

When vasculitis appears in association with malignant tumours, antigens deriving from the tumour itself play a part in the formation of immune complexes that are deposited on the vascular wall, causing inflammation. The clinical symptoms that arise from these arterial changes will depend on the vessel affected, its size and location, and the speed at which the obstruction develops. Even though they are rare, almost all forms of vasculitis have been associated with neoplastic diseases, especially Hodgkin's disease, lymphomas, hairy cell leukemia and lung cancer (Kurzrock & Cohen, 1993; Carsons, 1997; Lie, 1997). Approximately 5% of vasculitides are paraneoplastic in origin (Sánchez-Guerrero et al., 1990), but only a very small percentage cause cerebral infarction (Baumgartner et al., 1998).

Granulomatous angiitis of the central nervous system has only been reported in 7% of patients with lymphoproliferative neoplasms, although 77% of these patients develop focal neurological manifestations (Younger et al., 1997). In some cases, granulomatous angiitis affects the carotid artery, the middle cerebral artery or the anterior cerebral artery, and appears weeks after herpes zoster infection of the contralateral ophthalmic branch (Hilt et al., 1983).

The association between temporal arteritis, neoplastic disease and stroke is difficult to quantify given that these patients are usually of an advanced age, when other diseases are also prevalent (Haga et al., 1993). The association of neoplasia and temporal arteritis has been estimated at between 3.5% and 16% (Kurzrock & Cohen, 1993), and infarcts and transient ischemic attacks appear in 7% of these patients (Caselli & Hunder, 1997).

The second group of etiopathological mechanisms involved in paraneoplastic strokes are caused by the tumour releasing procoagulant substances responsible for hypercoagulability.

Non-bacterial thrombotic endocarditis is the most common cause of symptomatic cerebral infarcts in patients with cancer (Graus et al., 1985; Patchell & Posner,

1985) and is produced by growths of fibrin and platelets in the cardiac valves, particularly on the left (see colour Fig. 18.1). This disorder is often associated with cerebral intravascular thrombosis. In autopsy studies, non-bacterial thrombotic endocarditis appears in 1% to 2% of patients with cancer (Biller et al., 1982; Graus et al., 1985); a third of these patients have emboli in the brain. This paraneoplastic syndrome has been reported more often in very developed mucinous adenocarcinomas of the lung and stomach, but it can complicate any kind of neoplasm and appear at any early stage (Rogers et al., 1987).

Over 90% of cancer patients develop disseminated intravascular coagulation (Sletness et al., 1995), with increased fibrinogen degradation products, thrombocytosis, increased platelet adhesiveness and hyperfibrinogenemia. The triggering of this process is due to the release of procoagulant material from the tumour cells into blood circulation (Staszewski, 1997). The chronic form of disseminated intravascular coagulation produces a state of hypercoagulability in which fibrino-platelet thrombi occlude small cerebral arteries and venules, large intracranial venous sinuses or deposits on cardiac valves, leading to non-bacterial thrombotic endocarditis (Posner, 1995). This chronic form of disseminated intravascular coagulation is the second cause of symptomatic cerebral infarcts in patients with cancer (Patchell & Posner, 1985; Graus et al., 1985). The acute form of disseminated intravascular coagulation is associated with clinical hemorrhaging, consumption of coagulation factors and platelets, and an increase in fibrinolysis (Furui et al., 1983; Rogers, 1991). Disseminated intravascular coagulation is common in gastric and pancreatic mucinous adenocarcinomas, cancer of the lung, ovary and prostate, and in myeloproliferative syndromes (Graus et al., 1985; Cornuz et al., 1988; Posner, 1995). This process can complicate the evolution of the cancer at any stage, but appears more frequently in the advanced phases and in the presence of sepsis (Posner, 1995).

The association of migratory thrombophlebitis and neoplasms (Trousseau's syndrome) was one of the first paraneoplastic syndromes described (Prandoni et al., 1992). The mechanisms that affect hypercoagulability and thrombosis are complex and only partially elucidated. Fibrinopeptide A, a sensitive marker of thrombotic activity, appears in many developed neoplasms (Rickles & Edwards, 1983). Residues of sialic acid may be released by mucinous tumours and are responsible for the activation of the coagulation cascade. Other phospholipids and tissue factor, which activate hemostasia in normal situations following the disruption of the endothelium, may be released into the blood flow by the tumor itself or through abnormal vascularization arising from the growth of the tumour

(Staszewski, 1997). Platelet hyperactivity can also contribute to the increased risk of thrombosis in these patients, presumably due to factors released by the tumour or induced by its presence (Staszewski, 1997). It has been demonstrated in recent years that a large number of neoplasms are capable of releasing cytokines (IL-1, IL-6, IL-8, TNF, TGF and ICAM) which are responsible for the most common paraneoplastic syndromes, such as fever (Dinarello & Bunn, 1997), cachectic syndrome (Pucio & Nathanson, 1997) and hypercoagulability (Green & Silverstein, 1996). In addition, IL-6 is a powerful stimulant of thrombocytosis (Gastl et al., 1993). Deep venous thrombosis, both in the limbs and intracranial, pulmonary thromboembolism, and systemic embolizations due to non-bacterial thrombotic endocarditis are all consequence of this state of hypercoagulability (Staszewski, 1997).

On rare occasions, some tumours release paraproteins and monoclonal immunoglobulins, leading to a hyperviscosity syndrome that interferes with the polymerization of fibrin and causes coagulation disorders and symptomatic hemorrhages (O'Kane et al., 1994).

Clinical and diagnostic characteristics

Even though cerebrovascular manifestations in patients with cancer may be clinically similar and have the same etiopathology as the strokes that appear in the rest of the population (Chaturvedi et al., 1994), paraneoplastic strokes more commonly present specific clinical manifestations (Patchell & Posner, 1985; Rogers, 1991; 1994; Baumgartner et al., 1998).

In contrast to non-neoplastic patients, amongst whom cerebral infarcts are more prevalent than hemorrhages, in patients with cancer the frequency of hemorrhages is almost the same as the frequency of infarcts (Graus et al., 1985). Symptomatic cerebral infarction is more common in patients with lymphoma and carcinoma than it is in those with leukemia, amongst whom cerebral hemorrhage predominates.

The classic ischemic stroke, preceded or not by transient ischemic attacks, is a rare form of presentation in paraneoplastic strokes. The proportion of ischemic events in the vertebrobasilar territory and in the carotid artery is similar in patients with temporal arteritis, a fact that does not occur in arteriosclerotic disease. Neurological symptoms in these patients are usually the result of thrombotic obstruction of the vertebral and carotid arteries rather than of intracranial arteritis (Caselli & Hunder, 1997). In other forms of vasculitis, the clinical pattern may also be focal, but cerebral manifestations appear just as often as spinal signs and iso-lated lesions in cranial nerves (Younger et al., 1997). Cerebral infarcts with focal neurological manifestations also appear in non-bacterial thrombotic endocarditis, occasionally preceded by transient ischemic attacks.

More commonly, paraneoplastic strokes show a clinical picture different from those observed in stroke patients without cancer. Diffuse and progressive encephalopathy, either isolated or accompanied by focal neurological manifestations, is usual in disseminated intravascular coagulation, non-bacterial thrombotic endocarditis and in paraneoplastic vasculitis. This is due to the fact that cerebral infarctions in cancer patients are often multifocal, and the resulting multifocal manifestations are difficult to distinguish from those caused by encephalopathy. Many patients with paraneoplastic strokes progress towards stupor or coma (Rogers, 1991; Schwartzmann & Hill, 1982).

The clinical presentation of paraneoplastic cerebral venous thrombosis is very variable and includes severe, diffuse and progressive headache due to intracranial hypertension, partial or generalized seizures, transient ischemia or cerebral infarct of venous origin, and progressive ischemic encephalopathy (Ameri & Bousser, 1992; Russell & Enevoldson, 1993). This clinical pattern is usually more serious than the one caused by metastatic cerebral venous thrombosis or by a thrombosis induced by treatment (Hickey et al., 1982).

As we have indicated, the hemorrhagic presentation of paraneoplastic strokes is as common as ischemic forms (Fig. 18.2). Cerebral hemorrhage occurs more often in patients with leukemia than in those with lymphomas or solid tumours, and is more frequent in acute than in chronic leukemias and in myelogenous than in lymphocytic leukemias. Intracerebral hemorrhaging may present itself with the usual clinical pattern, although hemorrhages are more commonly smaller and cause symptoms of diffuse encephalopathy (Posner, 1995). Subdural hemorrhaging may be acute, subacute or chronic, with considerable clinical variability (Minette & Kimmel, 1989). Subarachnoid hemorrhaging is the rarest form of presentation of paraneoplastic hemorrhagic stroke (Graus et al., 1985).

In many cases the diagnostic process for paraneoplastic strokes is different from standard procedures for other types of stroke. Cerebral computed tomography and magnetic resonance imaging can be normal in ischemic events caused by disseminated intravascular coagulation (Schwartzman & Hill, 1982), or may show multiple images in several vascular territories in non-bacterial thrombotic endocarditis and vasculitis (Baumgartner et al., 1998).

Cerebral infarction due to disseminated intravascular coagulation should be diagnosed in patients with clinical manifestations coinciding with the characteristic hemato-

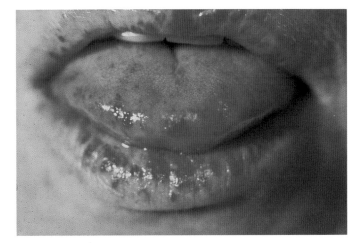

Fig. 28.1. This figure shows typical telangiectasis on the lips and the tongue of a woman 35 years old with Osler–Weber–Rendu disease. (By courtesy of Professor Panizzon, Department of Dermatology, CHUV, Lausanne, Switzerland.)

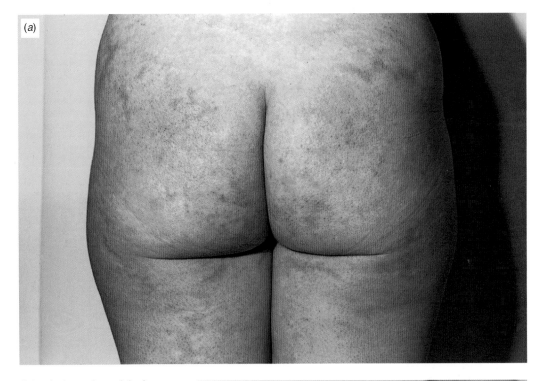

(a)

Fig. 33.1. Livedo racemosa involving the buttocks, and the feet and lower legs in two Sneddon syndrome patients (Courtesy of Professor J-M. Naeyaert, Ghent University Hospital.)

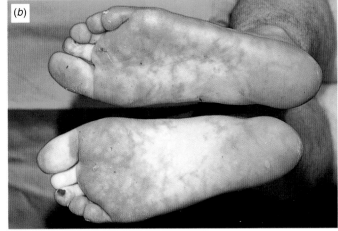

(b)

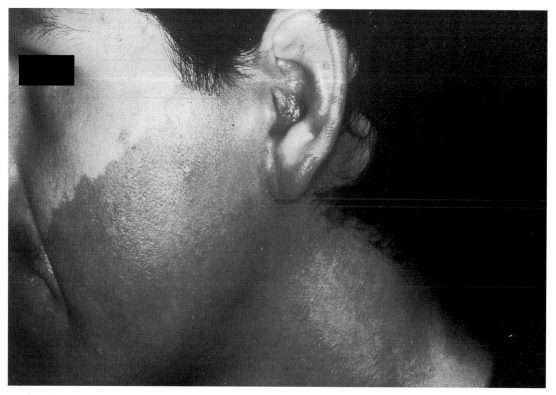

Fig. 48.2. Facial port wine angioma in Sturge–Weber syndrome.

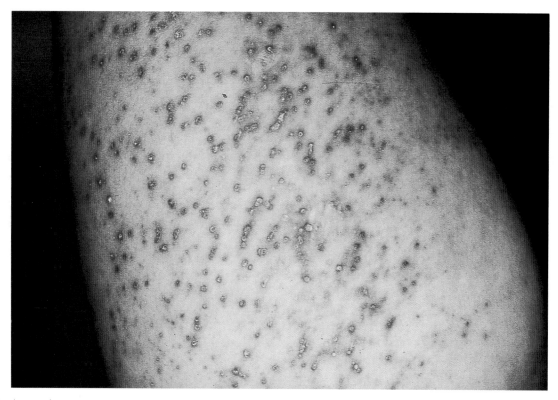

Fig. 48.4. Dark red papules of approximately 1–2 mm diameter on the trunk, in Angiokeratoma corporis diffusum (Fabry's disease). They can be rarely observed on face and distal part of the limbs.

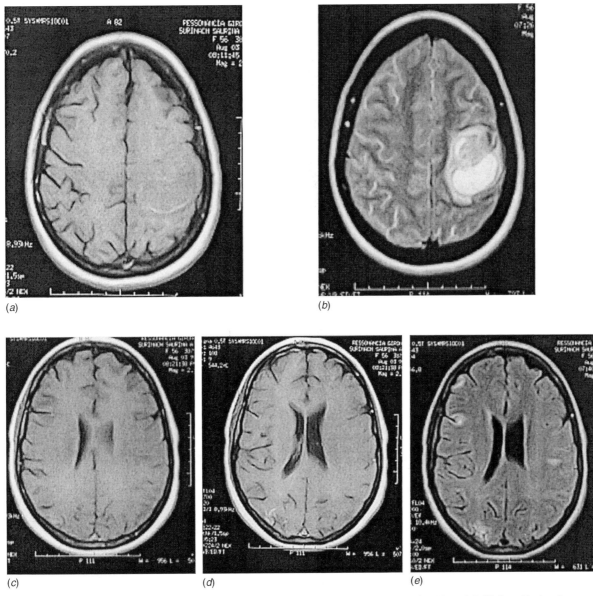

Fig. 18.2. Woman aged 70 admitted with intracerebral hemorrhage. Admitted a month previously with occipital infarct. During the current admission adenocarcinoma of the ovary was diagnosed. MR carried out in acute phase, section at the level of the corona radiata (above) and the semioval centre (below). Lobar, left parietal intraparenchymatous hematoma, in amplified images in T_1 (a) and T_2 (b). At the level of the corona radiata no changes in signal observed in amplified images in T_1 (c); images in T_1 with contrast (d) and FLAIR (e) show the presence of multiple ischemic cortical lesions, in the same stage and in different vascular areas.

logical profile. Systemic thrombosis, including deep vein thrombosis, pulmonary embolism and myocardial infarction, and systemic hemorrhages may occur together with the cerebral symptoms. Laboratory studies to confirm disseminated intravascular coagulation include determination of the number of platelets, prothrombin time, activated partial thromboplastin time, fibrinogen, fibrin split products, fibrinopeptide A and D-dimer assay. Results

of laboratory tests for coagulation function must be carefully interpreted in the clinical context, since abnormalities are not always clinically significant. Pleocytosis of cerebrospinal fluid helps in the diagnosis of vasculitis (Younger et al., 1997). Echocardiograms, including transesophageal echocardiograms, are usually normal in patients with non-bacterial thrombotic endocarditis, possibly due to the small size of the valve growths (Hofmann et al., 1990). The most useful test for diagnosing vasculitis and non-bacterial thrombotic endocarditis is the cerebral angiogram.

Treatment

Cerebral hemorrhages of paraneoplastic origin are difficult to treat. Surgical removal of hematomas during the course of coagulopathy is not indicated. Treatment with heparin and platelet concentrate or fresh plasma reverse the coagulopathy of consumption in some circumstances. Therapy with heparin and the administration of fresh plasma are usually more useful in preventing cerebral hemorrhaging in patients amongst whom hematological changes suggestive of disseminated intravascular coagulation are detected at an early stage (Rogers et al., 1987). Cytoreductive chemotherapy reduces the risk of cerebral hemorrhage in patients with chronic myeloproliferative processes (Wehmeier et al., 1991). However, in other patients, lysis of the blastos can exacerbate disseminated intravascular coagulation (Rogers, 1994).

Heparin is effective in preventing cerebral infarction amongst patients with non-bacterial thrombotic endocarditis and does not increase the risk of hemorrhagic complications (Rogers et al., 1987). Vasculitis responds to treatment with steroids and cytostatic agents (Inwards et al., 1991). Administering aspirin and cytostatics has also been shown to be effective in preventing the recurrence of thrombotic complications in patients with essential thrombocythemia (Michiels et al., 1993).

References

Ameri, A. & Bousser, M.G. (1992). Cerebral venous thrombosis. *Neurology Clinics*, **10**, 87–109.

Baumgartner, R.W., Mattle, H.P. & Cerny, T. (1998). Stroke and cancer. In *Cerebrovascular Disease: Pathophysiology, Diagnosis, and Management*, vol 2, ed. M.D. Ginsberg & J. Bogousslavsky pp. 1727–36. Massachusetts: Blackwell Science.

Biller, J., Challa, V.R., Toole, J.F. & Howard, V.J. (1982). Non-bacterial thrombotic endocarditis. A neurological perspective of clinicopathologic correlations of 99 patients. *Archives of Neurology*, **39**, 95–8.

Carsons, S. (1997). The association of malignancy with rheumatic and connective tissue diseases. *Seminars in Oncology*, **24**, 360–72.

Caselli, R.J. & Hunder, G.G. (1997). Giant cell (temporal) arteritis. *Neurology Clinics*, **15**, 893–902.

Chaturvedi, S., Ansell, J. & Recht, L. (1994). Should cerebral ischemic events in cancer patients be considered a manifestation of hypercoagulability? *Stroke*, **25**, 1215–18.

Cornuz, J., Bogousslavsky, J., Schapira, M., Regli, F. & Camenzind, E. (1988). Ischemic stroke as the presenting manifestation of localized systemic cancer. *Schweiz Archives of Neurology and Psychiatry*, **139**, 5–11.

Coull, B.M., Levine, S.R. & Brey, R.L. (1992). The role of antiphospholipid antibodies in stroke. *Neurology Clinics*, **10**, 125–43.

Dalmau, J.O., Posner, J.B. (1997). Paraneoplastic syndromes affecting the nervous system. *Seminars of Oncology*, **24**, 318–28.

Dinarello, C.A. & Bunn, P.A. Jr. (1997). Fever. *Seminars in Oncology*, **24**, 288–98.

Furui, T., Ichihara, K., Ikeda, A. Subdural hematoma associated with disseminated intravascular coagulation in patients with advanced cancer. *Journal of Neurosurgery*, **58**, 398–401.

Gastl, G., Plante, M., Finstad, C.L. et al. (1993). High IL-6 levels in ascitic fluid correlate with reactive thrombocytosis with epithelial ovarian cancer. *British Journal of Hematology*, **83**, 433–41.

Graus, F., Rogers, L.R. & Posner, J.B. (1985). Cerebrovascular complications in patients with cancer. *Medicine*, **64**, 16–35.

Green, K.B. & Silverstein, R.L. (1996). Hypercoagulability in cancer. *Hematology and Oncology Clinics of North America*, **10**, 506–7.

Haga, H.J., Eide, G.E., Brun, J., Johansen, A. & Langmark, F. (1993). Cancer in association with polymyalgia rheumatica and temporal arteritis. *Journal of Rheumatology*, **20**, 1335–9.

Harris, E.N., Gharavi, A.E. & Hughes, G.R.V. (1985). Antiphospholipid antibodies. *Clinical Rheumatic Diseases*, **11**, 591–608.

Hickey, W.F., Garnick, M.B., Henderson, I.C. & Dawson, D.M. (1982). Primary cerebral venous thrombosis in patients with cancer. A rarely diagnosed paraneoplastic syndrome. Report of three cases and review of the literature. *American Journal of Medicine*, **73**, 740–50.

Hilt, D., Buchholz, D., Krumholz, A., Weiss, H. & Wolinsky, J.S. (1983). Herpes zoster ophthalmicus and delayed contralateral hemiparesis caused by cerebral angiitis: diagnosis and management approaches. *Annals of Neurology*, **14**, 543–53.

Hofmann, T., Kasper, W., Meinertz, T., Geibel, A. & Just, H. (1990). Echocardiographic evaluation of patients with clinically suspected arterial emboli. *Lancet*, **336**, 1421–4.

Inwards, D.J., Piepgras, D.G., Lie, J.T., O'Neill, B.P., Scheithauer, B.W. & Habermann, T.M. (1991). Granulomatous angiitis of the spinal cord associated with Hodgkin's disease. *Cancer*, **68**, 1318–22.

Khamashta, M.A., Cervera, R., Asherson, R.A. et al. (1990). Association of antibodies against phospholipids with heart valve disease in systemic lupus erythematosus. *Lancet*, **335**, 1541–4.

Kurzrock, R. & Cohen, P.R. (1993). Vasculitis and cancer. *Clinical Dermatology*, **11**, 175–87.

Lie, J.T. (1997). Classification and histopathologic spectrum of central nervous system vasculitis. *Neurology Clinics*, **15**, 805–19.

McNeil, H.P., Chesterman, C.N. & Krilis, S.A. (1991). Immunology and clinical importance of antiphospholipid antibodies. *Advances in Immunology*, **49**, 193–280.

Michiels, J.J., Koudstaal, P.J., Mulder, A.H. & van Vliet, H.H. (1993).

Transient neurologic and ocular manifestations in primary thrombocythemia. *Neurology*, **43**, 1107–10.

Minette, S.E. & Kimmel, D.W. (1989). Subdural hematoma in patients with systemic cancer. *Mayo Clinic Procedure*, **64**, 637–42.

Mohri, H., Noguchi, T., Kodama, F., Itoh, A. & Ohkube, T. (1987). Acquired von Willebrand disease due to an inhibitor of human myeloma protein specific for von Willebrand factor. *American Journal of Clinical Pathology*, **87**, 663–8.

Nathanson, L. & Hall, T.C. (1997). Paraneoplastic syndromes. *Seminars in Oncology*, **24**, 265–68.

O'Kane, M.J., Wisdom, G.B., Desai, Z.R. & Archbold, G.P. (1994). Inhibition of fibrin monomer polymerization by myeloma immunoglobulin. *Journal of Clinical Pathology*, **47**, 266–8.

Patchell, R.A. & Posner, J.B. (1985). Neurologic complications of systemic cancer. *Neurology Clinics*, **3**, 729–50.

Posner, J.B. (1995). Neurologic complications of cancer. In *Contemporary Neurology series*, vol 45, ed. R.W. Reinhardt, pp. 199–229. Philadelphia: FA Davis.

Prandoni, P., Lensing, A.W.A., Buller, H.R. et al. (1992). Deep-vein thrombosis and the incidence of subsequent symptomatic cancer. *New England Journal of Medicine*, **327**, 1128–38.

Puccio, M. & Nathanson, L. (1997). The cancer cachexia syndrome. *Seminars in Oncology*, **24**, 277–87.

Rickles, F.R. & Edwards, R.L. (1983). Activation of blood coagulation in cancer: Trousseau's syndrome revisited. *Blood*, **62**, 14–41.

Rogers, L.R. (1991). Cerebrovascular complications in cancer patients. *Neurology Clinics*, **9**, 889–99.

Rogers, L.R. (1994). Cerebrovascular complications in cancer patients. *Oncology*, **8**, 23–30.

Rogers, L.R., Cho, E.S., Kempin, S. & Posner, J.B. (1987). Cerebral infarction from non-bacterial thrombotic endocarditis. *American Journal of Medicine*, **83**, 746–56.

Russell, R.W.R. & Enevoldson, T.P. (1993). Unusual types of ischemic stroke. In *Current Review of Cerebrovascular Disease*, ed. M. Fisher. & J. Bogousslavsky, pp. 63–77. Philadelphia: Current Medicine.

Sánchez-Guerrero, J., Gutiérrez-Urena, S., Vidaller, A. et al. (1990). Vasculitis as a paraneoplastic syndrome. Report of 11 cases and review of the literature. *Journal of Rheumatology*, **17**, 1458–62.

Schwartzman, R.J. & Hill, J.B. (1982). Neurologic complications of disseminated intravascular coagulation. *Neurology*, **32**, 791–7.

Sletness, K.E., Godal, H.C. & Wisloff, I. (1995). Disseminated intravascular coagulation (DIC) in adult patient with acute leukemia. *European Journal of Haematology*, **54**, 34–8.

Staszewski, H. (1997). Hematological paraneoplastic syndromes. *Seminars in Oncology*, **24**, 329–33.

Steingart, R.H. (1988). Coagulation disorders associated with neoplastic disease. *Recent Results in Cancer Research*, **108**, 37–43.

Wehmeier, A., Daum, I., Jamin, H. & Schneider, W. (1991). Incidence and clinical risk factors for bleeding and thrombotic complications in myeloproliferative disorders. *Annals of Hematology*, **63**, 101–6.

Younger, D.S., Calabrese, L.H. & Hays, A.P. (1997). Granulomatous angiitis of the nervous system. *Neurology Clinics*, **15**, 821–34.

19

Eales retinopathy

Thomas R. Hedges[1] and Louis R. Caplan[2]

[1]Department of Ophthalmology, New England Medical Center, Boston, MA, USA
[2]Beth Israel Deaconess Medical Center, Boston, MA, USA

Introduction

Henry Eales, in 1880, described a syndrome of recurrent vitreous hemorrhage associated with abnormal retinal veins and peripheral retinal capillary dropout in young men who also had epistaxis and constipation. During the ensuing years there has been considerable controversy as to whether the condition that Eales described is a specific disease entity or whether the retinopathy can be found in a variety of different conditions that affect the retinal vasculature. Although the retinal vascular disorder described by Eales may be inflammatory, some of the features are also consistent with non-inflammatory retinal vascular lesions. We prefer at present to consider this entity as Eales retinopathy rather than Eales disease.

Eales retinopathy

Patients have a variety of different visual symptoms. These include seeing floaters, cobwebs and clouds. Some patients notice only monocular scotomas. In many patients, visual acuity is diminished. Blindness also occurs on occasion.

Eales retinopathy is characterized by vascular sheathing with retinal veins being affected more than arteries (Gieser & Murphy, 1994; Raizman et al., 1998). Elliott (1975) used the term periphlebitis retinae to describe the venous sheathing, obstruction of veins, and retinal hemorrhages (Fig. 19.1) found in this condition. Overt inflammation in the form of vitritis or anterior uveitis is not consistently found. The other finding that is characteristic of Eales retinopathy is drop-out of capillaries especially in the peripheral portions of the retina indicating deficient arterial perfusion. (Fig. 19.2). Microaneurysms, beading of arteries, and arterio-venular shunts are sometimes seen adjacent to these regions of capillary drop-out. Areas of retinal ischemia may stimulate the development of neovascularization which can cause bleeding into the vitreous. Fibrosis and scarring can lead to retinal traction, retinal tears, and retinal detachment. Leakage of fluid from the affected retinal vessels causes retinal edema that sometimes extends into the macula with resulting visual loss. Fluid leakage can also cause superficial epiretinal scarring. Rarely, neovascularization of the iris may lead to increased intraocular pressure and glaucomatous complications.

In some patients, the retinal symptoms and findings are active during a period of 5 years (Geiser & Murphy, 1994; Pessin & Chung, 1995). In other patients the course of the visual symptoms is prolonged over decades. Acute visual loss can be due to vitreous hemorrhages; in that circumstance the visual loss often improves when the hemorrhage resolves.

Differential diagnosis of the retinopathy

This pathological sequence of retinal vascular insufficiency with the subsequent development of neovascularization and vitreous hemorrhages is common to many different retinal vasculopathies, of which diabetic retinopathy is the most common. Sickle cell disease (Goldberg, 1971) and Takayasu's arteritis (Karam et al., 1999) also cause capillary dropout, especially affecting the peripheral retina. Paucity of peripheral retinal circulation is also found in patients with carotid artery occlusion (Hedges, 1963; Mizener et al., 1997) in retinal artery and retinal vein occlusions, and occasionally in patients with hypertensive retinopathy. Neurosarcoidosis often causes vascular sheathing, often called 'candlewax drippings', and occasionally poor retinal vascular perfusion and neovascularization (Caplan et al., 1983; Duker et al., 1998). However, in most patients with sarcoidosis, ocular involvement is due to inflammation of the uvea, usually the iris. Conjunctival and lacrimal gland involvement is also very common. Iritis, conjunctivitis, and lacrimal gland inflammation are not described in patients with Eales retinopathy. Patients with multiple sclerosis often have perivascular sheathing if carefully sought, and occasionally also have uveitis. Multiple sclerosis patients do not develop ischemic neovascularization or hemorrhages. Behcet's disease rarely causes a form of retinopathy similar to that found in patients with sarcoidosis, but usually the retinopathy is characterized by prominent accumulation of cells in the vitreous and in the anterior chamber of the eye in the form of a hypopyon (Colvard et al., 1977). Segmental arteriolar occlusion and vascular sheathing occur in a syndrome of multiple branch retinal artery occlusions, encephalopathy, and deafness often referred to as Susac's syndrome. This entity is discussed in Chapter 41. The retinopathy of Susac's syndrome rarely is associated with retinal neovascularization or hemorrhages (O'Halloran et al.,1998; Bogousslavsky et al., 1989).

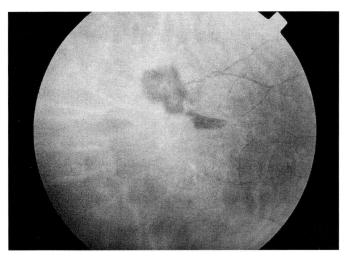

Fig. 19.1. Fundus photograph of retinal hemorrhage at the point where retinal vessels abnormally terminate abruptly in the retinal midperiphery.

Idiopathic retinal vasculitis, aneurysms, and neuroretinitis (IRVAN) and tuberculosis

Another entity, similar to Eales retinopathy, described as idiopathic retinal vasculitis, aneurysms, and neuroretinitis (IRVAN) occurs in patients of varying ages, who only rarely live or originate in geographic areas that harbour most patients with Eales disease. The IRVAN syndrome typically affects young healthy individuals and more women than men are involved. IRVAN differs from Eales retinopathy in the occurrence of more prominent regions of aneurysmal dilatation of retinal arteries, whereas Eales retinopathy is characterized more by venous sheathing and capillary dropout. Patients with IRVAN have not been known to develop systemic or neurological disease. They tend to develop loss of vision most often from macular edema rather than vitreous hemorrhages. However many patients with IRVAN have been treated with laser retinal photocoagulation before the vascular process has had time to develop vitreous hemorrhages (Chang et al., 1995).

Eales disease is usually separated from other retinal vascular pathologies that include ischemia and vitreous hemorrhages by epidemiology. There is a group of relatively healthy young men from India and neighbouring regions that develop during the third and fourth decades of life low grade peripheral retinal vasculitis. This condition usually presents in one eye with acute visual loss from vitreous hemorrhage. The opposite eye is usually affected within several months (Renie et al., 1983). This retinopathy is usually self-limited and can be controlled with systemic

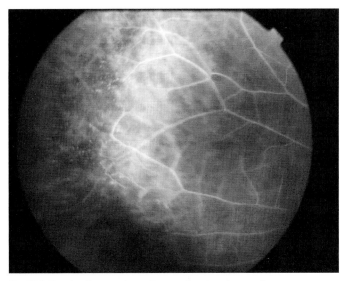

Fig. 19.2. Fundus fluorescein angiogram showing abnormal termination of midperipheral retinal arteries and veins with surrounding leakage of dye.

steroids and laser photocoagulation of affected areas of the retina. Some of the patients who have had this retinopathy were known to have active tuberculosis, a disorder very common in India. Most other patients undoubtedly had exposure to individuals with tuberculosis. Many have had positive tuberculin skin tests and many have received immunization with Bacille Calmette–Guérin (BCG) vaccine. Some have posited that the retinopathy in these patients is caused by a localized response to either the tubercle bacillus or to mycobacterial antigens (Raizman et al., 1998).

Ocular involvement from tuberculosis, on the other hand, which has been well studied and documented over many years, is not reported to cause the clinical picture shown by patients with Eales retinopathy (Deschene et al., 1997). Tuberculosis causes a spectrum of ocular complications including eyelid granulomas, orbital abscesses, dacryocystitis, conjunctivitis, keratitis, scleritis, and most importantly and frequently, uveitis. Posterior uveitis causes nodular choroiditis which is often followed by an exudative retinitis. Direct retinal involvement from tuberculosis may occur as miliary retinal tubercules or massive retinitis with vitriitis. Optic neuritis occurs in patients with tuberculous meningitis and also can occur in patients with active tuberculosis who do not clinically show meningitis.

Accompanying neurological findings

The only extraretinal manifestations in patients reported to have Eales retinopathy have related to the central nervous system (CNS). However, neurological involvement has not been common. In the largest series of patients thought to have Eales disease (947 cases), no CNS involvement was recognized by the authors (Doden & Adams, 1956). Others have reported CSF pleocytosis, seizures, myelopathy, chronic meningitis, brain vasculitis, demyelinating plaques, and strokes in occasional patients. These findings are most likely attributable to a vasculitis that affects the eye, brain, and spinal cord vasculature, predominantly veins.

Silverskiold (1947) described three young men who had Eales disease and a subacute onset of paraparesis accompanied by a CSF pleocytosis. Singhal and Dastur (1976) reported eight patients with Eales disease who had an acute or subacute onset of a myelopathy. White (1961) described two patients with Eales disease and a myelopathy.

CSF pleocytosis has been a relatively common finding. Among 17 patients considered to have Eales disease by White (1961), three had a lymphocytic pleocytosis without recognized brain or spinal cord involvement. Other patients have had cells in the spinal fluid with accompanying neurological signs (Silverskiold,1947; Singhal & Dastur, 1976). Herson and Squier (1978) described a patient who, at necropsy, had chronic meningitis and a vasculitis involving veins within the brain. This patient had progressive mental deterioration during a 6-year period. Another reported patient had a rapid clinical course characterized by brainstem and cerebellar signs followed by a myelopathy (Dastur & Singhal, 1976). Necropsy in this patient showed a widespread retinal and CNS vasculitis affecting mostly veins in the brainstem, cerebellum, and spinal cord

associated with demyelinating lesions. The cerebral hemispheres were spared, Silverskiold (1951) reported a patient thought to have multiple sclerosis clinically as well as a retinal vasculitis. Necropsy showed demyelinating plaques and perivascular inflammatory abnormalities. The inflammatory changes in the meninges and brain, especially around veins in these patients, is similar to that found in neurosarcoidosis which is also characterized by a retinal periphlebitis (Caplan et al., 1983).

Ballantyne and Michaelson (1937) reported a man with Eales type retinopathy who had an 8-year history of seizures and had additional neurological symptoms and signs (Singhal & Dastur, 1976). Renie et al. (1983) found sensory–neural hearing loss and vestibular abnormalities in most of 32 patients with Eales disease that had auditory and vestibular testing. It is not clear whether the disease affected the cochlea and vestibule or the VIIIth nerve. The findings are reminiscent of Cogan's syndrome and of microangiopathy of the brain, ear, and retina (Susac's syndrome).

Strokes

Occasional patients diagnosed with Eales disease have had strokes. Ludwig (1935) reported two patients with Eales who had sudden onset hemiplegia that developed after treatment with tuberculin. Another patient with Eales disease had a stroke during the puerperium (White,1961) Singhal and Dastur (1976) described a patient with Eales retinopathy who developed ocular symptoms at age 15 and, at age 42, had focal left-sided seizures followed by a left hemiparesis. This patient had a normal right carotid angiogram. Kutsal et al. (1987) reported a patient who had retinal symptoms at age 29 and 2 years later developed a left hemipareis with aphasia and dysphagia followed a month later by a right hemiparesis. CT scan showed multiple infarcts that involved both cerebral hemispheres including the lenticular nuclei, genu of the corpus callosum, and the cingulum. Angiography showed bilateral occlusion of the anterior cerebral arteries. No embolic source was identified.

Katz et al (1991) reported a 44-year-old man with a long history of Eales disease who developed a left hemiparesis. MRI showed an infarct in the right corona radiata adjacent to the upper border of the internal capsule. Carotid artery and cardiac studies were normal, and the spinal fluid was also normal. No etiology of the stroke was found in this normotensive patient who did not have atherosclerotic risk factors. Atabay et al. (1992) reported a 37-year-old man who had Eales disease and later developed dizziness.

Examination showed rotatory nystagmus, a left internuclear ophthalmoplegia, and bilateral extensor plantar reflexes. CT and MRI showed only an infarct in the right internal capsule but no brainstem lesion. CSF examination showed a high protein content (107 mg/dl) and oligoclonal bands but no cells. The patient was thought to have vasculitis as the cause of his stroke.

Gordon et al. (1988) described a 38-year-old man who developed retinal symptoms followed 6 months later by the sudden onset of dysarthria and right hemiparesis. This man was hypertensive and had smoked cigarettes for 20 years. The retina showed multiple peripheral venous occlusions with neovascularization and a large vitreous hemorrhage. On examination he had left facial weakness and slight weakness of the right limbs. CT showed infarcts in the left anterior thalamus and the right basal ganglia. Angiography showed right MCA occlusion.

In some patients with Eales retinopathy, strokes are probably caused by vasculitis. In other patients strokes are probably caused by atherosclerotic or other unrelated vascular disorders that are merely coincidental with the retinopathy.

References

Atabay, C., Endam, E., Kansu, T. & Eldem, B. (1992). Eales disease with internuclear ophthalmoplegia. *Annals of Ophthalmology*, **24**, 267–9.

Ballantyne, A.J. & Michaelson, I.C. (1937). A case of perivasculitis retinae associated with symptoms of cerebral disease. *British Journal of Ophthalmology*, **221**, 22–35.

Bogousslavsky, J., Gaio, J.M., Caplan, L.R. et al. (1989). Encephalopathy deafness and blindness in young women: a distinct retinocochleocerebral arteriolopathy. *Journal of Neurology, Neurosurgery and Psychiatry*, **52**, 43–6.

Caplan, L.R., Corbett, H.J., Goodwin, J. et al. (1983). Neuro-ophthalmological signs in the angiitic form of neurosarcoidosis. *Neurology*, **33**, 1130–5.

Chang, T.S., Aylward, G.W., Davis, J.L. et al. (1995). The retinal vasculitis study group. Idiopathic retinal vasculitis, aneurysms, and neuro-retinitis. *Ophthalmology*, **102**, 1089–97.

Colvard, D.M., Robertson, D.M. & O'Duffy, J. (1977). The ocular manifestations of Behcet's disease. *Archives of Ophthalmology*, **95**, 1813–17.

Dastur, D.K. & Singhal, B. (1976). Eales' disease with neurological involvement. Part 2. Pathology and pathogenesis. *Journal of Neurological Sciences*, **27**, 323–45.

Deschene, J., Seamone, C. & Cha, S.B. (1997). Tuberculosis and atypical mycobacteria. In *Duane's Clinical Ophthalmology*, ed. W. Tasman & E.A. Jaeger. Vol. 4, Chapter 58, pp. 1–8, Philadelphia: Lippincott-Raven.

Doden, W. & Adams, A. (1956). Ergebnisse neurologischer untersuchungen von kranken mit periphlebitis retinae. *Klinishe Monat für Augenheilkunde*, **129**, 305–17.

Duker, J.S., Brown, G.C. & McNamara, J.A. (1998). Proliferative sarcoid retinopathy. *Ophthalmology*, **95**, 1680–6.

Elliott, A.J. (1975). Thirty-year observation of Patients with Eales disease. *American Journal of Ophthalmology*, **80**, 404–8

Gieser, S.C. & Murphy, R.P. (1994). Eales disease In: *Principles and Practice of Ophthalmology*, ed. D.M. Albert & F.A. Jakobiecf, Vol. 2, pp. 791–5. Philadelphia: W.B. Saunders Co.

Goldberg, M.F. (1971). Natural history of untreated proliferative sickle retinopathy. *Archives of Opthalmology*, **85**, 428–33.

Gordon, M.F., Coyle, P.K. & Golub, B. (1988). Eales' disease presenting as stroke in the young adult. *Annals of Neurology*, **24**, 264–6.

Hedges, T.R. (1963). Ophthalmascopic findings in internal carotid occlusion. *American Journal of Ophthalmology*, **55**, 1007–12.

Herson, R.N. & Squier, M. (1978). Retinal perivasculitis with neurological involvement. A case report with pathological findings. *Journal of Neurological Science*, **36**, 110–1.

Karam, E.Z., Muci-Mendoza, R. & Hedges, T.R. III (1999). Retinal findings in Takayasu's arteritis. *Acta Ophthalmologica Scandinavica*, **77**, 209–13.

Katz, B., Wheeler, D., Weinreb, R.N. & Swenson, M.R. (1991). Eales' disease with central nervous system infarction. *Annals of Ophthalmology*, **23**, 460–3.

Kutsal, Y.G., Altioklar, K., Atasu, S., Kutluk, K. & Atmaca, L. (1987). Eales' disease with hemiparesis. *Clinical Neurology and Neurosurgery*, **89**, 282–6.

Ludwig, A. (1935). Zur diagnose der juvenilen glaskurperbustung. *Klinishe Monatsblader für Augenheilkunde*, **94**, 701–2.

Mizener, J.B., Podhajsky, P. & Hayreh, S.S. (1997). Ocular ischemic syndrome. *Ophthalmology*, **104**, 859–64.

O'Halloran, H.S., Pearson, P.A., Lee, W.B., Susac, J.O. & Berger, J.R. (1998). Microangiopathy of the brain, retina and cochlea (Susac Syndrome). *Ophthalmology*, **105**, 1038–44.

Pessin, M.S. & Chung, C. (1995). Eales's disease and Goenblad–Strandberg disease (*Pseudoxanthoma elasticum*). In *Stroke Syndromes*, ed. J. Bogousslavsky and L. Caplan, pp. 443–7. Cambridge: Cambridge University Press.

Raizman, M., Lashkari, K. & Haas, J.J. (1998). A 32 year-old-man with vitreous hemorrhage and lymphadenopathy. Case Records of the Massachusetts General Hospital, Case 4–1998. *New England Journal of Medicine*, **5**(338), 313–17.

Renie, W.A., Murphy, R.P., Anderson, K.C. et al. (1983) The evaluation of patients with Eales disease. *Retina*, **3**, 243–6.

Silverskiold, B.P. (1947). Retinal periphlebitis associated with paraplegia. *Archiv für Psychiatrie und Nervenkrankberten*, **57**, 351–7.

Silverskiold, B.P. (1951). Retinal periphlebitis and chronic disseminated encephalomyelitis. *Acta Psychiatrica et Neurologia Scandinavica* (Suppl) **74**, 55–7.

Singhal, B.S. & Dastur, D.K. (1976). Eales' disease with neurologic involvement. Part 1. Clinical features in 9 patients. *Journal of Neurological Science*, **27**, 313–21.

White, R.H.R. (1961). The aetiology and neurological complications of retinal vasculitis. *Brain*, **84**, 262–73.

20

Behçet's disease

Emre Kumral

Department of Neurology, School of Medicine, Ege University, Izmir, Turkey

Introduction

Behçet's disease (BD) is a multisystemic inflammatory disorder with unknown etiology, and neurologic involvement is one of the major clinical features (International Study Group for Behçet's disease,1990; Yazıcı, 1994). The most known triad of the disease, described as the components of this disease entity in 1937 by Behçet, includes recurrent oral and genital ulcerations and hypopyon iritis (Behçet, 1937). Since then, many other organ system involvements have been described such as mucocutaneous, ocular, articular, vascular, pulmonary, gastrointestinal, renal and nervous system, extending the borders of BD to a multisystem disorder (Serdaroğlu, 1998). Knapp has described the first clinical report of neurological involvement in BD (Knapp, 1941). Cavara and D'Ermo introduced the term 'neuro-Behçet's disease' (n-BD) to describe a patient with meningoencephalitis (Cavara & D'Ermo, 1954). It is well known that other neurological manifestations such as aseptic meningitis, myelitis, optic neuritis, peripheral neuritis, myositis, cerebral venous thrombosis, and arterial stroke may occur in n-BD (Wolf et al., 1965; Kawakita et al., 1967; O'Duffy et al., 1971; O'Duffy & Goldstein, 1976; Rougemont et al., 1982; Serdaroğlu et al., 1989, 1998).

The prevalence of Behçet's disease is higher in Japan (10–15:100000) and in Mediterranean countries (80–300:100000 in two areas in Turkey) when compared with Western countries (1:500000 in North America) (Yazıcı, 1994). Male gender and the association with the B51 split of HLA-5 were more frequent in Western than Eastern countries (Yazıcı et al., 1985). In Turkey and Japan, skin pathergy reaction is correlated with the presence of the disease; whereas no association between them could be found in Western countries (O'Duffy, 1990).

Etiology

The central pathological process in Behçet's disease is vasculitis. There is evidence suggesting a role of immunological mechanisms in this vasculitis. The clinical picture may be the consequence of the interaction of intrinsic (i.e. genetic) and extrinsic (i.e. some microorganisms) factors (Emmi et al., 1995; Mizuki & Ohno, 1996). Occurrence of the familial cases and association of the disease with HLA-B51, at least in some populations, has accelerated genetic studies. The suspected region of susceptibility gene(s) for the disease is between the tumour necrosis factor (TNF) and HLA-B or HLA-C genes (Mizuki & Ohno, 1996). Moreover, some pathogenetic microorganisms such as some streptococcal strains or herpes simplex virus type 1 or heat shock protein-65 (hsp 65) may induce specific immunopathological responses in genetically predisposed individuals. These factors may activate $\gamma\delta$Tcells, and subsequently the excreted inflammatory cytokines stimulate neutrophils and monocytes. The neutrophils of BD patients are responsible for the disruption of the endothelium and the uncontrolled inflammatory reaction in many tissues (Kansu, 1994).

Pathology

When the clinico-pathological and neuroradiological findings are combined, two different patterns of central nervous system involvement in Behçet's disease can be established: parenchymal (82% of cases) and neurovascular (18% of cases) involvements. The pathological process within the nervous parenchyma occurs mainly in the brainstem, basal ganglia, diencephalic structures (Fig. 20.1), internal capsules, and is also disseminated throughout the central nervous system (CNS) as a low grade inflammation. Neuropathological examination shows small foci of softening, lymphocytic perivascular infiltration, diffuse microglial activity, and small areas of demyelination (Shimizu, 1962; Totsuka & Midorikawa, 1972; Totsuka et al., 1979). Other pathological processes in the vascular system of the CNS are cerebral venous thrombosis, large-artery occlusion, aneurysm, hemorrhage. The visible lesions of parenchyma usually correspond well to a main vascular territory in this type of involvement. This type of vascular involvement should be called vasculo-BD (Akman-Demir et al., 1996; Wechsler et al., 1992). The large arterial lesion in vasculo-BD represents inflammation occuring in the media and adventitia. In the affected arteries, active arteritis occurs initially, followed by destruction of the media and fibrosis. Saccular aneurysms are probably produced by severe destruction of the media due to intense active inflammation (Matsumoto et al., 1991).

Neuro-Behçet's disease

Neurologic involvement is one of the most devastating manifestations of Behçet's disease. This involvement may occur primarily within the nervous parenchyma (neuro-Behçet) or secondarily in the cerebral vascular system (vasculo-Behçet) (Serdaroğlu, 1998). Meningoencephalitis of neuro-Behçet begins months or years after the mucocutaneous manifestations and often develops with exacerbations of the non-neurological symptoms. Neurologic deficits may be seen acutely or by gradual onset and usually progress in a halting manner with periods of acceleration and incomplete remission. The meningoencephalitis predominates in the brainstem and is characterized by a variety of symptoms that have fluctuating courses and include headache, pyramidal tract signs, cerebellar incoordination, pseudobulbar palsy, seizures and stupor (Wolf et al., 1965; Kawakita et al., 1967; O'Duffy & Goldstein, 1976; Rougemont et al., 1982; Tsutsui et al., 1998). Examination of the spinal fluid may reveal a mild pleocytosis with a preponderance of lymphocytes, a moderate increase in total protein, and an elevation of gamma globulins. Computer tomography scan (CT) may demonstrate focal areas of decreased density that may be enhanced after contrast injection (Herskovitz et al., 1988; Patel et al., 1989) Magnetic resonance imaging (MRI) may show focal regions of increased signal on T_2-weighted images, mainly in the brainstem, basal ganglia, and hypothalamus. These lesions do not conform to arterial territories and are often larger than those encountered in arteritis, and have a tendency to resolve over time, following treatment, although in chronic cases they are particularly associated with

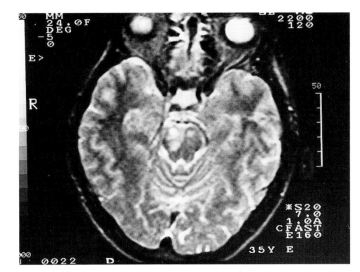

Fig. 20.1. MRI from 40-year-old man with Behçet's disease obtained following upper brainstem involvement. Multiple lesions are present in the upper brainstem.

brainstem atrophy (Montalban et al., 1990; Banna & El Ramahi, 1991; Wechsler et al., 1993).

In patients with vasculo-Behçet, neurologic abnormalities may develop due to the cerebral venous, large-artery or small-artery involvement, and a variety of clinical features such as pseudotumour cerebri, cerebral venous thrombosis, transient ischemic attacks, stroke, bulbar and pseudobulbar palsy may be seen (Shimizu et al., 1979; Uruyama et al., 1979; Bousser et al., 1980; Iragui & Maravi, 1986). The pathophysiology of vasculo-Behçet's disease is not clear and our knowledge is limited to the data derived from pathological and angiographic studies.

Vasculo-Behçet's disease

Central nervous system vasculature involvement is rare in Behçet's disease. The main vascular pathological process in the CNS is thrombosis of large venous sinuses which has special place and importance in Behçet's disease and may be considered as vasculo-BD. Arterial involvement is extremely rare, but does occur and can have a wide range of manifestations such as arterial malformations, intracranial hemorrhages, occlusive arterial disease.

Cerebral venous thrombosis

Thrombosis of cerebral large veins and sinuses is the most common feature of vasculo-BD, while thrombosis of the vena cava and portal vein may also occur in one third of

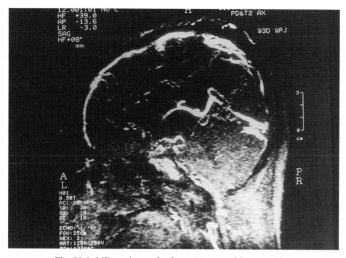

Fig. 20.2. MR angiography from 25-year-old man with neuro-Behçet's disease. Notice the lack of filling of the superior saggital and transverse sinuses.

these patients. It is well known that papilledema and pseudotumour cerebri or benign intracranial hypertension are reported frequently as a manifestation of cerebral venous thrombosis (CVT) in patients with Behçet's disease (Masheter, 1959; Kawakita et al., 1967; Bousser et al., 1980, 1985; Imaizumi et al., 1980; Pamir et al., 1981; Ben Itzhak et al., 1985; Wechsler et al., 1985; Wilkins et al., 1986; Serdaroğlu et al., 1989; Shakir et al., 1990). CT and MRI and/or angiography are important investigations to either disclose or rule out dural sinus thrombosis in patients presenting benign intracranial hypertension particularly in the context of Behçet's disease (Bousser et al., 1985; Ameri & Bousser, 1992; Harper et al., 1985).

Isolated intracranial hypertension is not the only manifestation of CVT in Behçet's disease. Most of the patients may present focal signs such as focal seizures or focal deficits, which can have highly variable patterns of onset: acute, mimicking an arterial stroke, or subacute, over days and sometimes weeks, mimicking meningoencephalitis (Bousser et al., 1985; Medejel et al., 1986; Ameri & Bousser, 1992). Such cases are often misdiagnosed as neuro-Behçet's disease, whereas the association of CVT with neuro-Behçet is rare (Serdaroğlu et al., 1989). The signs and symptoms of CVT in Behçet's disease are similar to the mode of onset in patients with CVT due to other causes. It most frequently affects, in order of decreasing frequency, the superior sagittal sinus (SSS), lateral sinuses, cortical veins, veins of the galenic system, and cavernous sinuses (Fig. 20.2). In most patients, thrombosis affects several sinuses, or sinuses together with cerebral veins, which explains the frequent association between signs of intra-

cranial hypertension and focal signs (Bousser at al., 1985; Ameri & Bousser, 1992).

Although CT is normal in 20% of patients with isolated intracranial hypertension, CT scan may show direct signs of SSS thrombosis in the majority of cases such as empty-delta signs or dense-triangle, localized or diffuse swelling, intense contrast enhancement of falx and tentorium, or a spontaneous hyperdensity or hypodensity, more or less suggestive of a venous infarct (Bousser et al., 1985; Ameri & Bousser, 1992). DSA is the gold method to reveal the thrombosis itself but it seems to be replaced by the magnetic resonance imaging (MRI), and angiography (MRA), the major advantage of these is non-invasiveness with higher sensivity to show CVT (Macchi et al., 1986; Montalban et al., 1990; Wechsler et al.,1992; Ameri & Bousser, 1992).

The neuro-Behçet form frequently occurs with exacerbations of the extraneurological and inflammatory signs, whereas CVT seems to belong to the vasculo-Behçet subgroup. The prognosis of patients with CVT is usually good, in which respect it again differs from neuro-Behçet meningoencephalitis. The treatment of choice is heparin or low-molecular weight heparin followed by long-term oral anticoagulants which can be combined with corticosteroid treatment for long-term supression of the immunopathological status (Bousser et al., 1985; Ameri & Bousser, 1992). In a previous series, worsening of a patient under anticoagulation was not related to treatment itself (Wechsler et al., 1992).

Ischemic Stroke

Ischemic cerebrovascular manifestations are less frequent in patients with Behçet's disease than in those with the aseptic meningitis and meningoencephalitis. Occlusions of the large cerebral arteries have been uncommonly reported, both clinically (Bienenstock & Margulies, 1961; Shimizu et al., 1979; Uruyama et al., 1979; Iragui & Maravi, 1986) and pathologically (Totsuka et al., 1979). In Japanese series, the incidence of intracerebral large-artery occlusive disease was around 0.15% (Shimizu et al., 1979; Uruyama et al., 1979), which is less than the 2.3% incidence for extracerebral large-artery involvement (Shimizu et al., 1979). In a series of 868 Behçet's patients, only two cases had cerebral artery occlusion (Uruyama et al., 1979). Shimizu et al. (1979) reported two cases of common carotid artery occlusion among 81 cases of vasculo-Behçet, investigated from a series of 1731 patients with Behçet's disease. In a study of 323 patients with Behçet's disease, two patients had supratentorial infarct in the centrum semiovale and internal capsule, and another three cases showed brainstem involvement with Wallenberg's syndrome, pseudobulbar signs and brief loss of consciousness. One case had cerebral angiogram with normal carotid and vertebral arteries (Serdaroğlu et al., 1989). In another case report, the patient presented transient ischemic attacks that preceded the mucocutaneous symptoms of the disease by several years. Angiography showed a high-grade stenosis of the left middle cerebral artery which became occluded during the procedure. In a few years, the patient developed almost total blindness of the left eye with fundoscopic signs of ischemic retinopathy due to an occlusion of the left internal carotid artery (Iragui & Maravi, 1986). A unique autopsy case was reported in which the patient had middle cerebral artery occlusion on angiogram that appeared after mucocutaneous lesions (Suga et al., 1990).

Behçet's disease is usually included among the systemic vasculitides (Allen, 1993) but documented cerebral arteritis is extremely rare and even a debatable mechanism for central nervous system involvement. However, some cases have been reported with typical appearance of arteritis with multiple segments of stenosis, occlusion, and dilatations of internal and external cerebral arteries (Kozin et al., 1977; Medejel et al., 1986; Zelenski et al., 1989). A previous clinico-pathological examination of Behçet's disease showed lymphocytic infiltration progressing from the adventitia toward the intima, possibly leading to thrombus formation (Totsuka & Midorikawa, 1972).

Some cases with CT signs of hemispheric infarction have been reported in which the patients have had arterial strokes but with no angiographic or pathological details concerning the underlying arterial lesions (Shakir et al., 1990). Zelenski et al. (1989) reported a single case with dramatic improvement of arterial lesions after 8 months of aggressive treatment with an initial course of intravenous nitrogen mustard and a long-term administration of chlorambucil and prednisolone.

Our recent study showed that one-third of the 55 patients with Behçet's disease had microembolic signals (MES) on transcranial Doppler examination, especially with a preponderance in the frequency of MES in patients with neurological involvement (Kumral et al., 1999). It is notable that MES were present in all patients with neurological involvement, including basal ganglia (four patients) and upper brainstem (one patient) involvement and cerebral venous thrombosis (one patient). The high prevalence of MES in the patient with cerebral venous thrombosis may be explained by generalized activation of the thrombotic system due to immunopathologic processes in the blood. It is probable that, in some patients with BD, an immunological mechanism propagates the formation of microthrombus, and thereafter yields to embolization of the distal vascular system. Previous studies showed an activation of blood coagulation such as shortening of prothrombin time, decreases in concentrations and activities of plasma antithrombin III and elevated levels of plasma thrombin–antithrombin-III complex. Moreover, increased plasma levels of protein C and total protein S levels, plasminogen activator activity, and decreased levels of alpha 2–plasmin inhibitor also indicated an activation of fibrinolysis in these patients (Fusegawa et al., 1991; Hampton et al., 1991).

Hemorrhagic Stroke

In Behçet's disease, subarachnoid and intracerebral hemorrhages are uncommon. A case with three recurrent massive intracranial hemorrhages had severe hypertension (Nagata, 1985). Postmortem examination showed the usual features of neuro-Behçet and concomitant hypertensive changes in the cerebral small penetrating arteries. The author accepted that the recurrent hemorrhages were more likely due to the hypertensive changes than to the perivascular lesions of Behçet's disease.

A rare case with a spinal subarachnoid hemorrhage due to a dissection of the extracranial vertebral artery in its V2 segment and an aneurysmal dilatation of a radiculomedullary brach in its intradural portion at the C5 level was reported (Bahar et al., 1993). Another case with a spinal subarachnoid hematoma was also found in a man with Behçet's disease. The hematoma was completely evacuated but there was no description of histological examination (Arias et al., 1987). In Behçet's disease, the aneurysm formation occurred most commonly in the aorta in either saccular or dissecting type (Matsumoto et al., 1991). In the affected arteries, active arteritis occurs initially followed by destruction of the media and fibrosis. Saccular aneurysms were probably produced by severe destruction of the media by active inflammation.

A few cases with single or multiple cerebral aneurysms have been reported (Shimizu et al., 1979; Godeau et al., 1980; Buge et al., 1987; Bartlett et al., 1988; Shakir et al., 1990). They are less frequent than systemic aneurysms with which they are frequently associated. They can be asymptomatic or can yield to subarachnoid, or intracerebral hemorrhage, or ischemic stroke (Buge et al., 1987). A unique case has been reported with multiple systemic arterial lesions and right-leg weakness of sudden onset. On angiography, she was found to have both an aneurysm of the left anterior communicating artery and a large arteriovenous malformation (Hassen Khoda et al., 1991). Another case with arteriovenous malformation was reported but it was a dural malformation draining into the right transverse sinus in a patient who had bilateral occlusion of lateral sinuses (Imaizumi et al., 1980).

Treatment of vascular manifestations

The long-term prognosis in neuro-Behçet's disease may not be as favourable as that observed in short-term follow-up. On seven-year follow-up of 42 patients with neuro-Behçet's disease, two had had dural sinus thrombosis and another two had gone through a Wallenberg-like brainstem syndrome, which could be attributable to the vascular events (Akman-Demir et al., 1996). The overall prognosis for patients with arterial involvement in Behçet's disease is far worse than that for patients with venous manifestations, because of aneurysm relapse, recurrence after vascular surgery, and rupture of the vascular wall. In a series of 24 patients with extracerebral arterial involvement, death occurred in six cases, mostly because of aneurysm rupture (Huong Du et al., 1993).

There has been no controlled trial of the therapy on cerebral ischemic events, although immunosuppressive agents are the main choice of drugs as well as in many immunopathological states. Corticosteroids control many symptoms, although they do not prevent end points such as blindness, recurrent central nervous system vasculature involvement or death (Yazıcı, 1994). Corticosteroids can be applied in oral or pulsed regimens especially in the acute phase. Some groups recommend chlorambucil but it is not widely utilized because of the side effects (O'Duffy, 1990). IVIg, plasma exchange, alpha-interferon, total nodal lymphoid irradiation, and transfer factor are not widely used (O'Duffy et al, 1996). For long-term suppression of the disease, steroids can be combined with azathioprine, colchicine and cyclophosphamide. Anticoagulants are utilized by some centres for occlusive large-artery involvement; however, their efficacy is still debatable (Wechsler et al., 1992; Yazıcı, 1994).

Conclusions

Cerebrovascular complications of Behçet's disease are more rare than parenchymal involvement of the central nervous system and aseptic meningitis. The most common vascular manifestation is CVT which is to account for about 11–35% of the neurological manifestations of Behçet's disease. It usually entails a good prognosis but it requires early and prolonged anticoagulation together with corticosteroid treatment. Cerebral arterial manifestations such as aneurysms, arteriovenous malformations, intracranial or spinal hemorrhages, arterial dissections, large-artery occlusions, and arteritis are extremely rare. They are usually associated with systemic arterial lesions and entail a severe prognosis. A combination of steroids, immunosuppressants and anticoagulants is required in occlusive cases.

References

Akman-Demir, G., Baykan-Kurt, B., Serdaroğlu, P. et al. (1996). Seven-year follow-up of neurologic involvement in Behçet's syndrome. *Archives of Neurology*, **53**, 691–4.

Allen, N.B. (1993). Miscellaneous vasculitic syndromes including Behçet's disease and cerebral nervous system vasculitis. *Current Opinion in Rheumatology*, **5**, 51–6.

Ameri, A. & Bousser, M.G. (1992). Cerebral venous thrombosis. *Neurologic Clinics*, **10**, 87–111.

Arias, M.J., Calero, E., Gil, J.F. & Paz, J. (1987). Spinal subarachnoid hematoma in Behçet's disease. *Neurosurgery*, **20**, 62–3.

Bahar, S., Çoban, O., Gurvit, I.H., Akman-Demir, G. & Gokyiğit, A. (1993). Spontaneous dissection of the extracranial vertebral artery with spinal subarachnoid haemorrhage in a patient with Behçet's disease. *Neuroradiology*, **35**, 352–4.

Banna, M. & El Ramahi, K. (1991). Neurologic involvement in Behçet's disease: imaging findings in 16 patients. *American Journal of Neuroradiology*, **12**, 791–6.

Bartlett, S.T., McCarthy W.J. III, Palmer, A.S., Flinn, W.R., Bergan, I.J., & Yao, J.S.T. (1988). Multiple aneurysms in Behçet's disease. *Archives of Surgery*, **123**, 1004–8.

Behçet, H. (1937). Ueber rezidivierende Aphtöse durch ein Virus verursachte Geschwüre am Mund am Auge und an den Genitalen. *Dermatologische Wochenschrift*, **36**, 1152–7.

Ben-Itzhak, J., Keren, S. & Simon, J. (1985). Intracranial venous thrombosis in Behçet's syndrome. *Neuroradiology*, **27**, 450–1.

Bienenstock, H. & Margulies, M. (1961). Behçet's syndrome: report of a case with extensive neurological manifestations. *New England Journal of Medicine*, **264**, 1342–5.

Bousser, M.G., Bletry, O., Launay, M., Portier, E., Guillard, A. & Castaigne, P. (1980). Thromboses veineuses cérébrales au cours de la maladie de Behçet. *Revue Neurologique*, **136**, 753–62.

Bousser, M.G., Chiars, J. & Bories, J. (1985). Cerebral venous thrombosis: a review of 38 cases. *Stroke*, **16**, 199–211.

Buge, A., Vincent, D., Rancurel, G., Dechy, H., Dorra, M., Betourne, C. (1987). Maladie de Behçet avec anévrysmes artériels multiples intracraniens. *Revue Neurologique*, **143**, 832–5.

Cavara, V. & D'Ermo, F. (1954). A case of Behçet's syndrome. XVII Concilium. *Acta Ophthalmologica*, **3**, 1489–505.

Cobby, M., Higgs, C.M. & Hall, C. (1988). Behçet's syndrome presenting as intracranial hypertension in a caucasian. *Journal of the Royal Society of Medicine*, **81**, 478–9.

Emmi, L., Salvati, G., Brugnolo, F. & Morchione, T. (1995). Immunopathological aspects of Behçet's disease (editorial). *Clinical Experimental Rheumatology*, **13**, 687–91.

Fusegawa, H., Ichikawa, Y., Tanaka, Y. et al. (1991). Blood coagulation and fibrinolysis in patients with Behçet's disease. *Rinsho Byori*, **39**, 509–16.

Godeau, P., Wechsler, B., Maaouni, A., Fagard, M. & Herreman, G.

(1980). Manifestations cardiovasculaires de la maladie de Behçet. *Annales de Dermatologie et de Vénéréologie*, **167**, 741–7.

Hampton, K.K., Chamberlain, M.A., Menon, D.K. & Davies, J.A. (1991). Coagulation and fibrinolytic activity in Behçet's disease. *Thrombosis and Haemostasis*, **66**, 292–4.

Harper, M.C., O'Neill, B.P., O'Duffy, J.D. & Forbes, G.S. (1985). Intracranial hypertension in Behçet's disease: demonstration of sinus occlusion with use of digital subtraction angiography. *Mayo Clinic Proceedings*, **60**, 419–22.

Hassen Khoda, R., Declemy, S., Batt, M., Daune, B., Avril, G., & Le Bas, P. (1991). Maladie de Behçet avec atteinte artérielle multiple et volumineux angiome intra-cérébrale. *Journal des Maladies Vasculaires*, **16**, 383–6.

Herskovitz, S., Lipton, R.B. & Lantos, G. (1988). Neuro-Behçet's disease. CT and clinical correlates. *Neurology*, **38**, 1714–20.

Huong du, L.T., Wechsler, B., Piette, J.C. et al. (1993). Long term prognosis of arterial lesions in Behçet's disease. In *Behçet's Disease*, ed. B. Wechsler & P. Godeau, pp. 557–62. Amsterdam: Excerpta Medica.

Imaizumi, M., Nukada, T., Toneda, S., & Abe, H. (1980). Behçet's disease with sinus thrombosis and arteriovenous malformation in brain. *Journal of Neurology*, **222**, 215–18.

International Study Group for Behçet's disease. (1990). Criteria for Behçet's disease. *Lancet*, **335**, 1078–80.

Iragui, V.J. & Maravi, E. (1986). Behçet's syndrome presenting as cerebrovascular disease. *Journal of Neurology, Neurosurgery and Psychiatry*, **49**, 838–40.

Kansu E. (1994). Endothelial cell dysfunction in Behçet's disease. *Rheumatology in Europe*, **23** (Suppl. 2), 30.

Kawakita, H., Nishimura, N., Satoh, Y. & Shibata, N. (1967). Neurological aspects of Behçet's disease. *Journal of the Neurological Sciences*, **5**, 417–39.

Knapp, P. (1941). Beitrag zur Symptomatologie und Therapie der rezidivierenden Hypopyoniritis und der begleitenden aphtözen Schleimhauterkrankungen. *Schweizerische Medizinische Wochenschrift*, **71**, 1288–90.

Kozin, F., Haughton, V. & Vernhard, G.C. (1977). Neuro-Behçet disease. Two cases and neuroradiologic findings. *Neurology*, **27**, 1148–52.

Kumral, K., Evyapan, D., Oksel, F., Keser, G. & Bereketoglu, M.A. (1999). Transcranial Doppler detection of microembolic signals in patients with Behçet's disease. *Journal of Neurology*, **246**, 592–5.

Macchi, P., Grossman, R.I., Gomori, J.M., Goldberg, H.I., Zimmerman, R.A. & Bilaniuk, L.T. (1986). High field MR imaging of cerebral venous thrombosis. *Journal of Computer Assisted Tomography*, **10**, 10–15.

Masheter, H.C. (1959). Behçet's syndrome complicated by intracranial thrombophlebitis. *Proceedings of the Royal Society of Medicine*, **52**, 1039–40.

Matsumoto, T., Uekusa, T. & Fukuda, Y. (1991). Vasculo-Behçet's disease: a pathologic study of eight cases. *Human Pathology*, **22**, 45–51.

Medejel, A., El Alaoui Faris, M., Al-Zemouri, K. et al. (1986). Les manifestations neurologiques de la maladie de Behçet. *Semaine des Hôpitaux*, **62**, 1325–8.

Mizuki, N. & Ohno, S. (1996). Immuno-genetic studies of Behçet's disease. *Revue de Rhumatologie (English Edition)*, **63**, 520–7.

Montalban, J., Codina, A., Alijotas, J., Ordi, J. & Khamashta, M. (1990). Magnetic resonance imaging in Behçet's disease. *Journal of Neurology, Neurosurgery and Psychiatry*, **53**, 442.

Nagata, K. (1985). Recurrent intracranial hemorrhage in Behçet's disease. *Journal of Neurology, Neurosurgery and Psychiatry*, **48**, 190–1.

O'Duffy, J.D. (1990). Behçet's syndrome. *New England Journal of Medicine*, **322**, 326–7.

O'Duffy J.D. & Goldstein, N.P. (1976). Neurological involvement in seven patients with Behçet's disease. *American Journal of Medicine*, **61**, 170–8.

O'Duffy, J.D., Carney, J.A. & Deodhar, S. (1971). Behçet's disease. Report of 10 cases, 3 with new manifestations. *Annals of Internal Medicine*, **75**, 561–9.

O'Duffy, J.D., Cohen, S., Jorizzo, J. et al. (1996). Alpha-interferon (IFN-a) treatment in Behçet's disease. *Revue Rhumatologie (English Edition)*, **63**, 560.

Pamir, M.N., Kansu, T., Erbengi, A. & Zileli, T. (1981). Papilledema in Behçet's syndrome. *Archives of Neurology*, **38**, 643–5.

Patel, D.V., Neuman, M.J. & Hier, D.B. (1989). Reversibility of CT and MR findings in Neuro-Behçet's disease. *Journal of Computed Assisted Tomography*, **13**, 669–73.

Rougemont, D., Bousser, M.G., Wechsler, B., Bletry, O., Castaigne, P. & Godeau, P. (1982). Manifestations neurologiques de la maladie de Behçet. *Revue Neurologique*, **138**, 493–505.

Serdaroğlu, P. (1998). Behçet's disease and the nervous system. *Journal of Neurology*, **245**, 197–205.

Serdaroğlu, P., Yazici, H., Özdemir, Ç., Yurdakul, S., Bahar, S. & Aktin, E. (1989). Neurologic involvement in Behçet's syndrome. A prospective study. *Archives of Neurology*, **46**, 265–9.

Shakir, R.A., Sulaiman, K., Kahn, R.A. & Rudwan, M. (1990). Neurological presentation of neuro-Behçet's syndrome: clinical categories. *European Neurology*, **30**, 249–53.

Shimizu, T. (1962). Epidemiological and clinico-pathological studies on neuro-Behçet's syndrome. *Advances in Neurological Science (Tokyo)*, **16**, 167–78.

Shimizu, T., Ehrlich, G.E., Inaba, G. & Hayashi, K. (1979). Behçet's disease. *Seminars in Arthritis and Rheumatism*, **8**, 223–60.

Suga, M., Sato, K., Nishimura, M. & Oda, M. (1990). An autopsy case of neuro-Behçet's disease with the middle cerebral artery occlusion on cerebral angiogram. *Rinsho Shinkeigaku*, **30**, 1005–9.

Totsuka, S. & Midorikawa, T. (1972). Some clinical and pathological problems in neuro-Behçet's syndrome. *Folia Psychiatrica et Neurologica (Japan)*, **28**, 275–84.

Totsuka, S., Hattori, T. & Yazari, M. (1979). Clinico-pathology of Neuro-Behçet's syndrome. In *Behçet's Disease. Clinical and Immunological Features*, ed. T. Kehner & C.G. Barnes, pp. 133–96. London: Academic Press.

Tsutsui, K., Hasegawa, M., Takata, M. & Takehara, K. (1998). Behçet's disease. *Journal of Rheumatology*, **25**, 326–8.

Uruyama, A., Sakuragi, S. & Sakai, F. (1979). Angio-Behçet syndrome. In *Behçet's Syndrome. Clinical and Immunological Features*, ed. T. Lehner & C.G. Barnes, pp. 176. London: Academic Press.

Wechsler, B., Bousser, M.G., Huong Du, L.T., Bletry, O., Le Hoang, P. & Godeau, P. (1985). Cerebral venous sinus thrombosis in Behçet's disease. *Mayo Clinic Proceedings*, **60**, 891–2.

Wechsler, B., Vidailhet, M., Piette, J.C. et al. (1992). Cerebral venous thrombosis in Behçet's disease-clinical study and long term follow-up of 25 cases. *Neurology*, **42**, 614–18.

Wechsler, B., Dell'Isola, B., Vidailhet, M. et al. (1993). Magnetic resonance imaging in 31 patients with Behçet disease and neurological involvement: prospective study with clinical correlation. *Journal of Neurology, Neurosurgery and Psychiatry*, **56**, 793–8.

Wilkins, M.R., Gove, R.I., Roberts, S.D. & Kendall, M.J. (1986).

Behçet's disease presenting as benign intracranial hypertension. *Postgraduate Medical Journal*, **62**, 36–41.

Wolf, S.M., Scrotland, D.L. & Phillips, L.L. (1965). Involvement of nervous system in Behçet's syndrome. *Archives of Neurology*, **12**, 315–25.

Yazı, H. (1994). Behçet's syndrome (the vasculitides). In *Rheumatology*, ed. J.H. Klippel, & P.A. Dieppe, pp. 6.20.1–6, London: Mosby Year Book Europe.

Yazı, H. & Moutsopoulos, H.H. (1985). Behçet's disease. In *Current Therapy in Allergy, Immunology and Rheumatology*, ed. L.M. Lichenstein & A.S. Fauci, pp. 194–7. Philadelphia: Decker.

Zelenski, J.D., Caparo, J.A., Holden, D. & Calabrese, L.H. (1989). Central nervous system vasculitis in Behçet's syndrome: angiographic improvement after therapy with cytotoxic agents. *Arthritis and Rheumatism*, **32**, 217–20.

21

Kohlmeier–Degos disease (malignant atrophic papulosis)

Serge Blecic[1] and Julien Bogousslavsky[2]

[1]Service de Neurologie, Hôpital Erasme, Brussels, Belgium
[2]Department of Neurology, University of Lausanne, Switzerland

Introduction

The first case of malignant atrophic papulosis (MAP) was probably reported by Kohlmeier in 1941, who attributed the cause of skin lesions and gastrointestinal perforations occurring in a young man, to a form of thromboangiitis obliterans (Kohlmeier, 1941). In 1942 Degos, examining another patient with the same symptomatology, suggested it could be a different entity which he named 'papulosquamous dermatitis' (Degos et al, 1942). Six years later, after the patient's autopsy, the term 'malignant atrophic papulosis' was definitively established (Degos et al., 1948).

MAP is a rare and clinically distinctive vasculopathy characterized mainly by cutaneous features with frequent gastrointestinal involvement. All systems can be affected (Degos et al., 1948; Burrow et al., 1991), but skin eruption is a constant and pathognomonic sign (Degos, 1979). The evolution is usually lethal, although a few patients with a benign form of MAP have been reported (Moulin, 1988; Shimazu et al., 1988). MAP occurs mainly in young adults but sometimes it may develop in childhood (Horner et al., 1976; Barabino et al., 1990).

The first symptom is general weakness and the illness evolves over many years (5–20). Death occurs mainly after gastrointestinal perforations or central nervous system (CNS) involvement (Degos et al., 1948; Dastur et al., 1981).

Although this entity is easily recognizable after clinical examination or after anatomo-pathological study, the etiology is unknown and the treatment remains uncertain.

Clinical manifestations

All organ systems can be involved in MAP. In all the cases clinical manifestations are the consequence of multifocal infarctions.

The dermatological involvement is constant and virtually pathognomonic of MAP but it can be absent in the early stage (Degos, 1979). Cutaneous lesions of MAP are scattered, whitish or skin coloured, as well as erythematous, papules with central atrophy showing a porcelain-like appearance, disseminated on the trunk and limbs with a size varying from 2 to 5 mm (Fig. 21.1). The eruption is always asymptomatic and evolves within a few days to a central atrophy leaving a flattened centre, sharply surrounded by an erythematous peripheral circle (Degos et al., 1942, 1948). (Fig. 21.2).

In some aspects, this eruption can resemble, especially in the early stages, the dermatological findings in systemic lupus erythematosus (SLE) (Doutre et al.,1987).

Gastrointestinal lesions are pathognomonic of MAP and in most of the cases are the cause of death (Degos et al., 1948; Degos, 1979).

The first gastrointestinal symptoms are often insidious, progressing to anorexia, diarrhoea and diffuse abdominal pain (Kohlmeier,1941; Degos et al., 1948).

Frequently, the symptoms worsen and lead to intestinal obstructions and hemorrhages due to perforations with peritonitis (Degos et al., 1948).

The diagnosis can easily be made by endoscopy (Casparie et al., 1991), or by laparoscopy (Shimazu et al., 1988), which reveal the same lesion (except with larger size), as those seen on the skin. More rarely, perforations can be limited within the seromuscular wall (Shimazu et al., 1988).

Because of the severe consequences of the gastrointestinal involvement, Casparie et al. emphasize the importance of routinely performing endoscopy in MAP, to detect silent or early perforation, even in patients without gastrointestinal complaints (Casparie et al., 1991).

Neurologic manifestations of MAP are mainly due to CNS involvement but a few cases of peripheral neuropathy

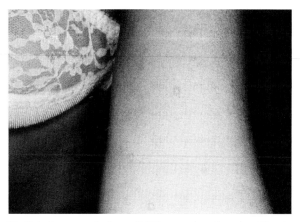

Fig 21.1. Cutaneous lesions of MAP on trunk and arm in a 35-year-old woman with MAP.

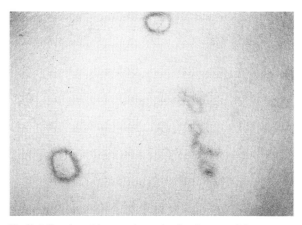

Fig 21.2. Papules with central atrophy showing porcelain appearance, surrounded by an erythematous peripheral circle, disseminated on the trunk.

have been reported. They can be the first manifestation of MAP, and they may precede skin or other systemic manifestations for many years, especially in children (Rosemberg et al., 1988; Barabino et al., 1990,). Neurological signs include mental dysfunction, motor and/or sensory deficits, ophthalmoplegia and cranial nerve dysfunction. The neurologic abnormalities result from multifocal infarctions or hemorrhages located in any part of the CNS, or peripheral nerves, resulting from involvement of small- or medium-sized arteries or cerebral veins (Dastur et al., 1981). Peripheral neuropathies are rarely encountered and result from demyelination (Horner et al., 1976). Label et al., in 1983, studied a patient with MAP who developed a polyradiculopathy with elevated CSF protein and hypoglycorrhachia, which was attributed, after autopsy, to multifocal infarctions and necrosis of CNS and peripheral nerve sheets. They suggested that MAP

should be added to the differential diagnosis of polyradiculopathy (Label et al., 1983).

Ophthalmological symptoms are common. They were reported in 35 out of 105 published observations. They consist of involvement of various eye structures with predominance in the conjunctiva, but also the sclera, retina, choroid, uvea, eyelids, pupils and optic tracts (Sotrel et al., 1983; Lee et al., 1984; Sibillat et al., 1986).

There are anecdotal reports of intrathoracic (Pierce & Smith, 1978), bladder (Lomholt et al.,1968) and heart involvement (Sotrel et al., 1983).

Pathology

MAP is an occlusive endarteriopathy which involves small and middle-sized arteries and veins. The appearance of the lesions is similar regardless of the tissues affected and has been classified as a proliferative vasculopathy (Degos et al., 1948; Sortee et al., 1982). Using refined microscopy, the lesions are characterized by intimal proliferation in the absence of an inflammatory reaction (Su et al., 1985). This process is confined to the intima of the vessels and always spares the media (Demitsu et al., 1992). Molenaar et al. (1987) identified three stages of lesion: early, intermediate and late, which can coexist.

Early lesions consist of cellular proliferation and edema of the intima with evidence for immune complex deposition; thrombosis is found occasionally and can be attributed to a secondary phenomenon. A decrease of edema and a proliferation of smooth muscle characterize the intermediate stage.

The late lesions consist of acellular intimal sclerosis with hyalinization and narrowing or obliteration of the vascular lumen (Molenaar et al., 1987). Although inflammation is often absent, it can sometimes be found in the early stages (Demitsu et al., 1992). In the other stages the lack of inflammatory cells helps to differentiate Degos' disease from other forms of vasculitis (Degos, 1979; Molenaar et al., 1987).

Electron microscopy confirms the presence of intimal proliferation with vacuolization and edema (Su et al., 1985), and intraluminal microvilosity 'paramyxovirus like' are often identified in the basal surfaces of the endothelial cells. The nature of these inclusions remains controversial. They are probably non-specific (Bioulac et al., 1980).

Etiology

The etiology of MAP remains unknown. Several hypotheses have been proposed but none of them has been confirmed.

The congenital hypothesis was proposed after the observations of several cases occurring in the same family. In one report, six relatives presented clinical features of MAP (Kisch & Bruynzeel, 1984). In another report, a mother and her daughter were both affected (Moulin et al., 1984). In the two reports, an autosomal dominant mode of inheritance was proposed but never confirmed.

An autoimmune mechanism has been proposed since the dermatologic lesions observed in SLE are in some aspects similar to those found in MAP (Black & Hudson, 1976; Doutre et al., 1987). This hypothesis was reinforced by the presence of antiphospholipid antibodies in a case of MAP (Asherson & Cevera, 1993).

These interesting findings should be confirmed by other analyses in future patients. However, the lack of inflammatory cells is a strong argument against the autoimmune hypothesis.

A viral etiology was suspected after observation of virus-like particles in endothelial cells (Degos et al., 1948). These findings were not confirmed and intracytoplasmic particles resembling paramyxovirus have subsequently been found to be the result of cellular degeneration (Stahl et al., 1978; Bioulac et al., 1980).

Treatment

No treatment is known to be successful.

Since an autoimmune process has been suspected, immuno-suppressive therapy was proposed, but the benefit has not been established yet (Asherson & Cevera, 1993).

In the early manifestations of artery occlusion, antifibrinolytic agents have been proposed but without benefit (Black & Hudson, 1976).

Reports concerning the use of antiplatelet therapy are inconsistent. Several observations did not show any evidence of beneficial effect (Pallesen & Rasmussen, 1979; Burrow et al., 1991), while Drucker in 1990, showed a real benefit in a patient who had several abnormalities of platelet adhesiveness and aggregation. During several months of treatment the patient was free of complications, but the patient worsened when treatment was discontinued (Drucker, 1990). However, this observation must be tempered by the fact that coagulation abnormalities are not a common feature in MAP.

Concerning the acute phases, Degos proposed anticoagulation with heparin to avoid artery occlusion (Degos, 1979), while surgery is commonly proposed in case of intestinal perforation (Pallesen & Rasmussen, 1979).

References

Asherson, R.A. & Cevera, R. (1993). Antiphospholipid syndrome. *Journal of Investigative Dermatology*, **100**, 21–7.

Barabino, A., Pesce, F., Gatti, R. et al. (1990). An atypical paediatric case of malignant atrophic papulosis (Kohlmeier–Degos disease). *European Journal of Pediatrics*, **149**, 457–8.

Bioulac, P., Doutre, M.S. & Beylot, C. (1980). La papulose atrophiante maligne de Degos.Etude ultrastructurale d' un nouveau cas. *Annales Anatomiques Pathologie Paris*, **25**, 111–24.

Black, M.M. & Hudson, P.M. (1976). Atrophie blanche lesions closely resembling malignant atrophic papulosis (Degos' disease) in systemic lupus erythematosus. *British Journal of Dermatology*, **95**, 649–52.

Burrow, J.N., Blumbergs, P.C., Iyper, P.V. & Hallpike, J.F. (1991). Kohlmeier–Degos disease: a multisystem vasculopathy with progressive cerebral infarction. *Australia and New Zealand Journal of Medicine*, **21**, 49–51.

Casparie, M.K., Meyer, J.W., van Huystee, B.E., Kneppelhout, J. & Mulder, C.J. (1991). Endoscopic and histopathologic features of Degos' disease. *Endoscopy*, **23**, 231–3.

Dastur, D.K., Singhal, B.S. & Shroff, H.J. (1981). CNS involvement in malignant atrophic papulosis (Kohlmeier–Degos disease) vasculopathy and coagulopathy. *Journal of Neurology, Neurosurgery and Psychiatry*, **44**, 156–60.

Degos, R., Delort, J. & Tricot, R. (1942). Dermatite papulosquameuse atrophiante. *Bulletin Société Francais Dermatologie et Syphiligraphie*, **49**, 148–50.

Degos, R., Delort, J. & Tricot, R. (1948). Papulose atrophiante maligne (syndrome cutanéo- intestinal mortel). *Bulletin et Memoires de la Société Medecin Hôpital Paris*, **64**, 803–6.

Degos, R. (1979). Malignant atrophic papulosis. *British Journal of Dermatology*, **100**, 21–35.

Demitsu, T., Nakajima, K., Okayuma, R. & Tadaki, T. (1992). Malignant atrophic papulosis (Degos' syndrome). *International Journal of Dermatology*, **31**, 99–102.

Doutre, M.S., Beylot, C., Bioulac, P., Busquet, M. & Conte, M. (1987). Skin lesion resembling malignant atrophic papulosis in lupus erythematosus. *Dermatologica*, **182**, 45–6.

Drucker, C.R. (1990). Malignant atrophic papulosis: response to antiplatelet therapy. *Dermatologica*, **180**, 90–2.

Horner, F.A., Myers, G.J., Stumpf, D.A., Oseroff, B.J. & Choi, B.H. (1976). Malignant atrophic papulosis (Kohlmeier–Degos disease) in childhood. *Neurology*, **26**, 317–21.

Kisch, L.S., Bruynzeel, D.P. (1984). Six cases of malignant atrophic papulosis (Degos' disease) occurring in a family. *British Journal of Dermatology*, **111**, 469–71.

Kohlmeier, W. (1941). Multiple Hautnekrausen bei Thrombangiitis obliterans. *Archiv Klinik Experimentale Dermatologie*, **181**, 783–92.

Label, L.S., Tandan, R. & Albers, J.W. (1983). Myelomalacia and hypoglycorrhachia in malignant atrophic papulosis. *Neurology*, **33**, 936–9.

Lee, D.A., Su, W.P., Liesegang, T.J. (1984). Ophthalmic changes of Degos' disease (malignant atrophic papulosis). *Ophthalmology*, **91**, 295–9.

Lomholt, G., Hjorth, N. & Fischerman, K. (1968). Lethal peritonitis from Degos' disease (malignant atrophic papulosis). *Acta Chirurgica Scandinavica*, **134**, 495–501

Molenaar, W.M., Rosman, J.B., Donker, A.J. & Houthoff, H.J. (1987). The pathology and pathogenesis of malignant atrophic papulosis (Degos' disease). *Pathology Research and Practice*, **182**, 98–106.

Moulin, G. (1988). Les formes bénignes de la papulose atrophiante maligne de Degos. *Annales Dermatologie et Vénéréologie*, **115**, 1289–90.

Moulin, G., Barutt, D., Franc, M.P. & Pierson, A. (1984). Papulose atrophiante de Degos familiale (mère-fille). *Annales Dermatologie et Vénéréologie*, **111**, 149–55.

Pallesen, R.M. & Rasmussen, N.R. (1979). Malignant atrophic papulosis (Degos syndrome). *Acta Chirurgica Scandinavica*, **145**, 279–83.

Pierce, R.N. & Smith, G.J. (1978). Intrathoracic manifestation of Degos' disease (malignant atrophic papulosis). *Chest*, **73**, 79–84.

Rosemberg, S., Lopez, M.B.S., Sotto, M.N. & Graudenz, M.S. (1988). Childhood Degos disease with proeminent neurological symptoms: report of a clinicopathological case. *Journal of Child Neurology*, **3**, 42–6

Shimazu, S., Imai, H. & Kokubu, S. (1988). Long term survival in malignant atrophic papulosis: a case report and review of the Japanese literature. *Nippon-Geka-Gakkai-Zasshi*, **89**, 1748–51.

Sibillat, M., Avril, M.F., Charpentier, P., Offret, H. & Bloch-Michel, E. (1986). Papulose atrophiante maligne (maladie de Degos): revue clinique a propos d' un cas. *Journal Francais d'Ophthalmologie*, **9**, 299–304.

Sortee, N.A., Murphy, G.F. & Mihm, M.C. Jr. (1982). Lymphocytes and necrosis of the cutaneous microvasculature in malignant atrophic papulosis: a refined light microscope study. *Journal of the American Academy of Dermatology*, **7**, 620–30.

Sotrel, A., Lacson, A.G. & Huff, K. (1983). Childhood Kohlmeier–Degos disease with atypical skin lesions. *Neurology*, **33**, 1146–51.

Stahl, D., Thomsen, K. & Hou-Jensen, K. (1978). Malignant atrophic papulosis. Treatment with Aspirin and Dipyridamole. *Archives of Dermatology*, **114**, 1687–9.

Su, W.P., Schroeter, A.L., Lee, D.A., Hsu, T. & Muller, S.A. (1985). Clinical and histological findings in Degos' syndrome (malignant atrophic papulosis). *Cutis*, **35**, 131–8.

22

Inflammatory bowel disease

Alexander Lossos and Israel Steiner

Department of Neurology, Hadassah University Hospital, Jerusalem, Israel

Inflammatory bowel disease

Inflammatory bowel disease (IBD) refers to an overlapping spectrum of idiopathic inflammatory intestinal disorders of complex pathogenesis. Ulcerative colitis and Crohn's disease are the two main forms of IBD characterized by chronic spontaneously relapsing course, and distinguished by the distribution of intestinal involvement, morphologic changes, and clinical and epidemiologic features (Podolsky, 1991). Ulcerative colitis (UC) is essentially a mucosal disease of the large intestine usually manifested with bloody diarrhoea. In contrast, Crohn's disease (CD), also known as granulomatous or regional enteritis, is a transmural process that may affect any portion of the alimentary tract, often in a patchy fashion, with diarrhoea, abdominal pain, intestinal obstruction, and malabsorption. The clinical, endoscopic and pathological features usually enable confident diagnostic distinction, although additional studies may be needed in overlap phenotypes (Panaccione & Sandborn, 1999).

The etiology of IBD is still obscure. Increasing epidemiologic and laboratory evidence suggests that multiple factors interact to trigger immunologically mediated intestinal inflammation (Sartor, 1995). Specific ethnic and geographic susceptibilities, a tendency for familial clustering and changing incidence rates argue for genetic and environmental influence. Laboratory animal models indicate interplay between intestinal commensal bacteria or their products with the mucosal immune compartment. Beneficial effect of immunosuppressive agents and association with autoimmune phenomena imply involvement of the immune system.

Extraintestinal manifestations

Inflammatory bowel disease is well recognized as a multisystemic disorder with a range of extraintestinal manifestations that may precede or follow the diagnosis of bowel involvement (Table 22.1). Large-scale case studies show that up to a third of patients with either form of IBD will have at least one such condition (Greenstein et al., 1976; Rankin et al., 1979). For convenience, these are categorized in relation to the intestinal disease activity and according to a specific form of IBD with which they tend to occur.

Peripheral arthritis mainly affects the large joints of the limbs and is usually transient and non-deforming. Clinical resemblance to the reactive arthritis associated with different enteric infections suggests a similar pathogenesis, possibly reflecting synovial exposure to arthritogenic bacterial antigens and inflammatory cell products (Levine & Lukawski-Trubish, 1995). Axial arthritis involving the spine or sacroiliac joints is strongly, but not uniformly, associated with HLA-B27, as are uveitis and erythema nodosum panniculitis. The close HLA-B27 restriction may imply a genetically determined spontaneous or infection-mediated mechanism (Levine & Lukawski-Trubish, 1995). Primary sclerosing cholangitis and IBD may be accompanied by antineutrophil cytoplasmic antibody, and both biliary tract and colon share antigenic epithelial-surface epitopes supporting a common pathophysiologic process (Hyams, 1994). Additional manifestations develop secondarily to chronic inflammation and bowel dysfunction with consequent malabsorption-induced metabolic and nutritional disturbances or represent treatment-related complications.

Until recently, non-vascular neurologic manifestations of IBD have received little attention in the subject reviews despite a substantial number of reported instances (Table 22.2). Accumulated evidence suggests that any part of the neuromuscular system may be affected by a wide range of disorders of putative immune-mediated origin or related to a definable nutritional or metabolic deficiency or iatrogenic cause. The documented frequency varies greatly, ranging from 0.2% to 35.7% in three different studies

Table 22.1. *Main extraintestinal manifestations of inflammatory bowel disease*

Skeletal: axial arthritis, oligoarticular arthritis, osteoporosis, clubbing

Hepatobiliary: primary sclerosing cholangitis, fatty liver, cholelithiasis, chronic active hepatitis, cirrhosis

Ocular: uveitis, episcleritis, scleritis, conjunctivitis, keratitis

Mucocutaneous: aphthous stomatitis, glossitis, cheilitis, erythema nodosum, pyoderma gangrenosum, erythema multiforme, cutaneous vasculitis

Renal: nephrolithiasis

Miscellaneous: thromboembolic phenomena, amyloidosis, nutritional deficiencies, anemia

Sources: Compiled from reviews by Hyams, 1994; Levine & Lukawski-Trubish, 1995.

Table 22.2. *Reported neurological complications in inflammatory bowel disease*

Cranial nerve: optic neuritis, ischemic optic neuropathy, deafness, Melkersson–Rosenthal syndrome

Peripheral nerve: multiple mononeuropathy, polyneuropathy, plexopathy, autonomic dysfunction

Muscle: orbital myositis, non-specific, granulomatous and interstitial myositis, polymyositis, dermatomyositis, vacuolar myopathy, vasculitis

Neuromuscular junction: myasthenia gravis

Central nervous system: cerebrospinal and retinal vascular disease, headache, seizures, meningitis, meningoencephalitis, demyelinating disease, asymptomatic cerebral white matter lesions, myelopathy

Sources: Compiled from reviews by Lossos et al., 1995; Pfeiffer, 1996; Wills & Hovell, 1996; Perkin & Murray-Lyon, 1998.

(Greenstein et al., 1976; Rankin et al., 1979; Elsebety & Bertorini, 1991). We have identified a rate of 3% from a retrospective cohort of 638 patients specifically searched for neurological problems (Lossos et al., 1995).

As with other extraintestinal manifestations, neurologic disorders may occur at any time during the course of IBD but tend to develop after the intestinal diagnosis. No strict correlation to the activity of intestinal disease is regularly observed, and symptoms may coincide with acute exacerbations or appear during periods of remission. Of note is a frequent association with other extraintestinal manifestations in up to a half of neurologically affected patients (Lossos et al., 1995).

Systemic thromboembolic phenomena

Since the original work by Bargen and Barker (1936), who identified 18 young patients with UC complicated by extensive arterial and venous thrombosis, there have been numerous contributions to the issue of thrombosis in IBD (Table 22.3). Earlier studies document a 1.2% to 7.1% frequency of clinically evident (Bargen & Barker, 1936; Graef et al., 1966) and a 33% to 39% frequency of autopsy diagnosed systemic thromboembolism (Sloan et al., 1950; Graef et al., 1966). More recent reports state a frequency of 0.2% to 1.3% (Rankin et al., 1979; Talbot et al., 1986) or fail to mention thrombotic events at all (Greenstein et al., 1976). Despite these discrepancies, it is a potentially ominous complication responsible for fatal outcome in up to a quarter of patients (Talbot et al., 1986) and ranked a third cause of death among IBD patients (Graef et al., 1966).

Thrombosis is usually venous, but various arterial sites may also be affected (Talbot et al., 1986). Deep venous thrombosis and pulmonary embolism account for the majority of events in adults, with a substantial number of multifocal and recurrent episodes (Jackson et al., 1997). Venous thrombosis in children with IBD is relatively less common (Lloyd-Still & Tomasi, 1989). Correlation to the intestinal disease activity is observed in up to 64% of patients (Talbot et al., 1986). However, thrombosis also develops during treatment-induced and spontaneous remissions, indicating a persistent procoagulant state (Jackson et al., 1997).

The mechanism of thrombosis in IBD is still not clear. Prolonged immobilization, surgery, indwelling catheters, dehydration and hypoalbuminemia are common during exacerbations but probably do not fully explain the observed association (Koenigs et al., 1987). A possible link to the basic disease process is suggested by the presence of mesenteric microvascular changes in CD and UC (Wakefield et al., 1989; Hamilton et al., 1995), by a protective influence of inherited bleeding disorders against development of IBD (Thompson et al., 1995), and by occasional beneficial response of intestinal disease to anticoagulation (Gaffney et al., 1995). Multiple attempts in search for an underlying defect revealed various alterations of coagulation factors, fibrinolysis, platelet number and activity, cellular procoagulant mediators, blood rheology, and vascular endothelial integrity. Elevated fibrinogen, fibrinopeptide A, factor V, VIII and thrombomodulin, increased levels of thrombin-antithrombin complexes, prothrombin fragment F1+2, D-dimer and plasminogen activator inhibitors, and decreased antithrombin III, protein C and protein S point to a sustained activation of

Table 22.3. *Main case-series of systemic thrombosis and cerebrovascular disorders in inflammatory bowel disease*

Study	Total number of cases			Cerebrovascular disorders	
	Number	IBD	Thrombosis (%)	Number (%)	Diagnosis
Autopsy					
Bargen & Barker (1936)	43	UC	14 (33%)	NS	
Sloan et al. (1950)	99	UC	33 (33%)	2 (2%)	1-Hemorrhagic encephalitis 1–NS
Graef et al. (1966)	100	UC	39 (39%)	2 (2%)	2-Cerebral venous thrombosis
Clinical					
Bargen & Barker (1936)	1500	UC	18 (1.2%)	NS	
Edwards & Truelove (1964)	624	UC	50 (8%)	NS	
Talbot et al. (1986)	7199	UC and CD	92 (1.3%)	9 (0.1%)	1-Cerebral arterial thrombosis 1-Retinal venous thrombosis 2-Transient ischemic attacks 5-NS
Lloyd-Still & Tomasi (1989)	180	UC and CD	6 (3.3%)	6 (3.3%)	1-Retinal artery thrombosis 1-Cerebral venous thrombosis 1-Cerebral arteritis 1-Hypertensive encephalopathy 2-NS
Elsebety & Bertorini (1991)	263	CD	NS	11 (4.2%)	11-NS
Lossos et al. (1995)	638	UC and CD	NS	4 (0.6%)	1-Cerebral arterial thrombosis 1-Transient ischemic attacks 2-Cerebral venous thrombosis
Jackson et al. (1997)	NS	UC and CD	52	4	NS

Notes: IBD: inflammatory bowel disease; UC: ulcerative colitis; CD: Crohn's disease; NS: Not specified.

coagulation cascade with increased thrombin generation and disturbed fibrinolysis (De Jong et al., 1989; Souto et al., 1995; Weber et al., 1999). Most of these alterations represent secondary phenomena of nonspecific inflammatory and hemostatic responses and therefore normalize with remissions or after treatment (Lake et al., 1978; Knot et al., 1983). Other abnormalities persist in quiescence and probably reflect an on-going disease process (Conlan et al., 1989; Souto et al., 1995). Enhanced consumption, reduction of vitamin K-dependent factors and treatment-related effect may also contribute to the observed changes (Koenigs et al., 1987; Weber et al., 1999).

Thrombocytosis and increased platelet activation and aggregation are well documented in IBD (Collins & Rampton, 1995). The proposed consequences of altered platelet function may be directly responsible for microvascular intestinal thrombosis and systemic hypercoagulability, and may indirectly mediate development of mucosal injury. Initial endothelial cell damage in the mesenteric vasculature may trigger platelet activation, but data sup-

porting this hypothesis remains controversial (Meucci et al., 1999). Vasculitis is another possible predisposing factor for systemic thrombosis, and several site-specific vasculitis variants occur in IBD. Skin, lung, bowel, muscle, retina and brain may be involved by a necrotizing or granulomatous inflammatory process affecting predominantly small or medium-size vessels (Wakefield et al., 1991; Hyams, 1994). Immune-mediated basis is suggested by the presence of circulating immune complexes (Conlan et al., 1989), autoantibodies (Panaccione & Sandborn, 1999) and by association with autoimmune diseases (Snook et al., 1989).

Additional procoagulant markers recently became the subject of investigation in IBD. Activated protein C resistance due to a mutation in clotting factor V is now recognized as the most common genetic cause of venous thrombosis in Caucasian population. The intriguing possibility of an association with IBD, providing the basis for increased thrombotic potential, was substantiated by one study (Liebman et al., 1998) but not confirmed by another (Jackson et al., 1997). Preliminary data of a similar study showed no significant association with the prothrombin G20210A mutation described with elevated plasma prothrombin and enhanced venous thrombosis (Liebman et al., 1999). Antiphospholipid antibodies are implicated in arterial and venous thrombosis in different clinical settings and antibodies to cardiolipin and to $\beta2$ glycoprotein I occur at high titers in IBD (Koutroubakis et al., 1998). However, since there is no specific correlation to thrombotic events, they probably represent an immunologic epiphenomenon. Hyperhomocysteinemia is another independent risk factor for thromboembolism, and patients with IBD appear to have elevated plasma total homocysteine probably due to cobalamin and folate deficiency (Cattaneo et al., 1998) or as a result of methylenetetrahydrofolate reductase C677T variant identified with increased prevalence in both UC and CD (Liebman et al., 1999; Mahmud et al., 1999).

To summarize the available data, spontaneous arterial and venous thrombosis in IBD seems to be of a multifactorial origin combining basic hypercoagulability with traditional vascular risk factors.

Neurovascular disorders

Cerebral and retinal vascular disorders occur in 0.1% to 4.2% of adults and children with IBD (Talbot et al., 1986; Lloyd-Still & Tomasi, 1989; Elsebety & Bertorini, 1991) and apparently constitute the most extensively covered neurological complication with more than 100 cases in the literature. Although most studies are retrospective and often present limited relevant information, a few general conclusions arise from several thorough reviews and case-series (Table 22.3). Affected patients are generally young with equal sex distribution and without recognizable vascular risk factors. Family history of autoimmune disorders is noted in some children (Lloyd-Still & Tomasi, 1989). Initial manifestations typically begin during a well-established intestinal disease or, less frequently, precede or occur at diagnosis. A tendency to concur with bowel exacerbations is noted in up to 70% of patients, while association with extracranial thrombosis or with other extraintestinal manifestations is less common (Talbot et al., 1986). In contrast to systemic thrombosis, the proportion of arterial events is higher with involvement of cerebral circulation, especially in CD (Markowitz et al., 1989; Johns, 1991); cerebral venous thrombosis is more frequent in UC (Wills & Hovell, 1996).

Vascular disease of the spinal cord is extremely rare in IBD with only two reported cases (Talbot et al., 1986; Slot et al., 1995). Both patients developed lower spinal cord ischemia with thrombosis of the distal aorta or its branches associated with active intestinal involvement by UC or CD. One of these patients was postpartum, smoking, and had elevated homocysteine level on methionine loading that responded to treatment with folic acid and pyridoxine.

Cerebral arterial manifestations

Cerebral arterial occlusive disease of the intracranial and extracranial circulation accounts for more than a half of cerebrovascular complications in IBD (Johns, 1991). Clinical and radiological features depend on the affected territory and are essentially identical to the non-IBD associated cerebral ischemic events. Transient ischemic attack (Schneiderman et al., 1979; Talbot et al., 1986; Lossos et al., 1995) and complete stroke, single (Silverstein & Present, 1971; Hilton-Jones & Warlow, 1985; Prior et al., 1987) or multiple (Jorens et al., 1990; Penix, 1998), are described. Neurological deficit may be significant but transient or may lead to a fatal outcome (Prior et al., 1987). Lacunar infarction of the subcortical structures (Hilton-Jones & Warlow, 1985; Jorens et al., 1990) and brainstem ischemia (Schneiderman et al., 1979; Talbot et al., 1986) are rare, whereas cortical involvement is common and may be responsible for epilepsy in pediatric IBD (Gormally et al., 1995; Akobeng et al., 1998).

Radiographic evaluation of the affected vessels has not been always performed. Studies with vascular imaging report occlusion of the intracranial and extracranial portions of the internal carotid artery (Silverstein & Present, 1971; Schneiderman et al., 1979; Prior et al., 1987; Penix, 1998), middle cerebral artery or its branches (Silverstein & Present, 1971; Gormally et al., 1995), and vessels of the posterior circulation (Schneiderman et al., 1979). In addition, central and branch retinal artery and posterior ciliary arteries may be involved independently (Schneiderman et al., 1979; Heuer et al., 1982; Lloyd-Still & Tomasi, 1989) or in association with cerebral thrombosis (Mayeux & Fahn, 1978).

Pathologically, examination of autopsy (Schneiderman et al., 1979; Prior et al., 1987) or endarterectomy material (Schneiderman, et al., 1979) showed massive clots without atheroma or vasculitis suggesting an *in situ* thrombosis with secondary vessel-to-vessel embolization. Potential cardioembolic source has been also demonstrated (Talbot et al., 1986), however, the relative impact of different cardiovascular causes is not possible to estimate on the basis of sporadic reports. Cerebral arterial thrombosis was occasionally related to hyperhomocysteinemia (Penix, 1998), antiphospholipid syndrome (Mevorach et al., 1996), anemia (Bar Dayan et al., 1995) or acquired protein C and S deficiency (Jorens et al., 1990). Otherwise, despite an apparent increase in the frequency of thrombotic risk factors in IBD patients (Hudson et al., 1996), instances of stroke with known predisposing conditions are usually excluded from further analysis (Talbot et al., 1986; Lossos et al., 1995) and the actual number of cerebral arterial events may be underestimated.

Cerebral venous thrombosis

From isolated descriptions, spontaneous cerebral venous thrombosis (CVT) seems to be more common in IBD than in the general population (Johns, 1991). Occlusion of intradural sinuses alone (Yerby & Bailey, 1980; Lloyd-Still & Tomasi, 1989; Garcia-Monco & Beldarrain, 1991; Johns, 1991; Musio et al., 1993; Lossos et al., 1995) or in combination with other venous channels (Harrison & Truelove, 1967; Borda et al., 1973; Averback, 1978; Sigsbee & Rottenberg, 1978; Markowitz et al., 1989; Papi et al., 1995) accounts for the majority of events. Isolated involvement of cortical (Harrison & Truelove, 1967; Derdeyn & Powers, 1998), deep cerebral (Mezoff et al., 1990; Vaezi et al., 1995), anastomotic (Schneiderman et al., 1979) or retinal veins (Talbot et al., 1986) occurs less often. Hemorrhagic infarction and intracerebral hemorrhage (Derdeyn & Powers, 1998) may follow CVT, further complicating neurological deficit.

As in CVT from other causes, clinical manifestations include a variable combination of headache, seizures, focal neurological deficit and impaired consciousness of subacute onset accompanied by signs of increased intracranial pressure. Diagnosis may be problematic and sometimes delayed particularly in view of a possible pseudotumour cerebri associated with corticosteroid treatment for IBD (Johns, 1991; Newton & Cooper, 1994). Angiographic confirmation, and more recently MRI, was obtained in most studies, or the diagnosis was based on clinical grounds (Mayeux & Fahn, 1978), surgery (Harrison & Truelove, 1967) or autopsy (Borda et al., 1973; Averback, 1978).

Most patients have no known CVT risk factors. Occasional association with oral contraceptives, pregnancy, early postoperative state and sepsis is cited (Johns, 1991; Musio et al., 1993). Additional possible predisposing conditions identified with IBD include antiphospholipid antibodies (Papi et al., 1995), transient protein S deficiency (Vaezi et al., 1995); infantile protein-losing enteropathy (Mezoff et al., 1990) and severe anemia (Markowitz et al., 1989; Musio et al., 1993).

Reported outcome of CVT in IBD is variable and cannot be accurately related to diverse treatment regimens sporadically applied over a period of 30 years (Harrison & Truelove, 1967). Partial or complete recovery is documented in a third of cases following treatment with anticoagulation, anticonvulsants, antiplatelet and antiedemic agents (Papi et al., 1995). Intestinal surgery is performed in some patients, basically to control bowel exacerbation (Markowitz et al., 1989; Johns, 1991). Fatal outcome due to CVT or related systemic thromboembolism is less common (Harrison & Truelove, 1967; Borda et al., 1973).

Cerebral vasculitis

Pathologically confirmed cerebral vasculitis is extremely rare in either form of IBD. The best-documented case concerns a young man with UC who developed seizures, coma and multiple low-density enhancing cerebral lesions on CT (Nelson et al., 1986). Antinuclear antibodies and rheumatoid factor were negative, skin and muscle biopsy showed mild perivascular infiltrate and inflammation, and brain biopsy demonstrated necrotizing vasculitis involving meningeal and cortical vessels. Treatment with prednisone and cyclophosphamide was followed by a full neurological recovery transiently complicated by systemic thrombosis and sepsis. A case similar with respect to the clinical features and management was associated with CD (Brohee et al., 1995). Other descriptions are based on cerebral angiography showing the typical segmental narrowing in the medium-to-small sized arteries (Edwards, 1977; Lloyd-Still & Tomasi, 1989) or on fluorescein angiography in case of retinal involvement (Garcia-Diaz et al., 1995). Reports of a presumed but unproven cerebral vasculitis rely on skin biopsy (Brohee et al., 1995) and on Takayasu arteritis-like large-size vessel stenosis also involving carotid and vertebral arteries in an adolescent with IBD, hypertension, reduced arterial pulses and a probable stroke (Yassinger et al., 1976).

Cerebral microangiopathy

Multifocal cerebral microangiopathy is a controversial, recently described condition identified by cranial MRI in 43% of young asymptomatic IBD patients in one study (Geissier et al., 1995) but not in another (Hart et al., 1998). Observed lesions were 1–7 in number, small hyperintense white matter foci on T_2-weighted images. The exact site of the lesions was not stated, but none showed contrast enhancement. A putative ischemic origin was suggested, although no correlation was found with various atherosclerotic and vasculitic markers except for elevated lipoprotein (a) in a subgroup with UC (Andus et al., 1995). An additional report in support of this condition describes a young man with mild, steroid-responsive central nervous system involvement associated with multiple subcortical hyperintense lesions that preceded the diagnosis of UC

(Dejaco et al., 1996). After excluding other possible causes, the authors suggested a microangiopathy based on the MRI characteristics. To further complicate the matter, others raise a possibility of inflammatory demyelinating process considering the known association of IBD with multiple sclerosis (Agranoff & Schon, 1995).

Miscellaneous disorders

Hemorrhagic disorders unrelated to venous thrombosis or to cerebral vasculitis (Edwards, 1977) are rarely described in IBD. There are two pathologically verified cases of acute hemorrhagic leukoencephalitis (AHL) with UC (Glotzer et al., 1964; Friedman, 1997). Both patients manifested fulminant course with fever, leukocytosis, focal neurological deficit and rapid deterioration of consciousness. Carotid angiogram in the earlier report showed cerebral mass effect, while brain MRI in the later demonstrated unilateral lobar white matter edema with multiple small hemorrhages, a discrete area of venous infarction, and a hemorrhagic swelling of the pons. The intestinal disease was well controlled in one patient but was active in another who also developed toxic megacolon, polyserositis and coagulopathy. He was treated with antibiotics, subtotal colectomy and later with amphotericin B for monilia stomatitis followed by a complete systemic and partial neurological recovery in face of multiple negative cultures. Diagnosis was established on brain biopsy and on autopsy showing fibrinoid necrosis of the small blood vessels, neutrophilic infiltrate and petechial hemorrhages in the white matter. Zones of perivascular demyelination and hemorrhagic infarction secondary to thrombosis and venous compression by the edematous tissue were mentioned in the autopsy case (Friedman, 1997). Although considered under demyelinating diseases, necrotizing venulitis with diapedesis of red blood cells is fundamental in AHL possibly related to a postinfectious immune-mediated process. An additional case of hemorrhagic encephalitis with UC is mentioned but not described (Sloan et al., 1950).

Disseminated intravascular coagulation (DIC) with generalized and focal cerebral and systemic manifestations was described in four patients with CD and one with UC (Ryan et al., 1977). Sepsis was the probable cause of DIC in three patients. Autopsy findings in the two cases with brain examination consisted of fibrin-rich thrombi in the small-sized vessels, ischemic changes and petechial hemorrhages. An additional patient with DIC and UC had basal ganglia infarction (Hilton-Jones & Warlow, 1985).

Finally, a child with UC, pulmonary vasculitis and hypertensive encephalopathy (Lloyd-Still & Tomasi, 1989) and a child with seizures, coma and cerebral ischemic changes in

the watershed distribution after surgery for UC (Hassan & Jenkins, 1998) are briefly mentioned in the literature.

Treatment

Treatment decisions are best made on an individual basis according to the current guidelines for cerebrovascular disease and taking into account extent and activity of bowel involvement, possible associated or previous extracranial thrombosis and risk of gastrointestinal hemorrhage. Whether IBD patients with known predisposing factors, prior thromboembolism or at time of acute intestinal exacerbation may benefit from prophylactic short- or long-term anticoagulation is unknown (Liebman et al., 1998), but screening and correction of vitamin deficiency implicated in hyperhomocysteinemia is probably warranted (Cattaneo et al., 1998).

References

Agranoff, D. & Schon, F. (1995). Are focal white matter lesions in patients with inflammatory bowel disease linked to multiple sclerosis (letter)? *Lancet*, **346**, 190–1.

Akobeng, A.K., Miller, V. & Thomas, A. G. (1998). Epilepsy and Crohn's disease in children. *Journal of Pediatric Gastroenterology and Nutrition*, **26**, 458–60.

Andus, T., Geissier, A., Herrmann, W. et al., (1995). Focal white matter lesions in the brain of ulcerative colitis patients are associated with increased serum concentration of lipoprotein (a) (abstract). *Gastroenterology*, **108**, 770.

Averback, P. (1978). Primary cerebral venous thrombosis in young adults: the diverse manifestations of an underrecognized disease. *Annals of Neurology*, **3**, 81–6.

Bar Dayan, Y., Levi, Y. & Shoenfeld, Y. (1995). Cerebral infarction in Crohn's disease. *Harefua*, **129**, 173–6.

Bargen, J.A. & Barker, N.W. (1936). Extensive arterial and venous thrombosis complicating chronic ulcerative colitis. *Archives of Internal Medicine*, **58**, 17–31.

Borda, I.T., Southern, R.F. & Brown, W.F. (1973). Cerebral venous thrombosis in ulcerative colitis. *Gastroenterology*, **64**, 116–19.

Brohee, P., Violon, P., Pirotte, B., Brotchi, J. & Hildebrand (1995). Treatment of central nervous system vasculitis associated with Crohn's disease: two case reports (abstract). *Journal of Neurology*, **242**(S2), 93.

Cattaneo, M., Vecchi, M., Zighetti, M.L. et al. (1998). High prevalence of hyperhomocysteinemia in patients with inflammatory bowel disease: a pathogenic link with thromboembolic complications? *Thrombosis and Haemostasis*, **80**, 542–5.

Collins, C.E. & Rampton, D.S. (1995). Platelet dysfunction: a new dimension in inflammatory bowel disease. *Gut*, **36**, 5–8.

Conlan, M.G., Haire, W.D. & Burnett, D.A. (1989). Prothrombotic abnormalities in inflammatory bowel disease. *Digestive Diseases and Sciences*, **34**, 1089–93.

De Jong, E., Porte, R.J., Knot, E.A.R., Verheijen, J.H. & Dees, J. (1989). Disturbed fibrinolysis in patients with inflammatory bowel disease. A study in blood plasma, colon mucosa, and faeces. *Gut*, **30**, 188–94.

Dejaco, C., Fertl, E., Prayer, D. et al. (1996). Symptomatic cerebral microangiopathy preceding initial manifestation of ulcerative colitis. *Digestive Diseases and Sciences*, **41**, 1807–10.

Derdeyn, C.P. & Powers, W.J. (1998). Isolated cortical venous thrombosis and ulcerative colitis. *American Journal of Neuroradiology*, **19**, 488–90.

Edwards, K.R. (1977). Hemorrhagic complications of cerebral vasculitis. *Archives of Neurology*, **34**, 549–52.

Elsebety, A.E. & Bertorini, T.E. (1991). Neurological complications in Crohn's disease (abstract). *Annals of Neurology*, **30**, 271.

Friedman, D.P. (1997). Neuroradiology case of the day. *Radiographics*, **18**, 246–50.

Gaffney, P.R., Doyle, C.T., Gaffney, A., Hogan, J., Hayes, D.P. & Annis, P. (1995). Paradoxical response to heparin in 10 patients with ulcerative colitis. *American Journal of Gastroenterology*, **90**, 220–3.

Garcia-Diaz, M., Mira, M., Nevado, L., Galvan, A., Berenguer, A. & Bureo, J.C. (1995). Retinal vasculitis associated with Crohn's disease. *Postgraduate Medical Journal*, **71**, 170–2.

Garcia-Monco, J.C. & Beldarrain, M.G. (1991). Superior sagittal sinus thrombosis complicating Crohn's disease. *Neurology*, **41**, 1324–5.

Geissier, A., Andus, T., Roth, M. et al. (1995). Focal white-matter lesions in brain of patients with inflammatory bowel disease. *Lancet*, **345**, 897–8.

Glotzer, D.J., Yuan, R.H. & Patterson, J.F. (1964). Ulcerative colitis complicated by toxic megacolon, polyserositis and hemorrhagic leukoencephalitis with recovery. *Annals of Surgery*, **159**, 445–50.

Gormally, S.M., Bourke, W., Kierse, B., Monaghan, H., McMenamin, J. & Drumm, B. (1995). Isolated cerebral thrombo-embolism and Crohn's disease. *European Journal of Pediatrics*, **154**, 815–18.

Graef, V., Baggenstoss, A.H., Sauer, W.G. & Spittell, J.A. (1966). Venous thrombosis occurring in nonspecific ulcerative colitis. A necropsy study. *Archives of Internal Medicine*, **117**, 377–82.

Greenstein, A.J., Janowitz, H.D. & Sachar, D.B. (1976). The extra-intestinal complications of Crohn's disease and ulcerative colitis: a study of 700 patients. *Medicine*, **55**, 401–12.

Hamilton, M.I., Dick, R., Crawford, L., Thompson, N.P., Pounder, R.E. & Wakefield, A.J. (1995). Is proximal demarcation of ulcerative colitis determined by the territory of the inferior mesenteric artery? *Lancet*, **345**, 688–90.

Harrison, M.J.G. & Truelove, S.C. (1967). Cerebral venous thrombosis as a complication of ulcerative colitis. *American Journal of Digestive Diseases*, **12**, 1025–8.

Hart, P.E., Gould, S.R., Macsweeney, J.E., Clifton, A. & Schon, F. (1998). Brain white-matter lesions in inflammatory bowel disease (letter). *Lancet*, **351**, 1558.

Hassan, K.O. & Jenkins, H.R. (1998). Multiple venous thrombosis in inflammatory bowel disease (letter). *Journal of Pediatric Gastroenterology and Nutrition*, **27**, 616–17.

Heuer, D.K., Gager, W.E. & Reeser, F.H. (1982). Ischemic optic neuropathy associated with Crohn's disease. *Journal of Clinical Neuro-ophthalmology*, **2**, 175–81.

Hilton-Jones, D. & Warlow, C.P. (1985). The causes of stroke in the young. *Journal of Neurology*, **232**, 137–43.

Hudson, M., Chitolie, A., Hutton, R.A., Smith, M.S.H., Pounder, R.E. & Wakefield, A.J. (1996). Thrombotic vascular risk factors in inflammatory bowel disease. *Gut*, **38**, 733–7.

Hyams, J.S. (1994). Extraintestinal manifestations of inflammatory bowel disease in children. *Journal of Pediatric Gastroenterology and Nutrition*, **19**, 7–21.

Jackson, L.M., O'Gorman, P.J., O'Connell, J., Cronin, C.C., Cotter, K.P. & Shanahan, F. (1997). Thrombosis in inflammatory bowel disease: clinical setting, procoagulant profile and factor V Leiden. *Quarterly Journal of Medicine*, **90**, 183–8.

Johns, D.R. (1991). Cerebrovascular complications of inflammatory bowel disease. *The American Journal of Gastroenterology*, **86**, 367–70.

Jorens, P.G., Hermans, C.R., Haber, I., Kockx, M.M., Vermylen, J. & Parizel, G.A. (1990). Acquired protein C and S deficiency, inflammatory bowel disease and cerebral arterial thrombosis. *Blut*, **61**, 307–10.

Knot, E., Ten Cate, J.W., Leeksma, O.C.H., Tytgat, G.N. & Vreeken, J. (1983). No evidence for a prethrombotic state in stable chronic inflammatory bowel disease. *Journal of Clinical Pathology*, **36**, 1387–90.

Koenigs, K.P., McPhedran, P. & Spiro, H.M. (1987). Thrombosis in inflammatory bowel disease. *Journal of Clinical Gastroenterology*, **9**, 627–31.

Koutroubakis, I.E., Petinaki, E., Anagnostopoulou, E. et al. (1998). Anti-cardiolipin and anti-β2–glycoprotein I antibodies in patients with inflammatory bowel disease. *Digestive Diseases and Sciences*, **43**, 2507–12.

Lake, A.M., Stauffer, J.Q. & Stuart, M.J. (1978). Hemostatic alterations in inflammatory bowel disease. Response to therapy. *Digestive Diseases*, **23**, 897–902.

Levine, J.B. & Lukawski-Trubish, D. (1995). Extraintestinal considerations in inflammatory bowel disease. *Gastroenterology Clinics of North America*, **24**, 633–46.

Liebman, H.A., Kashani, N., Sutherland, D., McGehee, W. & Kam, L. (1998). The factor V Leiden mutation increases the risk of venous thrombosis in patients with inflammatory bowel disease. *Gastroenterology*, **115**, 830–4.

Liebman, H., Sutherland, D. & Kashani, N. (1999). Thrombosis, factor V Leiden, and inflammatory bowel disease (letter). *Gastroenterology*, **116**, 778–9.

Lloyd-Still, J.D. & Tomasi, L. (1989). Neurovascular and thromboembolic complications of inflammatory bowel disease in childhood. *Journal of Pediatric Gastroenterology and Nutrition*, **9**, 461–6.

Lossos, A., River, Y., Eliakim, A. & Steiner, I. (1995). Neurologic aspects of inflammatory bowel disease. *Neurology*, **45**, 416–21.

Mahmud, N., Molloy, A., McPartlin, J. et al. (1999). Increased prevalence of methylenetetrahydrofolate reductase C677T variant in patients with inflammatory bowel disease, and its clinical implications. *Gut*, **45**, 389–94.

Markowitz, R.L., Ment, L.R. & Gryboski, J.D. (1989). Cerebral thromboembolic disease in pediatric and adult inflammatory bowel disease: case report and review of the literature. *Journal of Pediatric Gastroenterology and Nutrition*, **8**, 413–20.

Mayeux, R. & Fahn, S. (1978). Strokes and ulcerative colitis. *Neurology*, **28**, 571–4.

Meucci, G., Pareti, F., Vecchi, M., Saibeni, S., Bressi, C. & De Franchis, R. (1999). Serum von Willebrand factor levels in patients with inflammatory bowel disease are related to systemic inflammation. *Scandinavian Journal of Gastroenterology*, **34**, 287–90.

Mevorach, D., Goldberg, Y., Gomori, M. & Rachmilewitz, D. (1996). Antiphospholipid syndrome manifested by ischemic stroke in a patient with Crohn's disease. *Journal of Clinical Gastroenterology*, **22**, 141–3.

Mezoff, A.G., Cohen, M.B., Maisel, S.K. & Farrell, M.K. (1990). Crohn's disease in an infant with central nervous system thrombosis and protein-losing enteropathy. *Journal of Pediatrics*, **117**, 436–9.

Musio, F., Older, S.A., Jenkins, T. & Gregorie, E.M. (1993). Case report: cerebral venous thrombosis as a manifestation of acute ulcerative colitis. *American Journal of Medical Sciences*, **305**, 28–35.

Nelson, J., Barron, M.M., Riggs, J.E., Gutmann, L. & Schochet, S. (1986). Cerebral vasculitis and ulcerative colitis. *Neurology*, **36**, 719–21.

Newton, M. & Cooper, B.T. (1994). Benign intracranial hypertension during prednisolone treatment for inflammatory bowel disease. *Gut*, **35**, 423–5.

Panaccione, R. & Sandborn, W.J. (1999). Is antibody testing for inflammatory bowel disease clinically useful? *Gastroenterology*, **116**, 1001–2.

Papi, C., Ciaco, A., Acierno, G. et al. (1995). Severe ulcerative colitis, dural sinus thrombosis, and the lupus anticoagulant. *American Journal of Gastroenterology*, **90**, 1514–17.

Penix, L.P. (1998). Ischemic strokes secondary to vitamin B12 deficiency-induced hyperhomocystinemia. *Neurology*, **51**, 622–4.

Perkin, G.D. & Murray-Lyon, I. (1998). Neurology and the gastrointestinal system. *Journal of Neurology, Neurosurgery and Psychiatry*, **65**, 291–300.

Pfeiffer, R.F. (1996). Neurologic dysfunction in gastrointestinal disease. *Seminars in Neurology*, **16**, 217–26.

Podolsky, D.K. (1991). Inflammatory bowel disease. (First of two parts). *New England Journal of Medicine*, **325**, 928–37.

Prior, A., Strang, F.A. & Whorwell, P.J. (1987). Internal carotid artery occlusion associated with Crohn's disease. *Digestive Diseases and Sciences*, **32**, 1047–50.

Rankin, G.B., Watts, H.D., Melnyk, C.S. & Kelley, Jr, M.L. (1979). National cooperative Crohn's disease study: extraintestinal manifestations and perianal complications. *Gastroenterology*, **77**, 914–20.

Ryan, F.P., Timperley, W.R., Preston, F.E. & Holdsworth, C.D. (1977). Cerebral involvement with disseminated intravascular coagulation in intestinal disease. *Journal of Clinical Pathology*, **30**, 551–5.

Sartor, R.B. (1995). Current concepts of the etiology and pathogenesis of ulcerative colitis and Crohn's disease. *Gastroenterology Clinics of North America*, 24, 475–507.

Schneiderman, J.H., Sharpe, J.S. & Sutton, D.M.C. (1979). Cerebral and retinal vascular complications of inflammatory bowel disease. *Annals of Neurology*, **5**, 331–7.

Sigsbee, B. & Rottenberg, D.A. (1978). Sagittal sinus thrombosis as a complication of regional enteritis. *Annals of Neurology*, **3**, 450–2.

Silverstein, A. & Present, D.H. (1971). Cerebrovascular occlusions in relatively young patients with regional enteritis. *Journal of the American Medical Association*, **215**, 976–7.

Sloan, W.P., Bargen, J.A. & Gage, R.P. (1950). Life histories of patients with chronic ulcerative colitis: a review of 2000 cases. *Gastroenterology*, **16**, 25–38.

Slot, W.B., Van Kasteel, V., Coerkamp, E.G., Seelen, P.J. & Van Der Werf, S.D.J. (1995). Severe thrombotic complication in a postpartum patient with active Crohn's disease resulting in ischemic spinal cord injury. *Digestive Diseases and Sciences*, **40**, 1395–9.

Snook, J.A., De Silva, H.J. & Jewell, D.P. (1989). The association of autoimmune disorders with inflammatory bowel disease. *Quarterly Journal of Medicine*, **72**, 835–40.

Souto, J.C., Martinez, E., Roca, M. et al. (1995). Prothrombotic state and signs of endothelial lesion in plasma of patients with inflammatory bowel disease. *Digestive Diseases and Sciences*, **40**, 1882–9.

Talbot, R.W., Heppell, J., Dosois, R.R. & Beart Jr, R.W. (1986). Vascular complications of inflammatory bowel disease. *Mayo Clinic Proceedings*, **61**, 140–5.

Thompson, N.P., Wakefield, A.J. & Pounder, R.E. (1995). Inherited disorders of coagulation appear to protect against inflammatory bowel disease. *Gastroenterology*, **108**, 1011–15.

Vaezi, M.F., Rustagi, P.K. & Elson, C.O. (1995). Transient protein S deficiency associated with cerebral venous thrombosis in active ulcerative colitis. *American Journal of Gastroenterology*, **90**, 313–15.

Wakefield, A.J., Dhillon, A.P., Rowles, P.M. et al. (1989). Pathogenesis of Crohn's disease: multifocal gastrointestinal infarction. *Lancet*, **ii**, 1057–62.

Wakefield, A.J., Sankey, E.A., Dhillon, A.P. et al. (1991). Granulomatous vasculitis in Crohn's disease. *Gastroenterology*, **100**, 1279–87.

Weber, P., Husemann, S., Vielhaber, H., Zimmer, K-P. & Nowak-Gotttl, U. (1999). Coagulation and fibrinolysis in children, adolescents, and young adults with inflammatory bowel disease. *Journal of Pediatric Gastroenterology and Nutrition*, **28**, 418–22.

Wills, A. & Hovell, C.J. (1996). Neurological complications of enteric disease. *Gut*, **39**, 51–4.

Yassinger, S., Adelman, R., Cantor, D., Halsted, C.H. & Bolt, R.J. (1976). Association of inflammatory bowel disease and large vascular lesions. *Gastroenterology*, **71**, 844–6.

Yerby, M.S. & Bailey, G.M. (1980). Superior sagittal sinus thrombosis 10 years after surgery for ulcerative colitis. *Stroke*, **11**, 294–6.

23

Acute posterior multifocal placoid pigment epitheliopathy

Marc D. Reichhart, and Julien Bogousslavsky

Department of Neurology, University of Lausanne, Switzerland

General considerations

Acute posterior multifocal placoid pigment epitheliopathy (APMPPE) is a recently identified rare uveo-meningitis (Gass, 1968). Comparing their fundoscopic signs and clinical courses (Wright et al., 1978), a continuum probably exists between APMPPE (multifocal posterior pole lesions; spontaneous resolution) and Harada's disease (diffuse changes; recurrent disease). Gass first described the typical multifocal yellow–white placoid lesions at the level of the retinal pigment epithelium (RPE) in three young females with central vision loss, but there were further evidences that APMPPE is a choriocapillaritis (Deutman et al., 1972) or a choroid vasculitis (Spaide et al., 1991) with secondary RPE lesions. Its associations with erythema nodosum (Van Buskirk et al., 1971; Deutman et al., 1972) or cerebral vasculitis (see below) raise the question of a more systemic vasculitic syndrome. However, although a flu-like illness precedes the ocular manifestations of APMPPE, its etiopathogeny remains still unknown (postinfectious vs. idiopathic vasculitis). This syndrome has been described as a complication of infections with adenovirus type 5 (Azar et al., 1975), Mumps virus (Borruat, et al., 1998), *Borrelia burgdorferi* (Toenjes et al., 1989; Bodine et al., 1992), *Schistosoma mansoni* (Dickinson et al., 1990), possibly *Mycobacterium tuberculosis* (see Deutman et al., 1972), and after hepatitis B vaccine (Brézin et al., 1995). Conversely, APMPPE is also known to be associated with systemic-onset juvenile rheumatoid arthritis (Bridges et al., 1995), systemic lupus erythematosus (Matsuo et al., 1987; Kawaguchi et al., 1990), Crohn's disease (Gass, 1983), thyroiditis (Jacklin, 1977) and sarcoidosis (Foulds & Damato, 1986; Dick et al., 1988; Bodiguel et al., 1992). In one series (Priluck et al., 1981), urinary casts were found in patients with APMPPE, raising the hypothesis of a concomitant renal and choroidal (inflammatory) microvasculopathy. Finally, only one publication exists of a patient

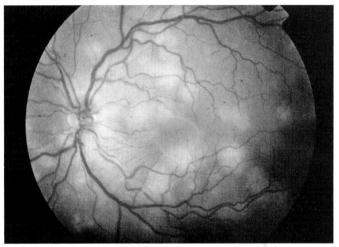

Fig. 23.1. Fundoscopic features of APMPPE: creamy white deeply located intraretinal well-lineated lesions (By courtesy of F-X. Borruat, MD.)

with APMPPE (and stroke) and histopathological signs of small-vessels vasculitis on muscle biopsy (Bewermeyer et al., 1993). HLA mapping of families with APMPPE emphasized HLA DR2 (and B7) to be associated with an increased risk of recurrent disease (Wolf et al., 1990a, b, Kim et al., 1995).

Clinical and paraclinical findings

APMPPE affects young adults (mean age, 26.5 years), and presents with acute/subacute visual blurring, scotomas, or metamorphopsia (Jones, 1995). Both eyes are involved, either simultaneously or sequentially within a few days, and recurrence is rare. Although the RPE changes are definitive, the visual prognosis is usually good (Williams & Mieler, 1989). The yellow/grey–white placoid lesions (see Fig. 23.1) are characteristically seen at the macula (thus affecting

Table 23.1. *Clinical pattern, radiological and CSF features, latencies, outcome and therapy of 11 APMPPE-associated strokes*

Reference (year)	Age, sex	Clinical pattern	CT, MRI and angiography	CSF WBC/ml, proteins mg/l	Stroke latency, outcome, therapy
Holt et al. (1976)	22 M	bilaterial MCA TIAs	multiple segmental narrowing (MSN) of MCA branches	177 1810	inaugural good CS
Sigelman et al. (1979)	18 M	L homonymous hemianopia	R occipital stroke; MSN of MCA branches	5 520 (33 IgG)	inaugural good no CS
Smith et al. (1983)	25 M	L hemianopic blurring and dysesthesia	R (thalamo-) occipital stroke MSN of MCA branches; R PCA occlusion	100 3000	7 wk good CS
Kersten et al. (1987)	30 M	vertigo, downbeat nystagmus/ocular flutter ataxia, tremor	Normal CT (2) and angiogram (on CS). Latency of 5 years after initial APMPPE symptoms	151 1440 pressure 20 cm	5 years good CS
Wilson et al. (1988)	24 M	coma, corticospinal tract sign, headache +	grey matter diffuse edema (necropsy); angiogram ND	0 (150 RBC) 660	6 wk died despite CS
Weinstein et al. (1988)	23 M	R hand clumsiness; L hemianopia	L basal ganglia and R occipital strokes (hemorrhagic conversion); MSN (MCA)	19 330	8/12 wk good CS
Hammer et al. (1989)	25 F	coma, hemiplegia	CT: ACA/MCA infarcts; angiogram ND	not done	3 wk died despite CS
Stoll et al. (1991)	54 M	dysarthria, L hemiparesis, ataxia	Multiple deep small infarcts, MSN of basal arteries	18 670	14 wk good CS + AZA
Bodiguel (1992)	35 M	dysarthria, R hemiparesis	deep small infarcts (internal capsule, corpus callosum). Normal angiogram	77 650 (+ IgG)	5 wk good CS
Bewermeyer (1993)	27 M	nystagmus, dysarthria, L hemiparesis	R pontine infarct; normal angiogram; muscle biopsy: signs of vasculitis	55 360	20 wk good CS + AZA
Comu et al. (1996)	23 F	stupor, R hemiplegia, aphasia; R MCA TIAs	B parieto-occipital and basal ganglia infarcts (one hemorrhage); normal angiogram	60 450	3 wk good CS + CYC

Notes: CS: corticosteroids; AZA: azathioprine; CYC: cyclophosphamide; B: bilateral; R: right; L: left; ND: not done.

the central vision), but never anterior to the equator. Fluorescein (or indocyanine green, see Dhaliwal et al., 1993; Howe et al., 1995) angiographic studies show typical choroidal hypofluorescence (see Fig. 23.1) underneath the active lesions (early stage) and further bright staining (late stage, Jones, 1995). Associated ocular findings include anterior/posterior uveitis, retinal vasculitis, papillitis, retinal serous detachment, edema, and hemorrhages, Marcus-Gunn pupil, and episcleritis (Williams & Mieler, 1989). One-

third of patients experience prodromic flu-like symptoms (fever, malaise, headache, dizziness, myalgia, arthralgia), and less frequently hearing loss, tinnitus, vertigo, fleeting rash, bowel upset, upper respiratory tract infection, or lymphadenopathy (Jones, 1995). In patients with APMPPE without evidences of CNS involvement, CSF analysis may show lymphocytic pleiocytosis (range, 56–70 WBC/ml, Bullock & Fletcher, 1977) and elevated protein levels (over 800 mg/L), but may be normal (Holt et al., 1976).

APMPPE-associated strokes

That stroke develops in patients with APMPPE supports strongly the hypothesis of a particular choroido-cerebral vasculitic syndrome. Indeed, cerebral angiographic studies showed typical multiple focal narrowing, whereas CSF analysis disclosed pleiocytosis or hyperproteinorachia in most of patients (Table 23.1). The first stroke patient with APMPPE (Holt et al., 1976) was a 22-year-old man who developed, 3 weeks after a flu-like episode, bilateral MCA TIAs (aphasia, right-side paresis; numbness/weakness of left arm). Tc-99 brain scan was normal (1973), but carotid angiograms showed 'attenuation, lumen irregularity, and abrupt termination of various small opercular branches and distal cortical vessels of the bilateral MCAs' and CSF analysis revealed frank pleicytosis (Table 23.1). The neurologic symptoms improved before the initiation of corticosteroids (3 weeks later). Shortly after, a CT-proven occipital infarct (controlateral hemianopia) in an 18-year-old (migrainous) man with APMPPE was published (Sigelman et al., 1979); again, carotid angiography showed multiple focal narrowing of MCA branches, whereas hyperproteinorachia with mild pleiocytosis were found in CSF. Until now, nine additional cases have been published (Smith et al., 1983; Kersten et al., 1987; Wilson et al., 1988; Weinstein et al., 1988; Hammer et al., 1989; Stoll et al., 1991; Bodiguel et al., 1992; Bewermeyer et al., 1993; Comu et al., 1996). The clinical patterns, neuroradiological and CSF findings, latencies (disease-onset-to stroke), and therapy as well as outcome of these 11 patients with APMPPE and stroke are shown on Table 23.1. First, APMPPE should be considered as a cause of stroke in every young adult (mean age, 28 years) presenting with blurring of vision after a flu-like episode, and careful fundoscopic examination should be performed. Except one case (5-year latency), the cerebrovascular insult appeared within 6 weeks after the first symptoms of APMPPE in all cases, and stroke was inaugural in two patients. Nearly half of cases involved the vertebro-basilar arteries (PCA infarcts with hemianopia secondary to (thalamo-)occipital strokes, three cases; vertebral or basilar infarcts, two cases). The pattern of small deep (lacunar) infarcts occurred in one-third (4/11) of patients, whereas recurrent bilateral MCA TIAs or strokes developed in two patients. Of the nine patients who came to angiography, more than half (5/9) showed typical signs of vasculitis (multiple segmental narrowing, MSN); half of the remaining normal angiograms (2/4) were performed while patients were on corticosteroids (CS). CSF analysis showed lymphocytic pleiocytosis (mild range, 18–77 WBC/ml, six cases; extreme range, 151–177 WBC/ml, two cases) with/without hyperproteinorachia in 80% (8/10) of patients; on the other hand, the remaining two cases without elevated WBC had mild hyperproteinorchia. Only one patient showed IgG intrathecal synthesis. On CS immunosuppressive therapy, the outcome was favourable in most patients (9/11). On the other hand, the pattern of fatal cerebral vasculitis with coma and corticospinal tract signs developed in two patients. In one of them (Wilson et al., 1988), necropsy confirmed signs of medium-sized artery granulomatous necrotizing (fibrinoid-like) vasculitis that resembled those of isolated angiitis of the CNS (multinucleated giant cells of Langhans' type). In one patient with stroke (Bodiguel et al., 1992), APMPPE was associated with sarcoidosis.

Conclusions

APMPPE, a particular choroido-cerebral vasculitic syndrome of various etiologies (postinfectious, systemic inflammatory diseases), should be considered as a cause of stroke in every young patient with a history of blurring of vision after a flu-like episode. Thorough ocular fundoscopy with further fluorescein (or indocyanine green) angiography, together with MRI and (MR-) angiography studies and CSF analysis should be performed. Muscle biopsy may be helpful. When the aforementioned infections or diseases (sarcoidosis) have been excluded (confirmed), prompt immunosuppressive therapy initiation (corticosteroids associated with azathioprine or cyclophosphamide) is mandatory.

References

Azar, P., Gohd, R.S., Waltman, D. & Gitter, K.A. (1975). Acute posterior multifocal placoid pigment epitheliopathy associated with adenovirus type 5 infection. *American Journal of Ophthalmology*, **80**, 1003–5.

Bewermeyer, H., Nelles, G., Huber, M., Althaus, C., Neuen-Jacob, E. & Assheuer, J. (1993). Pontine infarction in acute posterior multifocal placoid pigment epitheliopathy. *Journal of Neurology*, **241**, 22–6.

Bodiguel, E., Benhamou, A., Le Hoang, P. & Gautier, J-C. (1992). Infarctus cérébral, épithéliopathie en plaques et sarcoïdose. *Revue Neurologie (Paris)*, **148**, (12), 746–51.

Bodine, S.R., Marino, J., Camisa, T.J. & Salvate, A.J. (1992). Multifocal choroiditis with evidence of Lyme disease. *Annals of Ophthalmology*, **24**, 169–73.

Borruat, F-X., Piguet, B. & Herbort, C.P. (1998). Acute posterior multifocal placoid pigment epitheliopathy following mumps. *Ocular Immunology Inflammation*, **6**, 189–93.

Brézin, A.P., Massin-Korobelnik, P., Boudin, M., Gaudric, A., &

Lehoang, P. (1995). Acute posterior multifocal placoid pigment epitheliopathy after hepatitis B vaccine. *Archives of Ophthalmology*, **113**, 297–300.

Bridges, W.J., Saadeh, C. & Gerald, R. (1995). Acute posterior multifocal placoid pigment epitheliopathy in a patient with systemic-onset juvenile rheumatoid arthritis: treatment with cyclosporin A and prednisone. *Arthritis and Rheumatism*, **38**, 446–7.

Bullock, J.D. & Fletcher, R.L. (1977). Cerebrospinal fluid abnormalities in acute posterior multifocal placoid pigment epitheliopathy. *American Journal of Ophthalmology*, **84**, 45–9.

Comu, S., Verstraeten, T., Rinkoff, J.S. & Busis, N.A. (1996). Neurological manifestations of acute posterior multifocal placoid pigment epitheliopathy. *Stroke*, **27**, 996–1001.

Deutman, A.F., Oosterhuis, J.A., Boen-Tan, T.N. & Aan De Kerk, A.L. (1972). Acute posterior multifocal placoid pigment epitheliopathy. Pigment epitheliopathy or choriocapillaritis. *British Journal of Ophthalmology*, **56**, 863–74.

Dhaliwal, R.S., Maguire, A.M., Flower, R. W. & Arribas, N.P. (1993). Acute posterior multifocal placoid pigment epitheliopathy. An indocyanine green angiographic study. *Retina*, **13**, 317–25.

Dick, D. J., Newman, P.K., Richardson, J., Wilkinson, R. & Morley, A.R. (1988). Acute posterior multifocal placoid pigment epitheliopathy and sarcoidosis. *British Journal of Ophthalmology*, **72**, 74–7.

Dickinson, A.J., Rosenthal, A.R. & Nicholson, K.G. (1990). Inflammation of the retinal pigment epithelium: a unique presentation of ocular schistosomiasis. *British Journal of Ophthalmology*, **74**, 440–2.

Foulds, W.S. & Damato, B.E. (1986). Investigations and prognosis in the retinal pigment epitheliopathies. *Australian and New Zealand Journal of Ophthalmology*, **14**, 301–11.

Gass, J.D.M. (1968). Acute posterior multifocal placoid pigment epitheliopathy. *Archives of Ophthalmology*, **80**, 177–85.

Gass, J.D.M. (1983). Acute posterior multifocal placoid pigment epitheliopathy: a long-term follow up. In *Management of Retinal Vascular and Macular Disorder*, ed. S.L. Fine & L. Owens pp. 176–81. Baltimore, MD: Williams & Wilkins Co.

Hammer, M.E., Grizzard, W.S. & Travies, D. (1989). Death associated with acute multifocal placoid pigment epitheliopathy. *Archives of Ophthalmology*, **107**, 170–1.

Holt, W.S., Regan, C.D.J. & Trempe, C. (1976). Acute posterior multifocal placoid pigment epitheliopathy. *American Journal of Ophthalmology*, **81**, 403–12.

Howe, L.J., Woon, H., Graham, E.M., Fitzke, F., Bhandari, A. & Marshall, J. (1995). Choroidal hypoperfusion in acute posterior multifocal placoid pigment epitheliopathy. *Ophthalmology*, **102**, 790–8.

Jacklin, H.N. (1977). Acute posterior multifocal placoid pigment epitheliopathy and thyroiditis. *Archives of Ophthalmology*, **95**, 995–7.

Jones, N.P. (1995). Acute posterior multifocal placoid pigment epitheliopathy. *British Journal of Ophthalmology*, **79**, 384–9.

Kawaguchi, Y., Hara, M., Hirose, T. et al. (1990). A case of SLE complicated with multifocal posterior pigment epitheliopathy. *Ryumachi*, **30**, 396–402.

Kersten, D.H., Lessell, S. & Carlow, T.J. (1987). Acute posterior multifocal placoid pigment epitheliopathy and late-onset meningo-encephalitis. *Ophthalmology*, **94**, 393–6.

Kim, R.Y., Holz, F.G., Gregor, Z. & Bird, A.C. (1995). Recurrent acute multifocal placoid pigment epitheliopathy in two cousins. *American Journal of Ophthalmology*, **119**, 660–2.

Matsuo, T., Nakayama, T., Koyama, T. & Matsuo, N. (1987). Multifocal pigment epithelial damages with serous retinal detachment in systemic lupus erythematosus. *Ophthalmologica*, **195**, 97–102.

Priluck, I. A., Robertson, D.M. & Buettner, H. (1981). Acute posterior multifocal placoid pigment epitheliopathy. Urinary findings. *Archives of Ophthalmology*, **99**, 1560–2.

Sigelman, J., Behrens, M. & Hilal, S. (1979). Acute posterior multifocal placoid pigment epitheliopathy associated with cerebral vasculitis and homonymous hemianopia. *American Journal of Ophthalmology*, **88**, 919–24.

Smith, C.H., Savino, P.J., Beck, R.W., Schatz, N.J. & Sergott, R.C. (1983). Acute posterior multifocal placoid pigment epitheliopathy and cerebral vasculitis. *Archives of Neurology*, **40**, 48–50.

Spaide, R.F., Yanuzzi, L. A. & Slakter, J. (1991). Choroidal vasculitis in acute posterior multifocal placoid pigment epitheliopathy. *British Journal of Ophthalmology*, **75**, 685–7.

Stoll, G., Reiners, K., Schwartz, A., Kaup, F-G., Althaus, C. & Freund, H-J. (1991). Acute posterior multifocal placoid pigment epitheliopathy with cerebral involvement. *Journal of Neurology, Neurosurgery and Psychiatry*, **54**, 77–9.

Toenjes, W., Mielke, U., Schmidt, H.J., Haas, A. & Holzer, G. (1989). Akute multifokale plakoide Pigmentepitheliopathie mit entzuendlichem Liquorbefund. Sonderform einer Borreliose? *Deutsch Medicalische Wochenschrift*, **114**, 793–5.

Van Buskirk, E.M., Lessell, S. & Friedman, E. (1971). Pigmentary epitheliopathy and erythema nodosum. *Archives of Ophthalmology*, **85**, 369–72.

Weinstein, J.M., Bresnik, G.H., Bell, C.L., Roschmann, R.A., Brooks, B.R. & Strother, C.M. (1988). Acute posterior multifocal placoid pigment epitheliopathy associated with cerebral vasculitis. *Journal of Clinical Neuro-ophthalmology*, **8**, 195–201.

Williams, D.F. & Mieler, W.F. (1989). Long-term follow-up of acute multifocal posterior placoid pigment epitheliopathy. *British Journal of Ophthalmology*, **73**, 985–90.

Wilson, C.A., Choromokos, E.A. & Sheppard, R. (1988). Acute posterior multifocal placoid pigment epitheliopathy and cerebral vasculitis. *Archives of Ophthalmology*, **106**, 796–800.

Wolf, M.D., Folk, J.C. & Goeken, N.E. (1990a). Acute posterior multifocal pigment epitheliopathy and optic neuritis in a family. *American Journal of Ophthalmology*, **110**, 89–90.

Wolf, M.D., Folk, J.C., Panknen, C.A. & Goeken, N.E. (1990b). HLA-B7 and HLA-DR2 antigens and acute posterior multifocal placoid pigment epitheliopathy. *Archives of Ophthalmology*, **108**, 698–700.

Wright, B.E., Bird, A.C. & Hamilton, A.M. (1978). Placoid pigment epitheliopathy and Harada's disease. *British Journal of Ophthalmology*, **62**, 609–21.

24

Sweet's syndrome (acute febrile neutrophilic dermatosis)

B. Neundörfer and A. Druschky

Neurologische Klinik mit Poliklinik, Universität Erlangen-Nürnberg, Germany

Definition

In 1964, Sweet described for the first time a clinical picture in eight female patients which he termed acute febrile neutrophilic dermatosis. The illness commenced acutely with fever and leukocytosis. Erythematous pustules and plaques infiltrated with neutrophils were visible. Crow et al. (1969) were the first authors to call this disease 'Sweet's syndrome'. In the meantime, more than 500 cases have been described in the literature. In 1986, Su and Liu suggested a catalogue of diagnostic criteria with two obligatory (major criteria) and four facultative principal criteria (minor criteria). This catalogue was modified slightly by von den Driesch et al. in 1989 and by Su et al. in 1990, and in the meantime has become recognized throughout the world for establishing the diagnosis of this disease (see Table 24.1). For correct diagnosis of Sweet's syndrome, two obligatory (major) and two of the four facultative (minor) criteria must be fulfilled.

Epidemiology

Exact epidemiological data is not available. An annual incidence of 2: 1 000 000 was estimated in Scotland (Kemmett & Hunter, 1990). Prevalences of 1: 250 (Gunawardena et al., 1975) to 1: 1200 (von den Driesch, 1994) were found in dermatology outpatient departments. The disease occurs in patients of any age. The female sex predominates with a ratio of 2.3 to 3.7: 1 (von den Driesch, 1994). However, this predilection of one sex cannot be discerned in childhood.

Sweet's syndrome is mainly manifest in two subtypes: an idiopathic and a paraneoplastic form (Cohen & Kurzrock, 1993; von den Driesch, 1994). The former is observed especially in women in the fourth and fifth decade of life. It is frequently preceded by infection, especially of the upper airways. The latter accounts for up to 30% of patients

(Clemmensen et al., 1989). There are associations both with malignancies of the myeloproliferative system and solid tumours. The sex ratio is 1:1 in this subtype (Cohen et al., 1988).

Clinical picture

Multiple painful, sharply demarcated erythematous plaques located on the face, neck, thorax, back and on the limbs are characteristic (von den Driesch, 1994; Kemmett & Hunter, 1990; Su et al., 1990; 1995; Su & Liu, 1986; Sweet, 1964). In some cases, they are limited to the face (Cooper et al., 1983; Pachinger & Rauch, 1984). Locations in the region of the oral mucosa and in the genital region tend to be rare (Kemmett & Hunter, 1990; Lindskov, 1984; Mizoguchi et al., 1988). Swelling of lymph nodes occurs (Sitjas et al., 1993). Most patients run febrile or at least subfebrile temperatures (Kemmett & Hunter, 1990). One- to two-thirds of the patients complain of arthralgia or indeed suffer from arthritis (Kemmett & Hunter, 1990; Nolla et al., 1990; Smolle & Kresbach, 1990). The eyes are involved in about two-thirds of patients; these ophthalmological conditions are mainly conjunctivitis and episcleritis.

Histology

Dermal infiltration of mononuclear cells and neutrophilic leukocytes with leukocytoclasis is characteristic for Sweet's syndrome (von den Driesch, 1994; Jordaan, 1989; Su et al., 1995; Sweet, 1964). The vessels are dilated and the endothelia are swollen. Extravasation of erythrocytes is found in places. Edema in the upper corium leads to blisters. The infiltrates are arranged in ribbons. Perivascular accumulations of mononuclear cells are found in deeper layers of the

Table 24.1. *Essential components of sweet syndrome*

Major criteria

(i) Abrupt onset of tender, painful erythematous or violaceous plaques or nodules

(ii) Predominantly neutrophilic infiltration in dermis without leukocytoclastic vasculitis

Minor criteria

(i) Prodromal symptoms of fever or infection

(ii) Concurrent association with fever, arthralgia, conjunctivitis, or underlying malignancy

(iii) Laboratory finding or leukocytosis or erythrocyte sedimentation rate >50 mm/1 h

(iv) Good response to therapy with systemic steroids

Both major criteria and at least two of the minor criteria must be fulfilled to justify a diagnosis of Sweet syndrome.

Source: From Su et al. (1995).

corium. Lymphocytes followed by neutrophils are mainly observed in the early stage, whereas histiocytes predominate in the late stage. Vasculitis in the strict sense is only rarely seen (Delaporte et al., 1989; Dobbeler et al., 1980; Keller & Spira, 1986).

Clinical test parameters

Typical but by no means specific clinical test parameters are (von den Driesch, 1994; Su et al., 1995) an accelerated ESR, leukocytosis with moderate lymphopenia, anemia and raised C-reactive protein.

Concomitant diseases

A malignancy was found in about one-third of Sweet's syndrome cases. On the one hand, these were diseases of the hemoproliferative system such as acute and chronic leukemia as well as acute and chronic lymphatic leukemia, hairycell leukemia, polycythemia vera, non-Hodgkin lymphoma, Hodgkin lymphoma and other diseases of the hematopoietic system (von den Driesch, 1994). On the other hand, cases of solid tumours have been repeatedly described in association with Sweet's syndrome (Cohen et al., 1993; von den Driesch, 1994; Geelkerken et al., 1994). These are mainly breast, uterine, prostate, colon and rectal cancers. All other organs may also be affected.

An infection is not uncommonly found simultaneously with Sweet's syndrome and is caused by the most diverse pathogens such as yersinias, salmonellae, *Helicobacter*

pylori, *Mycobacteria leprae*, HIV, mycobacteria and cytomegalovirus (further references in: von den Driesch, 1994).

Further associated diseases (mainly autoimmune diseases) are Behçet's disease (Cho et al., 1989; Mizoguchi et al., 1988), Crohn's disease (Ly et al., 1995; Perales et al., 1997), ulcerative colitis (Hommel et al., 1993; Kemmett & Hunter, 1990; Sitjas et al., 1993; Sweet, 1964; van den Driesch, 1994), Sjögren syndrome (Bianconcini et al., 1991; Levenstein et al., 1991; Vatan et al., 1997), lupus erythematosus (Goette, 1985; Sequeira et al., 1986), thyroiditis (Alcalay et al., 1987; von den Driesch, 1994), rheumatoid arthritis (Delaporte et al., 1989; von den Driesch, 1994; Kemmett & Hunter, 1990). Sweet's syndrome has also been frequently described in pregnancy (see references in: von den Driesch, 1994). Finally, several cases with Sweet's syndrome after treatment with G-CSF (granulocyte colony stimulatory factor) have become known (Garty et al., 1996; Karp, 1992; Park et al., 1992; Petit et al., 1996; Shimizu et al., 1996).

Sweet's syndrome and the central nervous system

In 1983, Chiba described a 46-year-old male patient with Sweet's syndrome who suffered from convulsions and showed slowing in the EEG as well as cerebral atrophy in the CCT. The patient later developed myoclonus resistant to treatment as well as depression. The CSF was normal. In 1992, Dunn et al. reported on a 7-week-old boy with Sweet's syndrome and aseptic meningitis which developed following otitis media and an infection of the upper airways. Furukawa et al. (1992) as well as Martínez et al. (1995) each described a patient with slight meningitis (cell count 29/mm^3 (Furukawa et al., 1992) and 31/mm^3 (Martínez et al., 1995)) without neurological deficits in connection with a Sweet's syndrome.

The only case of cerebral ischemia with focal neurological deficits known so far in the literature was described by Druschky et al. in 1996. This was a 69-year-old man who had developed bronchitis 14 days before inpatient admission. He received antibiotic treatment for suspected meningitis. On inpatient admission, he showed the typical skin changes of Sweet's syndrome, meningism and a slight to moderately severe right hemiparesis. The ESR was enormously accelerated (100 m/h). Leukocytosis of 26 600/μl with 87.2% granulocytes and 7.7% lymphocytes was found with pleocytosis of 51 cells/mm^3 in the CSF. PCR for *Borrelia burgdorferi* and herpesvirus were negative. MRI and Doppler sonography were normal. A broad-scale antibiotic treatment (ceftriaxone, fosfomycin, penicillin) administered for 2 weeks remained unsuccessful. After confirmation of the diagnosis by the dermatological consultant on the basis of the typical histological finding, 100 mg methylprednisolone treatment was commenced. The patient then initially developed slight paresis of the left arm and the left leg in addition. Assuming that the patient had cerebral vasculitis, 250 mg prednisolone was then administered i.v. The skin changes regressed quickly under this treatment and the cell count in the CSF fell to $8/mm^3$ after 13 days. After 4 weeks, the motor deficit had markedly improved. A CCT and cerebral angiography had not shown any indications of vasculitis.

Pathogenesis and treatment

The pathogenesis of Sweet's syndrome is still unclear. It is assumed to be a hypersensitivity reaction to an unknown antigen. It still remains unresolved whether this is a reaction to an immune complex vasculitis, T-cell activation or an alteration in the function of neutrophils (von den Driesch, 1994).

The standard therapy is administration of prednisone or prednisolone at an initial dose of 0.5 to 1.5 mg/kg body weight with a subsequent slow reduction over 2 to 4 weeks. Fever and arthralgias mostly subside within two days and the skin eruptions within 7 days (von den Driesch, 1994; Su et al., 1995). Twenty to thirty per cent of patients suffer recurrences (Kemmett & Hunter, 1990; Sitjas et al., 1993). Potassium iodide, colchicine, dapsone, doxycycline, clofazimine and nonsteroid anti-inflammatories (indomethacin, naproxen) are recommended as alternatives (especially in the context of recurrences).

References

Alcalay, J., Filhaber, A., David, M. et al. (1987). Sweet's syndrome and subacute thyroiditis. *Dermatologica*, **174**, 28–9.

Bianconcini, G., Mazzali, F., Gardini, G. et al. (1991). Sindrome di Sweet (dermatosi neutrofila acuta febbrile) associata a sindrome di Sjögren. Un caso clinico. *Minerva Medica*, **82**, 869–76.

Chiba, S. (1983). Sweet's Syndrome with neurologic signs and psychiatric symptoms. *Archives of Neurology*, **40**, 829.

Cho, K.H., Shin, K.S., Sohn, S.J. et al. (1989). Behçet's disease with Sweet's syndrome-like presentation: a report of six cases. *Clinical and Experimental Dermatology*, **14**, 20–4.

Clemmensen, O.J., Menne, T., Brandrup, F. et al. (1989). Acute febrile neutrophilic dermatosis: a marker of malignancy? *Acta dermatologica-venereologica (Stockholm)*, **69**, 52–8.

Cohen, P.R. & Kurzrock, R. (1993). Sweet's syndrome and cancer. *Clinics in Dermatology*, **11**, 149–57.

Cohen, P.R., Talpaz, M. & Kurzrock, R. (1988). Malignancy-associated Sweet's syndrome: review of the world literature. *Journal of Clinical Oncology*, **6**, 1887–97.

Cohen, P.R., Holder, W.R., Tucker, S.B. et al. (1993). Sweet syndrome in patients with solid tumors. *Cancer*, **72**, 2723–31.

Cooper, P.H., Innes, D.J.J. & Greer, K.E. (1983). Acute febrile neutrophilic dermatosis (Sweet's syndrome) and myeloproliferative disorders. *Cancer*, **51**, 1518–26.

Crow, K.D., Kerdel-Vergas, F. & Rook, A. (1969). Acute febrile neutrophilic dermatosis: Sweet's syndrome. *Dermatologica*, **139**, 123–34.

Delaporte, E., Gaveau, D.J., Piette, F.A. et al. (1989). Acute febrile neutrophilic dermatosis (Sweet's syndrome): association with rheumatoid vasculitis. *Archives of Dermatology*, **125**, 1101–4.

Dobbeler, D., Laurent, R. & Achten, G. (1980). Dermal vessel injuries in acute febrile neutrophilic dermatosis (Sweet's syndrome): a ultrastructural study of two cases. *Journal of Cutaneous Pathology*, **7**, 179.

Druschky, A., von den Driesch, P., Anders, M. et al. (1996). Sweet's syndrome (acute febrile neutrophilic dermatosis) affecting the central nervous system. *Journal of Neurology*, **243**, 556–7.

Dunn, T.R., Saperstein, H.W., Biederman, A. et al. (1992). Sweet syndrome in a neonate with aseptic meningitis. *Pediatric Dermatology*, **9**, 288–92.

Furukawa, F., Toriyama, R. & Kawanishi, T. (1992). Neutrophils in cerebrospinal fluid of a patient with acute febrile neutrophilic dermatosis (Sweet's syndrome). *International Journal of Dermatology*, **31**, 670–1.

Garty, B.Z., Levy, I., Nitzan, M. et al. (1996). Sweet syndrome Associated with G-CSF treatment in a child with glycogen storage disease type Ib. *Pediatrics*, **97**, 401–3.

Geelkerken, R.H., Lagaay, M.B., van Deijk, W.A. et al. (1994). Sweet syndrome associated with liposarcoma: a case report. *Netherlands Journal of Medicine*, **45**, 107–9.

Goette, D.K. (1985). Sweet's syndrome in subacute cutaneous lupus erythematodes. *Archives of Dermatology*, **121**, 789–91.

Gunawardena, D.A., Gunarwardena, K.A., Ratnayaka, M.R.S. et al. (1975). The clinical spectrum of Sweet's syndrome (acute febrile neutrophilic dermatosis): a report of eighteen cases. *British Journal of Dermatology*, **92**, 363–73.

Hommel, L., Harms, M. & Saurat, J-H. (1993). The incidence of Sweet's syndrome in Geneva: a retrospective study of 29 cases. *Dermatology*, **187**, 303–5.

Jordaan, H.F. (1989). Acute febrile neutrophilic dermatosis: a histopathological study of 37 patients and a review of the literature. *American Journal of Dermatopathology*, **11**, 99–111.

Karp, D.L. (1992). The Sweet syndrome or G-CSF reaction? *Annals of Internal Medicine*, **117**, 875–6.

Keller, J. & Spira, I. (1986). Sweet-Syndrom mit Immunkomplexvaskulitis bei einem Kind. *H+G: Zeitschrift der Hautkrankheiten*, **61**, 1351–60.

Kemmett, D. & Hunter, J.A.A. (1990). Sweet's syndrome: a clinicopathologic review of twenty-nine cases. *Journal of the American Academy of Dermatology*, **23**, 503–7.

Levenstein, M.M., Fisher, B.K., Fisher, L.O.L. et al. (1991).

Simultaneous occurrence of subacute cutaneous lupus erythematosus and Sweet syndrome. A marker of Sjögren syndrome? *International Journal of Dermatology*, **30**, 640–3.

Lindskov, R. (1984). Acute febrile neutrophilic dermatosis with genital involvement. *Acta dermatologica-venereologica (Stockholm)*, **64**, 559–61.

Ly, S., Beylot-Barry, M., Beyssac, R. et al. (1995). Syndrome de Sweet associé à une maladie de Crohn. *La Revue de medecine interne*, **16**, 931–3.

Martínez, E., Fernández, A., Mayo, J. et al. (1995). Sweet's syndrome associated with cerebrospinal fluid neutrophilic pleocytosis. *International Journal of Dermatology*, **34**, 73–4.

Mizoguchi, M., Matsuki, M., Mochizuki, M. et al. (1988). Human leukocyte antigen in Sweet's syndrome and its relationship to Behçet's syndrome. *Archives of Dermatology*, **124**, 1069–73.

Nolla, J.M., Juanola, X, Valverde, J. et al. (1990). Arthritis in acute febrile neutrophilic dermatosis (Sweet's syndrome). *Annals of the Rheumatic Diseases*, **49**, 135.

Pachinger, W. & Rauch, H.J. (1984). Lokalisiertes Sweet-Syndrom. *Aktuelle Dermatologie*, **10**, 209–10.

Park, J.W., Mehrotra, B., Barnett, B.O. et al. (1992). The Sweet syndrome during therapy with granulocyte colony-stimulating factor. *Annals of Internal Medicine*, **116**, 996–8.

Perales, J.L.G., Ortí, R.T., Fayos, J.B. et al. (1997). Un caso de síndrome de Sweet Asociado a enfermedad de Crohn. *Gastroenterologia y Hepatologia*, **20**, 134–7.

Petit, Th., Francès, C., Marinho, E. et al. (1996). Lymphoedema-area-restricted Sweet syndrome during G-CSF treatment. The *Lancet*, **347**, 690.

Sequeira, W., Polisky, R.B. & Alrenga, B.P. (1986). Neutrophilic dermatosis (Sweet's syndrome): association with a hydralazin-induced lupus syndrome. *American Journal of Medicine*, **81**, 558–61.

Shimizu, T., Yoshida, I., Eguchi, H. et al. (1996). Sweet syndrome in a child with aplastic anemia receiving recombinant granulocyte colony-stimulating factor. *Journal of Pediatric Hematology/Oncology*, **18**, 282–4.

Sitjas, D., Puig, L., Cuatrecasas, M. et al. (1993). Acute febrile neutrophilic dermatosis (Sweet's syndrome). *International Journal of Dermatology*, **32**, 261–8.

Smolle, J., Kresbach, H. (1990). Acute febrile neutrophilic dermatosis (Sweet syndrome): a retrospective clinical and histological analysis. *Hautarzt*, **41**, 549–56.

Su, W.P.D. & Liu, H.N.H. (1986). Diagnostic criteria for Sweet's syndrome. *Cutis*, **37**, 167–74.

Su, W.P.D., Alegre V.A. & White, W.L. (1990). Myelofibrosis discovered after diagnosis of Sweet's syndrome. *International Journal of Dermatology*, **29**, 201–4.

Su, W.P.D., Fett, D.L., Gibson, L.E. et al. (1995). Sweet syndrome: acute febrile neutrophilic dermatosis. *Seminars in Dermatology*, **14**, 173–8.

Sweet, R.D. (1964). An acute febrile neutrophilic dermatosis. *British Journal of Dermatology*, **74**, 349–56.

Vatan, R., Sire, S., Constans, J. et al. (1997). Association syndrome de Goujerot-Sjögren primitif et syndrome de Sweet. À propos d'un cas. *La Revue de Medecine Interne*, **18**, 734–5.

von den Driesch, P. (1994). Sweet's syndrome (acute febrile neutrophilic dermatosis). *Journal of the American Academy of Dermatology*, **31**, 535–56.

von den Driesch, P., Schlegel, G.R., Kiesewetter, F. et al. (1989). Sweet's syndrome: Clinical spectrum and associated condition. *Cutis*, **44**, 193–200.

25

Nephrotic syndrome and stroke

Alfredo M. Lopez-Yunez and José Biller

Department of Neurology, Indiana University School of Medicine, Indianapolis, IN, USA

Background

When proteinuria is in excess of 3 to 3.5 grams per 24 hours (or $2g/day/m^2$), and is associated with hypoalbuminemia, edema, and hyperlipidemia, a nephrotic syndrome is said to be present. The first description of the nephrotic syndrome is attributed to Volhard and Fahr in the early part of this century (Arneil, 1971). The nephrotic syndrome may be idiopathic, or secondary to a number of systemic disorders affecting the renal glomeruli such as diabetes mellitus, systemic lupus erythematosus, amyloidosis (including multiple myeloma), light chain deposition disease, malaria, infections with hepatitis B, hepatitis C, or HIV, and as a side effect of non-steroidal anti-inflammatory drugs, gold, or penicillamine. Less common causes include the congenital nephrotic syndrome of the Finnish type, Fabry disease, Alport syndrome, nail-patella syndrome, polyarteritis nodosa, Wegener granulomatosis, Sjögren disease, Takayasu disease, Henoch–Schonlein purpura, sarcoidosis, mixed cryoglobulinemia, Hodgkin lymphoma, etc. (Olson & Schwartz, 1998).

The most common underlying renal condition causing idiopathic nephrotic syndrome in children between the ages of 6 months and 10 years is minimal change disease (minimal change nephrotic syndrome). In adults, the most common condition is membranous nephropathy, which may occur in association with malignancies. Another common underlying renal condition seen in patients with idiopathic nephrotic syndrome is focal segmental glomerulosclerosis and other proliferative and sclerosing glomerulonephritides. Approximately 80% of children with nephrotic syndrome and 25% of adults have idiopathic nephrotic syndrome. Of the adult cases, approximately 20% are secondary to diabetes mellitus or amyloidosis. Conditions like malaria represent a major cause of nephrotic syndrome in developing nations (Report of the International Kidney Study, 1984; Glassock, 1979).

Regardless of the etiology or age group, the end result of nephrotic syndrome is proteinuria of nephrotic magnitude (>3 to $3.5g/24h$), hypoalbuminemia, facial/periorbital and dependent edema, a predisposition to serious bacterial infections, potential for increased occurrence of cardiovascular disorders as a consequence of the atherogenicity of the associated hyperlipidemia (including abnormal lipoprotein (a) concentrations), and a predisposition to various thromboembolic phenomena in both the venous and the arterial circulation.

Patients with nephrotic syndrome should be referred to a nephrologist for further evaluation and have a thorough diagnostic work-up, including renal biopsy in all adult cases at presentation, and in highly selective pediatric cases.

Hypercoagulability in nephrotic syndrome

Numerous abnormalities in coagulation factors, the fibrinolytic system, and platelet function have been postulated to explain the hypercoagulability seen in patients with nephrotic syndrome. Mechanisms implicated in the development of thrombotic complications are summarized in Table 25.1.

Nephrotic syndrome causes a hypercoagulable state leading to both venous and arterial thromboses (Addis, 1948). Thrombotic events are most common in membranous nephropathy, involve predominantly the venous circulation, and are clinically silent in almost half of the patients (Cameron, 1984). In a review of 3377 pediatric patients with nephrotic syndrome, thromboembolic complications occurred in almost 2% of cases (Egli, 1974), and averaged 26% in eight series of adult patients (Llach, 1985).

Table 25.1. *Potential contributing factors for hypercoagulability in the nephrotic syndrome*

Platelet hyperaggregability
Thrombocytosis
↑ β-Thromboglobulin levels
↑ von Willebrand factor levels
↑ Release of β-thrombomodulin
↑ Platelet factor 4
↓ Sialoglycoprotein and other negative-charge sites

Increase procoagulant activity/decrease fibrinolysis
↑ Factor V and factor VIII levels
↓ Antithrombin-III
↓ Free protein-S
↑ α2–macroglobulin
↑ C4b-binding protein
Antiphospholipid antibodies/lupus anticoagulant
Factor V Leiden mutation
↑ Fibrinogen
↓ Factor XI
↓ Factor XII
↓Plasminogen
↑ tPA and PAI-1
↑ α_2 antiplasmin
↓ α_1-antitrypsin
Hemoconcentration and hyperviscosity
Infections

Thromboses are most frequently seen soon after diagnosis, but may occur at any stage during the course of the nephrotic syndrome. The most common thrombotic complications are venous, with renal vein thrombosis, femoral vein thrombosis, and pulmonary embolism accounting for more than a third of these complications. Cerebral venous thrombosis is infrequent, but is increasingly recognized in patients of all ages, and may be fatal (Cameron, 1984). Arterial thromboses occur less frequently and have been reported mostly in children.

Platelet hyperaggregability correlates with the degree of proteinuria. Thrombocytosis, increased levels of β thromboglobulin, increased levels of von Willebrand factor, increased release of β-thrombomodulin and platelet factor 4 have been described (Richman & Kasnic, 1982). Hyperlipidemia can lead to increased platelet aggregation. Hypoalbuminemia may also alter platelet function, as albumin is known to regulate the conversion of arachidonic acid from platelet phospholipids into mediators of aggregation. Finally, changes in platelet membranes have also been implicated in enhancing platelet aggregability. The presence of sialoglycoprotein with a pK of 2 ± 0.2 in the platelet membrane is important to prevent spontaneous platelet aggregation and interactions with the vessel wall by repelling negative charges at both surfaces. The number of these systemic negative charge sites is reduced in patients with nephrotic syndrome (George et al., 1984).

Nephrotic plasma has an increased fibrinogen concentration. Several abnormalities in the fibrinolytic system have been reported in these patients. Low levels of plasminogen, varying levels of α2-antiplasmin and tissue-type plasminogen activator (tPA) have been described. The levels of fibrin split products (D-dimers), tPA and plasminogen activator inhibitor-1 (PAI-1) are also elevated in patients with nephrotic syndrome, suggesting that concurrent activation of the coagulation and fibrinolytic pathways occurs in these patients (Malyszko et al., 1996). The lower-molecular-size molecules (<70kd) may be lost in the urine, while higher-molecular-size proteins (>300kd) are likely to be increased in plasma. In general, factor V, factor VIII, and α2–antiplasmin are increased in plasma, while factor IX, factor XI, factor XII, antithrombin-III, plasminogen, and α1–antitripsin are decreased. However, a direct correlation between these changes and the occurrence of thromboembolic complications is not fully established.

One of the most-studied changes in nephrotic syndrome is the decreased activity of naturally occurring anticoagulants. Plasma levels of antithrombin-III are decreased in patients with nephrotic syndrome, because of urinary loss (Lau et al., 1980b). However, significant reductions in antithrombin-III levels are only observed when albumin levels are <2g/dl, whereas hypercoagulability has been described with higher levels of albumin. This suggests that antithrombin-III urinary losses may contribute to thrombotic complications, but they are not sufficient to explain the occurrence of these complications in most patients.

Other abnormalities predisposing to thromboembolic complications include protein-C deficiency, protein-S deficiency, and the presence of antiphospholipid antibodies. The Factor V Leiden mutation also increases the risk (Petaja et al., 1995). Levels of free protein-S are low in the nephrotic syndrome. Protein-S exists in plasma in two forms: free, and bound to c4b-binding protein. The free form (molecular weight of 69kd) is a necessary cofactor for activated protein-C, that ultimately leads to the inactivation of factor VIIIa and factor Va. Abnormally low free protein-S has been described in patients with nephrotic syndrome. The role of these changes in the development of hypercoagulability is not entirely clear.

Hyperlipidemia may also contribute to the increased risk for thrombosis seen in the nephrotic syndrome. Several abnormalities in lipid metabolism are observed, including elevations in total cholesterol, very low density lipoprotein, intermediate-density lipoprotein, low-density lipoprotein (LDL), and lipoprotein(a) (Wheeler & Bernard, 1994). Hepatic overproduction of lipoproteins is thought to play a major role, along with defective receptor-mediated clearance of lipoproteins and paradoxical decrease in urinary apoprotein(a) excretion (Kostner et al., 1998). These abnormalities may lead to the development of atherosclerosis, endothelial dysfunction, or exacerbation of glomerular injury. Lipoprotein(a) is an LDL-like particle linked to a specific apolipoprotein. It has been correlated with increased risk for coronary artery disease (Kronenberg et al., 1996) and stroke (Peng et al., 1999). Lipoprotein(a) inhibits fibrinolysis by competing with the binding of plasminogen to fibrin and to the plasminogen receptor (Edelberg & Pizzo, 1991).

Finally, thrombotic risk varies according to the underlying cause of nephrotic syndrome and associated diseases. The incidence of thromboembolic complications is higher in membranous nephropathy. The coexistence of hypovolemia, overzealous diuretic therapy, corticosteroid therapy, cyclosporine use, infections, associated vascular risk factors, or prothrombotic states (i.e. the antiphospholipid antibody syndrome in lupus) also increase the risk for thrombosis.

Microalbuminuria

Substantial data suggest that microalbuminuria is an index of vascular damage, especially in hypertension and diabetes (Lydakis & Lip, 1998). Microalbuminuria is also an independent risk factor for stroke, regardless of stroke mechanism (Beamer et al., 1999). Screening for microalbuminuria may potentially detect patients at high risk for progression to nephrotic syndrome and for developing macrovascular complications such as stroke.

Microalbuminuria refers to a measurable increase in urine albumin excretion, which is still within normal total urine protein excretion levels. In normal urine, the biggest excreted protein fraction consists of Tamm-Horsfall protein, originated from renal tubular cells. Low-molecular-weight plasma proteins such as insulin and paratohormone are filtered through the glomerular basement membrane and then reabsorbed by the tubular cells. The appearance of any of these proteins in urine is indicative of tubular damage. Conversely, medium-sized (40–150 kd) plasma proteins are not filtered in the glomerulus and therefore, the appearance of these proteins (albumin, transferrin and HDL particles among others) in the urine indicates alteration of the glomerular barrier (Schnaper & Robson, 1996).

In arterial hypertension, the presence of low renal plasma flow and increased renal vascular resistance may lead to higher filtration fraction and increased albumin transmembrane escape. Hypertensive patients with microalbuminuria have shown higher glomerular filtration rates and higher plasma renin activity when compared with patients without microalbuminuria. Several studies in general unselected populations and in non-diabetic populations have also shown positive correlations between increased urinary albumin excretion and systolic and diastolic blood pressures (Agrawal et al., 1996; Cerasola et al., 1996; Redon, 1998).

A German study of 11343 non-diabetic hypertensive patients aimed to determine the degree of microalbuminuria (Luft & Agrawal, 1999). Microalbuminuria was present in 32% of men and 28% of women ($P<0.05$). In patients with microalbuminuria, 31% had coronary artery disease, 24% had left ventricular hypertrophy, 6% had suffered a stroke, and 7% had peripheral arterial disease. In patients without microalbuminuria, these rates were 22%, 14%, 4%, and 5%, respectively, lower in every category ($P<0.001$). Although this study did not include 'blinded' blood pressure determinations or a randomized subject selection process, the authors concluded that qualitative determinations of microalbuminuria may identify hypertensive patients with cardiovascular risk in a practice setting.

Microalbuminuria also precedes the development of overt diabetic nephropathy. At this early stage, the presence of widespread angiopathy is already evident (Jensen, 1991). The risk of progression from microalbuminuria to overt diabetic nephropathy within ten years may be as high as 80% (Mogensen & Christianson, 1994). This risk is modifiable by therapeutic intervention, mostly by improving blood glucose control and antihypertensive therapy. Urinary albumin excretion also occurs in non-insulin-dependent diabetes mellitus and may complicate about 25% of these patients (Standl & Stiegler, 1993). Macrovascular complications, including myocardial infarction, stroke, and peripheral vascular disease have also been positively correlated with the presence of microalbuminuria (Verges et al., 1997), and reductions in mortality and morbidity among hypertensive, type II diabetic patients, have been accomplished by intensified antihypertensive therapy directed at lowering microalbuminuria or macroproteinuria (Sawicki et al., 1995). Likewise, carotid bifurcation atherosclerosis as determined by intimal media thickness is also more frequent among diabetic patients with microalbuminuria (Visona et al., 1995). These data suggest that macrovascular complications in diabetes correlate with the degree of albuminuria and that

Table 25.2. *Mechanisms of cerebral infarction in nephrotic syndrome*

Mechanism
Hypercoagulability
Large vessel atherosclerotic occlusive disease
Cardioembolism
Non-atherosclerotic vasculopathies affecting cerebral and renal vessels

interventions directed at prevention may lower cardiovascular risk.

Associated cerebrovascular disorders

Cerebral infarction

Potential mechanisms of cerebral infarction in patients with nephrotic syndrome are summarized in Table 25.2.

Adults

Miller first reported the association of stroke and nephrotic syndrome (Miller et al., 1969), but the information was insufficient to exclude other causes of cerebral infarction. Few reports of cerebral infarction in adult patients with nephrotic syndrome have been published since this early observation. In 1990, Parag et al. evaluated a young man with nephrotic syndrome associated with left hemiparesis secondary to middle cerebral artery (MCA) thrombosis (Parag et al., 1990). On examination he also had anasarca and a superficial abdominal cellulitis. He had a serum albumin of 0.7 g/dl, a 24-hour protein of 10 g, hypercholesterolemia, elevated fibrinogen of 1440 mg/dl, and a decreased antithrombin-III level of 36%. Clinical course was complicated by a left femoral artery thrombosis. Treatment included embolectomy and heparin, but he eventually died from pulmonary edema. On autopsy, the kidney showed minimal change disease with fusion of podocytes on electron microscopy.

Marsh and colleagues reported two young patients with MCA distribution stroke and nephrotic syndrome (Marsh et al., 1991). The first patient, a 36-year-old man, with no vascular risk factors or family history of hypercoagulable disorder had a left MCA occlusion. There was no evidence for deep venous thrombosis, cardioembolic sources, or large vessel disease. He had severe hypoalbuminemia and proteinuria, hypocomplementemia, elevated fibrinogen

levels, and low free protein-S, with otherwise negative prothrombotic and rheumatologic work-up. No renal biopsy was obtained. He showed partial improvement after warfarin treatment. The second patient, a 34-year-old man, had a right MCA territory infarction. He also had a history of pulmonary embolism, cigarette smoking and a remote history of polysubstance abuse. Family history suggested arterial thrombotic events. Ancillary tests excluded cardioembolic and large vessel occlusive sources. He had an elevated erythrocyte sedimentation rate, hypoalbuminemia, marked proteinuria, elevated fibrinogen levels and normal rheumatologic and prothrombotic work-up (free protein-S not obtained). Renal biopsy showed membranous glomerulonephritis. He received prednisone and aspirin, but 4 months later, following recurrent pulmonary embolism, he received anticoagulant therapy.

Fritz et al. reported a 51-year-old man with a right MCA infarction. Aside from cigarette smoking, no other vascular risk factors were found. The patient had all the cardinal manifestations of nephrotic syndrome, including hyperlipidemia. Serum fibrinogen level was elevated, antithrombin-III and plasminogen levels were decreased. No renal biopsy was obtained. A diagnosis of associated hypercoagulable disorder was made but no information was given regarding treatment (Fritz & Braune, 1992). Fuh et al. found evidence of similar hemostatic abnormalities in seven patients diagnosed with stroke associated with nephrotic syndrome (Fuh et al., 1992).

Chaturvedi reported a fatal case of bilateral cerebral infarctions associated with membranous nephropathy in a 37-year-old woman with history of arterial hypertension and cigarette smoking. She presented with a left MCA infarction and also had occlusion of both the right axillary and radial arteries. Ancillary investigations showed elevated erythrocyte sedimentation rate, raised fibrinogen levels, and findings consistent with nephrotic syndrome. Treatment included intravenous heparin and thrombectomy of the right arm thrombi. Her course was complicated by bilateral cerebellar infarctions progressing rapidly to brain death, despite a suboccipital decompression. Autopsy disclosed left ventricular hypertrophy with no cardiac embolic source, and early membranous nephropathy with subepithelial intramembranous deposits on electron microscopy. No evidence for malignancy or cerebral vasculitis was found (Chaturvedi, 1993).

Low free protein-S levels were also described by Song and colleagues; they described a 39-year-old woman with history of membrano-proliferative glomerulonephritis who had dysarthria and a left hemiparesis. She exhibited mild anemia, hypoalbuminemia and a 24-hour proteinuria of 3.4 g. Platelet count and serum fibrinogen level were normal. Protein-C activity was elevated, plasma antigen level of total protein-S was 75% (normal 84–101%), and free protein-S content was 40% (normal 71–103%). CT scan of the brain showed multiple subcortical hypodensities involving the right frontal lobe. The patient received warfarin and showed partial improvement (Song et al., 1994).

An additional cause of stroke among patients with nephrotic syndrome is cardioembolism. Huang evaluated a diabetic patient with nephrotic syndrome without significant carotid atherosclerosis or cardiac disease who developed biventricular thrombi complicated by cerebral infarction (Huang & Chau, 1995). Two-dimensional echocardiography showed a left ventricular thrombus, an intramural right ventricular thrombus, normal chambers size, septum wall thickness and no regional wall motion abnormalities. He received warfarin, and eventually attained full neurologic recovery. The authors concluded that, in the absence of overt cardiac pathology, a hypercoagulable state associated with nephrotic syndrome was the likely cause of biventricular thrombi, a mechanism that has also been described in a patient with myeloproliferative disorder and ulcerative colitis (Chin et al., 1988).

More recently, de Gauna et al. evaluated a 45-year-old man with membranous nephropathy and nephrotic syndrome complicated by occlusion of the posterior inferior cerebellar artery resulting in a Wallenberg syndrome; he also had elevated fibrinogen levels (de Gauna et al., 1996).

Ahmed and Saeed (1995) described a 42-year-old man, who presented with chest pain, hemoptysis, and dyspnea, found to have a right lower lobe pulmonary artery thrombus on angiogram. He had thrombocytopenia, hypoalbuminemia, decreased antithrombin-III levels, hypercholesterolemia and elevated fibrinogen. Venous ultrasound of the lower extremities, venograms of the renal veins, and inferior vena cava showed thrombi. He received anticoagulants and prednisone, but two years later experienced a right MCA infarction. Prothrombin time was 12.4 s (INR not reported) and 24-h urine protein was 18 g. The authors reported no additional ancillary studies from the second admission, and attributed his cerebral infarction to an underlying hypercoagulable disorder and subtherapeutic anticoagulation; the possibility of paradoxical embolism was apparently not entertained.

Accelerated atherosclerosis involving the coronary arteries without evidence of hypercoagulability has also been described (Kallen et al., 1977). Leno and associates (Leno et al., 1992) evaluated a 30-year-old hypertensive man who had a fatal basilar artery thrombosis 10 months following diagnosis of membranoproliferative glomerulonephritis and hypercholesterolemia of 857 mg/dl. Aside from hyperlipidemia and an elevated erythrocyte sedimentation rate, there was no laboratory evidence to support diagnosis of thrombophilia, although free protein-S values were not reported. At autopsy, there was marked aortic atherosclerosis; the basilar artery was occluded by a fibrous plaque with superimposed fresh thrombus. The authors advised aggressive treatment of hyperlipidemia, a prominent feature among patients with nephrotic syndrome (Joven et al., 1990).

An unusual case of Capgras syndrome has been described in association with nephrotic syndrome. Capgras syndrome is a rare misidentification phenomenon whereby a patient believes that someone, usually a loved one, has been replaced by an identical looking impostor. Collins et al. (1990) reported a 31-year-old eclamptic woman with nephrotic syndrome who became agitated and disoriented and had the delusion that her husband had been replaced by an impostor. She also had severe hypertension, peripheral edema, hypoalbuminemia and proteinuria. Brain CT scan was normal. Renal biopsy showed IgA nephropathy. Symptoms subsided within 3 days. This observation, however, does not necessarily illustrate the association of nephrotic syndrome and cerebral infarction, but rather the possibility of a probable reversible leukoencephalopathy in the context of hypertensive encephalopathy and nephrotic syndrome.

Several vasculitides may also result in nephrotic syndrome, usually associated with membrano-proliferative and crescentic glomerulonephritis and involvement of intracranial and extracranial cerebral vessels. These include systemic lupus erythematosus, Wegener granulomatosis, Goodpasture syndrome, polyarteritis nodosa, and Takayasu disease (Arita et al., 1998). Finally, noninflammatory vasculopathies may play a pathogenic role as in the patient with Sneddon syndrome, mesangial glomerulonephritis with segmental IgA deposition, and lacunar infarctions reported by Ohtani and collaborators (Ohtani et al., 1995).

Children

Cerebral infarction may also complicate the course of children with nephrotic syndrome. Thromboses may be either venous or arterial and occur anywhere from <2% (Egli, 1974) up to one-third of patients (Hoyer et al., 1986). In 1984, the International Study of Kidney Disease in Children studied the mortality of children with nephrotic syndrome and minimal change on renal biopsy (Report of the International Study of Kidney Disease, 1984). Of 389 patients with minimal changes on renal biopsy, ten patients died, one had cerebral venous thrombosis, and none had a cerebral infarction. Although these data stress the low frequency of these complications, it should be remembered that cerebrovascular events might be asymptomatic, overlooked, or not uncommonly misinterpreted.

Thrombi involving the large vessels have been found on autopsy in 20% of patients affected by the congenital nephrotic syndrome of the Finnish-type (Huttunen, 1976). In 1935, Schwarz and Kohn reported a 13-year-old boy with a fatal right central retinal artery infarction and left hemiparesis secondary to a thrombotic occlusion of the right internal carotid artery. Thrombosis of the MCA and ACA (Habib et al., 1968), parietal-occipital infarctions (Raghu et al., 1981), and basilar artery thrombosis (Sakiyama et al., 1979) have also been reported. Most of these patients died within weeks of cerebral infarction.

While some reports provide insufficient information to allow further analysis of stroke mechanisms (Calcagno & Rubin, 1961; Kanfer et al., 1970; Egli et al., 1974; Kendall et al., 1971; Andrassy et al., 1980), others, including the patient reported by Raghu, suggest hemodynamic rather than thromboembolic mechanisms.

Congenital nephrotic syndrome may also follow focal segmental glomerulosclerosis in association with dysmorphic features and systemic involvement (Ehrich et al., 1995). Ehrich described five patients with steroid-resistant nephrotic syndrome associated with spondyloepiphyseal dysplasia, growth failure and lymphopenia. They also had episodic neurologic deficits including ataxia, dysarthria, hemiparesis, and amaurosis fugax. The authors hypothesized that these transient ischemic attacks are secondary to a generalized vascular defect involving the glomerular capillaries and the cerebral arteries. However, in the absence of definitive ancillary studies to allow exclusion of other causes of cerebral ischemia in these children, a sensible conclusion is that stroke mechanisms remain undetermined among these patients.

Igarashi et al. (1988) reported two children with cerebral infarction, one with congenital nephrotic syndrome, and one with minimal change nephrotic syndrome. The first patient, born at 34 weeks gestational age, required 4 weeks of hospitalization in an intensive care setting due to respiratory distress syndrome. He had motor and language developmental delay. At 9 months of age, congenital nephrotic syndrome resistant to prednisone and cyclophosphamide was diagnosed on the basis of severe proteinuria, hypoalbuminemia, and focal glomerulosclerosis with mesangial proliferation on renal biopsy. At age 3, he had partial seizures with secondary generalization prompting phenytoin treatment. Six months later, he developed right hemiparesis, lethargy, and head tilt. Ancillary studies disclosed anemia, thrombocytosis, hypoalbuminemia of 1.5 g/dl, total proteinuria of 3.4g/dl, borderline low antithrombin-III levels of 22.5 (normal 24.8–30.0), and

multiple bilateral hypodensities on brain CT. His course was complicated by cerebral edema leading to death six days later. Autopsy showed multiple, bilateral hemispheric infarctions and thrombosis of the small cerebral arteries. The second patient, an 11-year-old boy with a 9-year history of nephrotic syndrome had dysarthria and bifrontal headaches that progressed to aphasia and right-sided hemiparesis. Laboratory data was remarkable for thrombocytosis of 658000/mm³, albumin of 1.7, and antithrombin-III levels of 58%. He received prednisone and warfarin until the nephrotic syndrome remitted, but was left with a moderate right-sided hemiparesis and aphasia requiring special education classes.

In summary, cerebral infarction in children appears to be at least as frequent as in adults, and may be associated with a poor prognosis. A hypercoagulable disorder may occur in both congenital and acquired causes of nephrotic syndrome.

Cerebral venous thrombosis
Cerebral venous thrombosis has been recognized as a complication of the nephrotic syndrome since very early descriptions. The superior sagittal sinus is most commonly involved. In a review of 38 patients with cerebral venous thrombosis (Bousser et al., 1985) nephrotic syndrome was found in only one patient. Table 25.3 summarizes reported cases of cerebral venous thrombosis in adults with nephrotic syndrome.

In 1980, Barthélémy and collaborators described the first case of dural sinus thrombosis complicating a nephrotic syndrome with minimal glomerular changes. The patient, a 50-year-old man, had a relapse of his nephrotic syndrome. He presented with generalized weakness, diffuse headaches, orthostatic hypotension, hypoalbuminemia and proteinuria. He received albumin infusions, high doses of corticosteroids, and intravenous fluids with rapid progression of proteinuria, but persistence of orthostatic hypotension and headaches. Examination was remarkable only for papilledema. A lumbar puncture showed normal opening pressure, with 1 white blood cell, 120 red blood cells, and normal protein and glucose concentration. Cerebral angiography showed filling defects in the posterior aspect of the superior longitudinal sinus and the right lateral sinus. He received intravenous heparin followed by oral anticoagulation with complete resolution of his symptoms within 15 days. Repeat angioscintigraphy showed patency of the lateral and superior sagittal sinuses.

Levine et al. (1987) described two patients with cerebral venous thrombosis associated with a circulating anticoagulant, one of whom had mesangial proliferative glomerulonephritis. This 32-year-old man initially developed ankle

Table 25.3. *Cerebral venous thrombosis in adults with nephrotic syndrome*

Age (Yrs.)/ Gender	Presentation	Site of venous occlusion	Hematologic abnormalities	Neurologic outcome	Reference
50/M	Headaches, papilledema	SSS and LS	N/A	Complete recovery	Barthelémy, 1980
32/M	Headaches, papilledema, L IV CN palsy	SSS and SS	Lupus anticoagulant	Complete recovery	Levine, 1987
46/M	Superior vena cava syndrome	LS	N/A	Complete recovery	Tovi, 1988
20/M	Personality change, seizures	SSS	↓ AT-III	Expired	Burns, 1995
35/M	Headaches, L III CN palsy	ISS	↑ Fibrinogen	Residual deficits	Burns, 1995
42/F	Headaches, seizures, hemiparesis	LS	↓ Protein-S	Complete recovery	Laversuch, 1995
41/F	Headaches, aphasia, hemiparesis	SSS	N/A	Complete recovery	Urch, 1996
?/M	Aphasia, headaches	SSS and LS	N/A	Complete recovery	Urch, 1996
65/F	Headaches, progressing hemiparesis	SSS	↓ AT-III	Complete recovery	Akatsu, 1997
45/F	Hemiparesis, hemisensory deficit	SSS	↓ Protein-S	Complete recovery	Sung, 1999

Notes:
SSS: superior sagittal sinus.
ISS: inferior sagittal sinus.
SS: straight sinus.
LS: lateral sinus.
AT-III: antithrombin-III.
SLE: systemic lupus erythematosus.
N/A: not available.

edema, reduced creatinine clearance, thrombocytopenia and proteinuria. A week later, he had left-sided headaches, lightheadedness, vomiting and ataxia, associated with mild periorbital edema, papilledema and a left IVth nerve palsy. Platelet count was $34\,000/\text{mm}^3$. Thrombin clotting time, bleeding time, factor VIII, antithrombin-III, fibrin degradation products, ANA, VDRL and complement studies were normal. Protein-C and protein-S were not determined. Non-contrast CT showed hyperdensity areas along the straight sinus, the torcular region and the posterior aspect of the superior sagittal sinus. Cerebral angiogram confirmed filling defects in the anterior and posterior portions of the superior sagittal sinus and in the transverse sinus. The patient received prednisone 50 mg a day and intravenous heparin with gradual resolution of his neurologic deficits. Even though this report did not exclude all of the possible abnormalities associated with thrombotic tendency and nephrotic syndrome, it suggests that determinations of antiphospholipid antibodies and lupus anticoagulant are important in cases complicated by cerebrovascular events.

Cerebral venous thrombosis may also be asymptomatic and only become noticeable when the thrombotic process progresses to occlude the superior vena cava (Tovi et al.,

1988). Tovi described a 46-year-old man who had progressive swelling of the cervical area and right arm. He had venous engorgement of the chest wall and an undefined mass under the right sternocleidomastoid muscle, along with a perforation of his right tympanic membrane and an edematous mucosa lining of the middle ear. Fibrinogen was elevated at 1000 mg/ml, urinalysis showed microhematuria with urine protein of 300 mg/ml. Cervical ultrasound suggested thrombosis of the right internal jugular vein. Venography of the right arm detected occlusion of the brachial, axillary, subclavian veins and superior vena cava. He received intravenous heparin. A week later, he developed high fever and purulent discharge from the right ear requiring intravenous antibiotics and surgery. His symptoms resolved completely within 2 months. This patient did not show the typical findings of septic lateral sinus thrombosis including fever, headache, or otalgia. It is likely that the presence of nephrotic syndrome increased susceptibility to infection and to a hypercoagulable state leading to the asymptomatic extension of the thrombus as described.

Burns and associates reported two adult patients and one teenager with minimal change nephrotic syndrome complicated by cerebral venous thrombosis. All had a prior history of nephrotic syndrome that relapsed despite corticosteroid treatment. The first patient had a superior sagittal sinus thrombosis complicated by hemorrhagic infarction leading to death; the second had an inferior sagittal sinus thrombosis resulting in residual aphasia and right hemiparesis, and the last patient had cortical vein thrombosis leading to transient left hemiparesis. Initial presentations included headache and personality changes, but diagnosis was suspected only after seizures and focal neurologic deficits. Magnetic resonance imaging and CT scan with contrast were used for the diagnosis. Extensive prothrombotic workup performed in all of these patients showed low antithrombin-III levels in one, raised fibrinogen levels in all of them, and elevated von Willebrand factor in the last patient. Treatment consisted of anticoagulation, albumin replacement, and corticosteroids (Burns et al., 1995).

Laversuch and collaborators (1995) reported a case of protein-S deficiency associated with the nephrotic syndrome in a 42-year-old woman with history of systemic lupus erythematosus and hypertension. She initially presented with pulmonary embolism requiring oral anticoagulation. At that time, the C-reactive protein was elevated and renal biopsy showed membranous glomerulonephritis with increased glomerular cellularity and a strong staining for IgG, IgM and C3. Coagulation studies were within normal limits and antiphospholipid antibodies were negative. Three weeks after the event, she was readmitted with right-sided headaches, confusion, generalized seizures and left hemiparesis. At that time, protein-S level was 17%, antithrombin-III level was normal, 24-hour urinary protein was 7.6 g, and serum albumin was 25 g/dl. Antiphospholipid antibodies IgG were 'minimally elevated'. MRI showed thrombosis of the right transverse sinus extending inferiorly to the internal jugular vein with a venous infarct in the right temporal lobe. She received intravenous anticoagulation followed by warfarin, pulse methylprednisolone and cyclophosphamide. An asymptomatic extension of venous thrombosis to the superior sagittal sinus and left transverse sinus was seen on follow-up MRI. She remained neurologically stable for the 18-month follow-up period reported. Renal involvement as in this patient, and the presence of a lupus anticoagulant have been associated with an increased risk of cerebral venous thrombosis in patients with systemic lupus erythematosus; also, at least one-third of the reported cases of cerebral venous thrombosis associated with lupus had nephrotic syndrome (Vidailhet et al., 1990; Li & Chan, 1990; Kaplan et al., 1985; Parnass et al., 1987). Levels of protein-S were not mentioned in these reports. Lloyd et al. (1993) found low protein-S levels in 37 out of 78 patients

with lupus and an antiphospholipid antibody in 31 of them; the eight patients with low levels of free protein-S and high antiphospholipid antibodies had significantly more thrombotic events. This suggests that patients with systemic lupus at increased risk of cerebral venous thrombosis also have renal disease, particularly the nephrotic syndrome, and may have associated antiphospholipid antibodies or lupus anticoagulant.

Relapsing minimal change glomerulonephropathy was also present in two cases of superior sagittal sinus thrombosis and lateral sinus thrombosis. Both patients had severe headaches for a few days followed by confusion, aphasia, and right-sided hemiparesis (Urch & Pusey, 1996). The second patient also had a mastoiditis which may have contributed to the development of intracranial venous thrombosis. Both patients received corticosteroids and anticoagulation achieving complete recovery within weeks. Other ancillary studies were not reported.

Akatsu and collaborators (1997) described a 65-year-old woman who presented with anasarca and severe right-sided headache, followed by a complex partial seizure. She was a heavy smoker and was receiving estrogen and medroxyprogesterone replacement. She had no personal or family history of hypercoagulability. Initial studies showed hypoalbuminemia of 2 g/dl, hypercholesterolemia of 540 mg/dl, sedimentation rate of 83 mm/h, proteinuria of 16.8 g/24h, and normal PT, aPTT and platelet count. Initial brain CT was normal, but a repeat study at 24 hours showed a right parietal hemorrhagic infarction. She deteriorated within hours, presenting with generalized tonic-clonic seizures, lethargy and moderate left hemiparesis. MRI and contrast angiography confirmed the diagnosis of superior sagittal sinus thrombosis. Coagulation studies showed decreased antithrombin-III levels of 33% of normal, normal protein-C and protein-S levels, and negative fibrin-split products. She received 2850 units of antithrombin-III (reaching a level of 163%, 30 minutes after infusion), warfarin and enoxaparin 30 mg bid. She also received an empiric trial of cyclosporine for presumed membranous glomerulonephritis or minimal change disease. However, cyclosporine resulted in worsening of renal function and had to be discontinued. Once the neurologic status was stable, warfarin was discontinued and a renal biopsy showed minimal change disease. This case illustrated the difficulties in managing these complications in patients with nephrotic syndrome, especially when a renal biopsy cannot be performed rapidly. The combination of low molecular weight heparin with warfarin and the use of cyclosporine to reduce proteinuria were done on an empiric basis and their use remains controversial.

Acquired deficiency of free protein-S has been described in two additional patients with cerebral venous thrombosis and nephrotic syndrome (Sung et al., 1999). The first patient had a 2-month history of hypoalbuminemia and hypertension and presented with left hemiparesis and left hemisensory deficits. MRI and magnetic resonance venography showed thrombosis of the superior sagittal sinus with establishment of collateral circulation. Protein-S level was 71% (normal 75–136%), ANA was 1:320 with negative anticardiolipin antibodies and otherwise normal coagulation studies. A renal biopsy showed chronic tubulo-interstitial nephritis that responded well to prednisolone and aspirin. The second patient, a 16-year-old man with a seven-month history of nephrotic syndrome developed headaches, vomiting and a single generalized seizure. Neurologic examination was normal. Magnetic resonance studies showed thrombosis of the superior sagittal sinus, straight sinus and both lateral sinuses. Functional protein-S activity was 51%, antithrombin-III level was 56% (normal 76–135%), and plasminogen level was 66% (normal 74–134%) with otherwise negative workup. He received intravenous heparin, antithrombin-III replacement, and methylprednisolone. His renal and neurologic status improved. Following a review of 38 patients with cerebral venous thrombosis in the same institution, these authors found an association with nephrotic syndrome in 5.3% of them.

Children

Lau et al. (1980a) described a 2 year-old boy with relapsing nephrotic syndrome, complicated by superior sagittal sinus thrombosis. He first developed irritability and incoordination, followed by partial seizures with generalization. Coagulation studies showed increased factor V and factor VIII levels and marked reduction in factor XII level at 1% (normal 60–200%). He received heparin initially but wide variations in the activated partial thromboplastin time (aPTT) were observed during therapy. The authors attributed these fluctuations to significant urinary heparin excretion, confirmed by prolongation of the thrombin time using patient's urine that was reversed by protamine. The patient recovered uneventfully.

Divekar and associates (1996) reported similar difficulties in achieving adequate anticoagulation with intravenous heparin. They first administered prednisone to a 3-year-old boy with nephrotic syndrome. A week later, the boy developed generalized seizures, following severe episodes of watery diarrhoea and acute weight loss of 700 g. His examination showed papilledema and bilateral Babinski signs. CT confirmed thromboses of the superior sagittal sinus, straight sinus, left lateral sinus, and a left temporo-parietal infarction. He received fresh frozen plasma to replenish antithrombin-III (levels not reported), and intravenous heparin, followed by warfarin. Elevations in aPTT and prothromtin time (PT) were not sustained during the course of treatment. These findings were attributed to heparin urinary losses and to a possible interaction of warfarin and phenobarbital.

Only one of 389 patients with minimal change nephrotic syndrome studied by the International Study of Kidney Disease died as a consequence of multiple dural venous sinus thromboses (Report of the International Study of Kidney Disease, 1984). He was 2 years of age, and had an early relapse of proteinuria. Negrier et al. (1991) emphasized the potential role of decreased fibrinolysis mediated by factor XII in his report of a 2-year-old patient presenting with seizures. CT was consistent with superior sagittal sinus and cortical vein thromboses. Factor XII activity was 5%, levels of factors IX and XI were mildly decreased at 50% (normal 60–140%), with other coagulation tests in the normal range. He received intravenous heparin, followed by dipyridamole and aspirin, but had a fatal pulmonary embolism.

Cerebral venous thrombosis may also complicate congenital nephrotic syndrome. It may present as congenital hydrocephalus (Parchoux et al., 1981) or as neonatal seizures (Fofah & Roth, 1997). Fofah described a female newborn who developed respiratory distress despite absence of meconium below the vocal cords and normal Apgar scores. She was stabilized but on the fifth day developed poor feeding and jerking movements of the arms with left eye deviation. Studies showed nephrotic range proteinuria, hypoalbuminemia, hypocalcemia, undetectable levels of 25-hydroxy-vitamin D, hyperfibrinogenemia, and decreased protein-C functional activity. Ultrasound showed mild ventriculomegaly. MRI showed extensive thromboses involving the straight sinus, transverse sinus, superior sagittal sinus, and multiple cortical veins, as well as a small parietal-occipital hemorrhage. She received calcium and vitamin D supplementation, but no information was available regarding therapy for cerebral venous thrombosis. She showed partial recovery.

Other cases are summarized in Table 25.4. Most involved the superior sagittal sinus, and less commonly the lateral sinus, and straight sinus (Pillekamp et al., 1997; Purvin et al., 1987; Egli et al., 1974).

Intracranial hemorrhage

Intracranial hemorrhage is not a direct complication of the nephrotic syndrome. When present, a clear cause such as thrombocytopenia (Leung et al., 1998) or coexistent intracranial aneurysms (Nagayasu et al., 1986) is implicated.

Table 25.4. *Cerebral venous thrombosis in children with nephrotic syndrome*

Age (Yrs.)/ Gender	Presentation	Site of venous occlusion	Hematologic abnormalities	Neurologic outcome	Reference
12/M	Headaches	SS	N/A	Complete recovery	Egli, 1974b
2½/M	Seizures, hemiparesis, femoral artery/vein thromboses	SSS	↓Factor XII, ↑ Factor V and Factor VIII, ↓ AT-III	Complete recovery	Lau, 1980a
4 months/M	Hydrocephalus	LS (bilateral)	N/A	Partial recovery	Parchoux, 1981
4/F	Headaches, papilledema	SSS	N/A	Partial recovery	Purvin, 1987
2/M	Seizures, vomiting	SSS, CV	↑ Factor XII	Expired	Negrier, 1991
3/M	Vomiting, papilledema	SSS	N/A	Complete recovery	Freycon, 1992
17/M	Headaches, seizures	CV	↑ vWF	Complete recovery	Burns, 1995
3/M	Seizures, papilledema	SSS, LS	↓ AT-III	Complete recovery	Divekar, 1996
Newborn/F	Seizures	SSS, SS, LS	↓ Protein-S ↓ Protein-C	Partial recovery	Fofah, 1997
5/M	Vomiting, headaches, seizures	SSS	↓ AT-III	Complete recovery	Pillekamp, 1997
16/M	Headaches, seizures	SSS and SS	↓ Protein-S, anticardiolipin antibodies	Partial recovery	Sung, 1999

Notes:
SSS: superior sagittal sinus.
SS: straight sinus.
LS: lateral sinus.
CV: cortical veins.
AT-III: antithrombin-III.
SLE: systemic lupus erythematosus.
vWF: von Willebrand Factor.
N/A: not available.

Management guidelines

Management of patients with nephrotic syndrome associated with stroke focuses on etiological treatment of the nephrotic syndrome when possible; maintenance of normovolemia, anticoagulation, potential administration of antithrombin-III concentrates or fresh frozen plasma, and management of hyperlipidemia and proteinuria.

Although the nephrotic syndrome carries a high risk of thrombotic complications, there are no current prospective, randomized trials evaluating the efficacy of prophylactic anticoagulation in these patients. Nephrologists have empirically used this strategy in patients with serum albumin <2 g, marked coagulation abnormalities or membranous glomerulonephritis on biopsy. Options included the Kakkar protocol using subcutaneous low-dose heparin (Kakkar, 1974) and oral anti-vitamin K. Using a Markov-based decision-analysis model considering the consequences of recurrent embolic and bleeding events, Sarasin and Schifferli (1994) analysed the risk

benefit of prophylactic anticoagulation before any thromboembolic event, or anticoagulation started after the first clinical thromboembolic event in patients with membranous nephropathy. The authors found that the overall number of fatal thromboemboli prevented by the prophylactic use of oral anticoagulant therapy exceeded the number of fatal bleeding events for all ranges of nephrotic syndrome duration. Rostoker et al. (1995) studied the use of enoxaparin in the prevention of thromboembolic events among 55 adult patients with nephrotic syndrome. Enoxaparin was given at a dose of 40 mg daily. No thrombotic episodes occurred during therapy, as evidenced by renal vein ultrasonography, Doppler ultrasonography of the lower extremities, and lung ventilation-perfusion scintigraphy. There were no documented side effects and patients found self-administration of enoxaparin once daily to be tolerable. Cost–benefit analysis also favoured enoxaparin over no treatment. Even though Markov analysis cannot replace the need for a prospective, randomized trial, it seems reasonable that until those studies are conducted, prophylactic anticoagulation either with warfarin or enoxaparin might reduce the frequency of thromboembolic events among high risk nephrotic patients. However, its routine use in all nephrotic patients cannot be recommended.

Once the diagnosis of thrombotic cerebral infarction or cerebral venous thrombosis has been made, anticoagulant therapy should be started. A short course of heparin followed by warfarin constitutes the therapy of choice. Oral anticoagulation with warfarin should probably be continued for as long as the patient remains nephrotic (O'Meara & Levine, 1999). The International Normalized Ratio (INR) must be carefully monitored in these patients, as warfarin kinetics is affected by the nephrotic syndrome, and dose adjustments may be necessary with changes in serum albumin levels. In addition, concomitant use of other drugs, such as anticonvulsants, may also affect the INR. Patients with marked abnormalities in the anticoagulant proteins or coagulation factors might also benefit from fresh frozen plasma and antithrombin-III concentrates. Evidence in favour of this intervention is anecdotal at best, and its use should be individualized. Thrombolytic agents have been used in cases of renal vein thrombosis, but not in nephrotic patients with stroke.

Measures directed to avoid volume depletion and correction of hyperlipidemia should be started early in the course of the nephrotic syndrome. Low cholesterol diets (<300 mg) should usually be complemented with pharmacologic therapy given the severity of hyperlipidemia in these patients. Numerous reports have established the benefit of HMG-CoA reductase inhibitors in reducing LDL cholesterol and lipoprotein (a) levels in patients with the nephrotic syndrome (O'Meara & Levine, 1999). Some evidence also suggests that antiproteinuric treatment with angiotensin converting enzyme inhibitors may be accompanied by improvement in lipid parameters (Keilani et al., 1993). An innovative alternative is LDL apheresis (Takegoshi et al., 1990). Along with these interventions, it is important to modify risk factors such as diabetes, smoking, and obesity.

Notwithstanding, the management of the nephrotic syndrome with stroke should always include consultation with a nephrologist to assist in the management of the underlying disorder and diagnostic dilemmas such as indication and timing of renal biopsy.

Conclusions

The nephrotic syndrome, particularly in association with idiopathic membranous nephropathy, carries a high risk of thrombotic complications. Although most thrombotic complications occur outside the CNS (deep venous thrombosis, renal vein thrombosis, and pulmonary embolism), neurologists should remain attentive to the ever-present danger of intracranial arterial and venous pathology in these patients. While no consensus exists about the need for prophylactic anticoagulation, current recommendations are that once a diagnosis of thrombotic cerebral infarction or cerebral venous thrombosis is established, anticoagulation is the therapy of choice.

References

Addis, T. (1948). *Glomerular Nephritis. Diagnosis and Treatment.* p. 216. New York:Macmillan.

Agrawal, B., Wolf, K., Berger, & Luft, F.C. (1996). Effect of antihypertensive treatment on qualitative estimates of microalbuminuria. *Journal of Human Hypertension*, **10**, 551–5.

Ahmed, K. & Saeed, E. (1995). Nephrotic syndrome and pulmonary artery thrombosis. *American Journal of Nephrology*, **15**, 274–6.

Akatsu, H., Vaysburd, M., Fervenza, F., Peterson, J. & Jacobs, M. (1997). Cerebral venous thrombosis in nephrotic syndrome. *Clinical Nephrology*, **48**, 317–20.

Andrassy, K., Ritz, E. & Bommer, J. (1980). Hypercoagulability in the nephrotic syndrome. *Klinikalische Wochenschrift*, **58**, 1029–36.

Arita, M., Iwane, M., Nakamura, Y. & Nishio, I. (1998). Anticoagulants in Takayasu's arteritis associated with crescentic glomerulonephritis and nephrotic syndrome: a case report. *Angiology*, **49**, 75–8.

Arneil, G.C. (1971). The nephrotic syndrome. *Pediatric Clinics of North America*, **18**, 547–59.

Barthélémy, M., Bousser, M.G. & Jacobs, C. (1980). Thrombose veineuse cérèbrale au cours d'un syndrome néphrotique. *La Nouvelle Presse Médicale*, **9**, 367–9.

Beamer, N.B., Coull, B.M., Clark, W.M. & Wynn, M. (1999). Microalbuminuria in ischemic stroke. *Archives of Neurology*, **56**, 699–702.

Bousser, M.G., Chiras, J., Bones, J. & Castaigne, P. (1985). Cerebral venous thrombosis – a review of 38 cases. *Stroke*, **16**, 199–213.

Burns, A., Wilson, E., Harbor, M., Brunton, C. & Sweeny, T. (1995). Cerebral venous sinus thrombosis in minimal change nephrotic syndrome. *Nephrology Dialysis and Transplantation*, **10**, 30–4.

Calcagno, P.I. & Rubin, M.I. (1961). Physiologic considerations concerning corticosteroid therapy and complications in the nephrotic syndrome. *Journal of Pediatrics*, **58**, 686–709.

Cameron, J.S. (1984). Coagulation and thromboembolic complications in the nephrotic syndrome. *Advances in Nephrology Necker Hospital*, **13**, 75–114.

Cerasola, G., Cottone, S., Mule, G. et al. (1996). Microalbuminuria, renal dysfunction and cardiovascular complication in essential hypertension. *Journal of Hypertension*, **14**, 915–20.

Chaturvedi, S. (1993). Fuiminant cerebral infarctions with membranous nephropathy. *Stroke*, **24**, 473–5.

Chin, W.W., Tosh, A.V., Hecht, S.R. & Burger, M. (1988). Left ventricular thrombus with normal left ventricular function in ulcerative colitis. *American Heart Journal*, **116**, 65–6.

Collins, M.N., Hawthorne, M.E., Gribbin, N. & Jacobson, R. (1990). Capgras' syndrome with organic disorders. *Postgraduate Medical Journal*, **66**, 1064–7.

de Gauna, R.R., Alcelay, L.G., Conesa, M.J. & Asarta, A.P. (1996). Thrombosis of the posterior inferior cerebellar artery secondary to nephrotic syndrome. *Nephron*, **72**, 123.

Divekar, A.A., Ali, U.S., Ronghe, M.D., Singh, A.R. & Dalvi, R.B. (1996). Superior sagittal sinus1thrombosis in a child with nephrotic syndrome. *Pediatric Nephrology*, **10**, 206–7.

Edelberg, J.M. & Pizzo, S.V. (1991). Lipoprotein(a) inhibits plasminogen activation in a template-dependent manner. *Blood Coagulation and Fibrinolysis*, **2**, 759–64.

Egli, F. (1974). Thromboembolien beim nephrotischen syndrom im kindesalter. University of Basel, 17–21. Thesis.

Egli, F., Elmiger, P. & Stalder, G. (1974). Thromboembolism in the nephrotic syndrome. *Pediatric Research*, **8**, 903–7.

Ehrich, J.H., Burchert, W., Schirg, E. et al. (1995). Steroid resistant nephrotic syndrome associated with spondyloepiphyseal dysplasia, transient ischemic attacks and lymphopenia. *Clinical Nephrology*, **43**, 89–95

Fofah, O. & Roth, P. (1997). Congenital nephrotic syndrome presenting with cerebral venous thrombosis, hypocalcemia, and seizures in the neonatal period. *Journal of Perinatology*, **17**, 492–4.

Freycon, M.T., Richard, O., Allard, D., Damon, G., Reynaud, J. & Freycon, F. (1992). Intracranial venous sinus thrombosis in nephrotic syndrome. *Pediatrie*, **47**, 513–6.

Fritz, C. & Braune, H.J. (1992). Cerebral infarction and nephrotic syndrome. *Stroke*, **23**, 1380–1.

Fuh, J.L., Teng, M.M., Yang, W.C. & Liu, H.C. (1992). Cerebral infarction in young men with nephrotic syndrome. *Stroke*, **23**, 295–7.

George, J.N., Nurden, A.T. & Phillips, D.R. (1984). Molecular defects in interactions of platelets with the vessel wall. *New England Journal of Medicine*, **311**, 1084.

Glassock, R.J. (1979). The nephrotic syndrome. *Hospital Practice*, **14**, 105–9, 115–18, 123–4.

Habib, R., Courtecuisse, V. & Bodaghi, E. (1968). Thrombose des arteres pulmonaires dans les syndromes nephrotiques de l'enfant. *Journal of Urology and Nephrology*, **74**, 349–62.

Hoyer, P.F., Gonda, S., Barthels, M., Krohn, H.P. & Brodehl, J. (1986). Thromboembolic complications in children with nephrotic syndrome: risk and incidence. *Acta Paediatrica Scandinavica*, **75**, 804–10.

Huang, T.Y. & Chau, K.M. (1995). Biventricular thrombi in diabetic nephrotic syndrome complicated by cerebral embolism. *International Journal of Cardiology*, **50**, 193–16.

Huttunen, N.P. (1976). Congenital nephrotic syndrome of Finnish type. Study of 75 patients. *Archives of Diseases in Children*, **51**, 344–8.

Igarashi, M., Roy, S.D. & Stapleton, E.B. (1988). Cerebrovascular complications in children with nephrotic syndrome. *Pediatric Neurology*, **4**, 362–5.

Izumi, M., Terao, S., Nakamori, T. et al. (1988). Cerebral infarction associated with nephrotic syndrome in a young adult: a case report. *No To Shinkei*, **50**(1), 119–24.

Jensen, T. (1991). Albuminuria – A marker of renal and generalized vascular disease in insulin-dependent diabetes mellitus. *Danish Medical Bulletin*, **38**, 134–44.

Joven, J., Villabona, C., Vilella, E., Masana, L., Alberti, R. & Vallés, M. (1990). Abnormalities of lipoprotein metabolism in patients with the nephrotic syndrome. *New England Journal of Medicine*, **323**, 579–84.

Kakkar, V. (1974). Low-dose heparin in the prevention of venous thromboembolism. In *Heparin: Structure, Function and Clinical Implications*, ed. R.A. Bradshaw & S. Wessler, pp. 323–40. New York: Plenum Press.

Kallen, R.J., Brynes, R.K., Aronson, A.J., Lichtig, C. & Spargo, H. (1977). Premature coronary atherosclerosis in a 5-year-old with corticosteroid-refractory nephrotic syndrome. *American Journal of Diseases in Children*, **131**, 976–80.

Kanfer, A., Kleinknecht, D., Broyer, M. & Josso, F. (1970). Coagulation studies in 45 cases of nephrotic syndrome without uremia. *Thrombosis et Diathesis Haemorrhagica*, **24**, 562–71.

Kaplan, R.E., Springate, J.E., Feld, L.G. & Cohen, M.E. (1985). Pseudotumor cerebri associated with cerebral venous thrombosis, internal jugular thrombosis and SLE. *Journal of Pediatrics*, **107**, 266–8.

Keilani, T., Schlueter, W.A. & Levine, M.L. (1993). Improvement of lipid abnormalities associated with proteinuria using fosinopril, an angiotensin-converting enzyme inhibitor. *Annals of Internal Medicine*, **118**, 246–51.

Kendall, A.G., Lohmann, R.C. & Dossetor, J.B. (1971). Nephrotic syndrome. A hypercoagulable state. *Archives of Internal Medicine*, **127**, 1021–7.

Kostner, K.M., Banyai, S., Banyai, M. et al. (1998). Urinary apolipoprotein (a) excretion in patients with proteinuria. *Annals of Medicine*, **30**, 497–502.

Kronenberg, F., Utermann, G. & Dieplinger, H. (1996). Lipoprotein(a) in renal disease. *American Journal of Kidney Diseases*, **27**, 1–25.

Lau, S.O., Bock, G.H., Edson, J.R. & Michael, A.F. (1980a). Sagittal sinus thrombosis in the nephrotic syndrome. *Journal of Pediatrics*, **97**, 948–50.

Lau, S.O., Tkachuk, J.Y., Hasegawa, D.K. & Edson, J.R. (1980b). Plasminogen and antithrombin III deficiencies in the childhood nephrotic syndrome associated with plasminogenuria and antithrombinuria. *Journal of Pediatrics*, **96**, 390–2.

Laversuch, C.J., Brown, M.M., Clifton, A. & Bourke, B.E. (1995). Cerebral venous thrombosis and acquired protein S deficiency: an uncommon cause of headache in systemic lupus erythematosus. *British Journal of Rheumatology*, **34**, 572–5.

Leno, C., Pascual, J., Polo, J.M. & Berciano, J. (1992). Nephrotic syndrome, accelerated atherosclerosis and stroke. *Stroke*, **23**, 921–2.

Leung, T.F., Tsoi, W.C., Li, C.K., Chik, K.W., Shing, M.M. & Yuen, P.M. (1998). A Chinese adolescent girl with Fechtner-like syndrome. *Acta Paediatrica*, **87**, 705–7.

Levine, S.R., Kieran, S., Puzio, K., Feit, H., Patel, S.C. & Welch, K.M.

(1987). Cerebral venous thrombosis with lupus anticoagulants. Report of two cases. *Stroke*, 1, 801–4.

Li, E.K. & Chan, M.S.Y. (1990). Is pseudotumor cerebri in SLE a thrombotic event? *Journal of Rheumatology*, 17, 983–4.

Llach, F. (1995). Hypercoagulability, renal vein thrombosis, and other thrombotic complications of nephrotic syndrome. *Kidney International*, 28, 429–39.

Lloyd, M.E., D'Cruz, D., McAlindon, A., Hunt, B. & Hughes, G.R.V. (1993). Free protein S levels in systemic lupus erythematosus. *Arthritis and Rheumatism*, 36, D247.

Luft, F.C. & Agrawal, B. (1999). Microalbuminuria as a predictive factor for cardiovascular events. *Journal of Cardiovascular Pharmacology*, 33 Suppl 1, S41–3.

Lydakis, C. & Lip, G.Y. (1998). Microalbuminuria and cardiovascular risk. *Quarterly Journal of Medicine*, 91, 381–91.

Malyszko, J., Malyszko, J.S., Pawlak, D. et al. (1996). Comprehensive study on platelet function, hemostasis, fibrinolysis, peripheral serotoninergic system and serum lipids in nephrotic syndrome. *Polish Journal of Pharmacology*, 48, 191–5.

Marsh, E.E., Biller, J., Adams, H.P., Jr & Kaplan, J.M. (1991). Cerebral infarction in patients with nephrotic syndrome. *Stroke*, 22, 90–3.

Miller, R.B., Harrington, J.T., Ramos, C.P., Relman, A.S. & Schwartz, W.B. (1969). Long-term results of steroid therapy in adults with idiopathic nephrotic syndrome. *American Journal of Medicine*, 46, 919–29.

Mogensen, C.E. & Christianson, C.K. (1994). Predicting diabetic nephropathy in insulin-dependent patients. *New England Journal of Medicine*, 311, 89–93.

Nagasayu, S., Hanakita, J., Miyake, H., Suzuki, T. & Nishi, S. (1986). A case of systemic lupus erythematosus associated with multiple intracranial aneurysms. *No Shinkei Geka*, 14, 1251–5.

Negrier, C., Delmas, M.C., Ranchin, B., Cochat, P. & Dechavanne, M. (1991). Decreased factor XII activity in a child with nephrotic syndrome and thromboembolic complications. *Thrombosis and Haemostasis*, 66, 512–13.

Ohtani, H., Imai, H., Yasuda, T. et al. (1995). A combination of livedo racemosa, occlusion of cerebral blood vessels, and nephropathy: kidney involvement in Sneddon's syndrome. *American Journal of Kidney Diseases*, 26, 511–15.

Olson, J.L. & Schwartz, M. (1998). The nephrotic syndrome: minimal change disease, focal segmental glomerulosclerosis, and miscellaneous causes. In *Heptinstall's Pathology of the Kidney*, 5th edn, ed. C. Jenette, J. Olson, M. Schwartz & F. Silva, pp. 196–99. Boston: Lippincott-Raven.

O'Meara, Y.M. & Levine, J.S. (1999). Management of complications of nephrotic syndrome. In *Therapy in Nephrology and Hypertension*, ed. H.R. Brady & C.S. Wilcox, p. 221. Philadelphia: WB Saunders.

Parag, K.B., Somers, S.R., Seedat, Y.K., Byrne, S., Da Cruz, C.M. & Kenoyer, G. (1990). Arterial thrombosis in nephrotic syndrome. *American Journal of Kidney Diseases*, 15, 176–7.

Parchoux, B., Cotton, J.B., Langue, J., Guibaud, P. & Labre, F. (1981). Syndrome nephrotique congenital: Thrombose d'une veine renale et hydrocephalie. *Pediatrie*, 34, 55–9.

Parnass, S.M., Goodwin, J.A., Patel, D.V., Levinson, D.J. & Reinhard, J. (1987). Dural sinus thrombosis: a mechanism of pseudotumor cerebri in systemic lupus erythematosus. *Journal of Rheumatology*, 41, 152–5.

Peng, D.Q., Zhao, S.P. & Wang, J.L. (1999). Lipoprotein(a) and apolipoprotein E epsilon 4 as independent risk factors for ischemic stroke. *Journal of Cardiovascular Risk*, 6, 1–6.

Petaja, J., Jalanko, H., Holmberg, C., Kinnunen, S. & Syrjala, M. (1995). Resistance to activated protein C as an underlying cause of recurrent venous thrombosis during relapsing nephrotic syndrome. *Journal of Pediatrics*, 127, 103–5.

Pillekamp, F., Hoppe, B., Roth, B. & Querfeld, U. (1997). Vomiting, headache and seizures with idiopathic nephrotic syndrome. *Nephrology Dialysis and Transplantation*, 12, 1280–1.

Purvin, V., Dunn, D.W. & Edwards, M. (1987). MRI and cerebral venous thrombosis. *Computerized Radiology*, 11, 75–9.

Raghu, K., Malik, A.K., Datta, B.N., Narang, A. & Mehta, S. (1981). Focal glomerulosclerosis with cerebral infarction in a young nephrotic patient. *Indian Pediatrics*, 18, 754–6.

Redon, J. (1998). Ambulatory blood pressure and the kidney. *Blood Pressure Monitoring*, 3, 157–61.

Report of the International Study of Kidney Disease in Children. (1984). Minimal change nephrotic syndrome in children: deaths during the first 5 to 15 years' observation. *Pediatrics*, 73, 497–501.

Richman, A.V. & Kasnic, G. Jr. (1982). Endothelial and platelet reactions in the idiopathic nephrotic syndrome: an ultrastructural study. *Human Pathology*, 13, 548–53.

Rostoker, G., Durand-Zaleski, I., Petit-Phar, M. et al. (1995). Prevention of thrombotic complications of the nephrotic syndrome by the low-molecular-weight heparin enoxaparin. *Nephron*, 69, 20–8.

Sakiyama, T., Suzuki, H., Nishiya, O., Mashiko, N., Kikkawa, Y. & Sato, K. (1979). A case with nephrotic syndrome associated with hypoplasia of thymus. Cerebral thrombosis during corticosteroid therapy. *Nippon Jinzo Gakkai Shi*, 9, 837–47.

Sarasin, F.B. & Schifferli, J.A. (1994). Prophylactic oral anticoagulation in nephrotic patients with idiopathic membranous nephropathy. *Kidney International*, 45, 578–85.

Sawicki, P.T., Mulhauser, I., Didjurgeit, U., Reimann, M., Bender, R. & Verger, M. (1995). Mortality and morbidity in treated type II hypertensive diabetic patients with micro or macroproteinuria. *Diabetic Medicine*, 12, 893–8.

Schnaper, H.W. & Robson, A.M. (1996). Nephrotic syndrome: Minimal change disease, focal glomerulosclerosis, and related disorders. In *Diseases of the Kidney*, 6th edn, ed. R. Schrier & C. Gottschalk, pp. 1747–9. Boston: Little, Brown & Co.

Schwarz, H. & Kohn, J.L. (1935). Lipoid nephrosis: clinical and pathologic study on 15 years' observation with special reference to prognosis. *American Journal of Diseases in Children*, 49, 579–93.

Song, K.S., Won, D.I., Lee, A.N., Kim, C.H. & Kim, J.S. (1994). A case of nephrotic syndrome associated with protein-S deficiency and cerebral thrombosis. *Journal of Korean Medical Science*, 9, 347–50.

Standl, E. & Stiegler, H. (1993). Microalbuminuria in a random cohort of recently diagnosed type II diabetic patients in the greater Munich area. *Diabetologia*, 36, 1017–20.

Sung, S.F., Jeng, J.S., Yip, P.K. & Huang, K.M. (1999). Cerebral venous thrombosis in patients with nephrotic syndrome – case reports. *Angiology*, **50**, 427–32.

Takegoshi, T., Haba, T., Hirai, J., Saga, T., Kito, H.C. & Mabuchi, H. (1990). A case of hyperlipidaemia, associated with systemic lupus erythematosus, suffering from myocardial infarction and cerebral infarction. *Japanese Journal of Medicine*, **29**, 77–84.

Tovi, F., Hirsch, M. & Gatot, A. (1988). Superior vena cava syndrome: presenting symptom of silent otitis media. *Journal of Laryngology and Otology*, **102**, 623–5.

Urch, C. & Pusey, C.D. (1996). Sagittal sinus thrombosis in adult minimal change nephrotic syndrome. *Clinical Nephrology*, **45**, 131–2.

Verges, B.L., Lagrost, L., Vaillant, G., et al. (1997). Macrovascular diseases associated with increased plasma apolipoprotein A-IV levels in NIDDM. *Diabetes*, **46**, 125–32.

Vidailhet, M., Piette, J-C., Wechsler, B., Bousser, M. & Brunet, P. (1990). Cerebral venous thrombosis in systemic lupus erythematosus. *Stroke*, **21**, 1226–31.

Visona, A., Lusiani, L., Bonanome, A. et al. (1995). Wall thickening of common carotid arteries in patients affected by noninsulin-dependent diabetes mellitus: relationship to microvascular complications. *Angiology*, **46**, 793–9.

Wheeler, D.C. & Bernard, D.B. (1994). Lipid abnormalities in the nephrotic syndrome: causes, consequences, and treatment. *American Journal of Kidney Diseases*, **23**, 331–46.

26

Kawasaki syndrome

Serge Blecic[1] and Julien Bogousslavsky[2]

[1]Service de Neurologie, Hôpital Erasme, Brussels, Belgium
[2]Department of Neurology, University of Lausanne, Switzerland

Introduction

'The muco-cutaneous lymph node syndrome' was first described by Kawasaki in 1967, and has been presented as an acute febrile exanthematous disease. The first report by Kawasaki and colleagues described the medical evolution of several Japanese children, who presented a syndrome associating fever and maculo papular skin involvement. Indeed, other reports found in a more recent literature confirmed Kawasaki syndrome has been found mainly in children and more rarely young adults (Kawasaki, 1967; Fujiwara et al., 1992; Hoshino et al., 1995). The characteristic of the disease is an involvement of skin and all mucous membranes (Kawasaki, 1967). The course of the disease follows always the same pattern. Practically all patients had fever at onset, followed within the first three days by a squamous skin, generalized erythema with sometimes peeling exanthema, conjunctivitis and generalized lymph nodes, all the signs mimicking those encountered in scarlet fever (Kawasaki, 1967). The skin of the trunk is more frequently affected than other areas. Following these symptoms, systemic generalization can occur, essentially due to a multiple artery involvement. Most patients have spontaneous lesion regression but some of them can suffer stroke, subarachnoid hemorrhage or myocardial infarction. The etiologic basis of this disease remains still unknown and consequently the treatment has not been established yet.

Clinical manifestations

Kawasaki syndrome is exclusively encountered in children and young adults (Kawasaki, 1967; Fujiwara et al., 1992; Hoshino et al., 1995). However, roughly 1.5 to 2% of the patients will develop within the month vascular involvement, which could be due to either coronary or Willis circle aneurysms leading to severe and even lethal complications. The most frequent complications previously described are myocardial infarctions. They are attributed to progressive occlusion of coronary arteries. The mechanism by which stroke can appear is twofold. It can be the consequence of middle- or small-sized cerebral artery thrombosis, or of single or multiple emboli, arising from a cardiac source, due, in most of the cases previously described, to cardiac akinesia following myocardial infarction, or of transient episodes of atrial fibrillation, also the consequence of a recent myocardial infarction. Asymptomatic cerebral infarction have also been reported either in patients with skin and mucous membrane involvement only or in patients with cardiac dysfunction due to coronary artery occlusion.

Neurological signs include mental dysfunction, motor and/or sensory deficits, ophthalmoplegia and cranial nerve dysfunction. The neurologic abnormalities result from multifocal infarctions or hemorrhages located in any part of the CNS (Hoshino et al., 1995)

Pathology and etiology

Kawasaki disease can affect all organs since it has been regarded as a pan-arteritis with involvement of medium- and small-sized arteries. Large artery involvement is exceptional since only one author reported a case of carotid involvement (Lauret, 1979). The mechanism of the disease remains unknown.

Kawasaki disease has been classified as a proliferative vasculopathy, and the lesions are characterized by intimal proliferation in the absence of an inflammatory reaction. Angiitis of coronary arteries is the most frequent finding, but cerebral arteries can also be affected. Pathologically, involvement of both artery intima and media are encountered (Roesplung et al., 1984; Yonesaka et al., 1992)

Early lesions consist of intima cellular proliferation accompanied by a slight edema without evidence for immune complex deposition. The second stage is marked by aneurysmal formation due to rupture of both intima and media layers. The third stage is an occlusive endarteriolopathy, favoured in the late stages by increase in platelet aggregation and adhesiveness. The late lesions consist of an acellular intimal sclerosis with hyalinization and narrowing or obliteration of the vascular lumen. Mild inflammation can sometimes be found in the early stages. Pathological examination of eye and mouth mucous membrane or of skin lesion did not provide evidence of either of viral inclusion or bacterial presence. An autoimmune mechanism has been advocated but the lack of increase in antibody level and the absence of lymphocytic infiltration do not support this hypothesis (Kawasaki, 1967; Marcella, 1983; Laxer et al., 1984; Fujiwara et al., 1992; Ferro, 1998).

Treatment

No treatment is known to be successful, since until now no diagnostic clue has been proposed. As an increase in platelet aggregation and adhesiveness have been suggested to be the cause of secondary occlusions, one can assume antiplatelet therapy could be useful. However, reports concerning the use of antiplatelet therapy are inconsistent and, moreover, the use of that kind of medication should be carefully proposed regarding the risk of brain hemorrhage, since one of the major mechanism of the disease is aneurysm development (Lapointe et al., 1984).

References

Ferro, J.M. (1998). Vasculitis of the central nervous system. *Journal of Neurology*, **245**(12), 766–76.

Fujiwara, S., Yamano, T., Hattori, M., Fujiseki, Y. & Shimada, M. (1992). Asymptomatic cerebral infarction in Kawasaki disease. *Pediatric Neurology*, **8**(3), 253–6.

Hoshino, K., Morroka, K., Imai, H., Takagi, K., Arimoto, K. & Saji, T. (1995). Neurological involvements with transient gait disturbance in subacute phase of Kawasaki disease: a case report. *No To Hattatsu*, **27**(4), 315–19.

Kawasaki, T. (1967). Mucocutaneous lymph node syndrome. Clinical observation of 50 cases. *Japan Journal of Allergy*, **16**, 178–222.

Lapointe, J.S., Nugent, R.A., Graeb, D.A. & Robertson, W.D. (1984). Cerebral infarction and regression of widespread aneurysms in Kawasaki's disease: case report. **14**(1), 1–5.

Lauret, P. (1979). Kawasaki disease complicated by thrombosis of the internal carotid artery. *Annals of Dermatology and Venereology*, **106**(11), 901–5.

Laxer, R.M., Dunn, H.G. & Fiedmark, O. (1984). Acute hemiplegia in Kawasaki disease and infantile polyarteritis nodosa. *Developmental Medicine and Child Neurology*, **26**(6), 814–18.

Marcella, J.J. (1983). Kawasaki syndrome in an adult: endomyocardial histology and ventricular function during acute and recovery phases of illness. *Journal of the American College of Cardiology*, **2**(2), 374–8.

Roesplung, O., Tardieu, M., Losay, J. & Leroy, D. (1984). Hémiplégie aigue compliquant une maladie de Kawasaki. *Revue Neurologie*, **140**(8–9), 507–9.

Yonesaka, S., Takahashi, T., Matubara, T. et al. (1992). Histopathological study on Kawasaki disease with special reference to the relation between the myocardial sequelae and regional wall motion abnormalities of the left ventricule. *Japan Circulation Journal*, **56**(4), 352–8.

27

Epidermal nevus syndrome

Bhuwan P. Garg

Department of Neurology, Indiana University, Indianapolis, IN, USA

Epidermal nevus

Nevus is a hamartoma or malformation of skin in its broadest sense. An epidermal nevus is a benign hamartoma of the epidermis that may often involve the papillary dermis. Epidermal nevi arise primarily from the embryonic ectoderm though mesoderm may also be involved (Rogers et al., 1996). The nevi are usually present at birth. Rogers et al. (1989) reported that 60% of the nevi were present at birth, 81% by 1 year, and 96% were evident by 7 years of age. Nevus size may enlarge with age in proportion to, or in excess of, body growth. Disproportionate extension of nevi with age is rare when the nevus is present on the head and neck. Also, nevi present at birth enlarge much less often irrespective of their location. There is no racial or gender predilection and the nevi occur with equal frequency in males and females. Although most epidermal nevi are sporadic, autosomal dominant transmission has been described (Meschia et al., 1992; Rogers et al., 1996).

Solomon et al. (1968) and Solomon and Esterly (1975) used the term epidermal nevus in a generic sense to encompass lesions such as nevus verrucosus, epithelial nevi, systematized nevi, linear nevus comedonicus, acanthosis nigricans, ichthyosis hystrix, ichthyosis cornea, ichthyosis linearis neuropathica, linear sebaceous nevus, nevus sebaceous of Jadassohn, and nevus unius lateris. Nevus verrucosus is often a solitary lesion, grey to yellow-brown in colour and velvety, granular, warty, or papillomatous in appearance. Nevus unius lateris is a single linear or spiral lesion, limited to one side of the body. This lesion may be in a continuous or interrupted pattern and may affect multiple sites. The nevus follows the long axis on the extremities and is in groups or spiral streaks when present on the trunk. The term systematized epidermal nevus is used when this lesion is present on large parts of the body and is called ichthyosis hystrix when the histology

of the lesion shows epidermolytic hyperkeratosis (Hurwitz, 1983). The most common clinical variant of epidermal nevi is nevus unius lateris occurring frequently as a unilateral linear verrucous lesion. Next in frequency are whorled ichthyosis hystrix, acanthosis nigricans, and linear sebaceous nevi. Almost one-third of patients may have a combination of these nevi (Solomon & Esterly, 1975; Hurwitz, 1983). Hyperplasia of both epidermis and dermis is present in all types of epidermal nevi, while involvement of skin appendages may vary. The nevus may be composed primarily of keratinocytes, hair follicle elements, sweat glands, or sebaceous glands. Skin biopsy may show a variety of histologic patterns in a given patient, although most often one pattern predominates. Interaction of the dermis with epidermis and the role of dermal induction in epidermal nevi is not understood though the nevus tends to recur if only the epidermal component is removed (Solomon & Esterly, 1975).

Epidermal nevus syndrome

Epidermal nevus syndrome refers to the association of any epidermal nevus with extracutaneous abnormalities. The most common extracutaneous abnormalities are neurologic, skeletal, and ocular, although other organs may also be involved. In general, head and neck nevi are associated with neurologic abnormality and skeletal abnormalities are seen more commonly when nevi are present on the trunk or limbs (Solomon & Esterly, 1975; Grebe et al., 1993). This association of an epidermal nevus with nervous system abnormalities constitutes the neurologic type of epidermal nevus syndrome. A wide variety of abnormalities have been described in the neurologic type of epidermal nevus syndrome. These include mental retardation, early onset seizures including infantile spasms, hemiparesis, cerebral vascular abnormalities, cranial nerve disorders, especially involving the VI, VII, and VIII nerves, hemimegalencephaly, cerebral gyral malformations, and epilepsy (Solomon & Esterly, 1975).

Skeletal abnormalities may be seen in 60–70% of patients with epidermal nevus syndrome. These are most often associated with nevi on the trunk and limbs and include vertebral anomalies, kyphosis, scoliosis, short limbs, syndactyly, and other bony deformities, as well as hemihypertrophy, bone cysts, and spina bifida. Kyphoscoliosis is the most common abnormality, often becoming manifest in adolescence. Other limb deformities besides syndactyly include genu valgum, equinovarus, and bone hypoplasia. Vitamin D-resistant rickets has also been reported (Aschinberg et al., 1977; Besser, 1976; Golitz & Weston, 1979; Marden & Venters, 1966; Mollica et al., 1974; Paller, 1987; Rogers et al., 1989; Solomon & Esterly, 1975; Sugarman & Reed, 1969).

Up to one half of the patients with epidermal nevus syndrome have ocular abnormalities such as microophthalmia, macroophthalmia, coloboma of the lid, iris, and retina, and conjunctival lipodermoids. Nystagmus and congenital blindness have been described (Alfonso et al., 1987; Brodsky et al., 1997; Diven et al., 1987). Cardiac and vascular abnormalities including ventricular septal defect, coarctation of aorta, patent ductus arteriosus, aneurysms, and arterio-venous malformations have been reported (Eichler et al. 1989; Grebe et al., 1993; Rogers et al., 1989).

Other cutaneous abnormalities also may be seen in patients with epidermal nevus syndrome and include café-au-lait spots, congenital hypopigmented macules, capillary hemangiomas, and melanocytic nevi (Eichler et al., 1989; Rogers et al., 1989; Solomon & Esterly, 1975). Happle (1987) has proposed that mosaicism may explain the varied cutaneous manifestations. The observation that most epidermal nevi follow the lines of Blaschko, which probably represent migration tracks of clones of genetically identical cells, is in favour of this hypothesis.

Nevus sebaceous

Of the epidermal nevi, nevus sebaceous described by Jadassohn in 1895 is probably the most common nevus associated with the neurologic type of epidermal nevus syndrome (Holden & Dekaban, 1972). The sebaceous nevus is often present on the face and scalp. It reportedly occurs in 0.3% of births (Wagner & Hansen, 1995) although Solomon and Esterly's (1975) estimate of the overall incidence of epidermal nevi at 1:1000 live births is probably more accurate. The nevus sebaceous (sometimes called

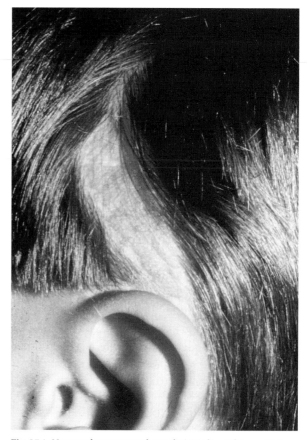

Fig. 27.1. Nevus sebaceous on the scalp just above the ear. Note alopecia in the area of the nevus. (Photograph courtesy of Patricia Treadwell MD, Department of Dermatology, Indiana University School of Medicine, Indianapolis, Indiana.)

the linear sebaceous nevus) occurs sporadically with no racial, or gender predilection. Familial occurrence is rare (Benedetto et al., 1990; Sahl, 1990). Nevus sebaceous is usually congenital; rarely late appearance in childhood has been reported. Rogers (1992) reviewed 233 cases of epidermal nevi and found 104 cases of nevus sebaceous. In 103 of these 104 cases of nevus sebaceous the lesion was noted at birth, and in 102 of them the nevus involved the head. The nevus was on the scalp in 58 instances, on the face in 38, and ear in one case. The nevus itself is most often isolated, slightly raised and yellowish orange, with a waxy appearance of the skin. The nevus is often linear or oval in shape. There is alopecia when the lesion is in the scalp (Fig. 27.1). The nevus evolves with age and three stages may be recognized (Lantis et al., 1968; Mehregan & Pinkus, 1965). In the first stage in infancy the lesion is characterized by a localized yellowish–orange patch of alopecia. The surface of the skin is most often smooth but may be rough, depressed, or verrucous. At this stage histological examination shows multiple small underdeveloped sebaceous glands and immature hair follicles; apocrine glands are rare. By puberty (second stage) the sebaceous glands mature and become hyperplastic. Androgenic stimulation may have a role in this enlargement. The hair follicles continue to remain immature and rudimentary while apocrine glands (usually present in axilla, and groin, and a few on the breast and eyelids but seen in almost half of the sebaceous nevi) begin to mature and occasionally may be cystic or hyperplastic. The third stage is characterized by onset of neoplastic transformation in puberty or adulthood. Benign or malignant tumours may arise in 10–31% of nevi. Nodular non-aggressive type of basal cell epithelioma or syringocystadenoma papilliferum are most common. Other tumour types include squamous cell carcinoma, apocrine carcinoma, adnexal carcinoma, syringoma, keratocanthoma, apocrine cystadenoma, and osteoma. Metastatic spread usually does not occur in the pediatric age group but rarely may be seen in adults. Neoplasms probably develop more often in sebaceous nevus than in other epidermal nevi. Local excision of the nevus before puberty is therefore recommended (Hurwitz, 1983; Mostafa & Satti, 1991; Rogers et al., 1996; Solomon & Esterly, 1975).

Neurologic abnormalities

Epidermal nevus syndrome characterized by the presence of an epidermal nevus and malformation in at least one extracutaneous organ system was found in 65% of 300 patients with epidermal nevus. In this study by Solomon, one-third of the patients with the epidermal nevus syndrome had CNS involvement (Micali et al., 1995). In another study 40% of patients with epidermal nevus syndrome had neurologic involvement. The most common neurologic abnormality in this study was epilepsy, present in 33.3%, followed by mental retardation of varying severity in 30.8% of patients (Holden & Dekaban, 1972). Others have found a much higher incidence of nervous system involvement (Baker et al., 1987; Barth et al., 1977; Clancy et al., 1985; Eichler et al., 1989; Solomon & Esterly, 1975; Zaremba, 1978). Baker and colleagues (1987) found that cerebral hemiatrophy and hemimegalencephaly were present in 7% each, while gyral malformation was seen in 3% of patients. Gurecki et al., (1996) studied 23 patients with epidermal nevus syndrome, who had biopsy proven epidermal nevus and adequate data on neurologic and anatomical studies. Seizures were present in 50% of patients and mental retardation in 50% of patients for whom information was available. Only 9 of the 19 patients for whom data were available had normal cognition in this study. Five of the 23 patients had hemiparesis, 9 cranial nerve abnormalities, 6 patients each hemiatrophy and vascular anomalies, and 5 patients each had hemimegalencephaly and gyral abnormalities. Widespread use of MRI has resulted in an increasing appreciation of the role of cortical malformations in patients with neurological symptoms. Studies prior to the general availability of MRI probably underestimated the prevalence of gyral and other cortical malformations in the neurologic type of epidermal nevus syndrome.

We reviewed data on 63 patients with epidermal nevus syndrome with severe neurologic abnormalities (Pavone et al., 1991). From this group, 17 patients in whom adequate data were available and who had hemimegalencephaly were studied further. Nevus was ipsilateral to the hemimegalencephaly in all. Macrocephaly was present in four and microcephaly in one patient. Mental retardation and seizures of various types were common. Morphological and microscopic studies revealed pachygyria, polymicrogyria, irregularly thickened cortex, heterotopic nodules in the white matter, giant neurons and giant astrocytes, and areas of astrocytic proliferation. Sakuta et al., (1989, 1991) reported clinical and neuropathologic findings in a 5-year-old boy. In addition to the hemimegalencephaly and increased white matter volume, there was cerebral polymicrogyria with pachygyria, heterotopic neurons, and prominent astrogliosis. Hypertrophic neurons with increased dendrites and spines were seen on Golgi staining. Hemimegalencephaly limited to the temporal lobe has also been described (Kwa et al., 1995). This clinical syndrome may be called the hemimegalencephalic variant of the neurologic type of epidermal nevus syndrome.

Vascular abnormalities

Strokes and vascular abnormalities have been reported in patients with epidermal nevus syndrome. We (Dobyns & Garg, 1991) reported one patient in whom cranial CT showed an infarct in the distribution of the right middle cerebral artery. There was ipsilateral atrophy and ventriculomegaly. We reviewed data on our patient and on three additional patients in whom the neurologic manifestations were due to vascular abnormalities. Two of the four patients had a clinically recognizable stroke. In the other two patients cerebral angiogram revealed vascular dysplasia. In all four patients the facial or scalp epidermal nevus was ipsilateral to the vascular and brain abnormalities. The neurologic abnormalities could best be explained on the basis of either hemorrhage or ischemia of the underlying brain.

Arteriovenous malformation and leptomeningeal angioma have been found in some patients with the epidermal nevus syndrome (Mollica et al., 1974; Solomon & Esterly, 1975). Patients with absent dural sinuses and with dysplastic and partially thrombosed left carotid artery and branches have been reported. Coarctation of aorta has been found in some patients. Vascular abnormalities may also be the underlying mechanism in some patients with epidermal nevus syndrome reported to have cerebral atrophy, hypoplasia or hemiatrophy although adequate information is often lacking.

We believe that an underlying vascular dysplasia may be the cause of neurologic abnormalities in patients with the neurologic type of epidermal nevus syndrome who do not have the hemimegalencephalic variant. Others have disputed this hypothesis, though there are no documented reports implicating other mechanisms. Differences in the extent and location of the vascular dysplasia (which may predispose to occlusion, ischemia, and infarcts ipsilateral to the nevus) may be an adequate explanation for the wide variety of neurologic manifestation seen in these patients (Dobyns & Garg, 1991).

Clinical investigations

Generally, the diagnosis of an epidermal nevus is not in doubt. If there are any doubts, a skin biopsy should be obtained. The biopsy may also help in further characterizing the nevus type although as mentioned earlier there is considerable variability in the histologic patterns. In all children who have an epidermal nevus, a thorough physical examination must be carried out to discover any associated abnormality in other organ systems. The organs most commonly involved are the central nervous system, eyes, and the skeletal system, though others may also be involved. In children with involvement of the nervous system an imaging study such as CT or MRI should be considered. MRI is usually the study of choice. Cerebral angiographic evaluation may be necessary in selected cases. Neuropsychiatric testing may be helpful in the management of children with mental retardation or learning disabilities.

Genetics

Epidermal nevus syndrome, sometimes also referred to as the Schimmelpenning–Feuerstein–Mims syndrome, is a sporadic condition. Autosomal dominant cases have been described (Meschia et al., 1992; Sahl, 1990). It should be dis-

tinguished from other phacomatoses, Proteus syndrome, and encephalocraniocutaneous lipomatosis. Parents should be counselled accordingly. Treatment of the nevus with dermabrasion, diathermy, laser treatment, and cryotherapy is associated with a fairly high risk of recurrence of the nevus. Focal resection of the epidermal nevus before puberty is advised because of the increased risk of tumour development. Resection must be complete as the nevus tends to recur if only the epidermal component is removed.

References

Alfonso, I., Howard, C., Lopez, P., Palomino, J. & Gonzalez, C. (1987). Linear nevus sebaceous syndrome: a review. *Journal of Clinical Neuro-ophthalmology*, **7**, 170–7.

Aschinberg, L., Solomon, L., Zeis, P., Justice, P. & Rosenthal, I. (1977). Vitamin D-resistent rickets associated with epidermal nevus syndrome: demonstration of a phosphaturic substance in the dermal lesions. *Journal of Pediatrics*, **91**, 56–60.

Baker, R., Ross, P. & Baumann, R. (1987). Neurologic complications of the epidermal nevus syndrome. *Archives of Neurology*, **44**, 227–32.

Barth, P., Valk, J., Kalsbeck, G. & Blom, A. (1977). Organoid nevus syndrome (linear nevus sebaceus of Jadassohn): clinical and radiological study of a case. *Neuropädiatrie*, **8**, 418–28.

Benedetto, L. (1990). Familial nevus sebaceus. *Journal of the American Academy of Dermatology*, **23**, 130–2.

Besser, F. (1976). Linear sebaceous nevi with convulsions and mental retardation (Feuerstein-Mims' Syndrome), vitamin-D-resistent rickets. *Proceedings of the Royal Society of Medicine*, **69**, 518–20.

Brodsky, M., Kincannon, J., Nelson-Adesokan, P. & Brown, H. (1997). Oculocerebral dysgenesis in the linear nevus sebacous syndrome. *Ophthalmology*, **104**, 497–503.

Clancy, R., Kurtz, M., Baker, D., Sladky, J., Honig, P. & Younkin, D. (1985). Neurologic manifestations of the organoid nevus syndrome. *Archives of Neurology*, **42**, 236–40.

Diven, D., Solomon, A., McNeely, M. & Font, R. (1987). Nevus sebaceous associated with major ophthalmologic abnormalities. *Archives of Dermatology*, **123**, 383–6.

Dobyns, W. & Garg, B. (1991). Vascular abnormalities in epidermal nevus syndrome. *Neurology*, **41**, 276–8.

Eichler, C., Flowers F. & Ross, J. (1989). Epidermal nevus syndrome: case report and review of clinical manifestations. *Pediatric Dermatology*, **6**, 316–20.

Golitz, L. & Weston, W. (1979). Inflammatory linear verrucous epidermal nevus. Association with epidermal nevus syndrome. *Archives of Dermatology*, **115**, 1208–9.

Grebe, T., Rimsza, M., Richter, S. Hansen, R. & Hoyme, E. (1993). Further delineation of the epidermal nevus syndrome: two cases with new findings and literature review. *American Journal of Medical Genetics*, **47**, 24–30.

Gurecki, P., Holden, K., Sahn, E., Dyer, D. & Cure, J. (1996). Developmental neural abnormalities and seizures in epidermal nevus syndrome. *Developmental Medicine and Child Neurology*, **38**, 716–23.

Happle, R. (1987). Lethal genes surviving by mosaicism: a possible explanation for sporadic birth defects involving the skin. *Journal of the American Academy of Dermatology*, **16**, 899–906.

Holden, K. & Dekaban, A. (1972). Neurological involvement in nevus unius lateris and nevus linearis sebaceus. *Neurology*, **22**, 879–87.

Hurwitz, S. (1983). Epidermal nevi and tumors of epidermal origin. *Pediatric Clinics of North America*, **30**, 483–94.

Kwa, V., Smitt, J., Verbeeten, B. & Barth, P. (1995). Epidermal nevus syndrome with isolated enlargement of one temporal lobe: a case report. *Brain and Development*, **17**, 122–5.

Lantis, S., Thew, M. & Heaton, C. (1968). Nevus sebaceus of Jadassohn: part of a new neurocutaneous syndrome? *Archives of Dermatology*, **98**, 117–23.

Marden, P. & Venters H. (1966). A new neurocutaneous syndrome. *American Journal of Diseases in Children*, **112**, 79–81.

Mehregan, A. & Pinkus, H. (1965). Clinical studies: life history of organoid nevi: special reference to nevus sebaceus of Jadassohn. *Archives of Dermatology*, **91**, 574–88.

Meschia, J., Junkins, E. & Hofman, K. (1992). Brief Clinical Report. Familial systematized epidermal nevus syndrome. *American Journal of Medical Genetics*, **44**, 664–7.

Micali, G., Bene-Bain, M., Guitart, J. & Solomon, L. (1995) Genodermatoses, In *Pediatric Dermatology*, ed. L. Schachner & R. Hansen, 2nd edn, vol. 1, p. 397, New York: Churchill Livingston.

Mollica, F., Pavone, L. & Nuciforo, G. (1974). Linear sebaceous nevus syndrome in a newborn. *American Journal of Diseases in Children*, **128**, 868–71.

Mostafa, W. & Satti, M. (1991). Epidermal nevus syndrome: a clinicopathologic study with six-year follow-up. *Pediatric Dermatology*, **8**, 228–30.

Paller, A. (1987). Epidermal nevus syndrome. *Neurologic Clinics*, **5**, 451–7.

Pavone, L., Curatolo, P., Rizzo, R. et al. (1991). Epidermal nevus syndrome: a neurological variant with hemimegalencephaly, gyral malformation, mental retardation, seizures, and facial hemihypertrophy. *Neurology*, **41**, 266–71.

Rogers, M. (1992). Epidermal nevi and the epidermal nevus syndromes: a review of 233 cases. *Pediatric Dermatology*, **9**, 342–4.

Rogers, M., McCrossin I. & Commens C. (1989). Epidermal nevi and the epidermal nevus syndrome. *Journal of the American Academy of Dermatology*, **20**, 476–88.

Rogers, M., Fischer, G., & Hogan, P. (1996). Nevoid conditions of epidermis, dermis, and subcutaneous tissue. In *Cutaneous Medicine and Surgery. An Integrated Program*, ed. K. Arndt, P. LeBoit, J. Robinson & B. Wintroub, vol. 2, pp. 1787. Philadelphia: W.B. Saunders Company.

Sahl, Jr, S. (1990). Familial nevus sebaceus of Jadassohn: occurrence in three generations. *Journal of the American Academy of Dermatology*, **22**, 853–4.

Sakuta, R., Aikawa, H., Takashima, S., Yoza, A. & Ryo, S. (1989). Epidermal nevus syndrome with hemimegalencephaly: a clinical report of a case with acanthosis nigricans-like nevi on the face and neck, hemimegalencephaly, and hemihypertrophy of the body. *Brain and Development*, **11**, 191–4.

Sakuta, R., Aikawa, H., Takashima, S. & Ryo, S. (1991). Epidermal nevus syndrome with hemimegalencephaly: neuropathological study. *Brain and Development*, **13**, 260–5.

Solomon, L. & Esterly, N. (1975). Epidermal and other congenital organoid nevi. *Current Problems in Pediatrics*, **6**, 1–56.

Solomon, L., Fretzin, D. & Dewald, R. (1968). The epidermal nevus syndrome. *Archives of Dermatology*, **97**, 273–85.

Sugarman, G. & Reed, W. (1969). Two unusual neurocutaneous disorders with facial cutaneous signs. *Archives of Neurology*, **21**, 242–7.

Wagner, A. & Hansen, R. (1995) Neonatal skin and skin disorders, In *Pediatric Dermatology*, ed. L. Schachner & R. Hansen, 2nd edn, vol. 1, p. 288, New York: Churchill Livingstone.

Zaremba, J. (1978). Jadassohn's naevus phakomatosis: 2. a study based on a review of thirty-seven cases. *Journal of Mental Deficiency Research*, **22**, 103–23.

28

Pulmonary arteriovenous fistulas

Gérald Devuyst and Julien Bogousslavsky

Department of Neurology, University of Lausanne, Switzerland

Introduction

Pulmonary arteriovenous fistulas may be congenital or acquired, solitary or multiple, microscopic or massive. The association of pulmonary arteriovenous fistulas with stroke is known as the Osler–Weber–Rendu disease although, but exceptionally, stroke can be linked to a pulmonary arteriovenous fistula without an Osler–Weber–Rendu disease.

Pulmonary arteriovenous fistulas (PAVFs) occur in approximately 15% of patients with Osler–Weber–Rendu disease also called hereditary hemorrhagic telangiectasia (Gammon et al., 1990). The Osler–Weber–Rendu (O–W–R) disease is an inherited autosomal dominant disorder characterized by cutaneous, mucosal and visceral vascular malformations which may spontaneously rupture, provoking hemorrhages. A family history of patients (Roman et al., 1978) and the clinical manifestations as well as the age at presentation are highly variable although occasional patients are asymptomatic (McCue et al., 1984). Telangiectases of the skin are the most frequent clinical manifestations, concerning mainly the face, lips and hands (Roach, 1995; Haitjema et al., 1996; Albucher et al., 1996), less frequently on the trunk and legs, associated with telangiectases of mucosal surfaces on the anterior tongue or of the nasal cavity which are responsible for the epistaxis that often precedes other clinical manifestations of the disease (Roach, 1995; Haitjema et al., 1996; Albucher et al., 1996). Visual loss from telangiectases is uncommon although 10% and one-third of patients have retinal vascular malformations and conjunctival telangiectases, respectively (Roach, 1995; Haitjema et al., 1996; Albucher et al., 1996). Other localization of telangiectases such as in lungs, gastrointestinal tract, genitourinary system, liver, coronary arteries and pericardium can produce hemoptysis, hematemesis, melena, hematuria, hepatic dysfunction, coronary artery aneurysm or coronary arteriovenous malformation and cardiac tamponade. Telangiectases are not frequently observed during the first decade of life, while they enlarge and multiply after (Roach, 1995).

Neurological complications of the O–W–R disease are noted in 8 to 12% of the patients (Roach, 1995; Peery, 1987) and mainly consist of infectious complications (brain abscess, meningitis) or hemorrhages resulting from arteriovenous malformation (AVM) rupture in brain or medulla (Adams et al., 1977) and, in a lesser extent, ischemic lesions of the brain (Chateau et al., 1968; Sisel et al., 1970; Néau et al., 1987; Lowe et al., 1992). The typical vascular lesions consist of direct arteriovenous connections without an intervening capillary bed. Larger arteriovenous malformations, consisting of thin-walled vascular spaces with single or multiple feeding arteries, occur mostly in the lungs, liver and brain.

Genetics

The prevalence of the O–W–R disease is estimated at one to two cases per 100 000 people (Garland & Anning, 1950), but it might be higher (Porteous et al., 1992). A much higher prevalence occurs in certain areas, e.g. the Danish island of Fyn (Vase et al., 1985), the Dutch Antilles (Jessurun et al., 1993), and parts of France (Plauchu et al., 1989). The O–W–R disease is an hereditary syndrome with an autosomal dominance and a high penetrance evaluated to 97% (Plauchu et al., 1989). The homozygote state is probably lethal (Snyder & Doan, 1944). The gene responsible for the O–W–R disease has been localized, in 1994, to the chromosome 9 (9q33–q34) in some families, next to the chromosome coding for endoglin – a receptor for transforming growth factor TGF-beta – and linked to chromosome 12q in other families (Marchuk, 1998; Haitjema et al., 1996;

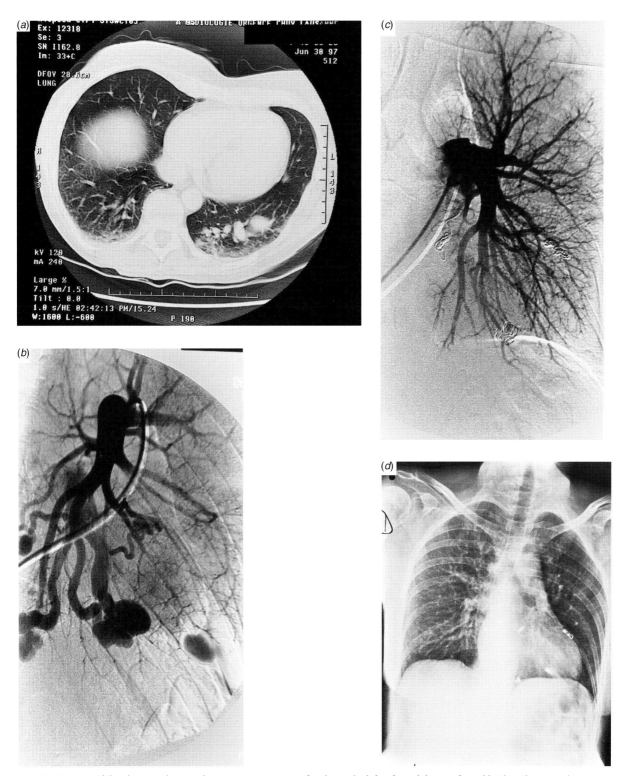

Fig. 28.2. CT scan of the chest (*a*) shows pulmonary arteriovenous fistulas in the left inferior lobe, confirmed by the selective pulmonary angiography (*b*) in a woman 42 years old with Osler–Weber–Rendu disease. After coil embolization of the fistulas, the angiographic control (*c*) revealed their correct exclusion. (*d*) The chest plane film demonstrates several coils located in the segments of the left inferior lobe (By courtesy of S. Wicky and P. Capasso, University Hospital, Department of Radiology, Lausanne, Switzerland.)

Albucher et al., 1996). Endoglin is an endothelial glycoprotein associated with the growth factor TGF-beta that provokes the endothelial response to this factor, including angiogenesis, remodelling and tissue repair. The abnormal endoglin which cannot link to the TGF-beta factor, could lead to the formation of telangiectases (McAllister et al., 1994a,b). Endoglin (CD105) is a cell surface component of the transforming growth factor-beta (TGF-beta) receptor complex highly expressed by endothelial cells. Mutations in the endoglin gene are responsible for the hereditary hemorrhagic telangiectasia type 1 (HHT1) also known as Osler–Weber–Rendu syndrome. This is an autosomal dominant vascular disorder probably caused by a haploinsufficiency mechanism displaying low levels of the normal protein. In contrast to the other mutations, the mutation on chromosome 9 seems to predispose to a high prevalence of pulmonary arteriovenous malformations (Heutink et al., 1994; McAllister et al., 1994a,b; Porteous et al., 1994) and this heterogeneity may be explained by the implication of different transforming growth factors in the pathophysiology. Moreover, a different pattern of inheritance, a different aspect of the lesions and the absence of hemorrhagic episodes suggest the existence of an unusual variant of primary telangiectasia described as hereditary benign telangiectasia (Grenz et al., 1998). Recently, germline mutations in one of two different genes, endoglin or ALK-1 which are both members of the transforming growth factor TGF-beta receptor family of proteins and expressed primarily on the surface of endothelial cells, have been evoked to cause O–W–R disease (Marchuk, 1998). The idea that endoglin modulates TGF-beta signalling through ALK-1 and the type I TGF-beta receptor, comes from biochemical studies but the factors that initiate vascular lesion formation still remain obscure. The endoglin promoter exhibited inducibility in the presence of TGF-beta I, suggesting possible therapeutic treatments in HHT1 patients, in which the expression level of the normal endoglin allele might not reach the threshold required for its functions. Isolation and characterization of the human endoglin promoter represent an initial step in elucidating the controlled expression of the endoglin gene.

Clinical features

Extra-neurological manifestations

Skin and mucosa
Telangiectases of the skin or mucosal surfaces (see colour Fig. 28.1) represent the most frequent clinical manifestations of the O–W–R disease but they are easily overlooked or misinterpreted (Haitjema et al., 1996). The preferential localizations of the telangiectases are nasal mucosa (in 68–100%), oral mucosa (58–79%), face (30–63%), trunk (13–89%), extremities (25–67%), conjunctiva/retina (45%) and digestive tract (prevalence unknown) (Haitjema et al., 1996). Cutaneous telangiectases usually appear in the third decade of life, increase in size and number with age (Peery, 1987; Hodgson & Kaye, 1963). Recurrent epistaxis occurs in 50% to 80% of patients with O–W–R disease (Peery, 1987; Hodgson & Kaye, 1963; Haitjema et al., 1995) and represents the first complaint in half of the symptomatic patients while blood transfusions are required in 10% to 30% of these patients (Reilly & Nostrant, 1984; Assar et al., 1991; McCaffrey et al., 1977). The characteristic lesion of the O–W–R disease is the telangiectasia which appears as a 1–2mm diameter lesion consisting in a dilated vessel directly connecting to an artery and a vein. Telangiectases probably develop from dilated postcapillary venules (Braverman et al., 1990).

Pulmonary arteriovenous fistulas
The O–W–R disease remains the first etiology of the pulmonary angiomas (Fig. 28.2). Pulmonary arteriovenous malformations (PAVMs) can be single or multiple and predominate mainly – 70% – in the lower lung fields (Albucher et al., 1996; Dines et al., 1983; Sluiter-Eringa et al., 1969; White et al., 1988). Thirty-six per cent of patients with single PAVM and 57% with multiple PAVMs are associated with the O–W–R disease (Roman et al., 1978; Peery, 1987; Adams et al., 1977; Lowe et al., 1992; White et al., 1988). PAVMs may enlarge with age or during pregnancy (Haitjema et al., 1996). PAVMs progressively increase in size until they become hemodynamically significant, which is the case during the third or fourth decade of life which corresponds to the beginning of the symptomatic (end-inspiratory bruit, cyanosis, clubbing, dyspnea and decreased exercise tolerance) period of the PAVMs. PAVMs are reported in 15% to 33% of patients with O–W–R disease and are usually fed by the pulmonary artery, draining through the pulmonary veins (Haitjema et al., 1996). When PAVMs reach a certain size, they can lead to a substantial right-to-left shunting, causing a significant hypoxemia or allowing systemic or cerebral paradoxical emboli. Other serious complications include a potentially life-threatening hemoptysis or hemothorax. One third of patients with PAVMs suffer from ischemic cerebral events while brain abscesses, caused by septic emboli, occur in 5% to 9% of patients with PAVMs (Adams et al., 1977; White et al., 1988).

Digestive tract
The exact prevalence of vascular malformations in the digestive tract is unknown despite the fact that blood loss via telangiectases in the gut appears in 10% to 40% of

patients with O–W–R disease (Reilly & Nostrant, 1984; Jahnke, 1970). The bleeding spot can be localized in the stomach or duodenum in half of the patients. Another digestive manifestation of the disease concerns large AVMs between the hepatic artery and vein; the shuntings caused by AVMs between the portal and hepatic veins may provoke hepatic encephalopathy following bleeding in the digestive tract, whereas AVMs between the hepatic artery and the portal vein may lead to portal hypertension with esophageal varices. Another type of liver involvement is represented by the cirrhosis of hereditary hemorrhagic telangiectasia (Haitjema et al., 1996).

Other clinical manifestations

Coronary artery aneurysm without stenosis (Tsuiki et al., 1991), coronary arteriovenous malformations (Gurevitch et al., 1998) and a cardiac tamponade (Kopel & Lage, 1998) have been described in relation with the O–W–R disease.

Neurological manifestations

The vascular cerebral complications of the O–W–R disease are mainly hemorrhagic and, in a lesser extent, ischemic among patients with PAVMs (Albucher et al., 1996). The prevalence of the cerebral vascular malformations is between 5 and 11% (Haitjema et al., 1996; White et al., 1988). In the literature's review of Roman et al. (1978) spanning 93 years and 91 patients, the authors reported that the most common neurological disorders in O–W–R patients resulted from the presence of a PAVM. In this series, 41% of the patients with O–W–R disease and PAVMs had neurological manifestations (Yeung et al., 1995). Fayad et al. (1995) noticed that the presence of PAVMs, but not cerebral vascular malformations, increased the risk for cerebral infarcts and brain abscess in a prospective study of 135 patients with O–W–R disease using brain MRI and pulmonary angiography.

Hemorrhagic complications

We can consider four types of cerebral vascular malformations in patients with O–W–R disease: telangiectases, cavernous angiomas, arteriovenous malformations, and aneurysms (Haitjema et al., 1996) but the confusion between these definitions in the literature makes comparison of the reported studies difficult (Haitjema et al., 1996). The molecular factors predisposing to each of these four types of vascular malformations are still unknown. Spontaneous carotid-cavernous fistulae have also been observed in patients with O–W–R disease (Roach, 1995). Cerebral telangiectases are defined as vascular lesions consisting of capillary-sized vessels, while cavernous angiomas are represented by thin-walled sinusoidal vessels of widely varying size; AVMs contain arteries and veins but no recognizable capillaries (Haitjema et al., 1996). Roman et al. (1978) classified cerebral vascular malformations as telangiectases or cavernous angiomas in 47%, AVMs in 22%, aneurysms in 8% and spinal vascular malformations in 22% in their literature review including 77 patients with O–W–R disease and CVMs. CVMs can be located anywhere in the brain, spinal cord or meninges, but fortunately most of them are clinically asymptomatic (Adams et al., 1977; Boczko, 1964). Roman et al. (1978) have reported that more than one type of CVMs may coexist in a given patient. For this reason, the O–W–R disease must be taken into consideration in patients with multiple and different CVMs. Intracranial aneurysms have been identified less often than arteriovenous malformations and are saccular, with loss of the muscularis layer at the neck of the aneurysm and degeneration of the elastica within the aneurysmal sac (Grollmus & Hoff, 1973). Because the prevalence of intracranial aneurysms is low in patients with O–W–R disease, it is difficult to establish that this disease is associated with an increased risk of developing aneurysms than that expected. Seventeen patients with spinal-cord AVM, typically situated posteriorly in the lumbar and lower thoracic regions of the cord, which can produce subarachnoid hemorrhage, localized cord hemorrhage or cord compression, have been detailed by Roman et al. (1978). Headache, seizure, dizziness attributed to hypoxemia or polycythemia (Roach, 1995) and ischemia of surrounding tissue as a result of steal (Roman et al., 1978; Stein & Mohr, 1988; Mohr et al., 1989) can also accompany CVMs. A much higher frequency of classic migraine – approximately 50% – has been found in the series of Steele et al. (1993) and could be explained by either cerebral or pulmonary vascular anomalies (Roach, 1995). The yearly bleeding risk associated with each type of CVMs (telangiectases, cavernous angiomas, AVMs, and aneurysms) is unknown (Adams et al., 1977) and it is unclear if the natural course of these CVMs in patients with O–W–R disease differs from that in other patients (bleeding risk of 1% to 4%). However, it seems that telangiectases occasionally give rise to intracerebral hemorrhages in patients with O–W–R disease (Haitjema et al., 1996).

Ischemic complications

Three different mechanisms have been proposed to explain ischemic stroke, more rarely reported than brain hemorrhages in O–W–R patients, occurring in O–W–R patients with PAVMs (Albucher et al., 1996). First, a hyperviscosity consecutive to the respiratory right-to-left shunting (hypoxemia) could induce a polyglobulia and arterial thrombi *in situ*. These arterial thrombi could consequently embolize in the brain circulation (Albucher et al., 1996). Secondly, a gaseous brain embolism could occur, resulting from a communication between a pulmonary vessel and the respiratory airways. Generally, a gaseous embolism is concomitant to a cough effort and is accompanied by an hemoptysia. This was the case in the observations of Chateau et al. (1968) and Néau et al. (1987). Gaseous embolism to the brain could explain repeated transient neurological deficits occurring in conjunction with episodes of hemoptysis but this relationship is difficult to prove. Nevertheless, air bubbles within retinal vessels have been demonstrated in the case of Lindskog et al. (1950). Thirdly, a cerebral paradoxical embolism of thrombotic material from a deep venous thrombosis or from right cardiac chambers or from the PAVM itself (Sisel et al., 1970; Lowe et al., 1992; Reguera et al., 1990) could bypass the normal filtration of the pulmonary bed and directly pass into the left circulation. However, no deep venous thrombosis or *in situ* (PAVM) thrombosis has ever been demonstrated in the literature (Albucher et al., 1996) and cerebral paradoxical embolism is most often a presumed diagnosis due to a lack of proof of the presence of a potential venous source. The paradoxical mechanism of brain ischemia in patients with O–W–R disease is also evoked to explain brain abscesses in these patients through septic emboli avoiding the pulmonary capillary bed, particularly during infectious diseases of the lung. The cases of Sisel et al. (1970) have shown that brain abscess and cerebral ischemia can succeed in the same patient with a delay of several years.

Symptoms by decreasing arterial oxygen saturation

The right-to-left shunting from a PAVM may contribute to decreased arterial oxygen saturation causing symptoms of headache, syncope, diplopia, vertigo, visual and auditory disturbances, dysarthria, focal or generalized seizure, paresthesias and pareses (Yeung et al., 1995).

Differential diagnosis and diagnostic evaluation

To know if PAVMs without O–W–R disease can be associated with cerebral paradoxical embolism remains an open question and uncertain. Only one case of stroke in a patient with a PAVM without O–W–R disease has been published in the literature until now.

To the best of our knowledge, there are no data concerning the optimal screening method to detect the presence of PAVMs. Diagnostic investigations can aim either at visualization of the PAVMs or at demonstration of the right-to-left shunting. A chest radiography alone is insufficient whereas information regarding the value of both computed tomographic scanning and MRI are lacking (Remy et al., 1992; Gutierrez et al., 1984). The right-to-left shunting can be demonstrated by measuring PaO_2 while the patient is breathing 100% oxygen, by evaluating the passage of technetium-labelled macroagregates of albumin through the lung, or by contrast echocardiography (Moser & Tenholder, 1986; Chilvers et al., 1988; Cotes, 1993). But because the exact diagnostic accuracy of the new radiographic methods (contrast MRA and thoracic CT) is undetermined and because the presence of PAVMs increases the risk of brain embolism or brain abscess, pulmonary angiography should be undertaken when a PAVM is suspected (Roach, 1995). Pulmonary angiography has traditionally been recognized as the definitive test for identification of PAVMs (Yeung et al., 1995). Although still limited, the new technique of contrast-enhanced MRA has already been successfully described for the evaluation of PAVMs (Kauczor, 1998).

Transcranial Doppler Ultrasound after contrast injection (c-TCD) is another interesting technique allowing the depiction of the right-to-left shunting through the PAVM as c-TCD has been shown to be a reliable technique to diagnose a right-to-left interatrial shunting through a patent foramen ovale (Devuyst, 1999). The study of Nemec et al. (1991) has found that c-TCD had 100% sensitivity for patent foramen ovale, but only 50% for intrapulmonary shunt. Intrapulmonary shunt is most of the time defined by the late appearance (Teague & Sharma, 1991) of contrast or a small amount of contrast in the left atrium and their direct visualization in the pulmonary veins during transesophageal echocardiography (Teague & Sharma, 1991; Di Tullio et al., 1993) or during c-TCD (Nemec et al., 1991; Karnick et al., 1992). However, no comparative studies addressing the screening methods to distinguish pulmonary from interatrial (patent foramen ovale) right-to-left shunting have been conducted to the best of our knowledge. Very recently, Horner et al. (1998) have presented preliminary results of their study comparing the sensitivity of c-TCD with contrast transesophageal echocardiography (c-TEE), computerized tomography (CT) of the chest and pulmonary angiography for the detection of PAVMs. Horner et al. (1998) observed that c-TCD correctly identified a right-to-left shunting in 32 of 34 (94%) c-TEE diagnosed PAVM patients but in none of the PAVM patients could the presence of a PAVM be demonstrated by chest-CT and/or pulmonary angiography. These authors (Horner et al., 1998) have also noticed that a higher count of contrast recorded on the brain circulation does not correlate with a more severe neurological deficit or higher presence of brain infarcts. Horner et al. (1998) concluded that c-TCD and c-TEE are most sensitive in the detection of mild degrees of right-to-left pulmonary shuntings in comparison to chest-CT and pulmonary angiography. Expecting confirmation of Horner's results in further studies on one hand and more accurate criteria to distinguish interatrial from pulmonary right-to-left shuntings by c-TCD on the other hand, we believe that c-TCD is a useful preliminary diagnostic procedure (particularly because it is non-invasive) to detect a potentially treatable right-to-left shunt in a patient with O–W–R disease. If a right-to-left shunt is depicted by c-TCD, definitive testing with c-TEE studies would exclude a patent foramen ovale and demonstrate the exact nature (pulmonary or interatrial) of the right-to-left shunt.

As for the diagnosis of PAVMs, to our knowledge, there are no comparative studies concerning the screening methods for cerebral vascular malformations reported in the literature. The optimal diagnostic approach varies according to the type of cerebral vascular malformation (Haitjema et al., 1996). Telangiectases can be diagnosed by MRI but not by angiography or computed tomography (Roman et al., 1978). Angiography and MRI are more sensitive to detect AVMs than computed tomography (Haitjema et al., 1996) whereas cavernous angiomas are best identified by MRI (Rigamonti et al., 1988). For screening purposes, MRI seems to be the first choice (ter Berg et al., 1993) and conventional angiography has been advocated for the depiction of AVMs when a doubt from MRI persists. Recently, Baba et al. reported two cases with an O–W–R disease accompanied by multiple hepatic arteriovenous malformations in whom brain MRI showed hyperintense basal ganglia lesions on T_1-weighted images. Although the precise mechanism of the high signal intensity in the basal ganglia on T_1-weighted images remains unproved, high blood levels of manganese such as observed in these two patients could explain the abnormal intensity of basal ganglia by the deposition of manganese. In patients with acquired hepato-cerebral degenerations, hyperintensity on T_1-weighted images in the basal ganglia is thought to be due to the deposition of manganese and/or reactive changes consecutive to the presence of manganese (Baba et al., 1998).

Treatment of neurological manifestations

As for the consequence of the rarity of the O–W–R disease and the absence of knowledge concerning the natural course of cerebral vascular malformations, the question of whether or not asymptomatic cerebral vascular malformations should be treated is still a matter of debate (Mohr et al., 1989). Because no data exist about comparative studies between conservative and surgical management of CVM in these patients, the therapeutic strategy will depend on the balance between the supposed risk of bleeding and the risks of surgical complications (ter Berg et al., 1993; Fisher, 1989; Aminoff, 1987; Iansek et al., 1983). The therapeutic alternatives for CVMs include surgery (Amin-Hanjani et al., 1998), embolization (Baroudet et al., 1997) (endovascular treatment), and stereotactic radiosurgery, using gamma-rays, that can be performed separately or in combination. The choice of the best therapy will depend on localization, angio-architecture of the lesion, size, experience and availability of the different treatments in each centre.

Because many neurological complications of the O–W–R disease (abscess, ischemic stroke) are related to the presence of PAVM fistula, resection or embolization of the fistula has been recommended. Resection of the PAVM represents a major surgical intervention, with loss of normal lung tissue surrounding the PAVM. Consequently, embolization of the feeding vessels of the PAVM is the therapy of choice, but long-term follow-up regarding this technique is lacking. Recanalization of the feeding vessels after embolization is seen in 5% to 10% of cases and can be treated by reembolization while the most severe complication of the embolization is pulmonary infarction, which occurs when normal branches of the pulmonary artery are occluded. Surgical resection of the PAVM is reserved if local anatomic considerations exclude embolization. The advent of minimally invasive surgical techniques such as PAVM resection under video-assisted thoracoscopy will offer both the advantages of a definitive therapy and a minimal morbidity rate (Temes et al., 1998) in the future.

References

Adams, H.P., Subbiah, B. & Bosch, E.P. (1977). Neurologic aspects of hereditary hemorrhagic telangiectasia. *Archives of Neurology*, **34**, 101–4.

Albucher, J.F., Carles, P., Giron, J. et al. (1996). Accidents vasculaires cérébraux ischémiques dans le cadre de la maladie de Rendu-Osler: 1 cas. *Revue Neurologie*, **152**(4), 283–7.

Amin-Hanjani, S., Robertson, R., Arginteanu, M.S. & Scott, R.M. (1998). Familial intracranial arteriovenous malformations. Case report and review of the literature. *Pediatric Neurosurgery*, **29**, 208–13.

Aminoff, M.J. (1987). Treatment of unruptured cerebral arteriovenous malformations. *Neurology*, 37, 815–19.

Assar, O.S., Friedman, C.M. & White, R.I. (1991). The natural history of epistaxis in hereditary hemorrhagic telangiectasia. *Laryngoscope*, 101, 977–80.

Baba, Y., Ohkubo, K., Hamada, K., Hokotate, H. & Najajo, M. (1998). Hyperintense basal ganglia lesions on T_1-weighted images in hereditary hemorrhagic telangiectasia with hepatic involvement. *Journal of Computer Assisted Tomography*, **22**(6), 976–9.

Baroudet, S., Houdart, E., Boissonnet, H. & Lot, G. (1997). Hémorrhagies cérébroméningées de la maladie de Rendu-Osler. Deux cas traités par embolisation. *Presse Medicin*, **26**, 1622–4.

Boczko, M.L. (1964). Neurological implications of hereditary hemorrhagic telangiectasia. *Journal of Nervous and Mental Diseases*, **139**, 525–36.

Braverman, T.M., Keh, A. & Jacobson, B.S. (1990). Ultrastructure and three-dimensional organisation of the telangiectases of hereditary hemorrhagic telangiectasia. *Journal of Investigative Dermatology*, **95**, 422–7.

Chateau, R., Boucharlat, J., Paramelle, B., Perret, J. & Wolf, R. (1968). Complication neurologique grave au cours d'un anévrisme artério-veineux pulmonaire. *Revue Neurologie*, **119**, 532–6.

Chilvers, R.J., Peters, A.M., George, P., Hughes, J.M.B. & Allison, D.J. (1988). Quantification of right to left shunt through pulmonary arteriovenous malformations using 99Tc^m albumin microspheres. *Clinical Radiology*, **39**, 611–14.

Cotes, J.E. (1993). Assessment of distribution of ventilation and of blood flow through the lungs. In *Lung Function: Assessment and Application in Medicine*, 8th edn. Boston, MA: Blackwell Scientific Publications Inc.

Devuyst, G. (1999). New trends in Neurosonology. In *Current Review of Cerebrovascular Disease*, ed. M. Fisher & J. Bogousslavsky, pp. 65–76. Philadelphia: Current Medicine, Inc.

Dines, D.E., Seward, J.B. & Bernatz, P.E. (1983). Pulmonary arteriovenous fistulas. *Mayo Clinic Proceedings*, **58**, 176–81.

Di Tullio, M., Sacco, R.L., Venketasubramanian, N., Sherman, D., Mohr, J.P. & Homma, S. (1993). Comparison of diagnostic techniques for the detection of a patent foramen ovale in stroke patients. *Stroke*, **24**, 1020–4.

Fayad, P.B., Fulbright, R.K., Chaloupka, J.C., Awad, I.A. & Whirte, R.I. Jr. (1995). A prospective neurological and magnetic resonance imaging evaluation of hereditary hemorrhagic telangiectasia. *Stroke*, **26**, 160 (abstract).

Fisher, W.S. (1989). Decision analysis: a tool of the future: an application to unruptured arteriovenous malformations. *Neurosurgery*, **24**, 129–35.

Gammon, R.B., Miksa, A.K. & Keller, F.S. (1990). Osler–Weber–Rendu disease and pulmonary arteriovenous fistulas. Deterioration and embolotherapy during pregnancy. *Chest*, **98**, 1522–24.

Garland, H.G. & Anning, S.T. (1950). Hereditary haemorrhagic telangiectasia: genetic and biographical study. *British Journal of Dermatology*, **62**, 289–310.

Grenz, H., Peschen, M., Wiek, K., Schopf, E. & Vanscheidt, W. (1998). Hereditary benign telangiectasia: a rare form of primary telangiectasia with successful treatment with flash-lamp-pumped pulsed dye laser. *Vasa*, **27**(3), 192–5.

Grollmus, J. & Hoff, J. (1973). Multiple aneurysms associated with Osler–Weber–Rendu disease. *Surgical Neurology*, **1**, 91–3.

Gurevitch, Y., Hasin, Y., Gotsman, M.S. & Rozenman, Y. (1998). Coronary arteriovenous malformations in a patient with hereditary hemorrhagic telangiectasia. *Angiology*, **7**, 577–80.

Gutierrez, E.R., Glazer, H.S., Levitt, R.G. & Moran, J.E. (1984). NMR imaging of pulmonary arteriovenous fistulae. *Journal of Computer Assisted Tomography*, **8**, 750–2.

Haitjema, T., Disch, E., Overtoom, T.T.C., Westermann, C.J.J. & Lammers, J.W.J. (1995). Screening of family members of patients with hereditary hemorrhagic telangiectasia. *American Journal of Medicine*, **99**, 519–24.

Haitjema, T., Westerman, C.J.J., Overtoom, T.T.C. et al. (1996). Hereditary hemorrhagic telangiectasia (Osler–Weber–Rendu disease). *Archives of Internal Medicine*, **156**, 714–19.

Heutink, P., Haitjema, T., Breedveld, G.J. et al. (1994). Linkage of hereditary haemorrhagic telangiectasia to chromosome 9q34 and evidence for locus heterogeneity. *Journal of Medical Genetics*, **31**, 933–6.

Hodgson, C.H. & Kaye, R.L. (1963). Pulmonary arteriovenous fistula and hereditary hemorrhagic telangiectasia: a review and report of 35 cases of fistula. *Diseases of the Chest*, **43**, 449–55.

Horner, S., Schuchlenz, S., Harb, S. et al. (1988). Contrast transcranial Doppler monitoring in stroke patients with pulmonary right-to-left shunts. *Stroke* (Abstract of the World Congress on Cerebral Embolism), 2240.

Iansek, R., Elstein, A.S. & Balla, J.I. (1983). Application of decision analysis of management of cerebral arteriovenous malformation. *Lancet*, **ii**, 1132–5.

Jahnke, V. (1970). Ultrastructure of hereditary telangiectasia. *Archives of Otolaryngology*, **91**, 262–5.

Jessurun, G.A., Kamphuis, D.J., van der Zande, E.H. & Nossent, J.C. (1993). Cerebral arteriovenous malformations in the Netherlands Antilles: high prevalence of hereditary hemorrhagic telangiectasia-related single and multiple cerebral arteriovenous malformations. *Clinical Neurology and Neurosurgery*, **95**, 193–8.

Karnik, R., Stöllberger, C., Valentin, A., Winkler, W.B. & Slany, J. (1992). Detection of patient foramen ovale by transcranial contrast Doppler ultrasound. *American Journal of Cardioligy*, **69**, 560–2.

Kauczor, H.U. (1998). Contrast-enhanced magnetic resonance angiography of the pulmonary vasculature. A review. *Investigative Radiology*, **33**(9), 606–17.

Kopel, L. & Lage, S.G. (1998). Cardiac tamponade in hereditary hemorrhagic telangiectasia. *American Journal of Medicine*, **105**, 252–3

Lindskog, G.E., Liebow, A., Kausel, H. & Janzen, J. (1950). Pulmonary arteriovenous aneurysm. *Annals of Surgery*, **132**, 591–610.

Lowe, B.B., Biller, J., Landas, S.K. & Hoover, W.W. (1992). Diagnosis of pulmonary arteriovenous malformation by ultrafast chest computed tomography in Rendu–Osler–Weber syndrome with cerebral ischemia: a case report. *Angiology*, **43**(6), 522–8.

McAllister, K.A., Grogg, K.M., Gallione, C.J. et al. (1994a). Endoglin, a TGF-β binding protein of endothelial cells, is the gene of haemorrhagic telangiectasia type 1. *Nature Genetics*, **8**, 345–51.

McAllister, K.A., Lennon, E., Bowles-Biesecker, B. et al. (1994b). Genetic heterogeneity in hereditary haemorrhagic telangiectasia: possible correlation with clinical phenotype. *Journal of Medical Genetics*, **31**, 927–32.

McCaffrey, T.V., Kern, E.B. & Lake, C.E. (1977). Management of epistaxis in hereditary hemorrhagic telangiectasia: review of 80 cases. *Archives of Otolaryngology*, **103**, 627–30.

McCue, C.M., Hartenberg, M. & Nance, W.E. (1984). Pulmonary arteriovenous malformations related to Rendu–Osler–Weber syndrome. *American Journal of Medical Genetics*, **19**, 19–27.

Marchuk, D.A. (1998). Genetic abnormalities in hereditary hemorrhagic telangiectasia. *Current Opinion in Hematology*, **5**(5), 332–8.

Mohr, J.P., Stein, B.M. & Hilal, S.K. (1989). Arteriovenous malformations. In *Handbook of Clinical Neurology*, ed. J.E. Toole, vol. 10, pp. 361–93. Amsterdam, The Netherlands: Elsevier Science Publishers.

Moser, R.J. & Tenholder, M.E. (1986). Diagnostic imaging of pulmonary arteriovenous malformations: evaluation with roentgenographic, sonographic and radionuclide imaging. *Chest*, **89**, 586–9.

Néau, J.P., Boissonnot, L., Boutaud, P., Fontanel, J.P., Gil, R. & Lefèvre, J.P. (1987). Manifestations neurologiques de la maladie de Rendu–Osler–Weber. A propos de 4 observations. *Revue Medicin Interne*, **8**, 75–8.

Nemec, J.J., Marwick, T.H., Lorig, R.J. et al. (1991). Comparison of transcranial Doppler ultrasound and transesophageal contrast echocardiography in the detection of interatrial right-to-left shunts. *American Journal of Cardiology*, **68**, 1498–502.

Peery, W.H. (1987). Clinical spectrum of hereditary hemorrhagic, telangiectasia (Osler–Weber–Rendu disease). *American Journal of Medicine*, **8**, 989–97.

Plauchu, H., de Chadarevian, J.P., Gideau, A.J. & Robert, J.M.L. (1989). Age-related clinical profile of hereditary hemorrhagic telangiectasia in an epidemiologically recruited population. *American Journal of Medical Genetics*, **32**, 291–7.

Porteous, M.E.M., Burn, J. & Proctof, S.J. (1992). Hereditary haemorrhagic telangiectasia: a clinical analysis. *Journal of Medical Genetics*, **29**, 527–30.

Porteous, M.E.M., Curtis, A., Williams, O., Marchuk, D., Bhattacharya, S.S. & Burn, J. (1994). Genetic heterogeneity in hereditary haemorrhagic telangiectasia. *Journal of Medical Genetics*, **31**, 925–6.

Reguera, J.M., Colmenero, J.D., Guerrero, M., Pastor, M. & Martin-Palanca, A. (1990). Paradoxical cerebral embolism secondary to pulmonary arteriovenous fistula. *Stroke*, **21**(3), 504–5.

Reilly, P.J. & Nostrant, T.T. (1984). Clinical manifestations of hereditary hemorrhagic telangiectasia. *American Journal of Gastroenterology*, **79**, 363–7.

Remy, J., Remy-Jardin, M., Wattine, L. & Deffontaines, C. (1992). Pulmonary arteriovenous malformations: evaluation with CT of the chest before and after treatment. *Radiology*, **182**, 809–16.

Rigamonti, D., Hadley, M.N., Drayer, B.D. et al. (1988). Cerebral cavernous malformation: incidence and familial occurrence. *New England Journal of Medicine*, **319**, 343–7.

Roach, E.S. (1995). Congenital cutaneovascular syndromes. In *Stroke Syndromes*, ed. J. Bogousslavsky & L. Caplan, pp. 481–490. Cambridge: Cambridge University Press.

Roman, G., Fisher, M., Perl, D.P. & Posner, C.M. (1978). Neurological manifestations of hereditary hemorrhagic telangiectasia (Rendu–Osler–Weber disease): report of 2 cases and review of the literature. *Annals of Neurology*, **4**, 130–44.

Sisel, R.J., Parker, B.M. & Bahl, O.P. (1970). Cerebral symptoms in pulmonary arteriovenous fistula. A result of paradoxical emboli. *Circulation*, **46**, 123–8.

Sluiter-Eringa, H., Orie, N.G.M. & Sluiter, H.J. (1969). Pulmonary arteriovenous fistula: diagnosis and prognosis in noncomplainant patients. *American Review of Respiratory Diseases*, **100**, 177–88.

Snyder, L.H. & Doan, L.A. (1944). Is the homozygous form of multiple telangiectasia lethal? *Journal of Laboratory Clinical Medicine*, **29**, 1211–16.

Steele, J.G., Nath, P.U., Burn, J. & Porteous, M.E. (1993). An association between migrainous aura and hereditary haemorrhagic telangiectasia. *Headache*, **33**, 145–8.

Stein, B.M. & Mohr, J.P. (1988). Vascular malformations of the brain. *New England Journal of Medicine*, **319**, 368–9.

Teague, S.M. & Sharma, M.K. (1991). Detection of paradoxical cerebral echo contrast embolization by transcranial Doppler ultrasound. *Stroke*, **22**, 740–5.

Temes, R.T., Paramsothy, P.P., Endara, S.A. & Wernly, J.A. (1998). Resection of a solitary pulmonary arteriovenous malformation by video-assisted thoracic surgery. *The Journal of Thoracic and Cardiovascular Surgery*, **116**(5), 878–9.

ter Berg, J.W.M., Overtoom, T.T.C., Ludwig, J.W. et al. (1993). Unruptured intracranial arteriovenous malformations with hereditary hemorrhagic telangiectasia: neurosurgical treatment or not? *Acta Neurochirurgica (Wien)*, **121**, 34–42.

Tsuiki, K., Tamada, Y. & Yasui, S. (1991). Coronary artery aneurysm without stenosis in association with Osler–Weber–Rendu disease. A case report. *Angiology*, 55–8.

Vase, P., Holm, M. & Arendrup, H. (1985). Pulmonary arteriovenous fistulas in hereditary hemorrhagic telangiectasia. *Acta Medica Scandinavica*, **218**, 105–9.

White, R.I., Lynch-Nyhan, A., Terry, P. et al. (1988). Pulmonary arteriovenous malformations: techniques and long-term outcome of embolotherapy. *Radiology*, **169**, 663–9.

Yeung, M., Khan, K.A., Antecol, D.H., Walker, D.R. & Shuaib, A. (1995). Transcranial Doppler ultrasonography and transesophageal echocardiography in the investigation of pulmonary arteriovenous malformation in a patient with hereditary hemorrhagic telangiectasia presenting with stroke. *Stroke*, **26**, 1941–4.

29

Cerebrovascular complications of Rendu–Osler disease (hereditary hemorrhagic telangiectasia)

Jean-François Albucher and François Chollet

INSERM U455, Department of Neurology, Hôpital Purpan, Toulouse, France

Introduction

Rendu–Osler disease or Hereditary Hemorrhagic Telangiectasia (HTT) is a familial disorder transmitted as an autosomal dominant trait of high penetrance. Rendu–Osler disease is a generalized vascular dysplasia, characterized by the presence of arteriovenous malformations in multiple organs. Rendu–Osler disease is responsible for multiple telangiectasias of the skin, mucous membranes and viscera, associated with recurrent bleeding (Peery, 1987; Haitjema et al., 1996).

Neurological complications occur in 10% of the patients and are mainly represented by infectious complications (brain abscess) and cerebral or spinal cord hemorrhages. Neurological symptoms are often associated with arteriovenous fistula of the lung (50%). Ischemic strokes have been described but are not frequent in this disease.

The first patient presenting HHT was described for the first time by Babington in 1865. The case was reported by Rendu in 1896, and in 1901 and 1908 Osler and Weber achieved the description of the Rendu–Osler–Weber disease. The term 'Hereditary Haemhorragic Telengiectasia' was defined by Hanes in 1909. They clearly identified this hemorrhagic disease, as a familial disease characterized by recurrent visceral or mucous bleedings.

The frequency of Rendu–Osler disease is estimated at from 1 to 2/100 000 (Roman et al., 1978; Kadoya et al., 1994) but higher incidences have been reported in parts of France, Danish Islands and Dutch Antilles (Haitjema et al., 1996). People from all origins and either sex can be affected.

Telangiectasias which are the main lesions of HHT, correspond to capillary and postcapillary venule dilation (Peery, 1987). Telangiectasias of HHT patients have been described with an enlargement of the postcapillary venules and a possible direct connection with arterioles thus bypassing the capillary network. Hemorrhages from telengiectasias occur despite normal blood hemostasis and platelet functions tests, and are related to local abnormalities of the vessel walls (endothelial cell degeneration, defect in endothelial cell junctions, weakness of the perivascular connective tissue (Peery, 1987)). No definite and clear pathogenic mechanisms have been proposed to explain their development: defect in endothelial cell junctions, incomplete smooth-cell layer surrounding the vessels, and extravasation of erythrocytes have been suggested. Telangiectasias usually appear on skin and mucosal surfaces and especially the nose. Larger arteriovenous malformations occur mostly in the lungs, liver and in the brain, and their size can be more than a few centimetres in diameter.

Genetic aspects

Rendu–Osler disease is an autosomal dominant disorder with a high penetrance. The penetrance is estimated to be 95% by the age of 50 (Haitjema et al., 1996). Negative family history of recurrent bleeding was noticed in 15 to 30% of the patients. However, internal lesions without external bleeding and thus no apparent symptom may explain the skipping of members of one generation (Roman et al., 1978). The homozygous state is probably lethal and the presence of giant cerebral malformations has been proposed to explain fetal loss in woman affected by HHT.

The pathophysiological mechanisms and the genetic explanations of the Rendu–Osler disease remained unexplained for a long time.

In 1994, a gene responsible for Rendu–Osler disease was mapped on chromosome 9 by two different groups (Shovlin et al., 1994; McAllister et al., 1994). Genetic linkage has been established to chromosome 9q33–q34 for some families (McAllister et al., 1994). This locus was called OWR1 and corresponds to the endoglin's gene, a transforming growth factor β (TGF-β) binding protein.

Endoglin protein is a functional component of the endothelial membrane TGF-β receptor complex. Endoglin is an abundant membrane glycoprotein expressed at a high level on human endothelial cells of capillaries, arterioles and venules. Endoglin binds TGF-β1 and TGF-β3 with a high affinity but is unable to bind TGF-β2. In association with β-TGF, endoglin is implicated in differentiation and remodelling of vascular tissues and in programmed cell death. So it has been proposed that the perturbations of one or more of these processes may cause the vascular dysplasia observed in the HHT patients. The gene of the endoglin was considered a strong candidate gene for HHT.

Three different and independent mutations of the OWR1 locus were reported by McAllister et al. (1994) in HHT patients. HHT type 1 had been linked to endoglin gene mutation.

However, it has been shown that not all the families affected by Rendu–Osler disease had a systematic chromosome 9 disorder. In 1995 two other different HHT genes were mapped on chromosome 3p22 (HHT type 2) and chromosome 12q (HHT type 3) (Vincent et al., 1995). The genetic heterogeneity of HHT was then recognized. The region 3p22 corresponds to the location of an other TGF β receptor gene (TGF-β2 receptor). The TGF-β2 receptor can bind to β-glycan, which is a membrane proteoglycan. A structural analogy was found between the transmembrane domain and cytoplasmic portion of the β-glycan and endoglin.

These results suggest that mutations within distinct TGF-β receptor genes may be responsible for genetic heterogeneity. This genetic heterogeneity seems to correspond to a clinical hetrogeneity, since pulmonary arteriovenous malformations are found in families linked to chromosome 9 while they are absent in families linked to chromosome 12 (Vincent et al., 1995). HHT appears to be a disorder within members of the TGF-β receptor complex or other endothelial cell components of the TGF-β signal pathway.

On a second occasion when HHT type 1 was clearly associated with a mutation of the endoglin gene, molecular progress found that most of the mutations of the endogline gene involved truncations of the extracellular domain of the protein. However, a number of missense mutations have now been reported including a start codon mutation that is predicted to lead to a nill allele (Gallione et al., 1997). This nill allele leads to reduced message or endoglin levels (Marchuk, 1998). This suggests the possibility of a haploinsufficiency model for HHT-1 (Gallione et al., 1997).

Reduced expression of endoglin from the mutant allele induces a decreased activity of endoglin, which falls below a critical threshold, predisposing the development of vascular lesion in HHT-1 patients (Rius et al., 1998). The promoter region of human endoglin has recently been individualized (Rius et al., 1998). The characterization of the human endoglin promoter represents an initial step in understanding the expression of the endoglin gene. It is not irrational to expect a therapeutic approach of patients with HHT-1, because we know that the endoglin promoter exhibits inducibility in the presence of TGF-β1 and then increases endoglin production so that the normal endoglin allele can reach the threshold required for its function (Rius et al., 1998).

Clinical aspects

General manifestations

Hereditary hemorrhagic telangiectasia (HHT) is mainly characterized by the presence of multiple dermal, mucosal and visceral telangiectasias responsible for recurrent cutaneous or visceral bleedings. The association of familial history, recurrent epistaxis and telangiectasias can recall the HHT's clinical diagnosis.

Skin and mucosa telangiectasias

Telangiectasias are frequently found in skin or mucosal surfaces. During clinical examination, telangiectasias of the tongue and of the lips must be systematically chased. They can be easily overlooked or misinterpreted. The size of angiomas and telangiectasias increases progressively with years and induces a higher number of hemorrhages (Samson et al., 1982). Progressive outbreaks of telangiectasias with specific cutaneous localizations on lips, face and digits and mucous localizations on lips, tongue, palate and intestinal tractus occur over the years. After several years, obvious telangiactasias are frequent and they become constant after the age of 60 (Hodgson et al., 1959).

Principal clinical symptoms are epistaxis, hemoptysis, hematuria and melena.

Epistaxis

Recurrent epistaxis is the most constant symptom and is present in 50 to 80% of the affected patients (Haitjema et al., 1996). Epistaxis appears to be the first complaint in 50% of the affected patients and is often present in childhood. It can be severe, and blood transfusions are required in 10 to 30% of the patients. Chronic anemia, induced by chronic bleeding can be observed.

Pulmonary manifestations

Telangiectasias are often located in the lungs (15 to 20% of the patients have an angioma located in the lungs, Peery, 1987). In the family of 231 persons, reported in 1959 by Hodgson, 14 (15.4%) had a pulmonary fistula (Hodgson et al., 1959). In the prospective study of Fayad concerning 135 patients with HHT a pulmonary fistula was found in 91 of them (67%) (Fayad et al., 1995). So Rendu–Osler disease represents the main etiology of pulmonary angioma and conversely 50% of the HHT patients present a pulmonary angiovenous fistula. Pulmonary angiomas in HHT may be single or multiple and can involve all pulmonary segments but their first location is the inferior lobe in 70% of the cases. The angiomas increase gradually in size to become hemodynamically significant in young adults (Adams et al., 1977; Peery, 1987; Haitjema et al., 1996) and clinical manifestations of pulmonary arteriovenous fistulas usually occur during the third or fourth decade. They may enlarge during pregnancy. Pulmonary arteriovenous malformations can result in a subsequent right-to-left shunt responsible for chronic hypoxemia. They are the origin of hemoptysis and hemothorax. Their detection must be systematic in affected HHT patients. In a family screening program, a simple method using the measure of PaO_2 and chest radiography was proposed by Haitjema. Angiography was performed only when hypoxemia was found (Haitjema et al., 1995). With this method a pulmonary malformation was found in 33% of the affected patients.

Neurological complications

Neurological symptoms occur in 8 to 12% of the HHT patients and are mainly represented by infectious and hemorrhagic complications (Adams et al., 1977; Peery, 1987). Neurological complications occur mainly in patients with a pulmonary vascular malformation (Love et al., 1992). Roman has clearly shown, from the medical literature, that neurological complications in HHT patients resulted from pulmonary fistula, and conversely 41% of HHT patients with pulmonary malformation presented neurological events (Roman et al., 1978). Neurological complications are significantly more frequent in patients with pulmonary angioma than in HHT patients without pulmonary fistula (Fayad et al., 1995).

Infectious neurological complications

Infectious diseases are represented by meningitis and brain abscess (Samson et al., 1982). The incidence of brain abscess in patients with pulmonary fistula was estimated at 5 to 6% (Adams et al., 1977, Wilkins et al., 1983). Brain abscess may be the first event of HHT and of pulmonary angioma and may develop before the skin lesions are apparent. In every patient with recurrent brain abscess, Rendu–Osler disease must be suspected and a pulmonary vascular malformation chased (Wilkins et al., 1983). The right-to-left shunt in the lung angioma allows septic emboli to bypass the natural pulmonary filter.

Hemorrhagic neurological complications

Hemorrhagic intracranial complications may occur in 2 to 3% of the HHT patients (Baroudet et al., 1997). Hemorrhagic complications are induced by arteriovenous malformation of the brain and of the spinal cord (Kadoya et al., 1994). Arteriovenous malformations may involve all parts of the brain but have been rarely reported in the posterior fossa. Subarachnoid hemorrhages induced by cerebral aneurysms have also been reported. Carotid fistulae may also occur. Dural fistulae were also reported as in the observation 2 of Baroudet. Arteriovenous malformation may also be located in the medulla and may be responsible for medullary hematoma and for subarachnoid hemorrhage. In the series of 215 patients suffering from Rendu–Osler disease reported by Roman, six patients (2.6%) presented a cerebral aneurysm and 17 (7.9%) presented a cerebral arteriovenous malformation (Roman et al., 1978). In HHT the incidence of cerebral vascular malformation appears less important when compared with the high incidence of pulmonary malformations (50%).

Headaches, visual or auditory disturbances, diplopia, vertigo, focal or generalized seizures have been reported. They were often related to hypoxemia. Porto-systemic encephalopathy due to hepatic telangiectasias has also been reported.

Neurological symptoms occurred mainly in patients with pulmonary fistula and in his review of the literature Roman related that 41% of the HHT patients with pulmonary fistula presented neurological symptoms.

Ischemic strokes

Rendu–Osler disease is recognized as being responsible for hemorrhagic complications. Ischemic strokes have rarely been reported in HHT patients, and few cases have been described (Chateau et al., 1968; Sisel et al., 1970; Neau et al., 1987; Love et al., 1992; Yeung et al., 1995; Albucher et al., 1996; Abet et al., 1984). Cerebral infarction may be the first manifestation of Rendu–Osler disease (Albucher et al., 1996; Love et al., 1992) and may lead to the discovery of a pulmonary angioma. Middle cerebral artery is the most frequent site of embolism. Several authors had noticed that, in HHT patients with pulmonary fistula, the central nervous system is the most frequent site for emboli.

30

Cervicocephalic arterial dissections

Bahram Mokri

Department of Neurology, Mayo Clinic, Rochester, MN, USA

General considerations

Cervicocephalic arterial dissections are recognized with increasing frequency, partly due to increased familiarity of clinicians and radiologists with the clinical and radiological features of the disorder and partly due to increasing availability and utility of noninvasive neuroimaging techniques which are steadily improving in quality and accuracy. Furthermore, a broader clinical spectrum of the disease is emerging, and more monosymptomatic or minimally symptomatic cases are recognized (Hart & Easton, 1983; Mokri, 1994, 1997b; Saver & Easton, 1998). Many such cases would have gone undiagnosed or wrongly diagnosed only a decade or so ago as the symptoms would not have warranted subjecting the patients to invasive angiographic studies.

Although many cervicocephalic arterial dissections, particularly the extracranial ones, do not cause strokes, many do. These dissections are among the major causes of strokes in young and middle-aged persons (Bogousslavsky et al., 1987).

The dissections are called 'traumatic' when there is history of definite trauma, penetrating or blunt. Otherwise, dissections are called 'spontaneous' although a sizeable minority of the patients with 'spontaneous dissections' may have history of trivial traumas, which may or may not be of clinical significance.

Dissections of internal carotid artery (ICA) typically involve the extracranial segment of the vessel and very infrequently may extend intracranially or only involve the intracranial ICA. On the other hand, vertebral artery (VA) dissections can frequently extend intracranially, or begin intracranially, or even extend to the basilar artery.

Basilar artery or other intracranial artery dissections are quite uncommon (Mokri, 1994).

Incidence

Population-based incidence studies of spontaneous ICA dissections from Rochester, Minnesota (Schievink et al., 1993), and Dijon, France (Giroud et al., 1994), have revealed annual incidence rates of 2.6 and 2.9 per 100 000. In our practice, the frequency of spontaneous VA dissections is about one-third of spontaneous ICA dissections (Schievink et al., 1994b). Furthermore, some ICA or VA dissections may be asymptomatic or minimally symptomatic. There is little doubt that nowadays more cases of these dissections are diagnosed. Therefore, it is reasonable to assume that the true annual incidence of spontaneous cervicocephalic arterial dissections is about 5 per 100 000. No information is available about the true incidence of traumatic cervicocephalic arterial dissections, but these are likely less common than spontaneous ones.

Since many patients with cervicocephalic arterial dissections never develop strokes (Mokri, 1997b), the studies based on, or biased towards, cases with strokes will not reflect the true incidence of these dissections.

Pathology and pathogenesis

In dissections, typically an intimal defect occurs and allows penetration of the blood into the arterial wall. The intramural hematoma propagates within the media for variable distances by splitting the media. Consequently, one of the following may occur:

(i) Formation of an elongated intramural hematoma that often would push the true lumen to one side forming an elongated narrowing of the true lumen (Fig. 30.1(*a*)) that angiographically appears as an elongated and often irregular stenosis (Fig. 30.1(*b*)).

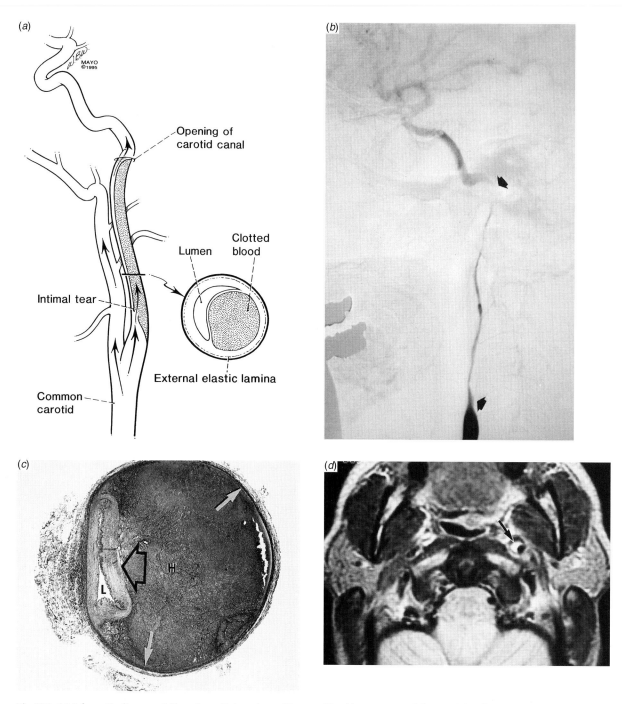

Fig. 30.1. (*a*) Schematic diagram of dissection of internal carotid artery. Blood has penetrated the arterial wall, causing an elongated intramural hematoma that has resulted in compression of the true lumen and creation of an elongated stenosis. (From Mokri, 1997b. By permission of Mayo Foundation.) (*b*) Carotid angiogram shows a tight, elongated stenosis (string sign). Proximally the arterial lumen is tapered to the stenosis (lower arrow), and distally there is a fairly abrupt reconstitution of the lumen (upper arrow). (From Mokri, 1997a). By permission of Academic Press.) (*c*) Cross-section of internal carotid artery involved by dissection (elastic van Gieson stain). A large intramural hematoma (*H*) has squeezed and narrowed the true lumen (L, large open arrow). External elastic lamina surrounds both the true lumen and the intramural clot (small arrows). (*d*) Magnetic resonance image at the level of dissection, showing hyperintense, crescent-shape intramural hematoma (arrow) surrounding a small area of flow void corresponding to the narrowed lumen of the internal carotid artery. (From Mokri, 1997b. By permission of Lippincott Williams & Wilkins.)

(a)

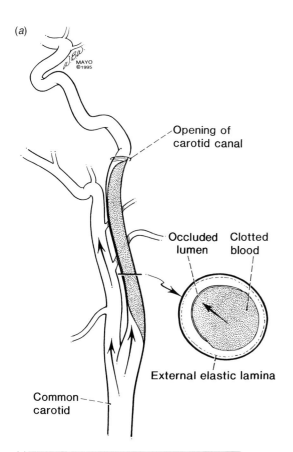

Opening of
carotid canal

Occluded   Clotted
lumen   blood

External elastic lamina

Common
carotid

(b)

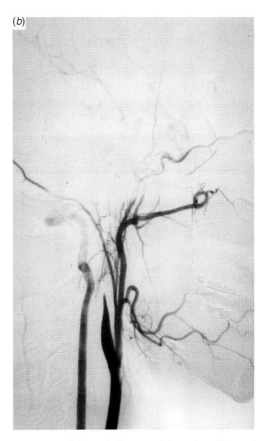

(c)

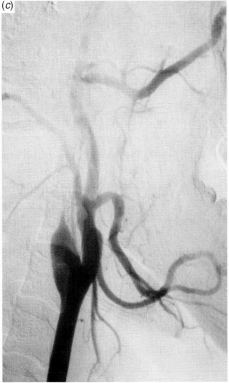

Fig. 30.2. (a) Schematic diagram of dissection of internal carotid artery. The intramural hematoma has caused complete occlusion of the true lumen. (From Mokri, 1997b. By permission of Mayo Foundation.) On angiography, a tapered flame-like (b) or radish-tailed (c) occlusion of the artery may be noted. ((b) and (c) from Mokri, 1987). By permission of Mayo Foundation.)

In extreme cases when the elongated narrowing is quite tight, the angiographic appearance is referred to as 'string sign' (Fisher et al., 1978; Houser et al., 1984). Proximally, these stenoses have a tapered appearance whereas distally a fairly abrupt reconstitution of the lumen is noted. Axial MR images that cut through the involved segments show findings that correspond to what is noted pathologically (Fig. 30.1(c)), demonstrating the intramural hematoma as a high signal crescent or donut surrounding a small dark low-signal circle corresponding to the narrowed arterial lumen (Fig. 30.1(d)).

(ii) Large intramural hematomas may seriously compress and completely occlude the arterial lumen (Fig. 30.2(a)). The angiographic appearance is a tapered occlusion resembling 'candle flame' or 'radish tail' (Fig. 30.2(b) and (c)).

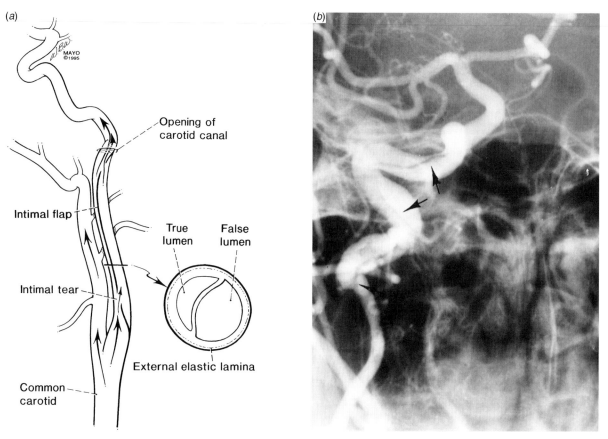

Fig. 30.3. (*a*) Schematic diagram of dissection of the internal carotid artery. The intramural hematoma is distally reconnected with the true lumen, creating a double lumen. (From Mokri, 1997b. By permission of Mayo Foundation.) (*b*) Angiography demonstrates the two parallel channels separated by a long intimal flap (arrows). (From Houser et al., 1984. By permission of the American Society of Neuroradiology.)

(iii) The false lumen created by the intramural hematoma may reconnect with the true lumen distally, creating parallel channels of circulation resembling a 'double-barrelled gun.' The two channels are separated by an elongated intimal flap (Fig. 30.3).

(iv) The intramural hematoma may expand outwards toward the adventitia creating an aneurysmal sac ('dissecting aneurysm') which is formed within the media and connected with a true lumen (Fig. 30.4). These may harbor thrombi and lead to distal embolization creating strokes or cerebral or retinal ischemic episodes.

(v) Commonly, a combination of the above changes is noted. Particularly frequent is occurrence of stenosis and dissecting aneurysm concomitantly in the same artery.

(vi) The changes that are noted in the extracranial segment of the vertebral artery are essentially similar to what is noted in the extracranial internal carotid artery (elongated stenosis, dissecting aneurysm, stenosis), although the typical 'flamelike' stenosis of ICA dissections may not be noted in VA dissection.

(vii) In intracranial arteries, the changes vary somewhat:

(a) Arterial media is normally attenuated and simplified intracranially. Therefore, the intracranial dissections may appear subintimal or subadventitial.

(b) With intracranial dissections, the intramural hematoma may break through the wall of the dissected vessel and cause subarachnoid hemorrhage. Rupture of a spontaneous dissection or dissecting aneurysm of the extracranial ICA or VA would be extremely unusual.

(viii) In traumatic extracranial ICA or VA dissections, exactly the same changes noted in spontaneous dissections may occur. However, particularly when there is penetrating trauma puncturing the artery, periarterial bleeding may occur that subsequently may

(*a*)

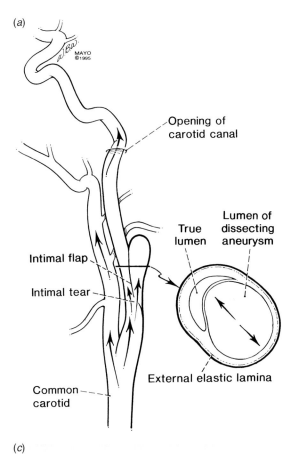

Opening of
carotid canal

True
lumen

Lumen of
dissecting
aneurysm

Intimal flap

Intimal tear

External elastic lamina

Common
carotid

(*b*)

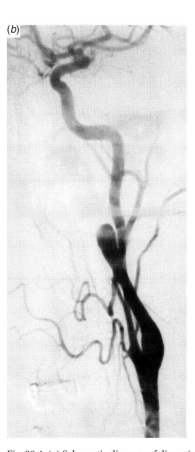

(*c*)

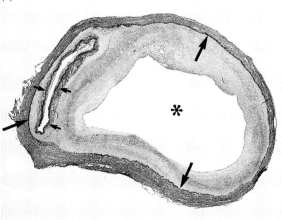

Fig. 30.4. (*a*) Schematic diagram of dissection of internal carotid artery. Outward extension of dissection has created a dissecting aneurysm. (From Mokri, 1997b. By permission of Mayo Foundation.) (*b*) Angiography shows a fingerlike dissecting aneurysm next to a mildly stenosed segment of the internal carotid artery and separated from it by a small intimal flap. (From Mokri, 1987). By permission of Mayo Foundation.) (*c*) Cross-section through the involved area demonstrates both the aneurysmal sac (asterisk) and the true lumen surrounded by the external elastic lamina (larger arrows). The true lumen is delineated by the internal elastic lamina (small arrows). Elastic van Gieson stain. (From Mokri, 1997b. By permission of Lippincott, Williams & Wilkins.)

become encapsulated. These encapsulated hematomas when connected with the arterial lumen are called 'pseudoaneurysms' or 'pulsating hematomas.' These should not be mistaken with dissecting aneurysms. The wall of a dissecting aneurysm is formed of blood vessel elements, and the wall of pseudoaneurysms is formed of the encapsulating connective tissue elements (Fig. 30.5). Furthermore, the term 'false aneurysm' should not be utilized for dissecting aneurysms (a common error) (Mokri, 1994).

Etiology

In most patients with cervicocephalic arterial dissections, the etiology of the dissection remains undetermined. Table

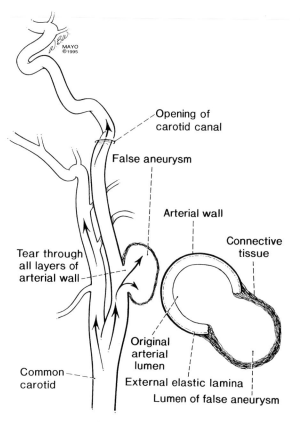

Fig. 30.5. Schematic diagram of a false aneurysm or 'pseudoaneurysm.' The aneurysmal wall is composed of connective tissue elements. (From Mokri, 1997b. By permission of Mayo Foundation.)

30.1 is a list of possible etiologic factors. Essentially, two major groups of etiologic factors are recognized or presumed: (i) trauma and (ii) arterial disease.

Trauma

Major trauma

The role of major trauma to the head or neck in production of ICA and VA dissections is well recognized. In case of ICA dissections, hyperflexion and rotation of the neck, such as might be seen in connection with automobile accidents, may stretch the ICA against the transverse processes of C2 and C3 vertebrae and cause an intimal tear and arterial dissection. Abrupt and severe neck flexion may even directly compress the ICA between the angle of the mandible and the upper cervical column (Zelenock et al., 1982) and thus lead to arterial dissection (Fig. 30.6). Furthermore, a prominent styloid process may also injure the ICA during abrupt or steady and severe rotations of the neck (Sundt et al., 1986; Montalbetti et al., 1995). Such injuries are not infrequent with motor vehicle accidents which seem to be the

Table 30.1. *Etiologic factors in cervicocephalic arterial dissections*

Trauma
  Definite – 'traumatic dissections'
  Trivial – many cases of 'spontaneous dissections'

Arterial disease
  Direct evidence
    Fibromuscular dysplasia
    Cystic medial necrosis
    Known heritable connective tissue disorders
    Marfan syndrome
    Type IV Ehlers–Danlos syndrome
    Osteogenesis imperfecta
    Pseudoxanthoma elasticum

  Indirect evidence
    Abnormal or deficient elastin or fibrillin in cultured dermal
      fibroblasts
    Multivessel dissections
    Higher incidence of intracranial aneurysms in patients with
      ICA dissections
    Familial occurrence of ICA dissections and intracranial
      aneurysms
    Familial occurrence of ICA dissections
    High prevalence of ICA dissections and cerebral aneurysms
      in siblings of patients with ICA dissections
    Possible role of a disorder of the neural crest
      Familial occurrence of bicuspid aortic valve and arterial
        dissections
      Occurrence of a familial syndrome of arterial dissections
        with lentiginosis
    α_1-Antitrypsin deficiency
    Migraine
    Recent infection
    Arterial redundancy
    Hypertension

Note: ICA, internal carotid artery.

leading cause of blunt injury to the ICA and traumatic ICA dissections (Mokri et al., 1988b; New & Momose, 1969; Scherman & Tucker, 1982) (Table 30.2).

Traumatic dissections of the VA are primarily related to injuries associated with rotations of the neck rather than to flexion and extension. With forceful, sudden, or extreme rotations, the artery may be distorted (i) by skeletal muscle and fascial bends at the junction of the first and second portions of the VA; (ii) by adjacent osteophytes as the artery travels upward in the transverse foramina, particularly at C4–5 and C5–6; and (iii) by the sliding motion of the atlantoaxial joint (Fig. 30.7). Chiropractic manipulations, therefore, tend to cause more vertebral artery traumas and dissections than ICA dissections (Table 30.3). Mechanical

Table 30.2. *Cause of injury sustained by 18 patients with traumatic dissection of the internal carotid*

Cause of injury	Number of cases
Motor vehicle accident	11
Automobile accident	10
Cycle accident	1
Sports accident	3
Football	1
Waterskiing	1
Skydiving	1
Other causes	4
Ear surgery[a]	1
Fistfight	1
Fall, blunt injury to lateral aspect of neck	1
Neck injury while handling cattle	1

Note:

[a] Injury caused during attempts to stop unexpected bleeding; however, there was no penetrating injury to the carotid artery.

Source: From Mokri et al. (1988b). By permission of the American Association of Neurological Surgeons.

torsion and stretch that occur with neck rotation are more prominent at C1–2 levels than others, explaining why dissections produced by chiropractic manipulations usually occur at this level (Hart, 1988).

Intracranial arteries obviously are more protected against such traumas.

Histologic examinations in some of the patients with definitely traumatic arterial dissections have shown evidence of a primary arterial disease, likely rendering the blood vessel more susceptible to development of dissection (Mokri et al., 1997b).

Trivial trauma

Many patients with cervicocephalic arterial dissections give history of minimal or trivial trauma. A variety of traumas such as forceful coughing, sports activities, blowing the nose, sexual activity, sustained head turning, sleeping with head in awkward position, prolonged neck extension (painting a ceiling, working under a car), etc. have been reported (Hart & Easton, 1983; Saver & Easton, 1998). Some of the reported events may be of no clinical

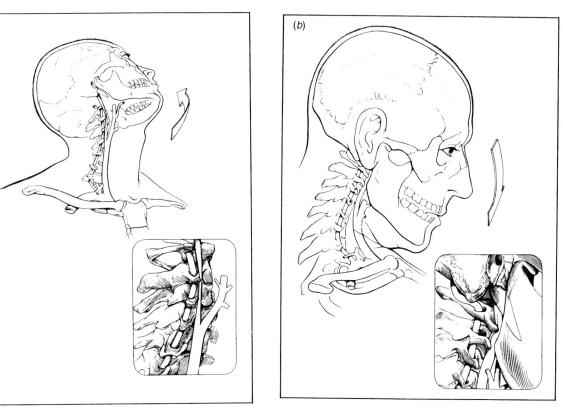

Fig. 30.6. (*a*) Hyperextension and rotation of the neck may cause stretching of the cervical segment of the internal carotid artery against the transverse processes of C2 and C3 (stretch injury). (*b*) Severe neck flexion may compress the internal carotid artery directly between the upper cervical vertebrae and angle of the mandible (impingement injury). (From Zelenock et al., 1982. By permission of the American Medical Association.)

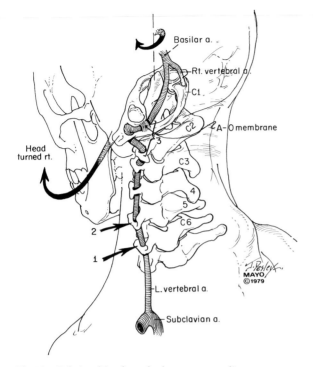

Fig. 30.7. Relationship of vertebral artery to osteoligamentous structures of the neck. The artery might be compressed or distorted by skeletal muscles and fasciobends at the junction of its first and second portions, two osteophytes in the transverse foramina, particularly at C4 to C6, and free sliding motion of the atlantoaxioid joint. A-O, atlanto-occipital. (From Krueger & Okazaki, 1980. By permission of Mayo Foundation.)

Table 30.3. *Associated trauma in 20 patients (21 episodes) with vertebral artery dissection*

Associated trauma[a]	Number
Chiropractic neck manipulation	8
Fell and caught neck while getting into a car	1
Neck stretched and pressed in a magnetic resonance imaging scanner	1
Slept in an unusual position on a couch	1
Fell while cross-country skiing and then hyperextended neck at movie for 2 hours	1
Fell headfirst into snow while sledding	1
Strained neck playing volleyball and on a waterslide	1
During injection for angiography	1
Neck hyperextended for a long period	1
Hypextension of the neck at work	1
During aerobics with vigorous head turn	1
Ski accident	1
Struck on the back of the neck with a piece of lumber	1
During climax of sexual intercourse	1

Note:
[a] Trivial or otherwise.
Source: From Hicks et al. (1994). By permission of the American Academy of Ophthalmology.

significance, while others might have played an etiologic role, especially when coupled with presence of an underlying arterial disease which could subject the vessel to the development of dissection.

Arterial disease

Direct evidence of arterial disease

Angiographic evidence of fibromuscular dysplasia or histologic evidence of cystic medial necrosis has been noted in some of the patients with cervicocephalic arterial dissections (Boström & Liliequist, 1967; Brice & Crompton, 1964; O'Dwyer et al., 1980; Thapedi et al., 1970). Up to 15% of the patients with ICA dissections have angiographic changes of FMD in carotid, vertebral, or renal arteries (Anderson et al., 1980; Garcia-Merino et al., 1983; Kramer, 1969; Mokri et al., 1986; Ringel et al., 1977). Some patients with known genetic disorders of collagen and elastin (Marfan's syndrome, type IV Ehlers–Danlos syndrome, osteogenesis imperfecta, and pseudoxanthoma elasticum) have developed cervical artery dissections (Schievink et al., 1994a).

Indirect evidence

Presence of abnormality or deficiency of elastin or fibrillin or both in cultured dermal fibroblasts of some of the patients with spontaneous cervical artery dissections (Mokri et al., 1994), and occurrence of multivessel dissections (unilateral or bilateral ICA dissections plus unilateral or bilateral VA dissections with renal artery or other visceral artery dissections) (Mokri et al., 1985, 1991) suggest the presence of an underlying arterial disease. Furthermore, there is higher incidence of intracranial aneurysms in patients with ICA dissections (Schievink et al., 1992), familial association of intracranial aneurysms and cervical artery dissections (Schievink et al., 1991), and familial occurrence of spontaneous ICA dissections (Mokri et al., 1987), which all point to a possibility of an underlying arterial disease that at least in some cases may be familial. Furthermore, a disorder of neural crest may play a role in pathogenesis of some of the patients with ICA dissections. There is familial occurrence of spontaneous ICA dissections and congenitally bicuspid aortic valve (Schievink & Mokri, 1995), and also occurrence of a familial syndrome of arterial dissections, and lentiginosis (Schievink et al., 1995). Neural crest has a significant role in early cardiac development, and melanocytes and the media of the aorta and muscularis of cervicocephalic arteries are of neural crest origin (Le Douarin, 1982; Le Lievre & Le Douarin, 1975). Experimentally, a correlation has been found between neural crest lesions and abnormalities of collagen and elastin in the arterial wall (Rosenquist et al., 1990).

α_1-Antitrypsin plays a crucial role in maintaining the integrity of connective tissues. A deficiency of this enzyme has been observed in a few patients with intracranial aneurysms and with cervical artery dissections (Schievink et al., 1994).

The pathogenetic role of migraine remains unsettled. Some studies have shown a significantly higher incidence of migraine in patients with ICA dissections (D'Anglejan-Chatillon et al., 1989).

Recent infection has been blamed by some authors as a trigger factor in pathogenesis of cervical artery dissections (Grau et al., 1997).

Redundancy of ICAs with the presence of coils, loops, or kinks is significantly higher in patients with ICA dissections (Barbour et al., 1994). The role of hypertension remains unsettled, and the role of cigarette smoking and the use of contraceptives has not been substantiated. Atherosclerosis does not seem to be a risk factor. Indeed the disease is less common in the older atherosclerotic patients.

Age and sex

Spontaneous ICA and VA dissections occur most frequently in the middle-aged or younger persons. The overall mean age for spontaneous ICA dissections is in the mid 40's and for the spontaneous VA dissections is in the very low 40's. Some reports point to a slightly higher incidence in men and others to a slightly higher incidence in women, and some point to no significant sex preponderance (Mokri, 1997b). Basically, there is no significant or meaningful sex difference. Overall, approximately 70% of the patients are younger than 50 years, there is no significant sex preponderance, and the mean age of the women as a group is a few years less than that of the men. Less than 5% of the patients are younger than 30 years, and only 8% are older than 60 years (Mokri, 1997a). This 'window of vulnerability' from age 30 to 60 years has been persistent in our patient population throughout the years with a peak incidence at the fifth decade of life.

Spontaneous cervicocephalic arterial dissections in the pediatric age group (18 years or younger) are rare. In the Mayo Clinic series, this accounted for less than 5% of the group (Schievink et al., 1994c). The intracranial arterial dissections are relatively more common in children and adolescents than in adults. The data on the traumatic dissections are less clear and understandably more susceptible to doubt and criticism. In our series, the mean age of the patients with traumatic ICA dissections was approximately 32 years (Mokri et al., 1988b), and two-thirds were men. For traumatic vertebral artery dissections, the mean age has been in mid 30's, and males have somewhat predominated (Hicks et al., 1994).

The number of patients with intracranial dissections (intracranial segment of the vertebral artery excluded) is too small to allow a meaningful statement regarding age and gender distribution. However, since intracranial dissections are relatively more common in the pediatric age group, they display a somewhat younger mean age as a group.

Clinical manifestations

Spontaneous ICA dissections

Initial manifestations and overall manifestations of the disease based on data from 190 patients (with 225 ICAs involved by dissection) seen at the Mayo Clinic are summarized in Tables 30.4 and 30.5.

Although the manifestations may vary, most of the patients with spontaneous ICA dissections present with one of the following syndromes:

(i)   Hemicranial and ipsilateral oculosympathetic palsy (OSP) (Mokri et al., 1979; West et al., 1976).

(ii) Hemicranial and delayed focal cerebral ischemic symptoms (transient ischemic attacks, stroke or both) (Hart & Easton, 1983; Mokri, 1977b; Saver & Easton, 1998; Mokri et al., 1986).

(iii) A syndrome of hemicrania and lower cranial nerve palsies (Mokri et al., 1992, 1996).

Furthermore, the following ought to be recognized:

(i)   Overlap or any combination of above three syndromes may occur.

(ii) More than one-fifth of all the patients also report a subjective bruit (pulsatile swishing noise in the ear, matching the heart beat).

(iii) In a significant minority of the patients (more than 13% in our series), ICA dissections may occur asymptomatically, being detected in the course of an evaluation for a contralateral ICA dissection or a VA dissection. The asymptomatic dissection may be noted as a residuum of a remote dissection or as a recent and concurrent dissection.

Table 30.4. *Initial manifestations in 196 symptomatic spontaneous dissections of the internal carotid artery (of 190 patients)*

	Number	%
Headache and/or face pain	123	63
Focal cerebral ischemic symptoms	41	21
Subjective bruit	8	4
Neck pain	7	4
Amaurosis fugax	6	3
Lower cranial nerve palsies	4	2
Syncope	3	
Ocular motor palsies	2	
Oculosympathetic palsy	1	
Scintillating scotomas	1	

Source: From Mokri (1997b). By permission of Lippincott Williams & Wilkins.

(iv) Monosymptomatic presentations (headache only, neck pain only, bruit only, OSP only, etc) or minimally symptomatic cases are not rare, yet most simply used to go undiagnosed. Nowadays some of them are diagnosed thanks to increasing reliability, availability, and utility of non-invasive neuroimaging techniques.

As noted in Tables 30.4 and 30.5, pain (headache, neck pain, or face pain) is the most common manifestation of the disease (as the initial symptom in more than two-thirds of the patients and as one of the overall symptoms in more than 80% of the patients).

Although the dissection is in the cervical segment of the artery, the neck pain which is typically in the anterolateral aspect of the neck on one side is much less common than headache. The headache is typically focal and unilateral (Silbert et al., 1995). When unilateral, it is always ipsilateral to the involved ICA. The most common headache is focal unilateral frontal/orbital/periorbital pain (Table 30.6).

Focal cerebral ischemic manifestations (TIAs or stroke or both) occur in approximately two-thirds of the symptomatic patients. Typically, but not always, they occur following a unilateral headache after a delay period which may range from minutes to several days or even longer. The mechanism of the focal ischemic event in the majority of cases is likely embolic (artery to artery embolization), but in some it is hemodynamic and related to tight stenosis or occlusion of the involved ICA.

OSP or incomplete Horner's syndrome occurs in more than one-third of the patients. Ipsilateral anhidrosis is absent except for a limited area of anhidrosis in the ipsilateral forehead.

Cranial nerve palsies occur in approximately 10% of the

Table 30.5. *Clinical manifestations in 225 spontaneous dissections of the internal carotid artery (of 190 patients)*

	Number	% of all cases	% of all symptomatic cases
Headache and/or face pain	141	63	72
Focal cerebral ischemic symptoms	121	54	62
Oculosympathetic palsy	71	32	36
Subjective bruit	42	19	21
Objective bruit	35	16	18
Neck pain	35	16	18
Asymptomatic[a]	29	13	
Cranial nerve palsies	23	10	12
Lower cranial nerve palsies	10		
Cranial nerve V palsy	7		
Ocular motor palsies	5		
Palsy of nerve chorda tympani	3		
Cranial nerve VIII palsy	1		
Ischemic optic neuropathy	1		
Amaurosis fugax	22	10	11
Syncope	11	5	5.5
Scalp tenderness	9	4	4.5
Dysgeusia[b]	8	3.5	4
Neck swelling	4		
Scintillating scotomas	4		

Notes:
[a] Detected during workup for a contralateral dissection of the internal carotid artery or a vertebral artery dissection, or detected as a concomitant dissection residual of a remote dissection.
[b] Includes some patients with lower cranial nerve palsies.
Source: From Mokri (1997b). By permission of Lippincott Williams & Wilkins.

patients (Mokri et al., 1996). Lower cranial nerve palsies, particularly 12th nerve palsy, are the most common. These palsies are always ipsilateral to the involved ICA. The mechanism of the palsies is a likely compromise of the nutrient arteries of the involved cranial nerves rather than mechanical stretch or compression of the nerves (Mokri et al., 1996).

Migraine and ICA dissection
Several issues surround migraine and ICA dissection.
(i) ICA dissection may mimic migraine or resemble 'migraine stroke.'

Table 30.6. *Location of headache in
60 patients with spontaneous dissection of
the internal carotid artery*

	Number	%
Diffuse bilateral	3	5
Diffuse unilateral	6	10
Focal unilateral	51	85
Orbital/periorbital	36	60
Ear, mastoid process	23	38
Frontal	22	37
Temporal	16	27
Angle of mandible	8	13
Lateral nose, midfacial	6	10
Occipital	5	8

Source: From Mokri (1997b). By permission of
Lippincott Williams & Wilkins.

(ii) Sometimes patients may report development of migraine headaches or resolution or improvement of migraine headaches following ICA dissections (Silbert et al., 1995).

(iii) Migraine has been considered as a risk factor predisposing the ICA to the development of dissection (D'Anglejan-Chatillon et al., 1989).

Hypertension and ICA dissection

A higher incidence of hypertension has been reported in some of the series of ICA dissections (Mokri et al., 1986). Patients with ICA dissection who show hypertension fall in one of the following three groups: (i) patients with previously known hypertension, (ii) patients who are found to be hypertensive at the time of evaluation of dissection and remain hypertensive, (iii) patients without a history of hypertension who are found to be hypertensive at the time of the dissection and remain hypertensive for some time, up to a few months and sometimes requiring treatment. Later, they become normotensive and remain so, even without use of antihypertensive medications.

Traumatic ICA dissections

The clinical manifestations of traumatic ICA dissections are essentially the same as spontaneous dissections, but the circumstances of trauma may modify the overall clinical picture, create diagnostic problems, and even derail the clinician to entirely miss the diagnosis. The following points are important to keep in mind.

(i) Focal brain ischemic symptoms may develop immediately after the accident or be delayed for hours,

Table 30.7. *Time intervals between accident and onset of
symptoms in 18 patients with traumatic dissection of the
internal carotid artery*

Interval	Number of cases	Accident to onset of symptoms	
		Time range	Mean time
Immediately	3		
Hours	6	0.5–18	7
Days	3	3, 4, 20	
Months	2	2, 3	
Years	4	6.5–14	9

Source: From Mokri et al. (1988b). By permission of the American Association of Neurological Surgeons.

days, or weeks. Sometimes a traumatic dissecting aneurysm may be left behind, and this may lead to embolization and focal brain ischemic symptoms even years after the accident (Table 30.7).

(ii) As the result of the injury (motor vehicle accident is one of the most common causes of traumatic ICA dissections), patients might have other injuries including multiorgan visceral injuries and head injury and may even be in coma. In such cases the diagnosis may be delayed or completely missed. Focal neurologic deficits may easily be attributed to 'head trauma' or 'contusion.' Adequate utilization and interpretation of neuroimaging and vascular imaging studies and their careful correlations with the clinical observations should be helpful to establish the diagnosis.

(iii) In about one-half of the patients with traumatic ICA dissections (despite presence of multiorgan injury in some of the patients), signs of direct injury to the neck may be absent (Yamada et al., 1967). Furthermore, in many of those who do have such signs, only mild abrasions or bruises of the neck area may be noted. Some of the patients may have fractures of mandible, neck, or skull base. Some may have suffered laryngeal trauma.

Despite relatively high frequency of cervical trauma, fortunately, damage to the cervical ICA as the result of blunt injury is surprisingly uncommon.

Spontaneous VA dissections

Pain, often an occipital headache or posterior neck pain or both, is the most common clinical manifestation and the most common initial symptom of vertebral artery dissections. Headache has been reported in 50 to 86% of the patients (Silbert et al., 1995; Caplan et al., 1985; Chiras et

Table 30.8. *Clinical manifestations in 25 patients with spontaneous dissection of the vertebral artery*

Findings (subtotal)	Number of patients
Headache with or without neck pain, with delayed (5 hr–2 wk) ischemic symptoms in VB distribution	13
Brainstem stroke	10
LMS	3
LMS plus[a]	5
Non-specific[b]	2
VB TIA	3
VB distribution transient ischemic symptoms associated with or followed by headache with or without neck pain	3
TIA	3
Ischemic symptoms alone	4
Stroke	2
TIA	1
Both	1
Other	2
Focal unilateral headache	1
Severe occipital headache and stiffness (SAH)	1
Asymptomatic (symptoms related to ICA dissection)	3

Notes:

ICA, internal carotid artery; LMS, lateral medullary syndrome; SAH, subarachnoid hemorrhage; TIA, transient ischemic attack; VB, vertebrobasilar.

[a] One or more of the following: hemiparesis, diplopia, brief loss of consciousness, facial weakness, unilateral tinnitus.

[b] Quadriplegia, decerebrate posturing, pinpoint pupils, ocular bobbing, and bilateral cranial nerve deficits in one patient; hemiparesis, cranial nerve deficits, cerebellar signs, and homonymous visual field defect in the other patient.

Source: From Mokri et al. (1988a). By permission of the American Academy of Neurology.

al., 1985; Hinse et al., 1991; Mas et al., 1987; Mokri et al., 1988a). It is often unilateral but can be bilateral.

Focal brain ischemic symptoms occur in the distribution of vertebrobasilar system (Caplan et al., 1985; Chiras et al., 1985; Hinse et al., 1991; Mas et al., 1987; Mokri et al., 1988a). Sometimes they occur without headache, but often they follow the headaches after a delayed period of time. Less commonly, they occur in conjunction with the headaches or rarely may precede the headache. Clinical manifestations in 25 patients with spontaneous VA dissections are listed in Table 30.8. Sometimes VA dissections may extend to the basilar artery or cause basilar artery thrombosis with serious consequences.

In contrast with spontaneous ICA dissections, it is not unusual for spontaneous VA dissections to involve the intracranial segment of the vessel or extend from extracranial VA to the intracranial VA. Since the media of the vessel intracranially is attenuated, intracranial dissections may cause subarachnoid hemorrhage (Caplan et al., 1988; Alom et al., 1986) while extracranial dissections rarely, if ever, rupture.

Similar to ICA dissections, VA dissections may occur asymptomatically or be monosymptomatic or minimally symptomatic.

A rare but interesting manifestation of VA dissection is myelopathy or cervical radiculopathy (Pullicino, 1994; Bergqvist et al., 1997; Hundsberger et al., 1998). Among 110 patients with VA dissections seen at the Mayo Clinic (Crum & Mokri, 1998), 2 had these findings: – 1 had C5-6 radiculopathy, and 1 had upper thoracic myelopathy.

Vertebrobasilar ischemic symptoms in VA dissections may be unilateral or bilateral or be related to dysfunction of brain stem, occipital lobes, cerebellum, or any combination of these. Sometimes basilar artery thrombosis may occur secondarily, or, rarely, dissection of the VA may extend to the basilar artery. The most common defined clinical syndrome is a lateral medullary syndrome (Wallenberg's syndrome). Occurrence of lateral medullary syndrome in a young person, especially when preceded by a posterior headache or neck pain, should strongly suggest VA dissection (Mokri, 1994; Caplan et al., 1985).

Traumatic VA dissections

Similar to ICA dissections, the patients may have had severe multiorgan trauma or be comatose. Some may have cervical fractures. These factors may introduce elements of delay and confusion in diagnosis. However, chiropractic manipulations, the most commonly reported trauma in connection with VA dissections (Krueger & Okazaki, 1980; Hicks et al., 1994; Mehalic & Farhat, 1974; Okawara & Nibbelink, 1974), ordinarily are not associated with other types of trauma, and the diagnosis should be uncomplicated. Presentations of such traumatic dissections of the vertebral artery are similar to the spontaneous ones.

Intracranial dissections

Intracranial arteries have attenuated and much thinner medial layers. Therefore, all intracranial dissections carry the risk of subarachnoid hemorrhage.

Intracranial VA dissections

The intracranial segment of the VAs is the most common intracranial artery involved by dissection. Indeed, a significant minority of VA dissections are only intracranial. Furthermore, extracranial dissections may extend intracranially. Sometimes, angiographic studies may show intracranial dissection in one vertebral artery and extracranial dissection in the other. In the same patient sometimes both VAs show intracranial or extracranial plus intracranial dissections. The clinical manifestations of intracranial VA dissections are identical to those of extracranial dissections, except that intracranial dissections may cause subarachnoid hemorrhage (Caplan et al., 1988; Alom et al., 1986). Some of the patients present either with the clinical picture of subarachnoid hemorrhage or subarachnoid hemorrhage plus ischemic manifestations in the vertebrobasilar distribution.

Intracranial ICA dissection

In contrast with intracranial VA dissections, intracranial ICA dissections are uncommon (Chang et al., 1975; Giedke et al., 1975; Hochberg et al., 1975; Nass et al., 1982; Pessin et al., 1989). Such dissections may occur merely intracranially, or as an intracranial extension of an extracranial ICA dissection. The dissection may extend to the MCA and cause stenosis or occlusion of this vessel. Clinical manifestations are similar to extracranial ICA dissections, but the intracranial dissections carry risk of subarachnoid hemorrhage. Headache is the most common clinical presentation. Hemiparesis is common and when the artery on the dominant side is involved, dysphasia is noted. Some of the patients, especially the children and adolescents, may also develop seizures.

Basilar artery and other intracranial artery dissections

These dissections are rare (Pozzati et al., 1995; Alexander et al., 1979; Berger & Wilson, 1984; Berkovic et al., 1983; Hayman & Anderson, 1966; Hosoda et al., 1991). Subarachnoid hemorrhage may occur but only in a significant minority of the patients. Basilar artery dissection may involve only this vessel, or it may be an extension of dissection from one of the VA. Furthermore, basilar artery dissection itself may extend distally to the posterior cerebral or superior cerebellar arteries.

Dissections of the middle cerebral artery (Sasaki et al., 1991; Grosman et al., 1980) may also occur in isolation or may be the result of extension of dissection from an intracranial ICA. Similarly, posterior cerebral artery dissection may occur in isolation or as extension of dissection from the basilar artery (Berger & Wilson, 1984; Maillo et al., 1991). The clinical manifestation in all of these dissections may include focal cerebral ischemic manifestations in the distribution of the involved vessel with or without head-

Table 30.9. *Angiographic findings in 90 internal carotid arteries (of 70 patients) with spontaneous dissection and 29 (of 21 patients) with traumatic dissection*

| | Group | | | |
| | Spontaneous | | Traumatic | |
Angiographic findings	Number	%	Number	%
Luminal stenosis	69	77	13	45
Aneurysm	35	39	17	59
Intimal flaps	25	28	7	24
Slow ICA–MCA flow	22	24	3	10
Occlusion	15	17	8	28
Distal branch occlusions (emboli)	11	12	3	10

Notes: ICA, internal carotid artery; MCA, middle cerebral artery.

ache and with or without manifestations of subarachnoid hemorrhage. Because of its size and the magnitude and nature of its territory, basilar artery dissection may cause profound and serious neurologic deficits. In cerebral artery dissections, dense focal neurologic deficits and seizures are not uncommon. Sometimes these intracranial dissections may present merely as a subarachnoid hemorrhage.

Diagnostic studies

Cerebral angiography

ICA dissections

Common angiographic abnormalities in ICA dissections include luminal stenosis (usually irregular, elongated, and tapered) (Fig. 30.1(b)), dissecting aneurysms (Fig. 30.4(b)), abrupt or fairly abrupt reconstitution of the lumen distal end of the dissection (Fig. 30.1(b), upper arrow), intimal flaps (Fig. 30.3(b), arrows), slow ICA-middle cerebral artery flow, occlusion (usually beginning about 1 to 2 cm above the bifurcation and tapering to a complete occlusion with a flame-like or radish-tail appearance) (Fig. 30.2(b) and (c), and distal branch occlusions (a sign of distal embolization) (Fisher et al., 1978; Houser et al., 1984). The frequencies of these angiographic abnormalities for spontaneous and traumatic ICA dissections are listed in Table 30.9. In traumatic ICA dissections, aneurysms and occlusions are somewhat more frequent, and in spontaneous dissections luminal stenoses appear relatively more common.

VA dissections

The common angiographic features of vertebral artery dissections include stenosis (often elongated, irregular, and

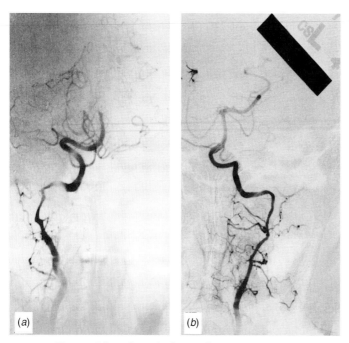

Fig. 30.8. Bilateral vertebral artery dissection. (*a*) and (*b*) Vertebral arteriograms. Note elongated, tapered, and irregular stenoses. From Mokri et al., 1988a. By permission of the American Academy of Neurology.)

Table 30.10. *Angiographic findings in 25 patients with spontaneous dissections of the vertebral artery (involving 35 arteries)*

	Vertebral arteries	
	Number	%
Stenosis (often irregular and tapered)	28	80
Stenosis only	25	
Stenosis + dissecting aneurysm	2	
Stenosis + intraluminal clot	1	
Level of stenosis		
C1–2 segment	17	
C1–2 segment + distal intradural segment[a]	6	
Distal intradural segment	4	
Proximal vertebral	1	
Aneurysm	5	14
Fusiform, just proximal or distal to level of dural penetration	3	
Saccular, midcervical	2	
Occlusion	4	11
At C1–2 level	2	
Proximal	2	
Intimal flap only	1	

Note:
[a] Extending to basilar artery in 1 patient.
Source: From Mokri et al. (1988a). By permission of the American Academy of Neurology.

sometimes tapered), dissecting aneurysms, occlusion, and intimal flaps (Table 30.10) (Figs. 30.8 and 30.9).

Basilar artery and other intracranial artery dissections

Basilar artery dissection on angiogram may appear as an elongated stenosis, double lumen, dissecting aneurysm or occlusion (Pozzati et al., 1995; Alexander et al., 1979; Berger & Wilson, 1984; Berkovic et al., 1983; Hayman & Anderson, 1966; Hosoda et al., 1991). Dissections of the smaller vessels such as posterior cerebral arteries or middle cerebral arteries have a much less specific angiographic appearance. Typically, a nonspecific segment of stenosis or an occlusion is seen. The stenosis may or may not show luminal irregularities or may or may not be associated with areas of luminal expansion or dilatation (Sasaki et al., 1991; Grosman et al., 1980; Maillo et al., 1991). It is not unusual that entities such as 'vasculitis' or meningeal infection or inflammation (supposedly compressing from outside and compromising the integrity of the lumen) enter into the differential diagnosis. Overall, often it becomes visually impossible to make an angiographic diagnosis of dissection in these small vessels with a reasonable certainty.

Magnetic resonance imaging (MRI) and angiography (MRA)

MRI and MRA are emerging as extremely useful diagnostic tests. The techniques and quality of images have steadily improved. With modern MRA techniques (such as bolus gadolinium injection), stenoses, some of the luminal irregularities, and many of the aneurysms can be seen. More subtle luminal irregularities and small aneurysmal dilatations could be missed when compared with high-quality conventional arteriograms. Cross-sectional MR images at the level of dissection frequently reveal specific MRI abnormalities consisting of a dark small circle of flow void (which is smaller than the normal calibre of the original lumen) representing the narrowed lumen. This is surrounded by a bright hyperintense crescent-shaped or donut-shaped zone that represents the intramural hematoma (Fig. 30.1(*d*)). The MRI abnormalities which could be quite specific can be seen in internal carotid artery, vertebral artery, and basilar artery dissections. However, for the smaller intracranial vessels, the diagnostic role of MRI and MRA remains limited, and the diagnosis of these dissections remains a challenge.

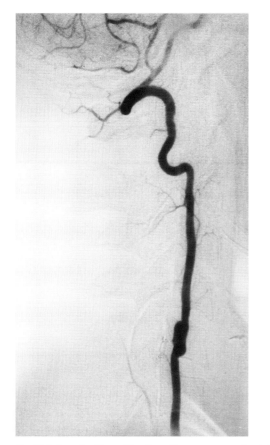

Fig. 30.9. Saccular finger-like dissecting aneurysm of vertebral artery at C5 level.

Doppler sonography

This is a simple and non-invasive technique (Sturzenegger et al., 1995; Hennerici et al., 1989). It has fairly limited value in diagnosis of ICA dissections and is even less helpful in vertebral artery dissections. It can be useful in monitoring the evolution and resolution of ICA dissections.

Treatment

Patients with cervicocephalic arterial dissections have been treated in a variety of ways, including symptomatic management and observation, antiplatelet therapy, anticoagulant therapy, surgical treatments, and placement of stents (Hart & Easton, 1983; Mokri, 1994, 1997b; Saver & Easton, 1998; Bogousslavsky et al., 1987). No controlled studies have been done to address the efficacy of any of these treatment modalities. The focal brain ischemic symptoms that may occur in these patients are likely embolic in the majority but are hemodynamic in a significant minority. Most

patients, especially those with extracranial dissections, do well regardless of the treatment that is administered. Mortality is fortunately uncommon for extracranial dissections that constitute the large majority of the patients with cervicocephalic arterial dissections. Many of these patients never develop strokes. Therefore, it is difficult to address with a high degree of confidence the feasibility and effectiveness of various treatment modalities.

Anticoagulation therapy

This treatment is expected to reduce the likelihood of stroke in patients with cervicocephalic arterial dissections. Sometimes stroke is the initial manifestation of the disease, but frequently, especially for extracranial dissections, it may be delayed for hours, days, or weeks after the onset of the initial manifestations. When there is a residual dissecting aneurysm, particularly in traumatic extracranial dissections, there is a risk of embolization even years later. At the time of diagnosis of recent dissections in patients without cerebral ischemic manifestations, it would be very difficult if not virtually impossible to predict which patient will or will not develop TIAs or stroke, minutes, hours, days, or weeks later. Therefore, one common practice has been to treat the patients with anticoagulants for about three months and follow by antiplatelet therapy for another three months (Hart & Easton, 1983). In urgent cases, initially treatment with heparin is started with a subsequent switch to warfarin. When a patient with dissection is diagnosed several weeks during the course of his illness and has not exhibited any cerebral ischemic symptoms, some physicians prefer to treat the patients with antiplatelet agents only and continue with observation.

Because intracranial dissections are associated with a risk of subarachnoid hemorrhage (sometimes as high as 20%, depending upon the involved vessel), anticoagulation therapy of intracranial dissections will call for far more caution than hesitation. Despite the power of the modern neuroimaging techniques, many have recommended a spinal fluid examination in these patients before initiation of anticoagulation therapy to make certain of the absence of subarachnoid hemorrhage (Saver & Easton, 1998). Anticoagulation therapy is contraindicated in subarachnoid hemorrhage or in hemorrhagic infarction (an unusual event in cervicocephalic arterial dissections). Furthermore, this treatment is not advised when there is massive brain infarct.

Surgical treatments

For the management of dissections and dissecting aneurysms, a number of surgical procedures have been carried out (Mokri, 1997b) including removal of the intramural hematoma, resection of the involved segment of the vessel with interposition of vein graft, graduated luminal dilatation, surgical resection of a residual dissecting aneurysm of extracranial arteries, repair, clipping, or wrapping of intracranial dissecting aneurysms, resection of cerebral artery (such as MCA) dissecting aneurysm with restoration of distal blood flow through bypass procedures, and STA-MCA bypass. The enthusiasm for surgical intervention, however, has decreased.

We have not attempted removal of intramural clots but have seen patients who developed carotid occlusions after such attempts. Although enthusiasm for surgical intervention has decreased, limited indications remain including: (i) when there is residual dissecting aneurysm that has been a source of embolization and when this aneurysm is technically accessible to resection (Sundt et al., 1986); (ii) when there is subarachnoid hemorrhage from a leaking intracranial dissection or dissecting aneurysm if technically feasible and if the patient's overall status would allow, and (iii) dissection that has caused tight stenosis of the ICA and recurrent hemodynamic focal cerebral ischemic manifestations, in which case an ipsilateral superficial temporal artery-middle cerebral artery bypass can restore adequate circulation and 'buy time' until the dissection is healed and the vessel is recanalized (Mokri, 1994). When this occurs, the bypass may become non-functional.

Placement of stents

This is a promising technique (Perez-Cruet et al., 1997; Mase et al., 1995; Marotta et al., 1998; Halbach et al., 1993; Lefkowitz et al., 1996). It allows immediate restoration of the true arterial lumen and decreases the size of the dissecting aneurysms that on follow-up angiography reveal continued improvement.

Outcome

For the VA dissections and extracranial ICA dissections, the prognosis is typically good. Although some patients die, considering the broad spectrum of clinical presentation, the asymptomatic cases and monosymptomatic or minimally symptomatic cases, the overall mortality rate is decidedly less than 5%. More than three-fourths of the patients have complete or excellent recoveries. Less than 5% are left with marked neurologic deficits (Hart & Easton, 1983; Mokri, 1994, 1997b; Saver & Easton, 1998). Angiographically on follow-up, over three-fourths of the stenoses either improve or completely resolve, and most

dissecting aneurysms become smaller or resolve. If an artery is completely occluded, it can recanalize but very infrequently. In about 90% of cases, such arteries remain occluded.

The outcome for the traumatic ICA dissections is somewhat different from the spontaneous ones. In traumatic dissections, although prognosis is still good, significantly fewer aneurysms resolve or become smaller, and fewer stenoses resolve or improve while more stenoses tend to progress to occlusion. Traumatic ICA dissections are more likely to leave the patients with neurologic deficits. Although extracranial ICA dissections whether spontaneous or traumatic mostly carry a good prognosis, the outcome for the traumatic group is less favourable (Mokri, 1990).

For intracranial dissections, the prognosis is less favourable. Of ten basilar artery dissecting aneurysms reported by Pozzati et al. (1995), six had presented with subarachnoid hemorrhage and four with ischemic brainstem manifestations. One died of subarachnoid hemorrhage, two remained severely disabled, three had residual neurologic deficits, and only four were in good clinical condition. Intracranial ICA-middle cerebral artery and other cerebral artery dissections also carry prognoses that are much less favourable than cervical arterial dissections. All may cause subarachnoid hemorrhage. Although difficulty in establishing a diagnosis of intracranial cerebral artery dissection and lack of specific angiographic findings have likely biased the reported cases towards the fatal cases (particularly in the older literature) (Grosman et al., 1980), it is generally believed that these dissections carry a significantly less favourable prognosis than extracranial dissections with higher rates of mortality and morbidity.

Recurrence

Recurrence of dissection in a previously dissected and healed cervical artery can occur but is very rare. What is usually noted is occurrence of dissection in other cervical arteries or in the renal arteries of the same patient.

Intracranial dissections are not frequent enough to allow follow-up of a cohort of reasonable size for study. Besides, many such dissections cannot be diagnosed antemortem with certainty due to their often nonspecific angiographic appearance.

For vertebral and extracranial ICA dissections, the rate of recurrence has been studied (Schievink et al., 1994b; Leys et al., 1995). The risk of recurrence was essentially small. It was maximal for the first month (2%), and subsequently much less (1% per year for all age groups) (Schievink et al.,

1994b). After the fifth decade of life, both rate of occurrence and rate of recurrence of dissection decreased. The 10-year rate of recurrence for all age groups was 12%; for patients younger than 45 years (the mean age of the cohort) the rate was 17%, and for those older than 45 years it was only 6%. Recurrent dissections are likely more frequent in patients who have underlying arterial disease or a family history of arterial dissections (Schievink et al., 1996).

References

Alexander, C.B., Burger, P.C. & Goree, J.A. (1979). Dissecting aneurysms of the basilar artery in 2 patients. *Stroke*, **10**, 294–9.

Alom, J., Matias-Guiu, J., Padro, L., Molins, M., Romero, F. & Codina, A. (1986). Spontaneous dissection of intracranial vertebral artery: clinical recovery with conservative treatment. *Journal of Neurology, Neurosurgery and Psychiatry*, **49**, 599–600.

Andersen, C.A., Collins, G.J. Jr, Rich, N.M. & McDonald, P.T. (1980). Spontaneous dissection of the internal carotid artery associated with fibromuscular dysplasia. *American Surgeon*, **46**, 263–6.

Barbour, P.J., Castaldo, J.E., Rae-Grant, A.D. et al. (1994). Internal carotid artery redundancy is significantly associated with dissection. *Stroke*, **25**, 1201–6.

Berger, M.S. & Wilson, C.B. (1984). Intracranial dissecting aneurysms of the posterior circulation: report of six cases and review of the literature. *Journal of Neurosurgery*, **61**, 882–94.

Bergqvist, C.A., Goldberg, H.I., Thorarensen, O. & Bird, S.J. (1997). Posterior cervical spinal cord infarction following vertebral artery dissection. *Neurology*, **48**, 1112–15.

Berkovic, S.F., Spokes, R.L., Anderson, R.M. & Bladin, P.F. (1983). Basilar artery dissection. *Journal of Neurology, Neurosurgery and Psychiatry*, **46**, 126–9.

Bogousslavsky, J., Despland, P.A. & Regli, F. (1987). Spontaneous carotid dissection with acute stroke. *Archives of Neurology*, **44**, 137–40.

Boström, K. & Liliequist, B. (1967). Primary dissecting aneurysm of the extracranial part of the internal carotid and vertebral arteries. A report of three cases. *Neurology*, **17**, 179–86.

Brice, J.G. & Crompton, M.R. (1964). Spontaneous dissecting aneurysms of the cervical internal carotid artery. *British Medical Journal (Clinical Research edition)*, **2**, 790–2.

Caplan, L.R., Zarins, C.K. & Hemmati, M. (1985). Spontaneous dissection of the extracranial vertebral arteries. *Stroke*, **16**, 1030–8.

Caplan, L.R., Baquis, G.D., Pessin, M.S. et al. (1988). Dissection of the intracranial vertebral artery. *Neurology*, **38**, 868–77.

Chang, V., Rewcastle, N.B., Harwood-Nash, D.C. & Norman, M.G. (1975). Bilateral dissecting aneurysms of the intracranial internal carotid arteries in an 8-year-old boy. *Neurology*, **25**, 573–9.

Chiras, J., Marciano, S., Vega Molina, J., Toubol, J., Poirier, B. & Bories, J. (1985). Spontaneous dissecting aneurysm of the extracranial vertebral artery (20 cases). *Neuroradiology*, **27**, 327–33.

Crum, B.A. & Mokri, B. (1998). Clinical spectrum of vertebral artery dissections: impact of magnetic resonance imaging. *Annals of Neurology*, **44**, 493.

D'Anglejan-Chatillon, J., Ribeiro, V., Mas, J.L., Youl, B.D. & Bousser, M.G. (1989). Migraine – a risk factor for dissection of cervical arteries. *Headache*, **29**, 560–1.

Fisher, C.M., Ojemann, R.G. & Roberson, G.H. (1978). Spontaneous dissection of cervico-cerebral arteries. *Canadian Journal of Neurological Sciences*, **5**, 9–19.

Garcia-Merino, J.A., Gutierrez, J.A., Lopez-Lozano, J.J., Marquez, M., Lopez, F. & Liano, H. (1983). Double lumen dissecting aneurysms of the internal carotid artery in fibromuscular dysplasia: case report. *Stroke*, **14**, 815–8.

Giedke, H., Kriebel, J. & Sindermann, F. (1975). Dissecting aneurysm of the petrous portion of the internal carotid artery. Case report and review of previous cases. *Neuroradiology*, **10**, 121–4.

Giroud, M., Fayolle, H., Andre, N. et al. (1994). Incidence of internal carotid artery dissection in the community of Dijon. *Journal of Neurology, Neurosurgery and Psychiatry*, **57**, 1443.

Grau, A.J., Brandt, T., Forsting, M., Winter, R. & Hacke, W. (1997). Infection-associated cervical artery dissection. *Stroke*, **28**, 453–5.

Grosman, H., Fornasier, V.L., Bonder, D., Livingston, K.E. & Platts, M.E. (1980). Dissecting aneurysm of the cerebral arteries. *Journal of Neurosurgery*, **53**, 693–7.

Halbach, V.V., Higashida, R.T., Dowd, C.F. et al. (1993). Endovascular treatment of vertebral artery dissections and pseudoaneurysms. *Journal of Neurosurgery*, **79**, 183–91.

Hart, R.G. (1988). Vertebral artery dissection (editorial). *Neurology*, **38**, 987–9.

Hart, R.G. & Easton, J.D. (1983). Dissections of cervical and cerebral arteries. *Neurology Clinics*, **1**, 155–82.

Hayman, J.A. & Anderson, R.M. (1966). Dissecting aneurysm of the basilar artery. *Medical Journal of Austria*, **2**, 360–1.

Hennerici, M., Steinke, W. & Rautenberg, W. (1989). High-resistance Doppler flow pattern in extracranial carotid dissection. *Archives of Neurology*, **46**, 670–2.

Hicks, P.A., Leavitt, J.A. & Mokri, B. (1994). Ophthalmic manifestations of vertebral artery dissection. Patients seen at the Mayo Clinic from 1976 to 1992. *Ophthalmology*, **101**, 1786–92.

Hinse, P., Thie, A. & Lachenmayer, L. (1991). Dissection of the extracranial vertebral artery: report of four cases and review of the literature. *Journal of Neurology, Neurosurgery and Psychiatry*, **54**, 863–9.

Hochberg, F.H., Bean, C., Fisher, C.M. & Roberson, G.H. (1975). Stroke in a 15-year-old girl secondary to terminal carotid dissection. *Neurology*, **25**, 725–9.

Hosoda, K., Fujita, S., Kawaguchi, T. et al. (1991). Spontaneous dissecting aneurysms of the basilar artery presenting with a subarachnoid hemorrhage. *Journal of Neurosurgery*, **75**, 628–33.

Houser, O.W., Mokri, B., Sundt, T.M. Jr, Baker, H.L. Jr & Reese, D.F. (1984). Spontaneous cervical cephalic arterial dissection and its residuum: angiographic spectrum. *American Journal of Neuroradiology*, **5**, 27–34.

Hundsberger, T., Thomke, F., Hopf, H.C. & Fitzek, C. (1998). Symmetrical infarction of the cervical spinal cord due to spontaneous bilateral vertebral artery dissection. *Stroke*, **29**, 1742.

Kramer, W. (1969). Fibromuscular hyperplasia and extracranial aneurysm of the internal carotid artery associated with a typical parapharyngeal syndrome [French]. *Revue Neurologique (Paris)*, **120**, 239–44.

Krueger, B.R. & Okazaki, H. (1980). Vertebral-basilar distribution infarction following chiropractic cervical manipulation. *Mayo Clinic Proceedings*, **55**, 322–32.

Le Douarin, N.M. (1982). *The Neural Crest*. Cambridge: Cambridge University Press.

Lefkowitz, M.A., Teitelbaum, G.P. & Giannotta, S.L. (1996). Endovascular treatment of a dissecting posteroinferior cerebellar artery aneurysm: case report. *Neurosurgery*, **39**, 1036–8.

Le Lievre, C.S. & Le Douarin, N.M. (1975). Mesenchymal derivatives of the neural crest: analysis of chimaeric quail and chick embryos. *Journal of Embryology and Experimental Morphology*, **34**, 125–54.

Leys, D., Moulin, T.H., Stojkovic, T., Begey, S. & Chavot, D. (1995). Follow-up of patients with history of cervical artery dissection. *Cerebrovascular Diseases*, **5**, 43–9.

Maillo, A., Diaz, P. & Morales, F. (1991). Dissecting aneurysm of the posterior cerebral artery: spontaneous resolution. *Neurosurgery*, **29**, 291–4.

Marotta, T.R., Buller, C., Taylor, D., Morris, C. & Zwimpfer, T. (1998). Autologous vein-covered stent repair of a cervical internal carotid artery pseudoaneurysm: technical case report. *Neurosurgery*, **42**, 408–12.

Mas, J.L., Bousser, M.G., Hasboun, D. & Laplane, D. (1987). Extracranial vertebral artery dissections: a review of 13 cases. *Stroke*, **18**, 1037–47.

Mase, M., Banno, T., Yamada, K. & Katano, H. (1995). Endovascular stent placement for multiple aneurysms of the extracranial internal carotid artery: technical case report. *Neurosurgery*, **37**, 832–5.

Mehalic, T. & Farhat, S.M. (1974). Vertebral artery injury from chiropractic manipulation of the neck. *Surgical Neurology*, **2**, 125–9.

Mokri, B. (1987). Dissections of cervical and cephalic arteries. In *Occlusive Cerebrovascular Disease: Diagnosis and Surgical Management*, ed. T.M. Sundt, Jr, pp. 38–59. Philadelphia: W.B. Saunders.

Mokri, B. (1990). Traumatic and spontaneous extracranial internal carotid artery dissections. *Journal of Neurology*, **237**, 356–61.

Mokri, B. (1994). Dissections of cervical and cephalic arteries. In *Sundt's Occlusive Cerebrovascular Disease*, 2nd edn, ed. F.B. Meyer, pp. 45–70. Philadelphia: W.B. Saunders.

Mokri, B. (1997a). Spontaneous dissections of cervicocephalic arteries. In *Primer on Cerebrovascular Diseases*, ed. K.M.A. Welch, L.R. Caplan, D.J. Reis, B.O.K. Siesyö & B. Weir, pp. 390–396. San Diego: Academic Press.

Mokri, B. (1997b). Spontaneous dissections of internal carotid arteries. *The Neurologist*, **3**, 104–19.

Mokri, B., Sundt, T.M. Jr & Houser, O.W. (1979). Spontaneous internal carotid dissection, hemicrania, and Horner's syndrome. *Archives of Neurology*, **36**, 677–80.

Mokri, B., Stanson, A.W. & Houser, O.W. (1985). Spontaneous dissections of the renal arteries in a patient with previous sponta-

neous dissections of the internal carotid arteries. *Stroke*, **16**, 959–63.

Mokri, B., Sundt, T.M. Jr, Houser, O.W. & Piepgras, D.G. (1986). Spontaneous dissection of the cervical internal carotid artery. *Annals of Neurology*, **19**, 126–38.

Mokri, B., Piepgras, D.G., Wiebers, D.O. & Houser, O.W. (1987). Familial occurrence of spontaneous dissection of the internal carotid artery. *Stroke*, **18**, 246–51.

Mokri, B., Houser, O.W., Sandok, B.A. & Piepgras, D.G. (1988a). Spontaneous dissections of the vertebral arteries. *Neurology*, **38**, 880–5.

Mokri, B., Piepgras, D.G. & Houser, O.W. (1988b). Traumatic dissections of the extracranial internal carotid artery. *Journal of Neurosurgery*, **68**, 189–97.

Mokri, B., Houser, O.W. & Stanson, A.W. (1991). Multivessel cervicocephalic and visceral arterial dissections: pathogenic role of primary arterial disease in cervicocephalic arterial dissections. *Journal of Stroke and Cerebrovascular Diseases*, **1**, 117–23.

Mokri, B., Schievink, W.I., Olsen, K.D. & Piepgras, D.G. (1992). Spontaneous dissection of the cervical internal carotid artery: presentation with lower cranial nerve palsies. *Archives of Otolaryngology – Head and Neck Surgery*, **118**, 431–5.

Mokri, B., Roche, P.C., O'Brien, J.F., Schievink, W.I. & Piepgras, D.G. (1994). Abnormalities of elastin in spontaneous internal carotid and vertebral artery dissections [abstract]. *Annals of Neurology*, **36**, 263.

Mokri, B., Silbert, P.L., Schievink, W.I. & Piepgras, D.G. (1996). Cranial nerve palsy in spontaneous dissection of the extracranial internal carotid artery. *Neurology*, **46**, 356–9.

Mokri, B., Meyer, F.B. & Piepgras, D.G. (1997). Primary arteriopathy in traumatic cervicocephalic arterial dissections (abstract). *Annals of Neurology*, **42**, 433.

Montalbetti, L., Ferrandi, D., Pergami, P. & Savoldi, F. (1995). Elongated styloid process and Eagle's syndrome. *Cephalalgia*, **15**, 80–93.

Nass, R., Hays, A. & Chutorian, A. (1982). Intracranial dissecting aneurysms in childhood. *Stroke*, **13**, 204–7.

New, P.F. & Momose, K.J. (1969). Traumatic dissection of the internal carotid artery at the atlantoaxial level, secondary to nonpenetrating injury. *Radiology*, **93**, 41–9.

O'Dwyer, J.A., Moscow, N., Trevor, R., Ehrenfeld, W.K. & Newton, T.H. (1980). Spontaneous dissection of the carotid artery. *Radiology*, **137**, 379–85.

Okawara, S. & Nibbelink, D. (1974). Vertebral artery occlusion following hyperextension and rotation of the head. *Stroke*, **5**, 640–2.

Perez-Cruet, M.J., Patwardhan, R.V., Mawad, M.E. & Rose, J.E. (1997). Treatment of dissecting pseudoaneurysm of the cervical internal carotid artery using a wall stent and detachable coils: case report. *Neurosurgery*, **40**, 622–5.

Pessin, M.S., Adelman, L.S. & Barbas, N.R. (1989). Spontaneous intracranial carotid artery dissection. *Stroke*, **20**, 1100–3.

Pozzati, E., Andreoli, A., Padovani, R. & Nuzzo, G. (1995). Dissecting aneurysms of the basilar artery. *Neurosurgery*, **36**, 254–8.

Pullicino, P. (1994). Bilateral distal upper limb amyotrophy and watershed infarcts from vertebral dissection. *Stroke*, **25**, 1870–2.

Ringel, S.P., Harrison, S.H., Norenberg, M.D. & Austin, J.H. (1977). Fibromuscular dysplasia: multiple 'spontaneous' dissecting aneurysms of the major cervical arteries. *Annals of Neurology*, **1**, 301–4.

Rosenquist, T.H., Beall, A.C., Modis, L. & Fishman, R. (1990). Impaired elastic matrix development in the great arteries after ablation of the cardiac neural crest. *Anatomical Record*, **226**, 347–59.

Sasaki, O., Koike, T., Tanaka, R. & Ogawa, H. (1991). Subarachnoid hemorrhage from a dissecting aneurysm of the middle cerebral artery. *Journal of Neurosurgery*, **74**, 504–7.

Saver, J.L. & Easton, J.D. (1998). Dissections and trauma of cervicocerebral arteries. In *Stroke: Pathophysiology, Diagnosis, and Management*, ed. H.J.M. Barnett, J.P. Mohr, B.M. Stein & F.M. Yatsu, 3rd edn, pp. 769–786. New York: Churchill Livingstone.

Scherman, B.M. & Tucker, W.S. (1982). Bilateral traumatic thrombosis of the internal carotid arteries in the neck: a case report with review of the literature. *Neurosurgery*, **10**, 751–3.

Schievink, W.I. & Mokri, B. (1995). Familial aorto-cervicocephalic arterial dissections and congenitally bicuspid aortic valve. *Stroke*, **26**, 1935–40.

Schievink, W.I., Mokri, B., Michels, V.V. & Piepgras, D.G. (1991). Familial association of intracranial aneurysms and cervical artery dissections. *Stroke*, **22**, 1426–30.

Schievink, W.I., Mokri, B. & Piepgras, D.G. (1992). Angiographic frequency of saccular intracranial aneurysms in patients with spontaneous cervical artery dissection. *Journal of Neurosurgery*, **76**, 62–6.

Schievink, W.I., Mokri, B. & Whisnant, J.P. (1993). Internal carotid artery dissection in a community. Rochester, Minnesota, 1987–1992. *Stroke*, **24**, 1678–80.

Schievink, W.I., Michels, V.V. & Piepgras, D.G. (1994a). Neurovascular manifestations of heritable connective tissue disorders. *Stroke*, **25**, 889–903.

Schievink, W.I., Mokri, B. & O'Fallon, W.M. (1994b). Recurrent spontaneous cervical-artery dissection. *New England Journal of Medicine*, **330**, 393–7.

Schievink, W.I., Mokri, B. & Piepgras, D.G. (1994c). Spontaneous dissections of cervicocephalic arteries in childhood and adolescence. *Neurology*, **44**, 1607–12.

Schievink, W.I., Prakash, U.B., Piepgras, D.G. & Mokri, B. (1994d). Alpha 1-antitrypsin deficiency in intracranial aneurysms and cervical artery dissection. *Lancet*, **343**, 452–3.

Schievink, W.I., Michels, V.V., Mokri, B., Piepgras, D.G. & Perry, H.O. (1995). A familial syndrome of arterial dissections with lentiginosis. *New England Journal of Medicine*, **332**, 576–9.

Schievink, W.I., Mokri, B., Piepgras, D.G. & Kuiper, J.D. (1996). Recurrent spontaneous arterial dissections. Risk in familial versus nonfamilial disease. *Stroke*, **27**, 622–4.

Silbert, P.L., Mokri, B. & Schievink, W.I. (1995). Headache and neck pain in spontaneous internal carotid and vertebral artery dissections. *Neurology*, **45**, 1517–22.

Sturzenegger, M., Mattle, H.P., Rivoir, A. & Baumgartner, R.W. (1995). Ultrasound findings in carotid artery dissection: analysis of 43 patients. *Neurology*, **45**, 691–8.

Sundt, T.M. Jr, Pearson, B.W., Piepgras, D.G., Houser, O.W. & Mokri, B. (1986). Surgical management of aneurysms of the distal extracranial internal carotid artery. *Journal of Neurosurgery*, **64**, 169–82.

Thapedi, I.M., Ashenhurst, E.M. & Rozdilsky, B. (1970). Spontaneous dissecting aneurysm of the internal carotid artery in the neck. Report of a case and review of the literature. *Archives of Neurology*, **23**, 549–54.

West, T.E.T., Davies, R.J. & Kelly, R.E. (1976). Horner's syndrome and headache due to carotid artery disease. *British Medical Journal*, **1**, 818–20.

Yamada, S., Kindt, G.W. & Youmans, J.R. (1967). Carotid artery occlusion due to nonpenetrating injury. *Journal of Trauma*, **7**, 333–42.

Zelenock, G.B., Kazmers, A., Whitehouse, W.M. Jr et al. (1982). Extracranial internal carotid artery dissections. Noniatrogenic traumatic lesions. *Archives of Surgery*, **117**, 425–32.

31

Cerebral amyloid angiopathies

Didier Leys[1], Catherine Masson[2] and Luc Buée[3]

[1]Clinique Neurologie, Hôpital Roger Salengro, Lille, France
[2]Service de Neurologie, Hôpital Beaujon, Lichy, France
[3]INSERM U422, Lille, France

Introduction

Cerebral amyloid angiopathies (CAA) are defined as the deposition of amyloid in the wall of the cerebral vessels (Glenner, 1980). Their presentation is variable, ranging from asymptomatic deposition in normal vessels, to a severe involvement of the wall of cerebral vessels (Mandybur, 1986; Vonsattel et al., 1991). CAA is probably a frequent cause of lobar cerebral hemorrhages, and contributes to the pathogenesis of cerebral infarcts and leukoencephalopathies (Erkinjuntti & Hachinski, 1993; Greenberg et al., 1993). They often remain undiagnosed in the absence of a neuropathological examination (Greenberg, 1998). Dementia is frequent, because of the association of stroke lesions and leukoencephalopathies (Pasquier & Leys, 1997; Leys et al., 1999).

'Amyloid' is used to describe deposits of proteins with specific physical characteristics: β-pleated sheet configuration, apple green birefringence under polarized light after Congo red staining, fibrillary structure and insolubility (Glenner, 1980; Castano & Frangione, 1988). They are fluorescent under ultraviolet light after thioflavin S or T stains (Stokes & Trickey, 1973; Richardson, 1985). The amyloid properties are linked to the physical configuration of the protein, irrespective of its biochemical nature (Glenner, 1980). Therefore, biochemistry is the basis of the classification of CAA. An overproduction, or an abnormal degradation of circulating precursor proteins, causes most amyloid angiopathies. A genetic abnormality leading to the production of variant precursor proteins is possible (Stone, 1990). A tissue, or organ, affinity often exists for each protein. Immunocytochemical studies are crucial to characterize the type of amyloid. The two types of cerebral amyloid deposition frequently associated with CAA are amyloid-β (Aβ) and cystatin C.

We will not consider as CAA, amyloid deposition due to malformations, radiation necrosis, plasmocytomas or pseudotumoral lesions called amyloidomas.

Aβ cerebral amyloid angiopathies

The peptide deposited in the main type of CAA (Glenner & Wong, 1984) was called amyloid peptide, then A-4 or βA4, and finally Aβ. Aβ is the 40–43 amino acid proteolysis product of a large precursor, the amyloid β-protein precursor (APP), with features of a cell surface receptor (Kang et al., 1987). APP has several isoforms generated by alternative splicing from a single gene located on chromosome 21. The predominant transcripts are APP695, APP751, and APP770. They differ in that APP751 and APP770 contain exon 7, which encodes a Kunitz serine protease inhibitor domain. APP695 is a predominant form in neuronal tissue, whereas APP751 is the predominant variant elsewhere. Van Nostrand et al. (1989) presented evidence that protease nexin-II, a protease inhibitor that is synthesized and secreted by various cultured extravascular cells, is identical to APP751. This angiopathy is restricted to the brain and has been reported in various conditions. Aβ deposits are found in cerebral vessel walls of patients with sporadic CAA, the most frequent CAA, hereditary cerebral hemorrhage with amyloidosis, Dutch type (HCHWA-D), Alzheimer disease (Fig. 31.1) and Down's syndrome (Fig. 31.2). Despite similarities between the vascular amyloid and the Aβ in the cerebral extracellular amyloid deposits (senile plaques) of AD, some features distinguish Aβ in CAA, especially the prominence of the Aβ species ending at amino acid position 39–40 (Suzuki et al., 1994; Alonzo et al., 1998) and the tendency of particular mutant forms of Aβ to accumulate preferentially in vessels (Hendriks et al., 1992). Cystatin C is found to colocalize with Aβ in cerebral vessel walls of

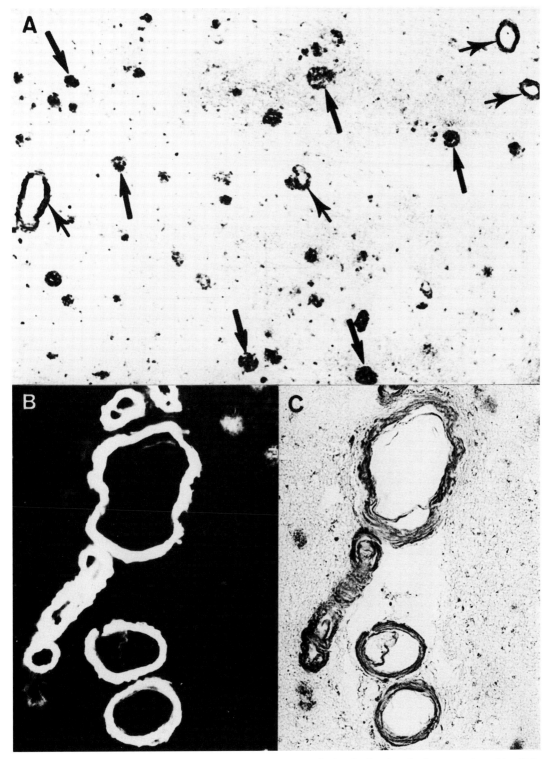

Fig. 31.1. (*a*) Aβ immunochemistry in Alzheimer's disease using an antibody raised against the first ten amino acids of Aβ peptide. Note the labelling of both senile plaques (broad arrows) and congophilic amyloid angiopathy (thin arrows) (×80). (*b*),(*c*) Double labelling of cerebral amyloid angiopathy by thioflavin S under fluorescence lighting conditions (*b*) and the Aβ antibody. Note the strong staining observed in vessel walls (×240).

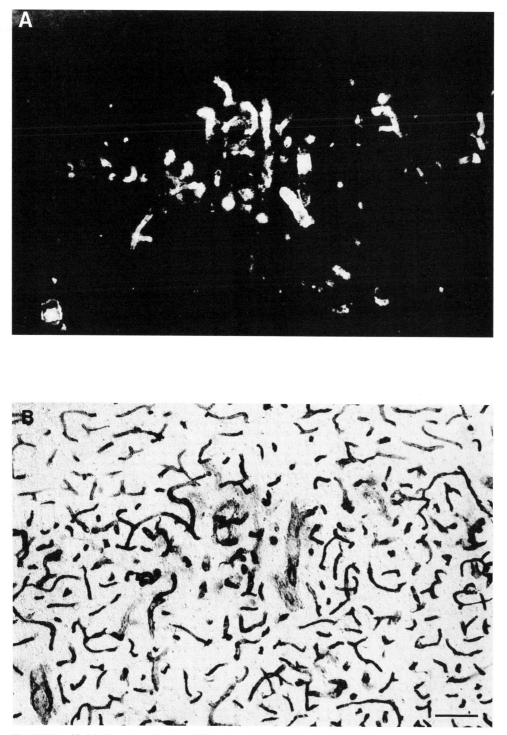

Fig. 31.2. Double labelling of cerebral amyloid angiopathy by thioflavin S under fluorescence lighting conditions (*a*) and an antibody raised against a component of the vascular basement membrane (heparan sulfate proteoglycan) (*b*) in layer IV-C of the primary visual cortex. Note the staining of congophilic amyloid angiopathy in the middle of the figure (*a*). This antibody mostly labels the entire vascular bed, including a few relatively large radial vessels, arterioles and capillaries. It indicates that CAA stained by thioflavin is localized in the highly vascularized layer IV-C. These affected capillaries are poorly labelled by the vascular basement membrane antibody compared to other capillaries (top and bottom of the figure).

patients with AD, HCHWA-D and sporadic CAA, but not in senile plaques (Nagai et al., 1998).

Sporadic Aβ cerebral amyloid angiopathies

Epidemiology

Most Aβ CAA are sporadic, and are found at autopsy in normal elderly subjects, Alzheimer's disease (AD) or Down's syndrome (Vinters, 1992). They have also been reported in dementia pugilitica, and postanoxic encephalopathy (Salama et al., 1986).

Depending on selection criteria of patients, and of staining methods, the prevalence of sporadic CAA largely varies between studies. All studies suggest that CAA is not rare in the elderly. In population-based studies, the annual incidence rate of lobar hemorrhages ranges from 30 to 40 per 100 000 over the age of 70 years (Schutz et al., 1990; Broderick et al., 1993). CAA accounts for approximately one-third of them (Schutz et al., 1990; Broderick et al., 1993). The question of the clinical impact of CAA in patients under antithrombotic therapies remains unknown. In a general hospital, 30% of autopsied patients over 80 years had amyloid deposits in their cerebral vessels. The prevalence of Aβ CAA is higher in women (Wildi & Dago-Akribi, 1968), and increases with age: 2.3% between 65 and 74 years (Greenberg, 1998), 12.1% over 85 years (Greenberg & Hyman, 1997) and up to 75% over 90 years (Yamada et al., 1987). In AD patients the prevalence of CAA ranges from 25% to 100% (Greenberg & Hyman, 1997; Glenner et al., 1981; Mandybur, 1975; Vonsattel et al., 1991); 5.1% of them having CAA-related intracerebral hemorrhage (Greenberg & Hyman, 1997). In Down's syndrome, CAA is rare before the age of 40.

Neuropathology

CAA involves small and medium arteries, and veins of the cortex and leptomeninges. Capillaries of the cerebral cortex can also be affected in severe cases. The deposits involve the external layers of the vessels (Okasaki et al., 1979). Progressively, the arterial wall appears eosinophilic and thickened, while muscle cells disappear. The lumen may be reduced or occluded. All cerebral vessels can be affected, but white matter and spinal cord vessels are spared. Surprisingly, the hippocampal vessels are rarely involved. Cystatin C is sometimes found to colocalize with Aβ and immunoreactivity can be present in white matter vessels (Wang et al., 1997).

Besides amyloid deposits, non-specific changes are seen in two-thirds of patients (Okasaki et al., 1979; Mandybur,

1975; Vonsattel et al., 1991). Associated lesions are more severe in familial or sporadic CAA, than in AD or in normal aging. They are similar to vascular changes seen in chronic arterial hypertension, including fibrinoid necrosis and microaneurysms. The severity of the amyloid deposition, and the presence of fibrinoid necrosis are consistently related to cerebral hemorrhage (Vonsattel et al., 1991). Another possible associated vessel lesion is vasculitis. Their cause remains unsettled, but a chronic inflammatory process leading to amyloid deposition is plausible. Conversely, amyloid may also be the causative agent of vasculitis (Yamada et al., 1987). CAA may be associated with brain lesions such as senile plaques, dystrophic neurites, and neurofibrillary tangles, i.e. abnormalities of the phosphorylation of Tau proteins (Delacourte et al., 1987; Buée et al., 1994). These vascular amyloid deposits may play a role in the constitution of senile plaques. Whether a continuum exists between CAA and AD remains a matter of discussion.

Clinical features

We know only the clinical presentation of patients who were autopsied or operated on for a hematoma. A marker of CAA during life would probably completely change the clinical spectrum of CAA.

Most sporadic CAA are silent and are just coincidental findings at autopsy.

Recurrent intracerebral hemorrhages are the most frequent features of CAA. Although no reliable statistics are available, CAA may account for 4 to 17% of all cerebral hemorrhages and even more in very old patients (Regli, 1989). Because of the possible coexistence of arterial hypertension, the hemorrhage cannot always be attributed with certainty to CAA. Cerebral hemorrhages associated with sporadic CAA do not occur before 55 years. They are lobar in location, and more frequent in frontal areas (Kase & Mohr, 1986a,b). This finding is classical and surprising, because CAA are more prominent in posterior areas. Cerebellar and pontine hemorrhages are rare. The clinical presentation is not specific, but headache, seizures (Kase & Mohr, 1986a), and recurrences (Cosgrove et al., 1985), are frequent.

Cerebral ischemia may be more frequent than cerebral hemorrhages (Okasaki et al., 1979). They usually consist of multiple, non-hemorrhagic, small, cortical infarcts. They are sometimes revealed by transient neurological deficits (Greenberg et al., 1993). However, transient episodes may also be due to epileptic seizures in patients with microbleedings.

Leukoencephalopathies have been reported in sporadic CAA. They may be asymptomatic, or associated with hemorrhages, infarcts or AD. Most leukoencephalopathies are not severe. Severe cases are rare (Gray et al., 1985; Roullet et al., 1986, 1988). They have no specificity. They may be similar to cases of Binswanger's disease, but they can occur in the absence of arterial hypertension. Hypoperfusion of the white matter supplied by long perforating arteries originating in leptomeningeal arteries involved by the CAA is the most likely explanation (Gray et al., 1985). In rare cases, the leukoencephalopathy may have a clinical and a radiological presentation suggestive of a tumour: such cases are usually diagnosed by a biopsy (Greenberg et al., 1993) and improve under corticosteroid therapy.

Dementia is frequent in CAA. Three types of dementia may be encountered (Pasquier & Leys, 1997): (i) vascular dementia due to the coexistence of multiple strokes (infarcts and hemorrhages) and leukoencephalopathy, (ii) AD, and (iii) dementia due to the coexistence of stroke, AD and leukoencephalopathies. Cases of dementia of rapid onset and course have been reported, either isolated (Probst & Ulrich, 1985) or in association with angiitis of the nervous system (Masson et al., 1998; Probst & Ulrich, 1985).

Genetics

While the ε4 allele of apoE has been identified as a risk factor for AD by promoting the aggregation and deposition of Aβ amyloid within the cortex (Strittmatter et al., 1993), apoE ε2 might play a major role in facilitating the deposition of Aβ amyloid in cerebral blood vessels. This may lead to amyloid angiopathy and cerebral hemorrhages (Greenberg & Hyman, 1997).

Diagnosis

Radiological findings have no specificity. The most useful radiological technique to approach a diagnosis of CAA is magnetic resonance imaging (MRI) with gradient-echo sequences. The major arguments supporting the diagnosis are: (i) lobar location of the intracerebral hemorrhage, sparing the basal ganglia, thalamus, pons and cerebellum, (ii) presence of one or more previous hemorrhages, as reported in three-quarters of CAA-related intracerebral hemorrhages (Greenberg, 1998). In addition, gradient-echo MRI may show the disease's progression with new hemorrhages (Hendricks et al., 1992).

Cerebral spinal fluid (CSF) abnormalities have no more specificity. A decreased level in the CSF of protease nexin-II (the secreted form of APP751), apolipoprotein E (Pirttila et al., 1996), and cystatin C (Kase & Mohr, 1986a) has been reported in some patients (Vinters et al., 1994). The contribution of CSF abnormalities to the diagnosis of CAA in patients with cerebral hemorrhage, has not be determined.

Neuropathological examination in case of surgery for a hematoma is the main way to make a diagnosis of CAA (Masson et al., 1998; Mandybur & Balko, 1992; Probst & Ulrich, 1985). The frequency of cerebral hemorrhage due to brain biopsy in patients with sporadic CAA reduces the indications to a very small number of patients. The biopsy is useful in pseudotumoural leukoencephalopathies and in cases where an associated angiitis is possible (Masson et al., 1998).

Genetical mutations reported in familial cases of CAA are absent in patients with sporadic CAA. Therefore, genetics is not useful for diagnostic purposes in the absence of a familial history.

Hereditary Aβ cerebral amyloid angiopathies

Hereditary cerebral hemorrhages with amyloidosis (Dutch type)

Hereditary cerebral hemorrhages with amyloidosis of the Dutch type (HCHWA-D) is an autosomal dominant disease characterized by cerebral hemorrhages occurring during the fourth and fifth decades (Wattendorf et al., 1982; Luyendijk et al., 1988; Haan et al., 1989).

Epidemiology
This rare disorder has been reported in four unrelated Dutch families originating from Schewingen (Wattendorf et al., 1982) and Katwijk (Luyendijk et al., 1988).

Neuropathology
Neuropathological findings are similar to those of sporadic AD, with the following differences (Wattendorf et al., 1982; Luyendijk et al., 1988; Haan et al., 1990a, c, 1994; Timmers et al., 1990; Maat-Schieman et al., 1992): (i) AD lesions are frequent, with only few neurofibrillary tangles, (ii) white matter changes occur early in the time-course of the disease (Durlinger et al., 1993); (iii) cerebral hemorrhages occur more frequently in posterior areas, (iv) a severe reduction of the lumen due to severe hyalinosis and sclerosis of the vessel walls is frequent.

Schmaier et al. (1993) provided biochemical evidence that protease nexin-II (the APP751 isoform) may serve as a cerebral anticoagulant. They suggested that this fact may explain the spontaneous intracerebral hemorrhages seen in patients with hereditary cerebral hemorrhage with amyloidosis of the Dutch type in which there is extensive accumulation of protease nexin-II in cerebral blood vessels.

Clinical features

HCHWA-D is characterized by recurrent cerebral hemorrhages occurring between 39 and 59 years (Wattendorf et al., 1982; Luyendijk et al., 1988; Haan et al., 1989). Patients who survive several hemorrhages develop stepwise dementia (Haan et al., 1990a, b, c). Progressive dementia without stroke, suggestive of AD, is also possible (Wattendorf et al., 1982; Haan et al., 1992). Migraine, transient neurological deficits and epileptic seizures are also frequent. The diagnosis is difficult in the absence of a clear family history.

Genetics

The underlying genetic defect is a point-mutation in the APP gene located on chromosome 21, leading to aberrant APP (Van Duinen et al., 1987; Van Broeckhoven et al., 1990; Levy et al., 1990; Bakker et al., 1991). The gene mutation leads to an amino acid modification at codon 693 (glutamic acid to glutamine change) (Levy et al., 1990; Bakker et al., 1991). The apolipoprotein ε4 (Haan et al., 1994) and ε2 alleles (Haan et al., 1995) do not influence the clinical expression of the codon 693 mutation (Hendriks et al., 1992). The penetrance of the gene is almost complete (Luyendijk et al., 1988).

Diagnosis

In patients with presumed HCHWA-D and familial AD (van Nostrand et al., 1992), a decreased level of protease nexin-II, and of Aβ amyloid in the CSF may be useful (Pirttila et al., 1996). However, direct evidence of the mutation by molecular genetics methods is possible (Bakker et al., 1991).

'Family 1302'

This peculiar family with hereditary CAA, was followed up over four generations (Hendriks et al., 1992): most patients suffered from early onset AD, but several patients had cerebral hemorrhages around 40 years of age. The cerebral Aβ CAA was identified in a patient who underwent surgery for a cerebral hemorrhage. This patient also had diffuse Aβ deposits and few senile plaques, without neurofibrillary tangles (Hendricks et al., 1992). Comparison of 'Family 1302' and HCHWA-D found an APP gene mutation in codon 692 (alanine to glycine change) (Hendricks et al., 1992). However, the clinical expression differs considerably

from that of HCHWA-D. The reason why the prominent lesions are on the brain vessels in HCHWA-D and on the brain tissue in 'Family 1302', remains unknown. However, De Jonghe et al. (1998) provided evidence that APP692 and APP693 have a different effect on Aβ secretion as determined by cDNA transfection experiments. While APP692 upregulates both Aβ-40 and Aβ-42 secretion, APP693 does not. These data corroborate the previous findings that increased Aβ secretion, and particularly increased secretion of Aβ-42, is specific for AD pathology and extracellular amyloid deposits. Thus, these data further support that 'Family 1302' is closer to AD than HCHWA-D.

Hereditary cystatin C cerebral amyloid angiopathies (Icelandic type)

Hereditary cystatin C amyloid angiopathy (HCAAA-I), previously called 'hereditary cerebral hemorrhages with amyloidosis, Icelandic type', is a rare autosomal dominant disorder limited to the brain. It has been reported in eight Icelandic families (Jensson et al., 1987b), and is caused by a point mutation (leucine (L) to glutamine (Q) change at codon 68) on the cystatin gene on chromosome 20, consisting of a L68Q substitution (Palsdottir et al., 1988). Cystatin C is a potent inhibitor of various cysteine proteases.

Abrahamson and Grubb (1994) produced normal and L68Q cystatin C in an *E. coli* expression system. They differ considerably in their tendency to dimerize and form aggregates. While wild-type cystatin C was monomeric and functionally active even after prolonged storage at elevated temperatures, L68Q cystatin C started to dimerize and lose biologic activity immediately after it was transferred to a nondenaturing buffer. The aggregation at physiologic concentrations was increased at 40°C compared to 37°C, by approximately 60%.

The first clinical signs occur between 20 and 30 years, and consist of hemorrhages that may involve the corticomedullary junction, and in the basal ganglia (Blöndal et al., 1989). Infarcts are rare. Vascular dementia is possible in survivors (Jensson et al., 1987b, Blöndal et al., 1989). Patients may remain stable for several years (Jensson et al., 1987b). In the family reported by Gudmundsson (Gudmundsson et al., 1972) the mean age at death was 44 years in the two first generations, decreasing to 29.6 and 22.5 years in the third and fourth generations. Death usually occurs before 50 years.

Autopsy findings consist of multiple and extensive intracerebral hemorrhages of different ages, and extensive amyloid depositions in the arterial walls of the cerebral and leptomeningeal vessels. The involvement of the most distal microcirculation (including capillaries) is usual. Areas of demyelination can also be observed (Blöndal et al., 1989; Gudmundsson et al., 1972), but not AD changes (Gudmundsson et al., 1972). Amyloid depositions may also be found in lymph nodes, spleen, salivary glands, seminal vesicles, testes and skin (Lofberg et al., 1987; Benedikz et al., 1990), but extracerebral deposits are silent.

Reduction to one-third of the normal level of cystatin C in cerebrospinal fluid, can be used as a diagnostic test (Jensson et al., 1987a). A specific diagnosis by polymerase chain reaction based analysis is available (Abrahamson et al., 1992).

A case of sporadic CAA with intracerebral hemorrhage has been reported in an elderly Croatian man who had a mutation in cystatin C similar to that of HCAAA-I.

Gelsolin-related amyloidosis (familial amyloidosis, Finnish type; AGel amyloidosis)

This is an autosomal dominant form of systemic amyloidosis where two mutations of the gelsolin gene have been described on chromosome 9 at codon 654 (aspartic acid 187 to asparagine change) and (aspartic acid 187 to tyrosine change) (Levy et al., 1990; De la Chapelle et al., 1992; Kiuru et al., 1999). As demonstrated by cDNA transfection, both mutant forms of gelsolin are abnormally processed and secreted as an aberrant 68 kDa gelsolin fragment in cell culture. This fragment contains the suggested amyloid forming sequence (Paunio et al., 1998).

AGel is deposited in both the grey and white matter vessels of the brain and spinal cord. Clinical signs, as dementia or mood disorders, and white matter lesions on MRI may be related to the Gelsolin-related CAA (Kiuru et al., 1999).

Transthyretin cerebral amyloid angiopathies (familial oculoleptomeningeal amyloidosis)

Familial oculoleptomeningeal amyloidosis (transthyretin CAA) is an autosomal dominant disorder with hemiplegic migraine, dementia, seizures, strokes, and visual deterioration (Goren et al., 1980; Uitti et al., 1988). Amyloid deposition can be found in leptomeningeal and retinal vessels. The cerebral vessels are usually spared, but superficial hemorrhages can occur when vessels of the superficial neocortex are involved. Transthyretin CAA may also be seen in type I familial amyloid neuropathy, but usually remains asymptomatic.

Amyloid angiopathies of undetermined biochemical nature

The Worster-Drought type (also called 'British type')

The Worster-Drought type CAA (Worster-Drought et al., 1940; Griffiths et al., 1982; Plant et al., 1990) is a rare autosomal dominant disorder characterized by progressive dementia, spasticity and ataxia, with diffuse white matter changes (Plant et al., 1990). The clinical onset occurs in the fifth decade and the mean duration of the disease is almost 10 years. Clinically obvious strokes are not frequent. Three families, two of them sharing a common ancestor, have been identified. At autopsy, patients have multiple cerebral hemorrhages and lacunes, amyloid angiopathy, and senile plaques in the hippocampus and cerebellum. Amyloid angiopathy affects the small vessels of less than 150 mm, in the cerebral parenchyma and in leptomeninges of the entire central nervous system, including the spinal cord, but not in other organs. Arteriolosclerotic lesions are frequently associated. Senile plaques are seen in the brain.

The biochemical nature of the amyloid deposit is unknown. It is likely that a process very reminiscent of that suggested for Aβ formation – fibrillar protein deposition (FBD) – is to blame. FBD shares features of Alzheimer's disease, including amyloid deposits, neurofibrillary tangles, neuronal loss, and progressive dementia. The cause of the disease was identified earlier this year as a mutation in a gene termed BRI. The mutant BRI codes for an abnormal protein dubbed ABri, a major component of plaques in FBD. The structure of ABri suggested that it was cleaved by the prohormone convertase, furin. Sam Sisodia and his colleagues from the University of Chicago and Rockefeller University report that furin constitutively processes both ABri and the normal protein product of BRI with subsequent secretion of carboxyl terminal peptides that encompass all or part of ABri. More significantly, furin generates more peptide product in the presence of the mutant BRI protein and the peptides thus produced assemble into irregular, short fibrils. Although the role of ABri peptides in the genesis of FBD is not known, it seems likely that the elucidation of this process can shed light on the role of abnormal protein aggregation in other neurodegenerative diseases such as Alzheimer's.

Other familial angiopathies

Other familial disorders with amyloid deposits of undetermined biochemical nature have also been reported (Haan & Roos, 1990; Haan et al., 1994).

Therapeutic strategies and prospects

There is no reason to treat CAA-related hemorrhages differently than other varieties of intracerebral hemorrhages. However, when a patient is suspected of CAA, surgery should be avoided anytime it is possible, because of a high risk of rebleeding, and a good spontaneous recovery (Regli, 1989).

CAA is the only major type of stroke without any prevention (Greenberg, 1998). Aspirin and anticoagulant should be avoided as much as possible in these patients. No treatment has been proven useful to prevent amyloid deposition and hemorrhages, although a clinical and radiological improvement has been reported after administration of corticosteroids and cyclophosphamide, alone or in association, in patients with a proven associated granulomatosous angiitis (Masson et al., 1998; Mandybur & Balko, 1992; Probst & Ulrich, 1985; Fountain & Lopes, 1999). Early treatment of febrile periods might reduce amyloid formation as suggested in HCAAA-I, where it might slow down the in vivo formation of L68Q cystatin C aggregates (Abrahamson & Grubb, 1994). Potential approaches to prevent CAA progression include: inhibitors of Aβ cleavage from APP, potentiators of Aβ clearance, antagonists of vasoactive cytokines, and inhibitors of Aβ binding to apolipoprotein E or the vascular extracellular matrix. The breakdown of amyloid-laden vessel walls might be prevented by inhibitors of Aβ toxicity, antioxidants or anti-inflammatory agents (Greenberg, 1998).

A better knowledge of the mechanisms leading to amyloid deposition is now necessary to determine how to block the pathological cascade of events. Biochemical analysis of the amyloid vessels, genetical studies of so-called 'sporadic cases', and determination of risk factors for amyloid deposition are the main research activities that will help to achieve this goal.

Acknowledgments

To Drs André Delacourte, Patrick R. Hof and André Défossez for helpful discussion. Supported by the Centre National de la Recherche Scientifique (CNRS), Institut National de la Santé et de la Recherche Médicale (INSERM, U422) and Ministère de l'éducation Nationale de la Recherche et de la Technologie (MENRT, EA 2691).

References

Abrahamson, M. & Grubb, A. (1994). Increased body temperature accelerates aggregation of the Leu-69>Gln mutant cystatin C, the amyloid forming protein in hereditary cystatin C amyloid angiopathy. *Proceedings of the National Academy of Sciences of the United States of America*, **91**, 1416–20.

Abrahamson, M., Jonsdottir, S., Olafsson, I., Jensson, O. & Grubb, A. (1992). Hereditary cystatine-C angiopathy. Identification of the disease causing mutation and specific diagnosis by polymerase chain reaction based analysis. *Human Genetics*, **89**, 337–80.

Alonzo, N.C., Hyman, B.T., Rebeck, G.W. & Greenberg S.M. (1998). Progression of cerebral amyloid angiopathy. Accumulation of amyloid β40 in already affected vessels. *Journal of Neuropathology and Experimental Neurology*, **57**, 353–9.

Bakker, E., van Broeckhoven, C., Haan, J. et al. (1991). DNA-diagnosis for hereditary cerebral hemorrhage with amyloidosis (Dutch type). *American Journal of Human Genetics*, **49**, 518–21.

Benedikz, E., Blöndal, H. & Gudmundsson, G. (1990). Skin deposits in hereditary cystatin C amyloidosis. *Virchow's Archiv. Pathological Anatomy and histopathology*, **417**, 325–31.

Blöndal, H., Gudmundsson, G., Benedikz, E. & Johannesson, G. (1989). Dementia in hereditary cystatin C amyloidosis. *Progress in Clinical and Biological Research*, **317**, 157–64.

Broderick, J., Brott, T., Tomsick, T. & Leach, A. (1993). Lobar hemorrhage in the elderly. The undiminishing importance of hypertension. *Stroke*, **24**, 49–51.

Buée, L., Vermersch, P., Hof, P.R., Défossez, A. & Delacourte, A. (1994). Alzheimer's vasculopathy. In *Vascular Dementia*, ed. D. Leys & Ph. Scheltens, pp. 155–66. Dordrecht, The Netherlands: ICG Publications.

Castano, E.M. & Frangione, B. (1988). Human amyloidosis, Alzheimer disease and related disorders. *Laboratory Investigation*, **58**, 122–32.

Cosgrove, G.R., Leblanc, R., Meagher-Villemure, K. & Ethier, R. (1985). Cerebral amyloid angiopathy. *Neurology*, **35**, 625–31.

De Jonghe, C., Zehr, C., Yager, D. et al. (1998). Flemish and Dutch mutations in amyloid beta precursor protein have different effects on amyloid beta secretion. *Neurobiology of Disease*, **5**, 281–6.

de la Chapelle, A., Tolvanen, R., Boysen, G. et al. (1992). Gelsolin-derived familial amyloidosis caused by asparagine or tyrosine substitution for aspartic acid at residue 187. *Nature Genetics*, **2**, 157–60.

Delacourte, A., Défossez, A., Persuy, P. & Peers, M.C. (1987) Observation of morphological relationships between blood vessels and degenerative neurites in Alzheimer's disease. *Virchow's Archives A*, **411**, 199–204.

Durlinger, E.T.L., Haan, J. & Roos, R.A.C. (1993). Hereditary cerebral hemorrhage with amyloidosis-Dutch type. *Neurology*, **43**, 1626–7.

Erkinjuntti, T. & Hachinski, V.C. (1993). Rethinking vascular dementia. *Cerebrovascular Diseases*, **3**, 3–23.

Fountain, N.B. & Lopes, B.S. (1999). Control of primary angiitis of the CNS with cerebral amyloid angiopathy by cyclophosphamide alone. *Neurology*, **52**, 660–2.

Glenner, G.G. (1980). Amyloid deposits and amyoïdosis. The β-fibrilloses. *The New England Journal of Medicine*, **302**, 1283–92.

Glenner, G.G. & Wong, C.W. (1984). Alzheimer's disease: initial report of the purification and characterization of a novel cerebrovascular amyloid protein. *Biochemical and Biophysical Research Communications*, **120**, 885–90.

Glenner, G.G., Henry, J.H. & Fujihara, S. (1981). Congophilic angiopathy in the pathogenesis of Alzheimer's degeneration. *Annals of Pathology*, **1**, 120–9.

Goren, H., Steinberg, M.C. & Farboody, G.H. (1980). Familial oculoleptomeningeal amyloidosis. *Brain*, **103**, 473–95.

Gray, F., Dubas, F., Roullet, E. & Escourolle, R. (1985). Leukoencephalopathy in diffuse hemorrhagic cerebral amyloid angiopathy. *Annals of Neurology*, **18**, 54–9.

Greenberg, S.M. (1998). Cerebral amyloid angiopathy. Prospects for clinical diagnosis and treatment. *Neurology*, **51**, 690–4.

Greenberg, S. & Hyman, B. (1997). Cerebral amyloid angiopathy and apolipoprotein E: bad news for the good allele? *Annals of Neurology*, **41**, 701–2.

Greenberg, S.M., Vonsattel, J.P., Stakes, J.W., Gruber, M. & Finklestein, S.P. (1993). The clinical spectrum of cerebral amyloid angiopathy: presentations without lobar hemorrhages. *Neurology*, **43**, 2073–9.

Griffiths, R.A., Mortimer, T.F., Oppenheimer, D.R. & Spalding, J.M.K. (1982). Congophilic angiopathy of the brain: a clinical and pathological report on two siblings. *Journal of Neurology, Neurosurgery and Psychiatry*, **45**, 396–408.

Gudmundsson, G., Hallgrimsson, J., Jonasson, T.A. & Bjarnason, O. (1972). Hereditary cerebral hemorrhage with amyloidosis. *Brain*, **95**, 387–404.

Haan, J. & Roos, R.A.C. (1990). Amyloid in central nervous system. *Clinical Neurology and Neurosurgery*, **92**, 305–10.

Haan, J., Roos, R.A.C., Briet, P.E., Herpers, M.J.H.M., Luyendijk, W. & Bots, G.T.A.M. (1989). Hereditary cerebral hemorrhage with amyloidosis-Dutch type. *Clinical Neurology and Neurosurgery*, **81**, 285–90.

Haan, J., Algra, P.R. & Roos, R.A.C. (1990a). Hereditary cerebral hemorrhage with amyloidosis-Dutch type: Clinical and CT analysis of 24 cases. *Archives of Neurology*, **47**, 649–53.

Haan, J., Lanser, J.B.K., Zijderveld, I., Does, I.G.F. & van der Roos, R.A.C. (1990b). Dementia in hereditary cerebral hemorrhage with amyloidosis-Dutch type. *Archives of Neurology*, **47**, 965–7.

Haan, J., Roos, R.A.C., Algra, P.R., Lanser, J.B.K., Bots, G.T.A.M. & Vegter-van der Vlis, M. (1990c). Hereditary cerebral hemorrhage with amyloidosis-Dutch type: magnetic resonance imaging findings of seven cases. *Brain*, **113**, 1251–67.

Haan, J., Bakker, B., Jennekens-Schinkel, A. & Roos, R.A.C. (1992).

Progressive dementia, without cerebral hemorrhage in a patient with hereditary cerebral amyloid angiopathy. *Clinical Neurology and Neurosurgery*, **94**, 317–18.

Haan, J., Olafson, I. & Jensson, O. (1994). Non-Alzheimer familial cerebral amyloid angiopathy. In *Vascular dementia*, ed. D. Leys & P. Scheltens, pp. 183–93. Dordrecht: ICG Publications.

Haan, J., Roos, R.A.C. & Bakker, E. (1995). No protective effect of apolipoprotein Eε2 allele in Dutch hereditary cerebral amyloid angiopathy. *Annals of Neurology*, **37**, 282.

Hendriks, L., van Duijn, C.M., Cras, P. et al. (1992). Presenile dementia and cerebral hemorrhage linked to a mutation at codon 692 of the β-amyloid precursor protein gene. *Nature Genetics*, **1**, 218–21.

Jensson, O., Gudmundsson, G., Arnason, A. et al. (1987a). Hereditary (gamma-trace) cystatin C amyloid angiopathy of the CNS causing cerebral hemorrhage. *Acta Neurologica Scandinavica*, **76**, 102–14.

Jensson, O., Palsdottir, A. & Gudmundsson, G. (1987b). An isolate of families in the South of Iceland suspected of hereditary cystatin C amyloid angiopathy. In *Amyloid and Amyloidosis*, ed. T. Isobe, S. Araki, F. Uchino, S. Kito & E. Tsubura, pp. 579–84. New York: Plenum Press.

Kang, J., Lemaire, H.G., Unterbeck, A. et al. (1987). The precursor of Alzheimer's disease amyloid A4 protein resembles a cell-surface receptor. *Nature*, **325**(6106), 733–6.

Kase, C.S. & Mohr, J.P. (1986a). General features of intracerebral hemorrhage. In *Stroke-Pathophysiology, Diagnosis and Management*, ed. H.L.M. Barnett, J.P. Mohr, B.M. Stein & F.M. Yatsu, pp. 497–523. New York: Churchill Livingstone.

Kase, C.S. & Mohr, J.P. (1986b). Supratentorial intracerebral hemorrhage. In *Stroke-Pathophysiology, Diagnosis and Management*, ed. H.L.M. Barnett, J.P. Mohr, B.M. Stein & F.M. Yatsu, pp. 525–47. New York: Churchill Livingstone.

Kiuru, S., Salonen, O. & Haltia, M. (1999). Gelsolin-related spinal and cerebral amyloid angiopathy. *Annals of Neurology*, **45**, 305–11.

Levy, E., Carman, M.D., Fernandez-Madrid, I.J. et al. (1990). Mutation of the Alzheimer's disease amyloid gene in hereditary cerebral hemorrhage with amyloidosis, Dutch type. *Science*, **248**, 1124–6.

Leys, D., Erkinjuntti, T., Desmond, D.W. et al. (1999). Vascular dementia: the role of stroke. *Alzheimer's Disease and Associated Disorders*, **13**(Suppl. 3), S38–S48.

Lofberg, H., Grubb, A.O., Nilsson, E.K. et al. (1987). Immunohistochemical characterization of the amyloid deposits and qualification of pertinent cerebrospinal fluid proteins in hereditary cerebral hemorrhage with amyloidosis. *Stroke*, **18**, 431–40.

Luyendijk, W., Bots, G.T.A.M., Vegter-Van der Vlis, M., Went, L.N. & Frangione, B. (1988). Hereditary cerebral hemorrhage caused by cortical amyloid angiopathy. *Journal of Neurological Sciences*, **85**, 267–80.

Maat-Schieman, M.L.C., Van Duinen, S.G., Haan, J. & Roos, R.A.C. (1992). Morphology of cerebral plaque-like lesions in hereditary cerebral hemorrhage with amyloidosis (Dutch). *Acta Neuropathologica (Berlin)*, **84**, 674–9.

Mandybur, T.I. (1975). The incidence of cerebral amyloid angiopathy in Alzheimer's disease. *Neurology*, **25**, 120–6.

Mandybur, T.I. (1986). Cerebral amyloid angiopathy: the vascular pathology and complications. *Journal of Neuropathology and Experimental Neurology*, **45**, 79–90.

Mandybur, T.I. & Balko, G. (1992). Cerebral amyloid angiopathy with granulomatosous angiitis ameliorated by steroid-cytoxan treatment. *Clinical Neuropharmacology*, **15**, 241–7.

Masson, C., Henin, D., Colombani, J.M. & Dehen, H. (1998). Un cas d'angéite cérébrale à cellules géantes associée à une angiopathie amyloide cérébrale. Evolution favorable sous traitement corticoide. *La Revue Neurologique (Paris)*, **154**, 695–8.

Nagai, A., Kobayashi, S., Shimode, K. et al. (1998). No mutations in cystatin C gene in cerebral amyloid angiopathy with cystatin C deposition. *Molecular and Chemical Neuropathology*, **33**, 63–78.

Okasaki, H., Reagan, T.J. & Campbell, R.J. (1979). Clinicopathologic studies of primary cerebral amyloid angiopathy. *Mayo Clinic Proceedings*, **54**, 22–31.

Palsdottir, A., Abrahamson, M., Thorsteinsson, L., et al. (1988). Mutation in cystatin C gene causes hereditary brain hæmorrhage. *Lancet*, **i**, 603–4.

Pasquier, F. & Leys, D. (1997). Why are stroke patients prone to develop dementia? *Journal of Neurology*, **244**, 135–42.

Paunio, T., Kangas, H., Heinonen, O. et al. (1998). Cells of the neuronal lineage play a major role in the generation of amyloid precursor fragments in gelsolin-related amyloidosis. *Journal of Biological Chemistry*, **273**, 16319–24

Pirttila, T., Mehta, P.D., Soininen, H. et al. (1996). Cerebrospinal fluid concentrations of soluble amyloid beta-protein and apolipoprotein E in patients with Alzheimer's disease: correlations with amyloid load in the brain. *Archives of Neurology*, **53**, 189–93.

Plant, G.T., Revesz, T., Barnard, R.O., Harding, A.E. & Gautier-Smith, P.C. (1990). Familial cerebral amyloid angiopathy with nonneuritic plaque formation. *Brain*, **113**, 721–47.

Probst, A. & Ulrich, J. (1985). Amyloid angiopathy combined with granulomatous angiitis of the central nervous system: report on two patients. *Clinical Neuropathology*, **4**, 250–9.

Regli, F. (1989). Cerebral amyloid angiopathy. In *Handbook of Clinical Neurology. Vascular Disease (part II)*, pp. 333–44. Amsterdam: Elsevier Science.

Richardson, E.P. Jr. (1985). Amyloid in the human brain. *Western Journal of Medicine*, **143**, 518–19.

Roullet, E., Baudrimont, M., Singer, B. et al. (1986). Angiopathie amyloide cérébrale: deux observations anatomo-cliniques. *Archives d'Anatomie et de Cytologie Pathologiques*, **34**, 95–8.

Roullet, E., Gray, F.F. & Dubas, F. (1988). Leuko-araiois in severe amyloid angiopathy. *Archives of Neurology*, **45**, 140–1.

Salama, J., Gherardi, R., Amiel, H., Poirier, J., Delaporte, P. & Gray, F. (1986). Post-anoxic delayed encephalopathy with leukoencephalopathy and nonhemorrhagic cerebral amyloid angiopathy. *Clinical Neuropathology*, **4**, 153–6.

Schmaier, A.H., Dahl, L.D., Rozemuller, A.J. et al. (1993). Protease nexin-2/amyloid beta protein precursor. A tight-binding inhibitor of coagulation factor IXa. *Journal of Clinical Investigation*, **92**, 2540–5.

Schutz, H., Bodeker, R.H., Damian, M., Krack, P. & Dorndorf, W. (1990). Age-related spontaneous intracerebral hematoma in a German community. *Stroke*, **21**, 1412–18.

Stokes, M.I. & Trickey, R.J. (1973). Screening for neurofibrillary tangles and argyrophilic plaques with Congo red and polarized light. *Journal of Clinical Pathology*, **26**, 241–2.

Stone, M.J. (1990). Amyloidosis: a final common pathway for protein deposition in tissues. *Blood*, **92**, 531–45.

Strittmatter, W.J., Saunders, A.M., Schmechel, D. et al. (1993). Apolipoprotein E: high-avidity binding to beta-amyloid and increased frequency of type 4 allele in late-onset familial Alzheimer disease. *Proceedings of the National Academy of Sciences of the United States of America*, **90**, 1977–81.

Suzuki, N., Iwatsubo, T., Odaka, A., Ishibashi, Y., Kitada, C. & Ihara, Y. (1994). High tissue content of soluble beta 1–40 is linked to cerebral amyloid angiopathy. *American Journal of Pathology*, **145**, 452–60

Timmers, W.F., Tagliavini, F., Haan, J. & Frangione, B. (1990). Parenchymal preamyloid and amyloid deposits in the brains of patients with hereditary cerebral hemorrhage with amyloidosis-Dutch type. *Neuroscience Letters*, **118**, 223–6.

Uitti, R.J., Donat, J.R., Rozdilsky, B., Schneider, R.J. & Koeppen, A.H. (1988). Familial oculoleptomeningeal amyloidosis: report of a new family with unusual features. *Archives of Neurology*, **45**, 1118–22.

Van Broeckhoven, C., Haan, J., Bakker, E. et al. (1990). Amyloid beta protein precursor gene and hereditary cerebral hemorrhage with amyloidosis (Dutch). *Science*, **248**, 1120–2.

van Duinen, S.G., Castano, E.M., Prelli, F., Bots, G.T., Luyendijk, W. & Frangione, B. (1987). Hereditary cerebral hemorrhage with amyloidosis in patients of Dutch origin is related to Alzheimer's disease. *Proceedings of the National Academy of Sciences of the United States of America*, **84**, 5991–4.

Van Nostrand, W.E., Wagner, S.L., Suzuki, M. et al. (1989). Protease nexin-II, a potent antichymotrypsin, shows identity to amyloid beta-protein precursor. *Nature*, **341**(6242), 546–9.

Van Nostrand, W.E., Wagner, S.L., Haan, J., Bakker, E. & Roos, R.A. (1992). Alzheimer's disease and hereditary cerebral hemorrhage with amyloidosis-Dutch type share a decrease in cerebrospinal fluid levels of amyloid β-protein precursor. *Annals of Neurology*, **32**, 215–18.

Vinters, H. (1992). Cerebral amyloid angiopathy and Alzheimer's disease: two entities or one? *Journal of Neurological Sciences*, **112**, 1–3.

Vinters, H.V., Secor, D.L., Read, S.L. et al. (1994). Microvasculature in brain biopsy specimens from patients with Alzheimer's disease: an immunohistochemical and ultrastructural study. *Ultrastructural Pathology*, **18**, 333–48.

Vonsattel, J.P., Myers, R.H., Hedley-Whyte, E.T., Ropper, A.H., Bird, E.D. & Richardson, E.P. (1991). Cerebral amyloid angiopathy without and with cerebral hemorrhages: a comparative histological study. *Annals of Neurology*, **30**, 637–49.

Wang, Z.Z., Jensson, O., Thorsteinsson, L. & Vinters, H.V. (1997). Microvascular degeneration in hereditary cystatin C amyloid angiopathy of the brain. *APMIS*, **105**, 41–7.

Wattendorf, A.R., Bots, G.T.A.M., Went, L.N. & Endtz, L.J. (1982). Familial cerebral amyloid angiopathy presenting as recurrent cerebral hemorrhage. *Journal of Neurological Sciences*, **55**, 121–35.

Wildi, E. & Dago-Akribi, A. (1968). Altérations cérébrales chez l'Homme âgé. *Bulletin Suisse de l'Académie Médicale des Sciences*, **24**, 107–32.

Worster-Drought, C., Greenfield, J.G. & McMenemy, W.H. (1940). A form of familial presenile dementia with spastic paralysis, (including the pathological examination of a case). *Brain*, **63**, 237–54.

Yamada, M., Tsukagoshi, H., Otomo, E. & Hayakawa, M. (1987). Cerebral amyloid angiopathy in the aged. *Journal of Neurology*, **234**, 371–6.

32

Moya-moya

Harold P. Adams, Jr.

Department of Neurology, University of Iowa College of Medicine, IN, USA

Introduction

An uncommon cause of hemorrhagic or ischemic stroke in children and young adults, moya-moya was first described by Japanese investigators in 1955. Most of the initial reports about moya-moya were from Japan but in the last 45 years, multiple cases with moya-moya have been identified around the world. The largely intracranial arteriopathy is associated with a progressive bilateral obliteration of the major arteries of the anterior circulation (distal internal carotid artery (ICA) and proximal portions of the anterior cerebral artery (ACA) and middle cerebral artery (MCA)). These vessels are replaced by a fine meshwork of small collateral vessels at the base of the brain that are the hallmark of moya-moya. The arteriographic appearance of these vessels which resembles a 'puff of smoke' is the source of the name moya-moya. In reality, the term moya-moya encompasses two relatively distinct clinical entities – moya-moya disease and moya-moya syndrome. The presence of the arterial changes consistent with the arteriopathy in a child or young adult in the absence of other conditions leads to the diagnosis of moya-moya disease. On the other hand, the arterial abnormalities have been associated with a large number of conditions – these findings are compatible with the diagnosis of moya-moya syndrome. The latter situation may be more common in young adults than in children. Differentiating moya-moya disease from moya-moya syndrome is important because the prognosis and treatment of the patient with the latter is modified to emphasize management of the underlying illness.

The progressive nature of the arteriopathic changes is another key feature of moya-moya. Based on arteriographic findings, six stages of the disease have been described (Suzuki, 1986) (Table 32.1). In general, the patients' clinical status corresponds to the advancement of the arteriographic changes. While approximately 10% of patients present with changes of unilateral moya-moya, a majority of these cases eventually will have bilateral abnormalities. The angiographic findings of moya-moya syndrome are akin to those of moya-moya disease (Natori et al., 1997). The presence of a unilateral process is more suggestive of moya-moya syndrome than moya-moya disease. The diagnosis of moya-moya should be made with caution when the findings are strictly one-sided.

Epidemiology of moya-moya

The incidence and prevalence of moya-moya is higher in Japan than in any other country in the world. Based on the marked differences between ethnic groups, a genetic factor is presumed to predispose to moya-moya disease. Wakai et al. (1997) estimated that approximately 3900 persons with moya-moya are treated annually in Japan. They estimated that the incidence rate and prevalence rate of moya-moya in Japan is approximately 0.35/100000 and 3.16/100000 respectively. Studies from Taiwan and Korea report rates of moya-moya that are lower than in Japan but higher than elsewhere in the world (Hung et al., 1997; Ikezaki et al., 1997a, b). Presumably most of the cases described in Asia represent moya-moya disease rather than moya-moya syndrome.

Based on a questionnaire mailed to European centers, Yonekawa et al. (1997) estimated that the incidence of moya-moya in Europe was approximately one-tenth of that reported in Japan. Although most of the patients were white, many of the clinical features of moya-moya reported in the European survey were similar to those described among the Japanese patients. A small Italian study reported similar results (Battisella & Carolla, 1997). Surveys in the United States and Canada also report very low rates

Table 32.1. *Stages of moya-moya as detected by arteriography*

Stage 1[a] Segmental narrowing of the distal portion of the internal carotid artery.

Stage 2 Initial appearance of the basal moya-moya. Segmental narrowing of the proximal portions of the anterior and middle cerebral arteries.

Stage 3 The basal moya-moya becomes very prominent. The proximal portions of the anterior and middle cerebral arteries are no longer visualized. Distal branches of the anterior and middle cerebral arteries may be visualized via collaterals from branches of the posterior cerebral artery.

Stage 4 The basal moya-moya begins to disappear. The proximal portion of the posterior cerebral artery becomes narrowed.

Stage 5 The basal moya-moya becomes less apparent. All the major intracranial arteries are no longer visualized.

Stage 6 The basal moya-moya is absent. Only meningeal–pial collaterals arising from branches of the external carotid artery supply the cerebral hemispheres.

Note:
[a] In most patients, the changes are bilateral.

(Peerless, 1997; Edwards-Brown & Quets, 1997; Numaguchi et al., 1997). Diverse racial backgrounds are reported among Americans who have moya-moya diagnosed (Edwards-Brown & Quets, 1997; Numaguchi et al., 1997). A higher rate of moya-moya in Hawaii than on the mainland of the United States was reported by Graham and Matoba (1997). They attributed the greater rate to the high concentration of persons of Japanese ancestry in Hawaii. They found the prevalence and incidence of moya-moya among Japanese–Americans in Hawaii to be similar to that reported in Japan, while rates among residents of Hawaii who were not of Japanese ancestry were quite low. The presentations of moya-moya in the United States and Canada also appear to differ from those reported in Japan. In a series of 39 cases with moya-moya, Peerless (1997) reported that 23 had hemorrhages. This finding raises the possibility that a majority of patients in North America have moya-moya syndrome secondary to an underlying illness rather than true moya-moya disease.

In Japan, Wakai et al. (1997) noted the highest frequency of moya-moya in two age groups: children aged under 14 and adults aged 25–49. Approximately 50% of patients had symptoms before the age of 10. Ikezaki et al. (1997a) found similar peaks in the Korean population but the mean age of patients was higher. In the United States and Canada, a majority of cases are diagnosed in young adults (Peerless, 1997; Edwards-Brown & Quets, 1997). The differences in the age groups between Japan and North America suggest

a different underlying condition. In Japan, the female to male ratio is approximately 1.6–1.8 to 1 (Wakai et al., 1997; Ikezaki et al., 1997b; Fukui, 1997). Ikezaki et al. (1997b) noted that hemorrhage as the presentation of moya-moya was more common among women than men. In Korea and Taiwan, the female to male ratio is approximately 1.3 to 1 (Hung et al., 1997; Ikezaki et al., 1997a, b). A predominance of cases in women also is reported from North America (Peerless, 1997; Numaguchi et al., 1997). In North America, young women usually have ischemic stroke as the initial complaint.

Approximately 10% of patients in Japan have a history of other family members with moya-moya (Wakai et al., 1997). Yamauchi et al. (1997) reported that 14 of 68 cases of moya-moya had a family history of the disease. A mother-to-child inheritance was observed in five cases. This phenomenon raises the possibility of a genetic mitochondrial process. Most patients with familial moya-moya become symptomatic in childhood. Several cases of moya-moya disease in identical twins have been reported (Fukui, 1997). A survey from Korea found that approximately 2% of cases were familial (Ikezaki et al., 1997b). The familial association among patients with moya-moya disease supports an underlying genetic predisposition to the arteriopathy. A familial aggregation of moya-moya syndrome has not been reported and this may explain the paucity of reports of familial cases from Europe or North America.

Pathology of moya-moya

Information about the pathological findings of moya-moya disease continues to mount. Pathological changes have been found in extracranial arteries, a finding that suggests that moya-moya disease is not an isolated intracranial vasculopathy. Bilateral occlusion or severe narrowing of the terminal portion of the ICA and the proximal portions of the ACA and MCA is the hallmark of moya-moya disease. The disease also involves the posterior circulation, most commonly in the posterior cerebral artery (PCA), but the findings are less pronounced. Branches of the external carotid artery, especially the superficial temporal artery (STA) and the middle meningeal artery (MMA), are affected (Aoyagi et al., 1996, 1997; Yang et al., 1997). Microscopic findings in the larger intracranial and extracranial arteries include segmental narrowing, thickening of the intima and media, proliferation of smooth muscle cells, and tortuosity of the internal elastic lamina (Yamashita et al., 1983; Ikeda, 1991; Li et al., 1991; Takebayashi et al., 1984). Li et al. (1991) described degeneration of the smooth muscle cells and fragmentation or absence of the internal elastic lamina.

Hosoda et al. (1997) found that organized mural thrombi in the narrowed arteries induce fibrous thickening of the intima and that leads to arterial occlusion. Inflammatory changes, calcification, and lipid depositions are absent in the arterial wall. Thus, moya-moya disease appears to be a pathologic entity distinct from vasculitis or atherosclerosis (Haltia et al., 1982). Ohtoh et al. (1988) examined the vessels in the posterior circulation of two patients who died of moya-moya. The changes described in the arteries in the anterior circulation were absent but a markedly increased thickness of the medial layer was noted. They attributed these changes, which mimic those of sustained, severe arterial hypertension, to increased pressure secondary to augmented collateral flow to the anterior portions of the cerebral hemispheres through the arteries of the posterior circulation.

The fine meshwork of the basal collateral vessels, which is the clinical hallmark of moya-moya, can involve frontal basal regions (ethmoidal moya-moya) or can be generalized (vault moya-moya) (Suzuki, 1986). Collateral vessels can arise from several branches of the external carotid artery including the MMA, STA, facial artery, temporal artery, or occipital artery. The ethmoidal arteries or the anterior falcine artery can serve as collaterals diverting blood from the ophthalmic artery to the hemisphere. In addition, pial or deep collateral vessels can arise from the tectal plexus, posterior choroidal artery, thalamoperforating arteries, or dorsal callosal branches of the posterior cerebral artery. Many of these vessels are leptomeningeal in location. Rather than new vessels these collateral channels appear to be normal arterioles that are dilated. Kono et al. (1990) found no increase in the number of meningeal vessels; rather, both the arteries and veins were dilated. On microscopic examination, the vessels had fibrous intimal thickening and attenuation of the internal elastic lamina. Microscopically, the small penetrating arteries at the base of the brain show fibrous thickening of the intima, a thin media, a fragmented internal elastic lamina, and microaneurysms (Yamashita et al., 1983). Many of these changes appear similar to those found among patients with chronic, severe arterial hypertension. Vessels that had ruptured were noted to be dilated and to have intramural fibrin deposits, a fragmented elastic layer, and a thin media while the non-ruptured vessels had more thickening of the wall and constriction of the lumen (Yamashita et al., 1983). The presence of dilated arteries correlates with younger ages of the patients and stenoses are more common among older patients. Takebayashi et al. (1984) noted severe damage of the lenticulostriate vessels that make the walls appears moth-eaten and that mimic those of severe hypertension. They also speculated that the changes of the walls of the deep penetrating arteries looked similar to those of a sustained vasospastic process.

The presumed cause of brain ischemia among patients with moya-moya usually is a gradually progressive hypoperfusion secondary to occlusion of the major blood vessels. The collateral channels are unable to maintain adequate blood supply to the brain and infarctions develop in a watershed distribution. Multiple small infarctions also occur in the basal ganglia and deep hemispheric white matter. Progressive cortical ischemia also can result from the borderline perfusion. Larger infarctions result from thromboembolic occlusion and usually are in the cortical distribution of the MCA or ACA. Infarctions in the posterior portions of the hemispheres or the posterior fossa are unusual.

The collateral vessels have microaneurysms or false aneurysms that can be the source of intracranial hemorrhage. Most hemorrhages are located deep in the cerebral hemispheres. Small collateral vessels adjacent to the lateral ventricles can be the source of primary intraventricular hemorrhage (IVH). In addition, saccular aneurysms, most commonly arising from the basilar artery or other collateral vessels have been detected among patients with moya-moya (Leblanc, 1992; Kawaguchi et al., 1996).

Pathogenesis of moya-moya disease and associated conditions

Considerable research has focused on the pathogenesis of moya-moya disease. Still, the cause of moya-moya disease remains elusive. An inherited metabolic abnormality that affects the endothelial or arterial smooth muscle cells is suspected. The factor's primary actions must induce narrowing and occlusion of the large intracranial arteries. The development of the small collaterals (moya-moya phenomenon) may be a secondary event and may be a reactive process in response to subacute ischemia.

Fibroblast growth factor is a mitogen for endothelial cells and may stimulate arterial growth. Increased immunoreactivity to fibroblast growth factor has been detected in specimens obtained from the dura or superficial temporal artery among patients with moya-moya (Hoshimaru et al., 1991; Suzui et al., 1994; Yamamoto et al., 1998). High levels of fibroblast growth factor are found in both the intimal and medial layers and in smooth muscle (Suzui et al., 1994). Levels of basic fibroblast growth factor are elevated in the cerebrospinal fluid among patients with moya-moya (Malek et al., 1997; Yoshimoto et al., 1996, 1997; Takahashi et al., 1993) Transforming growth factor beta-1, which may lead to neovascularization of vessels and angiogenesis, is also implicated as a contributing factor in the pathogenesis of moya-moya (Yamamoto et al., 1997; Hojo et al., 1998). The agent may stimulate elastin mRNA and protein levels in smooth muscle cells (Hojo et al., 1998). The smooth muscle cells obtained from the arteries of patients with moya-moya do not react to platelet-derived growth factor (Aoyagi et al., 1993, 1997). Masuda et al. (1993) detected increased generation of smooth muscle cells among patients with moya-moya disease by detecting the presence of proliferating cell nuclear antigen in cells. While these findings are important and imply a non-atherosclerotic mechanism for the thickening of the arterial wall in moya-moya, additional research on the pathophysiology of the arteriopathy is needed.

The familial occurrence of moya-moya disease and the much higher rates of the disease among persons of Japanese ancestry point towards a genetic predisposition (Graham & Matoba, 1997; Yamauchi et al., 1997) Recently, Inoue et al. (1997) reported that several alleles of the class II genes of the human leukocyte antigen (HLA) have been associated with moya-moya disease. Reports of patients with Down syndrome, von Recklinghausen's disease, and polycystic kidney disease and a moya-moya-like intracranial arteriopathy also suggest a genetic substrate for moya-moya (Cramer et al., 1996; Hattori et al., 1998; Pracyk & Massey, 1989). The two peaks of moya-moya disease in children and young adults suggest more than one genetic abnormality. Future research likely will determine one or more genetic abnormalities that are related to moya-moya disease. Already, Cramer et al. (1996) postulated that a protein encoded on chromosome 21 might be related to the pathogenesis of moya-moya disease. Several reports have associated moya-moya disease with renal artery stenosis; these findings suggest that the arteriopathy may not be restricted to the intracranial and extracranial vasculature (Halley et al., 1988; Jansen et al., 1990; Rupprecht et al., 1992; Nakano et al., 1993) This information also might provide additional clues about a genetic defect leading to a multisystem vascular disease as the cause of moya-moya disease.

The pathogenesis of moya-moya syndrome undoubtedly differs from that of moya-moya disease. Epidemiological variables and clinical presentations differ between the two groups of patients. Persons with moya-moya syndrome usually are young adults, who often have potential risk factors for stroke and a potential for intracranial hemorrhage. Moya-moya syndrome is associated with a large number of diseases. (Table 32.2) Such relationships are not described among the Asian populations with moya-moya disease. Many of the diseases associated with moya-moya

Table 32.2. *Possible relationships with moya-moya syndrome*

Neurofibromatosis	Tuberous sclerosis
Turner syndrome	Retinitis pigmentosa
Down syndrome	Pseudoxanthoma elasticum
Glycogen storage disease type I	Sickle cell disease
Thalassemia	Polycystic kidney disease
Eosinophilic granuloma	Protein C deficiency
Type II plasminogen deficiency	Protein S deficiency
Leptospirosis	Anaerobic meningitis
Epstein–Barr virus	Tuberculous meningitis
Tonsillitis	Pharyngitis
Proprionibacterium acnes	Vasculitis
Systemic lupus erythematosus	Sjogren syndrome
Periarteritis nodosa	Parasellar neoplasms
Kawasaki disease	Craniocerebral trauma
Oral contraceptive use	Alcohol use
Tobacco use	Cranial/basal irradiation
Atherosclerosis	Fibromuscular dysplasia
Renal artery stenosis	Dissecting aneurysm
Arteriovenous malformation	Saccular aneurysm

syndrome seem to have a chronic or subacute course leading to brain ischemia. The ischemia may serve as a potent stimulus for the growth and proliferation of the small vessels at the base of the brain that produces the radiological findings of moya-moya. Rather than a *de novo* arterial disease, many of the arterial changes may be secondary to the underlying illness, such as sickle cell disease, or to a relatively non-specific stimulus to improve blood flow to deep brain structures that are ischemic. Moya-moya syndrome can follow radiation therapy for treatment of an optic nerve glioma, particularly that associated with neurofibromatosis type 1 (Kestle et al., 1993; Bitzer & Topka, 1995). The interval from the radiation exposure until the appearance of the arterial changes has been 6–12 years (Bitzer & Topka, 1995). Interactions between abnormalities in coagulation and recent infections and the development of moya-moya also are reported (Tsuda et al., 1997; Holz et al., 1998; Andeejani et al., 1998; Yamada et al., 1997; Tanigawara et al., 1997). A mesh of small vessels at the base of brain (moya-moya syndrome) arteries can also be secondary to a gradual atherosclerotic occlusion of the major intracranial arteries. Reports from the United States correlate development of moya-moya in young women to the use of oral contraceptives and tobacco (Peerless, 1997; Bruno et al., 1988a; Levine et al., 1991). The large number of associated conditions suggests that the moya-moya syndrome changes may be an epiphenomenon rather than a specific consequence of the primary illness.

Clinical presentations

Patients with moya-moya disease or syndrome can have a number of presentations. No one finding is specific for either form of moya-moya. The presentations appear to be slightly different in children and adults and between moya-moya disease and moya-moya syndrome. Still, moya-moya is included in the differential diagnosis of either hemorrhagic or ischemic stroke in children and young adults.

Affected children commonly present with headaches, motor impairments or seizures (Yamashiro et al., 1984). The headaches have features of migraine and seizures are an important symptom in approximately 5–10% of children. Most seizures are generalized. Recurrent ischemic stroke or transient ischemic attacks (TIA), especially following hyperventilation have been reported (Hung et al., 1997; Battisella & Carollo, 1997). The occurrence of a transient episode of neurological dysfunction following vigorous exercise or hyperventilation in a child should prompt consideration of moya-moya. The infarctions are located in both cortical and subcortical structures and many of the subcortical lesions are small. The appearance on brain imaging is similar to that found among persons with lacunar strokes secondary to hypertension. Multiple small infarctions can lead to a progressive cognitive decline, mental retardation, or failure at school. This sequence of events is distressingly common among children with moya-moya disease.

Recurrent ischemic stroke or TIA also is a common presentation of moya-moya in young adults (Peerless, 1997; Bruno et al., 1988b; Chiu et al., 1998). Subarachnoid hemorrhage also occurs in young adults with moya-moya. As with childhood moya-moya disease, both small subcortical and larger branch cortical infarctions can occur. Ischemic lesions often are in the borderzones between the terminal perfusion beds of the ACA, MCA, and PCA (Bruno et al., 1988a,b). The lesions can be cortical or deep in the hemispheric white matter. Motor, sensory, and cognitive impairments are prominent. A progressive ischemic syndrome can lead to cortical atrophy particularly in the frontal lobes. The resulting clinical syndrome can present with prominent behavioural disturbances and disorders of executive function. In addition, a syndrome imitating multi-infarction dementia also occurs. Brainstem ischemia is an atypical feature (Hirano et al., 1998). With involvement of the posterior cerebral arteries, either children or adults can report visual phenomena (Noda et al., 1987; Miyamoto et al., 1986). Miyamoto et al. (1986) reported that 43 of 178 adult patients with moya-moya had visual symptoms including amaurosis fugax, visual field defects, decreased visual acuity, positive visual phenom-

ena, and diplopia. Seizures and headache are less common among adults than in children.

Intracranial hemorrhage is a presentation of moya-moya in adults. Hemorrhages are secondary to rupture of collateral or penetrating artery, small false aneurysms, or an associated saccular aneurysm or vascular malformation (Iwama et al., 1997a,b,c). Recurrent intracranial hemorrhages occur in a sizeable proportion of patients (Kaufman et al., 1988). Kawaguchi et al. (1996) concluded that recurrent hemorrhage happens at a rate of approximately 2% per patient–year. The locations of bleeding were: intracerebral in approximately 60% of cases, intraventricular in 30% and subarachnoid in 5% (Leblanc, 1992; Saeki et al., 1997; Aoki & Mizutani, 1984). The most common parenchymal locations are the basal ganglia and thalamus (Kawaguchi et al., 1996). The thalamic hemorrhages generally are associated with intraventricular extension (Aoki & Mizutani, 1984; Irikura et al., 1996). Caudate hemorrhage is described as a complication of moya-moya (Steinke et al., 1992). Vascular malformations have been described in association with moya-moya but a direct relationship between the two intracranial vascular diseases is not established (Lichtor & Mullan, 1987).

Several studies report that subarachnoid hemorrhage is rare in moya-moya unless an intracranial saccular aneurysm is present (Kawaguchi et al., 1996; Aoki & Mizutani, 1984; Adams et al., 1979). Although the number of patients with moya-moya and saccular aneurysms is relatively small, the disproportionately high rate of posterior circulation aneurysms raises a possible cause-and-effect relationship. An increase in blood flow through the vertebrobasilar circulation is presumed to stimulate growth of aneurysms in the posterior circulation (Nagamine et al., 1981; Muizelaar, 1988; Kodama et al., 1996; Iwama et al., 1997a,b,c). Small, false aneurysms located on the moya-moya collaterals deep in the brain or along the ventricular surface can also produce subarachnoid hemorrhage (Tanaka et al., 1980; Waga & Tochio, 1985; Konishi et al., 1985).

Several groups have reported cases with unilateral occlusive disease consistent with moya-moya (Kawano et al., 1994; Matsushima et al., 1994; Wanifuchi et al., 1996; Houkin et al., 1996a,b; Hirotsune et al., 1997). A sizeable proportion of these patients subsequently develop bilateral changes but some patients with unilateral disease do not have the progressive course typical of moya-moya disease. While both children and adults with moya-moya disease or moya-moya syndrome can present with unilateral symptoms, persons with unilateral arteriographic changes should be considered to have an atypical process (Houkin et al., 1996a). Houkin et al. (1996a) found that persons with unilateral moya-moya had lower levels of basic fibroblast growth factor than patients with bilateral changes. Persons with unilateral moya-moya do not have a family history of the disease. Thus, moya-moya disease should be diagnosed with caution if a patient has only unilateral clinical, brain imaging, or arterial disease.

Miyakawa et al. (1986) reported a young woman with recurrent stroke, including hemorrhage, secondary to moya-moya, who became pregnant. They successfully treated the woman with a cesarean section in order to avoid a hemorrhage secondary to the labour. More recently, another review of the management of pregnancy in women who have moya-moya concluded that there was no evidence that pregnancy or delivery is associated with an increased risk of stroke, including hemorrhage (Miyakawa et al., 1986). They recommended either cesarean section or vaginal delivery could be performed but that special attention be paid to avoid hypocapnia, hypotension, or hypertension. Although oral contraceptive use may be associated with progression of moya-moya, there is no evidence that pregnancy can cause worsening of the arteriopathy.

Evaluation and diagnosis

Vascular imaging

The diagnosis of moya-moya syndrome or disease requires visualization of the characteristic arterial findings. Accurate imaging of the intracranial vasculature is key to the diagnosis of moya-moya and, in most cases, this necessity means that the patient will need an arteriogram. While arteriography is an invasive study that is associated with some risk, Robertson et al. (1998) found the likelihood of complications among children with moya-moya to be quite low.

As described in Table 32.1, the arterial changes are located predominantly in the anterior circulation and usually are bilateral (Suzuki, 1986). The presence of a distal occlusion of an ICA with the finding of the typical basal network of fine calibre vessels is not sufficient for the diagnosis of moya-moya; in such a situation, a thromboembolic occlusion is likely. Similarly, segmental stenosis of the proximal MCA or ACA secondary to vasospasm should not be confused with moya-moya in a patient with subarachnoid hemorrhage. In the absence of intracranial bleeding, the narrowing is most likely due to moya-moya but accelerated intracranial atherosclerosis is a diagnostic alternative in adults. Several areas of sausage-like constriction and dilation of cortical arteries are not consistent with moya-moya; these findings are more suggestive with a vasculitis espe-

cially if the changes are most prominent in distal branches. Occlusions of branches of the MCA or ACA without the presence of more proximal narrowing are not typical for moya-moya even if pial or leptomeningeal collaterals are visualized. The collaterals often arise from ethmoidal vessels and other leptomeningeal vessels at the base of the brain. A myriad of these fine-calibre vessels is so typical of moya-moya that their absence should lead to questioning of the diagnosis. During the early stages of the disease, prominent leptomeningeal collateral vessels will arise from the PCA and its branches (Satoh et al., 1988; Miyamoto et al., 1984). The presence of these collaterals on a posterior circulation angiogram should raise the diagnosis of moya-moya, although these findings are non-specific. Any obstruction of the proximal portions of the major arteries of the anterior circulation can induce these changes. As the moya-moya progresses, the PCA can become involved in the arteriopathic process (Yamada et al., 1995a,b). Thus, the absence of conspicuous posterior collaterals should not be surprising in advanced stages of the disease.

Arteriography also can demonstrate intracranial saccular aneurysms of the major arteries, particularly in the posterior circulation. The aneurysms appear similar to other saccular aneurysms and they arise at bifurcations. The false microaneurysms found in the penetrating collateral arterioles are not seen by arteriography. Hoshimaru and Kikuchi (1992) evaluated the arteriographic findings of moya-moya in the external carotid artery and its branches. They found stenotic lesions in 13 of 66 cases but no occlusions were identified. The stenotic lesions are similar to those found on major intracranial arteries. These findings may influence decisions about using branches of the external carotid artery in operations to revascularize the cerebral hemisphere.

Several groups tested the usefulness of magnetic resonance angiography (MRA) in detecting the arteriographic abnormalities (Houkin et al., 1994; Yamada et al., 1995; Hasuo et al., 1998). Houkin et al. (1994) found that MRA can accurately detect the stenotic lesions of the distal ICA and proximal portions of the MCA and ACA in most patients. However, they reported that MRA had difficulty in visualizing the basal moya-moya vessels. Conversely, Yamada et al. (1995a,b) found that MRA was able to detect the moya-moya collaterals in 42 of 52 hemispheres that had vascular changes demonstrated by arteriography (81%). They concluded that the sensitivity and specificity of MRA in the diagnosis of moya-moya disease was 73% and 100%, respectively. Because magnetic resonance imaging (MRI) also images the vasculature of the brain, it provides clues about the presence and extent of the arterial disease. MRI can visualize both the absence of flow voids in the ICA,

MCA, and ACA in the suprasellar region and the characteristic collateral network in the basal ganglia (Fujisawa et al., 1987). Yamada et al. (1995a,b) noted that MRI also can detect dilated leptomeningeal and transdural collateral vessels and that the MRI findings correlate well with the extent of the arteriographic changes. Contrast enhancement increases the likelihood of finding these collaterals. The combination of MRI and MRA has a very high yield in detecting the vascular pathology of moya-moya; one report concluded that the two studies provided evidence for the diagnosis of moya-moya with a sensitivity of 92% and specificity of 100% (Yamada et al., 1995a,b).

Katz et al. (1995) concluded that spiral computed tomography (CT) angiography is superior to MRA in visualizing the major arteries at the circle of Willis and that this technology might be superior in the assessment of these vessels in cases of suspected moya-moya. This opinion was supported by the experience of Tsuchiya et al. (1994). They tested the ability of the CT angiography to detect the arterial changes of moya-moya in seven patients; the changes in the main trunks of the ACA and MCA were seen in all cases. Dilated leptomeningeal collaterals were found in four patients and the moya-moya vessels deep in the hemispheres were visualized in two. CT angiography also has been used to monitor the progress of the arterial disease and the patency of collaterals created by revascularization procedures (Kikuchi et al., 1996).

Transcranial Doppler (TCD) is used to assess the patency of the major intracranial arteries and search for the presence of major leptomeningeal collaterals (Muttaqin et al., 1993; Laborde et al., 1993; Takase et al., 1997; Muppala & Castaldo, 1994). Muttaqin et al. (1993) performed TCD in eight patients with moya-moya disease and found low flow velocities in the MCA in comparison to the ICA; these changes probably reflect the severe proximal MCA disease and correlate with poor opacification of the arterial segments by arteriography. At the same time, markedly elevated flow velocities in the PCA and ophthalmic arteries probably reflect the increased flows via these collaterals. Takase et al. (1997) found very high flow velocities at the narrowed sections of the MCA, ACA, and ICA but diminished flow distally. The changes on TCD correlate well with the arteriographic findings and evolve as the disease progresses (Laborde et al., 1993; Takase et al., 1997). As the arteries become obliterated, flow becomes very slow or stops. TCD is a non-invasive way to monitor progression of the arterial disease, especially in children, as tests may be less difficult technically. The relative thinness of the skull in children makes the test easier to perform. In addition, the shorter distances from the skull's surface to the circle of Willis makes the insonation technically clearer.

Duplex ultrasound of the neck may provide evidence of severe disease of the distal ICA or the MCA and ACA by showing no flow at the neck or a very high resistance to flow (Muppala & Castaldo, 1994). The absence of a stenotic or occlusive lesion at the carotid bifurcation and the finding of sluggish distal flow could provide important clues about the location of the distal occlusion and the possible presence of moya-moya. It is likely that this finding will prompt further investigation with MRA or arteriography. The results of the carotid duplex might be particularly helpful in screening a young adult with an ischemic stroke.

Imaging of the brain

Both CT and MRI assess the presence, extent, and location of the ischemic and hemorrhagic lesions of the brain. Takeuchi et al. (1982) reported the results of CT examinations in 18 patients with moya-moya disease. Findings included multiple hypodense lesions (infarctions) in the hemispheres, enlarged ventricles, and cerebral atrophy. The strokes are located predominantly in the deep nuclear structures and deep hemispheric white matter. With contrast enhancement, CT can demonstrate the vascular networks in the basal ganglia. CT also detects intracranial hemorrhages complicating moya-moya. MRI is more successful than CT in detecting ischemic lesions (Bruno et al., 1988b; Takanashi et al., 1993). Multiple small infarctions are found in the basal ganglia, internal capsule and subcortical white matter. The infarctions often will be detected in a border zone pattern between the terminal branches of the ACA and MCA. Takanashi et al. (1993) found that most ischemic lesions in younger children are in the cortical and immediate subcortical structures while adults have more deep white matter infarctions in the centrum semiovale and the basal ganglia. Ischemic cortical lesions located primarily in the anterior portions of the cerebral hemispheres also can be detected.

Electroencephalography and evoked potentials

The abnormalities detected by electroencephalography (EEG) are non-specific but more commonly noted among children. The EEG generally shows bilateral diffuse slow activity. A characteristic EEG finding is the 're-build-up' phenomenon, which is a gradual decrease in the frequency but an activation of the amplitude of electrical activity, induced by hyperventilation (Kurlemann et al., 1992; Kuroda et al., 1995). The changes in EEG appear to be related to a focal reduction in perfusion reserve that is induced by the hyperventilation causing vasoconstriction

(Kuroda et al., 1995). Abnormalities in visual evoked potentials are correlated with involvement of the PCA and performing the test might be an effective way to monitor for progression of the vasculopathy (Tashima-Kurita et al., 1989). Chen et al. (1989) evaluated the usefulness of brain-stem auditory-evoked potentials, visual-evoked potentials, and somatosensory-evoked potentials in the evaluation of 22 children with moya-moya disease. Findings on the tests included prolonged latencies, reduced amplitudes, and poor wave forms, which correlated well with the clinical, brain imaging, and arteriographic abnormalities.

Measurements of cerebral metabolism and blood flow

Changes in cerebral blood flow and metabolism can be assessed by position emission tomography (PET), single photon emission computed tomography (SPECT), xenon enhanced CT, and functional MRI. In a PET-based study, Taki et al. (1989) found decreased regional cerebral blood flow (rCBF) in hemispheric grey matter, white matter and the basal ganglia among nine adults with moya-moya disease. They also noted an increase in regional cerebral blood volume (rCBV) in the deep structures among patients with either ischemic or hemorrhagic symptoms but the cerebral metabolic rate for oxygen and the oxygen extraction fraction were not reduced. Similar findings were described among children with moya-moya disease (Ikezaki et al., 1994). These findings, detected among patients who did not have recent symptoms, suggest a border-line compensated status of circulation in the brain and suggests that vascular reserve is minimal. This conclusion is supported by the experience of Kuwabara et al. (1997a, b), who found severely decreased cerebrovascular responses to hypercapnia and decreased hemodynamic reserve capacity in both adults and children with moya-moya. Based on the results of xenon-enhanced CT studies, Obara et al. (1997) found markedly different patterns of rCBF in reaction to increased blood concentrations of carbon dioxide among patients with moya-moya when compared to persons with atherosclerotic occlusion of the ICA. They concluded that relative preservation of the rCBF might be secondary to the presence of more abundant collaterals among persons with moya-moya. Horowitz et al. (1995) concluded that detecting changes in rCBF on xenon-enhanced CT in response to challenges from carbon dioxide or acetazolamide was a useful way to predict which patients with moya-moya could benefit from revascularization procedures.

Several groups have reported on the usefulness of SPECT in the evaluation of patients with moya-moya (Takikawa et al., 1990; Ogawa et al., 1990a, b; Dietrichs et al., 1992; Inoue et al., 1993; Hoshi et al., 1994; Yamada et al., 1996; Miller et al., 1996; Nakagawara et al., 1997; Oyama et al., 1998; Ishikawa et al., 1998; Sato et al., 1999). Tests have been used to detect discrepancies in rCBF both at rest and in response to a challenge such as acetazolamide (Dietrichs et al., 1992). These tests show relative preservation of rCBF in the posterior portions of the hemisphere that corresponds to the relative conservation of the patency of the posterior cerebral arteries (Ogawa et al., 1990a,b). Detection of a diminution of rCBF in the posterior hemispheres foretells development of stenotic or occlusive lesions in the vertebrobasilar circulation (Yamada et al., 1996). Patients with moya-moya have significantly lower rCBF levels than controls, and these changes progress with age (Ogawa et al., 1990a,b; Oyama et al., 1998; Ishikawa et al., 1998). The disturbances in perfusion involve a more extensive area of the brain than that predicted by the arteriographic findings (Hoshi et al., 1994). Functional and metabolic studies of the brain using MRI techniques also are used to assess patients with moya-moya. In general, the results of these tests parallel those found with SPECT (Tzika et al., 1997; Shimizu et al., 1997; Tsuchiya et al., 1998).

The results of these studies, in aggregate, provide data that outline the presence, location, and severity of perfusion defects in children and adults with moya-moya. The changes in blood flow and metabolism appear more pronounced than the arteriographic or brain imaging abnormalities. The role of these tests in determining prognoses and developing treatment plans likely will increase. For example, sequential deterioration of rCBF in a clinically stable patient may prompt consideration of a revascularization procedure before the patient has an ischemic stroke (Takikawa et al., 1990; Nakagawara et al., 1997). The tests also can be used to measure hemodynamic responses to revascularization procedures.

Prognosis and treatment

As a rule, the prognosis is guarded for both children and adults with moya-moya disease or moya-moya syndrome. In particular, children with moya-moya disease have a very high risk for recurrent strokes that leads to cognitive declines and severe disability (Maki & Enomoto, 1988; Ueki et al., 1994). The impairments of mental functioning seem to be worst among those children who become symptomatic at early ages, who have bilateral disease, or who have had multiple strokes (Maki & Enomoto, 1988; Ishii et al.,

1984). Young adults with moya-moya also seem to be at high risk for recurrent strokes that can lead to progressive motor, sensory, and cognitive impairments. The neurological sequelae from the recurrent strokes can lead to disability or even long-term institutionalized care.

Because of the very bleak natural history of moya-moya disease and moya-moya syndrome, medical or surgical measures to prevent stroke or to lessen its consequences are critical. Determination of the efficacy of any therapy is difficult because of the low incidence and prevalence of moya-moya even in Japan, and the diversity of the presentations of the illness makes a clinical trial complex and hard to perform. In many ways, moya-moya would meet the definition of an orphan disease. The ability to recruit sufficient patients into a clinical trial to test an intervention is limited. In addition, many physicians have little experience dealing with the disease. Thus, little solid data will probably be available about the usefulness or lack of usefulness of any intervention to prevent the cerebrovascular complications of moya-moya.

No therapy has been tested for its ability in reversing or halting the progression of the primary arteriopathy. Thus, treatment is aimed at easing the hemorrhagic or ischemic sequelae of the arterial disease.

In general, treatment of acute ischemic stroke secondary to moya-moya is similar to management of stroke secondary to other diseases. Management includes measures to forestall medical or surgical complications and interventions, including rehabilitation, to maximize recovery. Because the patients are children and young adults who might live several years, rehabilitative and restorative efforts to limit disability are critical. Hypoxia, hypercarbia, and hypotension should be aggressively treated in an effort to limit the possibility of additional ischemia. In addition, hypertension should be aggressively managed because of the risk of cerebral hemorrhage. Because of the potential for intracranial bleeding, anticoagulants and thrombolytic agents might be contraindicated. While young patients with ischemic stroke secondary to moya-moya likely will be treated with thrombolytic agents in the future, no data are currently available about either the safety or effectiveness of such treatment.

Patients with an intracranial hemorrhage secondary to a rupture of a complicating saccular aneurysm should have the aneurysm treated as soon as possible (Adams et al., 1979; Kodama et al., 1996). Options include surgical clipping or intravascular placement of coils. Measures to avoid dehydration or extremes of blood pressure are important because vasospasm secondary to subarachnoid hemorrhage could worsen the already borderline perfusion from the moya-moya. Surgical management of the aneurysms can be difficult because they often are located in the posterior circulation (Muizelaar, 1988; Iwama et al., 1997a,b,c). The surgeon needs to take care to preserve the critical collateral circulation which may be quite prominent around the circle of Willis (Kodama et al., 1996). No surgical therapy is prescribed to treat the small aneurysms that arise on the penetrating collateral vessels. Treatment of intraventricular or intracerebral hemorrhage secondary to moya-moya is similar to that prescribed for hematomas of other causes. Because the hematomas usually are deep in the cerebral hemispheres, surgical evacuation of the lesions is difficult.

Management of the underlying or associated condition is a fundamental component of care of patients with moya-moya syndrome. Treating the concomitant disease likely will help slow the arterial process and it might lessen the likelihood of recurrent cerebrovascular events. For example, prevention of crises in children with sickle cell disease or halting use of oral contraceptives or smoking might help prevent recurrent stroke. Hypertension and other risk factors for stroke should be treated. Children should be instructed to avoid activities associated with hyperventilation.

Because antiplatelet agents are effective in lessening the risk of stroke among patients with TIA, these medications are prescribed in an attempt to forestall recurrent stroke. Still, no data are available about their usefulness. In addition, information is lacking about the relative effectiveness of aspirin, ticlopidine, clopidogrel or dipyridamole alone or in combination. In general, low doses of aspirin alone are prescribed first. If recurrent attacks occur, either ticlopidine or clopidogrel could be prescribed or dipyridamole could be added to the aspirin. Because dipyridamole has a vasodilating effect, it might have the potential of altering flow among patients with moya-moya. No information is known about either a flow-related benefit or adverse reaction to treatment with dipyridamole. Other vasodilating drugs have had limited success. Because patients with moya-moya do have a high risk for brain hemorrhage, the role of long-term anticoagulants appears to be minimal. Volume expansion therapy has the potential to improve rCBF but administration of low-molecular-weight dextran is not effective. No information is available about the use of pentoxifylline. An anecdotal report of success with forestalling recurrent stroke in two children following the administration of a calcium channel-blocking agent (nicardipine) is interesting (Hosnain et al., 1994).

Because of the limited success from medical interventions and because of the high probability of recurrent strokes, several surgical interventions are used to prevent stroke in children or adults with moya-moya (Quest &

Correll, 1985; Matsushima et al., 1989; Kobayashi et al., 1991; Karasawa et al., 1992; Yamada et al., 1992; Kinugasa et al., 1993; George et al., 1993; Aoki, 1993; Ross et al., 1994; Nariai et al., 1994; Kinugasa et al., 1994; Kawaguchi et al., 1996a; Touho et al., 1996; Mizoi et al., 1996; Houkin et al., 1996b; Kashiwagi et al., 1996; Dauser et al., 1997; Houkin et al., 1997a, b; Tenjin & Ueda, 1997; Ishikawa et al., 1997; Han et al., 1997; Hoffman, 1997; Nakashima et al., 1997; Choi et al., 1997; Iwama et al., 1997a; Sakamoto et al., 1997; Ikezaki et al., 1997a, c; Ohtaki et al., 1998; Okada et al., 1998; Kohno et al., 1998; Imaizumi et al., 1998; Iwama et al., 1998; Houkin et al., 1998). The primary aim of the operations is to prevent recurrent ischemic stroke although a few clinical studies assessed the value of the operations in preventing recurrent brain hemorrhage. The operations attempt to improve blood supply to the brain via surgical creation of new collaterals; areas with borderline perfusion would receive improved flow and could have a lower risk of recurrent brain ischemia. The operations might lower the risk of hemorrhage from the moya-moya vessels by reducing pressure in these small calibre collaterals by providing new channels for flow to the brain (Houkin et al., 1996b).

Information about the use of interventional radiologic techniques including angioplasty and stenting is sparse. However, angioplasty of multiple intracranial arteries is being done successfully in treatment of vasospasm after aneurysmal subarachnoid hemorrhage. Thus, angioplasty of the stenotic lesions of the distal ICA and the proximal portions of the MCA and ACA might be possible if the moya-moya is recognized early.

Creation of a STA to MCA anastomosis (extracranial/intracranial bypass (EC/IC bypass)) is used to treat either children or adults with moya-moya. A branch of the STA usually is attached surgically to a parietal or temporal branch of the posterior/inferior division of the MCA (Houkin et al., 1998). A branch of the STA also can be attached to distal branches of the ACA in order to improve blood supply to the medial portion of the frontal lobe (Iwama et al., 1997, 1998; Houkin et al., 1998). Unfortunately, the operation does not seem to slow progression of the stenosis or occlusion of the ICA or the proximal portions of the ACA or MCA. Thus, the primary response is to maintain sufficient flow in the distal vascular beds. This operation has shown success in treatment of patients with moya-moya. The procedure often is done bilaterally in staged operations. Quest and Correll (1985) reported that six of eight patients treated by STA/MCA anastomosis seemed to benefit from treatment. They treated patients who had either recurrent hemorrhagic or ischemic stroke. Improvement in the angiographic findings, including a regression of the moya-moya vessels has

followed the STA/MCA anastomosis operation (Kobayashi et al., 1991; George et al., 1993; Okada et al., 1998). Karasawa et al. (1992) noted a decline in the frequency of recurrent ischemic events (TIA or stroke) among 87 of 104 children with moya-moya disease who had revascularization operations. Children older than 7 who did not have a major preoperative stroke generally had good outcomes and normal intelligence on postoperative assessments. Houkin et al. (1997b) concluded that STA/MCA anastomosis remains the best way to improve blood flow to the frontal lobe in patients with moya-moya.

Because of the advanced state of the intracranial arterial disease, cortical branches of the MCA or ACA may be atretic and can not serve as the recipient vessel for a STA/MCA anastomosis. Thus, alterative operations to supply collaterals to the hemisphere have been developed including encephalo-duro-arterio-synangiosis (EDAS), encephalo-arterio-synangiosis (EAS), encephalo-duro-arterio-myo-synangiosis (EDAMS) and encephalo-myo-synangiosis (EMS). Although the details of the operations vary slightly as denoted by their different names, in general, they involve opening the dura and placing a piece of tissue with a vascular supply on the pial surface of the hemisphere. The tissue can be branches of the STA that are moved from the temporalis muscle or a piece of the temporalis muscle and its arterial supply (Nariai et al., 1994). The goal is to indirectly improve blood supply via angiogenesis and both donor and recipient vessels dilate after the operation (Nariai et al., 1994). Besides attaching a vessel to the pial surface of the lateral portion of the hemisphere to improve flow in the territory of the MCA, tissue also can be placed along the interhemispheric fissure to augment blood supply to the terminal bed of the territory of the ACA (Kinugasa et al., 1994; Nakashima et al., 1997). Adjacent meningeal arteries, including the MMA, also seem to participate in developing the new collateral vessels (Yamada et al., 1992).

The patients can be selected for surgery based on evidence of poor perfusion detected by blood flow studies (Kohno et al., 1998). Sequential studies have demonstrated improvements in metabolic activity and blood flow on the side of the brain with the revascularization procedure (Nariai et al., 1994; Kashiwagi et al., 1996). These operations appear to be safe in children and adults and the results of these procedures generally have been positive when using a reduction in the frequency of recurrent stroke as a measure of efficacy (Kinugasa et al., 1993; Ross et al., 1994; Tenjin & Udea, 1997; Han et al., 1997; Hoffman, 1997; Nakashima et al., 1997; Choi et al., 1997; Ikezaki et al., 1997c; Imaizumi et al., 1998).

The indirect operations can be combined with STA/MCA anastomosis in treatment of some patients; for example, the patient may have an anastomosis on one side of the brain and an indirect procedure on the other (Ishikawa et al., 1997; Sakamoto et al., 1997). The procedures have been performed in combination on the same side of the brain during a single operation (Houkin et al., 1997). Mizoi et al. (1996) concluded that the indirect revascularization procedures were superior to STA/MCA anastomosis in adults with moya-moya.

Transposition or transplantation of a piece of omentum to the pial surface of the hemisphere also has been used to treat patients with moya-moya (Touho et al., 1996; Ohtaki et al., 1998). Omental tissue was selected because of its potency in stimulating angiogenesis and improving vascularity of the brain. Omental tissue is placed on an extensive area of the surface of the brain. The tissue is placed along with a branch of the STA or in combination with an STA/MCA anastomosis (Ohtaki et al., 1998). This procedure has been successful in children who have not had a response to other revascularization operations (Touho et al., 1996).

Kawaguchi et al. (1996) recommended a technique of placement of multiple burr holes in the calvarium. The surgical procedure could stimulate neovascularization of the dural surface via branches of the MMA and the STA to improve blood supply to the brain. The procedure could be done safely in adults with moya-moya and they noted clinical improvement in their patients. A technique where part of the circulation of the MMA is diverted to serve as a source of blood supply to the pial surface of the brain also has been used (Dauser et al., 1997).

The responses to the revascularization procedures among patients who have presented with intracranial hemorrhage have not been as promising as among the persons who had primarily ischemic symptoms (Aoki, 1993; Choi et al., 1997; Ikezaki et al., 1997b; Okada et al., 1998). No operative procedure has been shown to be effective in prevention of rebleeding (Ikezaki et al., 1997b). Houkin et al. (1996b) reported that 5 of 35 patients had recurrent hemorrhage following a revascularization procedure during a mean period of follow-up of 6.4 years. Still, because the risk of recurrent stroke, including hemorrhage, seems to be extraordinarily high in persons with moya-moya, a recurrence rate of 14% in 6 years might be a clinically relevant reduction in the number of events.

The data about the ideal timing and the potential efficacy of the operative procedures are not derived from any clinical trials formally testing the usefulness of the surgery. Still, the experience to date suggests that either the direct or indirect revascularization procedures offer the best promise in preventing recurrent ischemic stroke. The operations should be performed early in the course of the

illness in order to lessen the risk of the disabling sequelae of recurrent brain ischemia including cognitive impairments and mental retardation. The superiority of either the direct approach of an anastomosis using a branch of the STA as a donor or the indirect approach based on synangiosis is not established. Similarly, data have not established the superiority of one indirect revascularization approach over another.

Conclusions

The term moya-moya encompasses two clinical scenarios, moya-moya disease and moya-moya syndrome. Moya-moya disease likely is a distinct entity that has a genetic basis. The differences in ages among affected patients suggest that more than one genetic or metabolic disturbance may cause moya-moya disease. Children affected at young ages by moya-moya disease might have a more serious metabolic derangement than may young adults. Moya-moya disease is most prevalent in populations in northeastern Asia. While moya-moya disease can occur in other ethnic groups, the rates of the true disease probably are sufficiently low that the diagnosis of moya-moya disease should be made with caution. The presentations and course of moya-moya disease have been described in detail. A hallmark of the disease is its relentlessly progressive nature with recurrent strokes leading to cognitive disabilities.

The group of persons with moya-moya syndrome is not defined well. Moya-moya syndrome remains a non-specific diagnosis based on the radiological findings that imitate those of moya-moya disease. In the future, a common thread may be identified that will denote the subset of patients with other intracranial arterial diseases who will develop the moya-moya syndrome. However, at present, the best approach is to assume that many of the radiological changes are epiphenomena induced by a progressive arterial process (of whatever cause) and chronic ischemia. The large number of associated conditions supports the concept that the development of the meshwork of fine collateral vessels deep in the cerebral hemispheres is in response to another vascular process. Clinical presentations probably are less stereotyped and the prognoses may differ with moya-moya syndrome than with moya-moya disease. The finding of a unilateral process at the time of presentation should raise consideration of moya-moya syndrome rather than true moya-moya disease. Moya-moya syndrome probably is relatively uncommon in children under the age of 10 but probably accounts for the majority of cases in adults. Moya-moya syndrome likely can occur in any ethnic group and most cases from Europe and North America probably will have moya-moya syndrome.

Moya-moya should be considered as the potential cause of any TIA, ischemic stroke, or hemorrhagic stroke in childhood. While moya-moya is not the most common cause of either hemorrhagic or ischemic stroke in young adults, it should be included in the etiologic differential diagnosis – especially if one of the associated conditions is identified or if no other obvious etiology of stroke is detected. Even if the moya-moya phenomenon is identified angiographically in a young person with a stroke, other potential causes should be sought.

While brain-imaging tests, especially MRI, can provide clues towards the diagnosis of moya-moya, arteriography remains the standard way to detect the arteriopathy. It remains the most definitive measure to assess the presence, location, and extent of the vascular abnormalities. Non-invasive studies of blood flow or metabolism can be used to monitor progress of the disease and to aid in selection of patients who might be treated with a revascularization procedure.

The acute management of ischemic stroke secondary to moya-moya probably does not differ greatly from the treatment of persons with stroke secondary to other causes. Antiplatelet aggregating agents should be prescribed. However, because of the perceived high risk of hemorrhage among persons with moya-moya, the use of anticoagulants or thrombolytic agents should be viewed with caution. Treatment of a hemorrhagic stroke in a patient with moya-moya should parallel that prescribed to patients with intracranial bleeding from other sources.

Management to control risk factors, such as hypertension or smoking, is fundamental for strategies to prevent ischemic stroke or recurrent ischemic stroke among patients with moya-moya. Direct or indirect revascularization procedures should be offered early in the course of the illness in order to prevent recurrent ischemic stroke.

References

Adams, H.P. Jr, Kassell, N.F., Wisoff, H.S. & Drake, C.G. (1979). Intracranial saccular aneurysm and moyamoya disease. *Stroke*, **10**, 174–9.

Andeejani, A.M., Salih, M.A., Kolawole, T. et al. (1998). Moyamoya syndrome with unusual angiogr aphic findings and protein C deficiency. Review of the literature. *Journal of Neurological Sciences*, **159**, 11–16.

Aoki, N. (1993). Cerebrovascular bypass surgery for the treatment of moyamoya disease. Unsatisfactory outcome in the patients presenting with intracranial hemorrhage. *Surgical Neurology*, **40**, 372–7.

Aoki, N. & Mizutani, H. (1984). Does moyamoya disease cause subarachnoid hemorrhage? Review of 54 cases with intracranial hemorrhage confirmed by computerized tomography. *Journal of Neurosurgery*, **60**, 348–53.

Aoyagi, M., Fukai, N., Matsushima, Y., Yamamoto, M. & Yamamoto, K. (1993). Kinetics of ^{125}I-PDGF binding and down-regulation of PDGF receptor in arterial smooth muscle cells derived from patients with moyamoya disease. *Journal of Cellular Physiology*, **154**, 281–8.

Aoyagi, M., Fukai, N., Yamamoto, M., Nakagawa, K., Matsushima, Y. & Yamamoto, K. (1996). Early development of intimal thickening in superficial temporal arteries in patients with moyamoya disease. *Stroke*, **27**, 1750–4.

Aoyagi, M., Fukai, N., Yamamoto, M., Matsushima, Y. & Yamamoto, K. (1997). Development of intimal thickening in superficial temporal arteries in patients with moyamoya disease. *Clinical Neurology and Neurosurgery*, **99**(Suppl. 2), S213–17.

Battisella, P.A. & Carollo, C. (1997). Clinical and neuroradiological findings of moyamoya disease in Italy. *Clinical Neurology and Neurosurgery*, **99**(Suppl. 2), S54–7.

Bitzer, M. & Topka, H. (1995). Progressive cerebral occlusive disease after radiation therapy. *Stroke*, **26**, 131–6.

Bruno, A., Adams, H.P. Jr, Biller, J., Rezai, K., Cornell, S. & Aschenbrener, C.A. (1988a). Cerebral infarction due to moyamoya disease in young adults. *Stroke*, **19**, 826–33.

Bruno, A., Yuh, W.T., Biller, J., Adams, H.P. Jr & Cornell, S.H. (1988b). Magnetic resonance imaging in young adults with cerebral infarction due to moyamoya. *Archives of Neurology*, **45**, 303–6.

Chen, Y.J., Kurokawa, T., Kitamoto, I. & Ueda, K. (1989). Multimodality evoked potentials in children with moyamoya disease. *Neuropediatrics*, **20**, 20–4.

Chiu, D., Sheddon, P., Bratina, P. & Grotta, J.C. (1998). Clinical features of moyamoya disease in the United States. *Stroke*, **29**, 1347–51.

Choi, J.U., Kim, D.S., Kim, E.Y. & Lee, K.C. (1997). Natural history of moyamoya disease. Comparison of activity of daily living in surgery and non surgery groups. *Clinical Neurology and Neurosurgery*, **99**(Suppl. 2), S11–18.

Cramer, S.C., Robertson, R.L., Dooling, E.C. & Scott, R.M. (1996). Moyamoya and Down syndrome. Clinical and radiological features. *Stroke*, **27**, 2131–5.

Dauser, R.C., Tuite, G.F. & McCluggage, C.W. (1997). Dural inversion procedure for moyamoya disease. Technical note. *Journal of Neurosurgery*, **86**, 719–23.

Dietrichs, E., Dahl, A., Nyberg-Hansen, R., Russell, D., Rootwelt, K. & Veger, T. (1992). Cerebral blood flow findings in moyamoya disease in adults. *Acta Neurologica Scandinavica*, **85**, 318–22.

Edwards-Brown, M.K. & Quets, J.P. (1997). Midwest experience with moyamoya disease. *Clinical Neurology and Neurosurgery*, **99**(Suppl. 2), S36–8.

Fujisawa, I., Asato, R., Nishimura, K. et al. (1987). Moyamoya disease: MR imaging. *Radiology*, **164**, 103–5.

Fukui, M. (1997). Current state of study on moyamoya disease in Japan. *Surgical Neurology*, **47**, 138–43.

George, B.D., Neville, B.G. & Lumley, J.S. (1993). Transcranial revascularization in childhood and adolescence. *Developmental Medicine and Child Neurology*, **35**, 675–82.

Graham, J.F. & Matoba, A. (1997). A survey of moyamoya disease in Hawaii. *Clinical Neurology and Neurosurgery*, **99**(Suppl. 2), S31–5.

Halley, S.E., White, W.B., Ramsby, G.R. & Voytovich, A.E. (1988). Renovascular hypertension in moyamoya syndrome. Therapeutic response to percutaneous transluminal angioplasty. *American Journal of Hypertension*, **1**(4 Pt. 1), 348–52.

Haltia, M., Iivanainen, M., Majuri, H. & Puranen, M. (1982). Spontaneous occlusion of the circle of Willis (moyamoya syndrome). *Clinical Neuropathology*, **1**, 11–22.

Han, D.H., Nam, D.H. & Oh, C.W. (1997). Moyamoya disease in adults. Characteristics of clinical presentation and outcome after encephalo-duro-arterio-synangiosis. *Clinical Neurology and Neurosurgery*, **99**(Suppl. 2), S151–5.

Hattori, S., Kiguchi, H., Ishii, T., Nakajima, T. & Yatsuzuka, H. (1998). Moyamoya disease with concurrent von Recklinghausen's disease and cerebral arteriovenous malformation. *Pathology, Research and Practice*, **194**, 363–9.

Hirano, T., Uyama, E., Tashima, K., Mita, S. & Uchino, M. (1998). An atypical case of adult moyamoya disease with initial onset of brain stem ischemia. *Journal of Neurological Sciences*, **157**, 100–4.

Hirotsune, N., Meguro, T., Kawada, S., Nakashima, H. & Ohmoto, T. (1997). Long-term follow-up study of patients with unilateral moyamoya disease. *Clinical Neurology and Neurosurgery*, **99**(Suppl. 2), S178–81.

Hoffman, H.J. (1997). Moyamoya disease and syndrome. *Clinical Neurology and Neurosurgery*, **99** (Suppl. 2), S39–44.

Hojo, M., Hoshimaru, M., Miyamoto, S. et al. (1998). Role of transforming growth factor-beta 1 in the pathogenesis of moyamoya disease. *Journal of Neurosurgery*, **89**, 623–9.

Holz, A., Woldenberg, R., Miller, D., Kalina, P., Black, K. & Lane, E. (1998). Moyamoya disease in a patient with hereditary spherocytosis. *Pediatric Radiology*, **28**, 95–7.

Horowitz, M., Yonas, H. & Albright, A.L. (1995). Evaluation of cerebral blood flow and hemodynamic reserve in symptomatic moyamoya disease using stable Xenon-CT blood flow. *Surgical Neurology*, **44**, 251–61.

Hoshi, H., Ohnishi, T., Jinnouchi, S. et al. (1994). Cerebral blood flow study in patients with moyamoya disease evaluated by IMP SPECT. *Journal of Nuclear Medicine*, **35**, 44–50.

Hoshimaru, M. & Kikuchi, H. (1992). Involvement of the external carotid arteries in moyamoya disease. Neuroradiological evaluation of 66 patients. *Neurosurgery*, **31**, 398–400.

Hoshimaru, M., Takahashi, J.A., Kikuchi, H., Nagata, I. & Hatanaka, M. (1991). Possible roles of basic fibroblast growth factor in the pathogenesis of moyamoya disease. An immunohistochemical study. *Journal of Neurosurgery*, **75**, 267–70.

Hosnain, S.A., Hughes, J.T., Forem, S.L., Wisoff, J. & Fish, I. (1994). Use of a calcium channel blocker (nicardipine HCl) in treatment of childhood moyamoya. *Journal of Child Neurology*, **9**, 378–80.

Hosoda, Y., Ikeda, E. & Hirose, S. (1997). Histopathological studies on spontaneous occlusion of the circle of Willis (cerebrovascular moyamoya disease). *Clinical Neurology and Neurosurgery*, **99**(Suppl. 2), S203–8.

Houkin, K., Aoki, T., Takahashi, A. & Abe, H. (1994). Diagnosis of moyamoya disease with magnetic resonance angiography. *Stroke*, **25**, 2159–64.

Houkin, K., Abe, H., Yoshimoto, T. & Takahashi, A. (1996a). Is 'unilateral' moyamoya disease different from moyamoya disease? *Journal of Neurosurgery*, **85**, 772–6.

Houkin, K., Kamiyama, H., Abe, H., Takahashi, A. & Kuroda, S. (1996b). Surgical therapy for adult moyamoya disease. Can surgical revascularization prevent the recurrence of intracerebral hemorrhage? *Stroke*, **27**, 1342–6.

Houkin, K., Ishikawa, T., Yoshimoto, T. & Abe, H. (1997a). Direct and indirect revascularization for moyamoya disease surgical techniques and peri-operative complications. *Clinical Neurology and Neurosurgery*, **99**(Suppl. 2), S142–5.

Houkin, K., Kamiyama, H., Takahashi, A., Kuroda, S. & Abe, H. (1997b). Combined revascularization surgery for childhood moyamoya disease. STA-MCA and encephalo-duro-arterio-myo-synangiosis. *Childs Nervous System*, **13**, 24–9.

Houkin, K., Ishikawa, T., Kuroda, S. & Abe, H. (1998). Vascular reconstruction using interposed small vessels. *Neurosurgery*, **43**, 501–5.

Hung, C.C., Tu, Y.K., Lin, L.S. & Shih, C.J. (1997). Epidemiological study of moyamoya disease in Taiwan. *Clinical Neurology and Neurosurgery*, **99**(Suppl. 2), S23–5.

Ikeda, E. (1991). Systemic vascular changes in spontaneous occlusion of the circle of Wills. *Stroke*, **22**, 1358–62.

Ikezaki, K., Matsushima, T., Kuwabara, Y., Suzuki, S.O., Nomura, T. & Fukui, M. (1994). Cerebral circulation and oxygen metabolism in childhood moyamoya disease. A perioperative emission tomography study. *Journal of Neurosurgery*, **81**, 843–50.

Ikezaki, K., Fukui, M., Inamura, T., Kinukawa, N., Wakai, N. & Ono, Y. (1997a). The current status of the treatment for hemorrhagic type moyamoya disease based on a 1995 nationwide survey in Japan. *Clinical Neurology and Neurosurgery*, **99**(Suppl. 2), S183–6.

Ikezaki, K., Han, D.H., Kawano, T., Inamura, T. & Fukui, M. (1997b). Epidemiological survey of moyamoya disease in Korea. *Clinical Neurology and Neurosurgery*, **99**(Suppl. 2), S6–10.

Ikezaki, K., Inamura, T., Kawano, T. & Fukui, M. (1997c). Clinical features of probable moyamoya disease in Japan. *Clinical Neurology and Neurosurgery*, **99**(Suppl. 2), S173–7.

Ikezaki, K., Han, D.H., Kawano, T., Kinukawa, N. & Fukui, M. (1997d). A clinical comparison of definite moyamoya disease between South Korea and Japan. *Stroke*, **28**, 2513–17.

Imaizumi, T., Hayashi, K., Saito, K., Osawa, M. & Fukuyama, U. (1998). Long-term outcomes of pediatric moyamoya disease monitored to adulthood. *Pediatric Neurology*, **18**, 321–5.

Inoue, Y., Momose, T., Machida, K., Honda, N. & Tsutsumi, K. (1993). Cerebral vasodilatory capacity mapping using technetium-99m-DTPA-HAS SPECT and acetalozamide in moyamoya disease. *Journal of Nuclear Medicine*, **34**, 1984–6.

Inoue, T.K., Ikezaki, K., Sasazuki, T., Matsushima, T. & Fukui, M.

(1997). Analysis of class II genes of human leukocyte antigen in patients with moyamoya disease. *Clinical Neurology and Neurosurgery*, **99**(Suppl. 2), S234–7.

Irikura, K., Miyasaka, Y., Kurata, A. et al. (1996). A source of haemorrhage in adult patients with moyamoya disease. The significance of tributaries from the choroidal artery. *Acta Neurochirurgica*, **138**, 1282–6.

Ishii, R., Takeuchi, S., Ibayashi, K. & Tanaka, R. (1984). Intelligence in children with moyamoya disease. Evaluation after surgical treatments with special reference to changes in cerebral blood flow. *Stroke*, **15**, 873–7.

Ishikawa, T., Houkin, K., Kamiyama, H. & Abe, H. (1997). Effects of surgical revascularization on outcome of patients with pediatric moyamoya disease. *Stroke*, **28**, 1170–3.

Ishikawa, T., Tanaka, N., Houkin, K., Kuroda, S., Abe, H. & Mitsumori, K. (1998). Regional cerebral blood flow in pediatric moyamoya disease. Age-dependent decline in specific regions. *Childs Nervous System*, **14**, 366–71.

Iwama, T., Hashimoto, N., Tsukahara, T. & Miyake, H. (1997a). Superficial temporal artery to anterior cerebral artery direct anastomosis in patients with moyamoya disease. *Clinical Neurology and Neurosurgery*, **99**(Suppl. 2), S134–6.

Iwama, T., Morimoto, M., Hashimoto, N., Goto, Y., Todaka, T. & Sawada, M. (1997b). Mechanism of intracranial bleeding in moyamoya disease. *Clinical Neurology and Neurosurgery*, **99**(Suppl. 2), S187–90.

Iwama, T., Todaka, T. & Hashimoto, N. (1997c). Direct surgery for major artery aneurysm associated with moyamoya disease. *Clinical Neurology and Neurosurgery*, **99**(Suppl. 2), S191–3.

Iwama, T., Hashimoto, N., Miyake, H. & Yonekawa, Y. (1998). Direct revascularization to the anterior cerebral artery territory in patients with moyamoya disease. Report of five cases. *Neurosurgery*, **42**, 1157–61.

Jansen, J.N., Donker, A.J., Luth, W.J. & Smit, L.M. (1990). Moyamoya disease associated with renovascular hypertension. *Neuropediatrics*, **21**, 44–7.

Karasawa, J., Touho, H., Ohnishi, H., Miyamoto, S. & Kikuchi, H. (1992). Long-term follow-up study after extracranial-intracranial bypass surgery for anterior circulation ischemia in childhood moyamoya disease. *Journal of Neurosurgery*, **77**, 84–9.

Kashiwagi, S., Yamashita, T., Katoh, S. et al. (1996). Regression of moyamoya vessels and hemodynamic changes after successful revascularization in childhood moyamoya disease. *Acta Neurologica Scandinavica Suppl.*, **166**, 85–8.

Katz, D.A., Marks, M.P., Napel, S.A., Bracci, P.M. & Roberts, S.L. (1995). Circle of Willis. Evaluation with spiral CT angiography, MR angiography, and conventional angiography. *Radiology*, **195**, 445–9.

Kaufman, M., Little, B.W. & Berkowitz, B.W. (1988). Recurrent intracranial hemorrhage in an adult with moyamoya disease. Case report, radiographic studies and pathology. *Canadian Journal of Neurological Sciences*, **15**, 430–4.

Kawaguchi, T., Fujita, S., Hosoda, K. et al. (1996). Multiple burr-hole operation for adult moyamoya disease. *Journal of Neurosurgery*, **84**, 468–76.

Kawaguchi, S., Sakaki, T., Kakizaki, T., Kamada, K., Shimomura, T. & Iwanaga, H. (1996a). Clinical features of the hemorrhage type moyamoya disease based on 31 cases. *Acta Neurochirurgica*, **138**, 1200–10.

Kawaguchi, S., Sakaki, T., Morimoto, T., Kakizaki, T. & Kamada, K. (1996b). Characteristics of intracranial aneurysms associated with moyamoya disease. A review of 111 cases. *Acta Neurochirurgica*, **138**, 1287–94.

Kawano, T., Fukui, M., Hashimoto, N. & Yonekawa, Y. (1994). Follow-up study of patients with 'unilateral' moyamoya disease. *Neurologia Medico-Chirurgica*, **34**, 744–7.

Kestle, J.R., Hoffman, H.J. & Mock, A.R. (1993). Moyamoya phenomenon after radiation for optic glioma. *Journal of Neurosurgery*, **79**, 32–5.

Kikuchi, M., Asato, M., Sugahara, S. et al. (1996). Evaluation of surgically formed collateral circulation in moyamoya disease with 3D-CT angiography. Comparison with MR angiography and X-ray angiography. *Neuropediatrics*, **27**, 45–9.

Kinugasa, K., Mandai, S., Kamata, I., Sugiu, K. & Ohmoto, T. (1993). Surgical treatment of moyamoya disease. Operative technique for encephalo-duro-arterio-myo-synagiosis, its follow-up, clinical results, and angiograms. *Neurosurgery*, **32**, 527–31.

Kinugasa, K., Mandai, S., Tokunaga, K. et al. (1994). Ribbon encephalo-duro-arterio-myo-synangiosis for moyamoya disease. *Surgical Neurology*, **41**, 455–61.

Kobayashi, H., Hayashi, M., Handa, Y., Kabuto, M., Noguchi, Y. & Aradachi, H. (1991). EC-IC bypass for adult patients with moyamoya. *Neurological Research*, **13**, 113–16.

Kodama, N., Sato, M. & Sasaki, T. (1996). Treatment of ruptured cerebral aneurysm in moyamoya disease. *Surgical Neurology*, **46**, 62–6.

Kohno, K., Oka, Y., Kohno, S., Ohta, S., Kumon, Y. & Sakaki, S. (1998). Cerebral blood flow measurement as an indicator for an indirect revascularization procedure for adult patients with moyamoya disease. *Neurosurgery*, **42**, 752–7.

Konishi, Y., Kadowaki, C., Hara, M. & Takeuchi, K. (1985). Aneurysms associated with moyamoya disease. *Neurosurgery*, **16**, 484–91.

Kono, S., Oka, K. & Sueishi, K. (1990). Histopathologic and morphometric studies of leptomeningeal vessels in moyamoya disease. *Stroke*, **21**, 1044–50.

Kurlemann, G., Fahrendorf, G., Krings, W., Sciuk, J. & Palm, D. (1992). Characteristic EEG findings in childhood moyamoya syndrome. *Neurosurgical Review*, **15**, 57–60.

Kuroda, S., Kamiyama, H., Isobe, M., Houkin, K., Abe, H. & Mitsumori, K. (1995). Cerebral hemodynamics and 're-build-up' phenomenon on electroencephalogram in children with moyamoya disease. *Childs Nervous System*, **11**, 214–19.

Kuwabara, Y., Ichiya, Y., Sasaki, M. et al. (1997a). Cerebral hemodynamics and metabolism in moyamoya disease. A positron emission tomography study. *Clinical Neurology and Neurosurgery*, **99**(Suppl. 2), S74–8.

Kuwabara, Y., Ichiya, Y., Sasaki, M. et al. (1997b). Response to hypercapnia in moyamoya disease. Cerebrovascular response to hypercapnia in pediatric and adult patients with moyamoya disease. *Stroke*, **28**, 701–7.

Laborde, G., Harders, A., Klimek, L. & Hardenack, M. (1993). Correlation between clinical, angiographic and transcranial Doppler sonographic findings in patients with moyamoya disease. *Neurological Research*, **15**, 87–92.

Leblanc, R. (1992). Cerebral amyloid angiopathy and moyamoya disease. *Neurosurgery Clinics of North America*, **2**, 625–36.

Levine, S.R., Fagan, S.C., Pessin, M.S. et al. (1991). Accelerated intracranial occlusive disease, oral contraceptives, and cigarette use. *Neurology*, **41**, 1893–901.

Li, B., Wang, C.C., Zhao, Z.Z., et al. (1991). A histological, ultrastructural and immunohistochemical study of superficial temporal arteries and middle meningeal arteries in moyamoya disease. *Acta Pathologica Japonica*, **41**, 521–30.

Lichtor, T. & Mullan, S. (1987). Arteriovenous malformation in moyamoya syndrome. Report of three cases. *Journal of Neurosurgery*, **67**, 603–8.

Maki, Y. & Enomoto, T. (1988). Moyamoya disease. *Childs Nervous System*, **4**, 204–12.

Malek, A.M., Connors, S., Robertson, R.L., Folkman, J. & Scott, R.M. (1997). Elevation of cerebrospinal fluid levels of basic fibroblast growth factor in moyamoya and central nervous system disorders. *Pediatric Neurosurgery*, **27**, 182–9.

Masuda, J., Ogata, J. & Yutani, C. (1993). Smooth muscle cell proliferation and localization of macrophages and T cells in the occlusive intracranial major arteries in moyamoya disease. *Stroke*, **24**, 1960–7.

Matsushima, T., Fujiwara, S., Nagata, S. et al. (1989). Surgical treatment for paediatric patients with moyamoya disease by indirect revascularization procedures (EDAS, EMS, EMAS). *Acta Neurochirurgica*, **98**, 135–40.

Matsushima, T., Inoue, T., Natori, Y. et al. (1994). Children with unilateral occlusion of stenosis of the ICA associated with surrounding moyamoya vessels – 'unilateral' moyamoya disease. *Acta Neurochirurgica*, **131**, 196–202.

Miller, J.H., Khonsary, A. & Raffel, C. (1996). The scintigraphic appearance of childhood moyamoya disease on cerebral perfusion imaging. *Pediatric Radiology*, **26**, 833–88.

Miyakawa, I., Lee, H.C., Haruyama, Y., Mori, N., Mikura, T. & Kinoshita, K. (1986). Occlusive disease of the internal carotid arteries with vascular collaterals (moyamoya disease) in pregnancy. *Archives of Gynecology*, **237**, 175–80.

Miyamoto, S., Kikuchi, H., Karasawa, J., Nagata, I., Ikota, T. & Takeuchi, S. (1984). Study of the posterior circulation in moyamoya disease. Clinical and neuroradiological evaluation. *Journal of Neurosurgery*, **61**, 1032–7.

Miyamoto, S., Kikuchi, H., Karasawa, J., Nagata, I., Ihara, I. & Yamagata, S. (1986). Study of the posterior circulation in moyamoya disease. Part 2. Visual disturbances and surgical treatment. *Journal of Neurosurgery*, **65**, 454–60.

Mizoi, K., Kayama, T., Yoshimoto, T. & Nagamine, Y. (1996). Indirect revascularization for moyamoya disease. Is there a beneficial effect for adult patients? *Surgical Neurology*, **45**, 541–8.

Muizelaar, J.P. (1988). Early operation of ruptured basilar artery aneurysm associated with bilateral carotid occlusion (moyamoya disease). *Clinical Neurology and Neurosurgery*, **90**, 349–55.

Muppala, M. & Castaldo, J.E. (1994). Unilateral supraclinoid internal carotid artery stenosis with moyamoya-like vasculopathy. Noninvasive assessments. *Journal of Neuroimaging*, **4**, 11–16.

Muttaqin, Z., Ohba, S., Arita, K. et al. (1993). Cerebral circulation in moyamoya disease. A clinical study using transcranial Doppler sonography. *Surgical Neurology*, **40**, 306–13.

Nagamine, Y., Takahashi, S. & Sonobe, M. (1981). Multiple intracranial aneurysms associated with moyamoya disease. Case report. *Journal of Neurosurgery*, **54**, 673–6.

Nakagawara, J., Takeda, R., Suematsu, K. & Nakamura, J. (1997). Quantification of regional cerebral blood flow and vascular reserve in childhood moyamoya disease using (123)IMP-ARG method. *Clinical Neurology and Neurosurgery*, **99**(Suppl. 2), S96–9.

Nakano, T., Azuma, E., Ido, M. et al. (1993). Moyamoya disease associated with bilateral renal artery stenosis. *Acta Paediatrica Japonica*, **35**, 354–7.

Nakashima, H., Meguro, T., Kawada, S., Hirotsune, N. & Ohmoto, T. (1997). Long-term results of surgically treated moyamoya syndrome. *Clinical Neurology and Neurosurgery*, **99**(Suppl. 2), S156–61

Nariai, T., Suzuki, R., Matsushima, Y. et al. (1994). Surgically induced angiogenesis to compensate for hemodynamic cerebral ischemia. *Stroke*, **25**, 1014–21.

Natori, Y., Ikezaki, K., Matsushima, T. & Fukui, M. (1997). 'Angiographic moyamoya' its definition, classification, and therapy. *Clinical Neurology and Neurosurgery*, **99**(Suppl. 2), S168–72.

Noda, S., Hayasaka, S., Setogawa, T. & Matsumoto, S. (1987). Ocular symptoms of moyamoya disease. *American Journal of Ophthalmology*, **103**, 812–16.

Numaguchi, Y., Gonzalez, C.F., Davis, P.C. et al. (1997). Moyamoya disease in the United States. *Clinical Neurology and Neurosurgery*, **99**(Suppl. 2), S26–30.

Obara, K., Fukuuchi, Y., Kobari, M., Watanabe, S. & Dembo, T. (1997). Cerebral hemodynamics in patients with moyamoya disease and in patients with atherosclerotic occlusion of the major cerebral arterial trunks. *Clinical Neurology and Neurosurgery*, **99**(Suppl. 2), S86–9.

Ogawa, A., Yoshimoto, T., Suzuki, J. & Sakurai, Y. (1990a). Cerebral blood flow in moyamoya disease. Part 1. Correlation with age and regional distribution. *Acta Neurochirurgica*, **105**, 30–4.

Ogawa, A., Nakamura, N., Yoshimoto, T. & Suzuki, J. (1990b). Cerebral blood flow in moyamoya disease. Part 2. Autoregulation and CO_2 response. *Acta Neurochirurgica*, **105**, 107–11.

Ohtaki, M., Uede, T., Morimoto, S., Nonaka, T., Tanabe, S. & Hashi, K. (1998). Intellectual functions and regional cerebral haemodynamics after extensive omental transplantation over both frontal lobes in childhood moyamoya disease. *Acta Neurochirurgica*, **140**, 1043–53.

Ohtoh, T., Iwasaki, Y., Namiki, T. et al. (1988). Hemodynamic characteristics of the vertebobasilar system in moyamoya disease. A histometric study. *Human Pathology*, **19**, 465–70.

Okada, Y., Shima, T., Nishida, M. et al. (1998). Effectiveness of superficial temporal artery-middle cerebral artery anastomosis in adult moyamoya disease. Cerebral hemodynamics and clinical course in ischemic and hemorrhagic varieties. *Stroke*, **29**, 625–30.

Oyama, H., Niwa, M. & Kida, Y. (1998). CBF change with aging in moyamoya disease. *Journal of Neurosurgical Sciences*, **42**, 33–6.

Peerless, S.J. (1997). Risk factors of moyamoya disease in Canada and the USA. *Clinical Neurology and Neurosurgery*, **99**(Suppl. 2), S45–8.

Pracyk, J.B. & Massey, J.M. (1989). Moyamoya disease associated with polycystic kidney disease and eosinophilic granuloma. *Stroke*, **20**, 1092–4.

Quest, D.O. & Correll, J.W. (1985). Basal arterial occlusive disease. *Neurosurgery*, **17**, 937–41.

Robertson, R.L., Chavali, R.V., Robson, C.D. et al. (1998). Neurologic complications of cerebral angiography in childhood moyamoya syndrome. *Pediatric Radiology*, **28**, 824–9.

Ross, I.B., Shevell, M.I., Montes, J.L. et al. (1994). Encephaloduroarteriosynagniosis (EDAS) for the treatment of childhood moyamoya disease. *Pediatric Neurology*, **10**, 199–204.

Rupprecht, T., Wenzel, D., Schmitzer, E., Hofbeck, M., Bowing, B. & Neubauer, U. (1992). Diagnosis of moyamoya disease with additional renal artery stenosis by colour coded Doppler sonography. *Pediatric Radiology*, **22**, 527–8.

Saeki, N., Nakazaki, S., Kubota, M. et al. (1997). Hemorrhagic type moyamoya disease. *Clinical Neurology and Neurosurgery*, **99**(Suppl. 2), S196–201.

Sakamoto, H., Kitano, S., Yasui, T. et al. (1997). Direct extracranial–intracranial bypass for children with moyamoya disease. *Clinical Neurology and Neurosurgery*, **99**(Suppl. 2), S128–33.

Sato, S., Shirane, R., Marouka, S. & Yoshimoto, T. (1999). Evaluation of neuronal loss in adult moyamoya disease by 123I-iomazenil SPECT. *Surgical Neurology*, **51**, 158–63.

Satoh, S., Shibuya, H., Matsushima, Y. & Suzuki, S. (1988). Analysis of the angiographic findings in cases of childhood moyamoya disease. *Neuroradiology*, **30**, 111–19.

Shimizu, H., Shirane, R., Fujiwara, S., Takahashi, A. & Yoshimoto, T. (1997). Proton magnetic resonance spectroscopy in children with moyamoya disease. *Clinical Neurology and Neurosurgery*, **99**(Suppl. 2), S64–7.

Steinke, W., Tatemichi, T.K., Mohr, J.P., Massaro, A., Prohovnik, I. & Solomon, R.A. (1992). Caudate hemorrhage with moyamoya-like vasculopathy from atherosclerotic disease. *Stroke*, **23**, 1360–3.

Suzui, H., Hoshimaru, M., Takahashi, J.A. et al. (1994). Immunohistochemical reactions for fibroblast growth factor receptor in arteries of patients with moyamoya disease. *Neurosurgery*, **35**, 20–4.

Suzuki, J. (1986). *Moyamoya Disease*. Berlin: Springer-Verlag.

Takahashi, A., Sawamura, Y., Houkin, K., Kamiyama, H. & Abe, H. (1993). The cerebrospinal fluid in patients with moyamoya disease (spontaneous occlusion of the circle of Willis) contains high levels of basic fibroblast growth factor. *Neuroscience Letters*, **160**, 214–16.

Takanashi, J., Sugita, K., Ishii, M. et al. (1993). Moyamoya syndrome in young children. MR comparison with adult onset. *American Journal of Neuroradiology*, **14**, 1139–43.

Takase, K., Kashihara, M. & Hashimoto, T. (1997). Transcranial Doppler ultrasonography in patients with moyamoya disease. *Clinical Neurology and Neurosurgery*, **99**(Suppl. 2), S101–5.

Takebayashi, S., Matsuo, K. & Kaneko, M. (1984). Ultrastructural studies of cerebral arteries and collateral vessels in moyamoya disease. *Stroke*, **15**, 728–32.

Takeuchi, S., Kobayashi, K., Tsuchida, T., Imamura, H., Tanaka, R. & Ito, J. (1982). Computed tomography in moyamoya disease. *Journal of Computer Assisted Tomography*, **6**, 24–32.

Taki, W., Yonekawa, Y., Kobayashi, A. et al. (1989). Cerebral circulation and metabolism in adults' moyamoya disease – PET study. *Acta Neurochirurgica*, **100**, 150–4.

Takikawa, S., Kamiyama, H., Abe, H., Mitsumori, K. & Tsuru, M. (1990). Hemodynamic evaluation of vascular reconstructive surgery for childhood moyamoya disease using single photon emission computed tomography. *Neurologia Medico-Chirurgica*, **30**, 389–95.

Tanaka, Y., Takeuchi, K. & Akai, K. (1980). Intracranial ruptured aneurysm accompanying moyamoya phenomenon. *Acta Neurochirurgica*, **52**, 35–43.

Tanigawara, T., Yamada, H., Sakai, N., Andoh, T., Deguchi, K. & Iwamura, M. (1997). Studies on cytomegalovirus and Epstein–Barr virus infection in moyamoya disease. *Clinical Neurology and Neurosurgery*, **99**(Suppl. 2), S225–8.

Tashima-Kurita, S., Matsushima, T., Kato, M. et al. (1989). Moyamoya disease. Posterior cerebral artery occlusion and pattern-reversal visual-evoked potential. *Archives of Neurology*, **46**, 550–3.

Tenjin, H. & Ueda, S. (1997). Multiple EDAS (encephalo-duro-arterio-synangiosis). Additional EDAS using the frontal branch of the superficial temporal artery (STA) and the occipital artery for pediatric moyamoya patients in whom EDAS using the parietal branch of the STA was insufficient. *Childs Nervous System*, **13**, 220–4.

Touho, H., Karasawa, J., Tenjin, H. & Ueda, S. (1996). Omental transplantation using a superficial temporal artery previously used for encephalopduroarteriosynangiosis. *Surgical Neurology*, **45**, 550–8.

Tsuchiya, K., Makita, K. & Furui, S. (1994). Moyamoya disease. Diagnosis with three-dimensional CT angiography. *Neuroradiology*, **36**, 432–4.

Tsuchiya, K., Inaoka, S., Mizutani, Y. & Hachiya, J. (1998). Echo-plan perfusion MR of moyamoya disease. *American Journal of Neuroradiology*, **19**, 211–16.

Tsuda, H., Hattori, S., Tanabe, S. et al. (1997). Thombophilia found in patients with moyamoya disease. *Clinical Neurology and Neurosurgery*, **99**(Suppl. 2), S229–33.

Tzika, A.A., Robertson, R.L., Barnes, B.D., et al. (1997). Childhood moyamoya disease. Hemodynamic MRI. *Pediatric Radiology*, **27**, 727–35.

Ueki, K., Meyer, F.B. & Mellinger, J.F. (1994). Moyamoya disease. The disorder and surgical treatment. *Mayo Clinic Proceedings*, **69**, 749–57.

Waga, S. & Tochio, H. (1985). Intracranial aneurysm associated with moyamoya disease in childhood. *Surgical Neurology*, **23**, 237–43.

Wakai, K., Tamakoshi, A., Ikezaki, K. et al. (1997). Epidemiological features of moyamoya disease in Japan: findings from a nation-wide study. *Clinical Neurology and Neurosurgery*, **99**(Suppl. 2), S1–5.

Wanifuchi, H., Takeshita, M., Aoki, N. et al. (1996). Adult moyamoya disease progressing from unilateral to bilateral involvement. *Neurologia Medico-Chirurgica*, **36**, 87–90.

Yamada, I., Matsushima, Y. & Suzuki, S. (1992). Childhood moyamoya disease before and after encephalo-duro-arterio-synangiosis. An angiographic study. *Neuroradiology*, **34**, 318–22.

Yamada, I., Himeno, Y., Suzuki, S. & Matsushima, Y. (1995a). Posterior circulation in moyamoya disease. Angiographic study. *Radiology*, **197**, 239–46.

Yamada, I., Suzuki, K. & Matsushima, Y. (1995b). Moyamoya disease. Comparison of assessment with MR angiography and MR imaging versus conventional angiography. *Radiology*, **196**, 211–18.

Yamada, I., Suzuki, S. & Matsushima, Y. (1995c). Moyamoya disease. Diagnostic accuracy of MRI. *Neuroradiology*, **37**, 356–61.

Yamada, I., Murata, Y., Umehara, I., Suzuki, S. & Matsushima, Y. (1996). SPECT and MRI evaluations of the posterior circulation in moyamoya disease. *Journal of Nuclear Medicine*, **37**, 1613–17.

Yamada, H., Deguchi, K., Tanigawara, T. et al. (1997). The relationship between moyamoya disease and bacterial infection. *Clinical Neurology and Neurosurgery*, **99**(Suppl. 2), S221–4.

Yamamoto, M., Aoyagi, M., Tajima, S. et al. (1997). Increase in elastin gene expression and protein synthesis in arterial smooth muscle cells derived from patients with moyamoya disease. *Stroke*, **28**, 1733–8.

Yamamoto, M., Aoyagi, M., Fukui, N., Matsushima, Y. & Yamamoto, K. (1998). Differences in cellular responses to mitogens in arterial smooth muscle cells derived from patients with moyamoya disease. *Stroke*, **29**, 1188–93.

Yamashiro, Y., Takahashi, H. & Takahashi, K. (1984). Cerebrovascular moyamoya disease. *European Journal of Pediatrics*, **142**, 44–50.

Yamashita, M., Oka, K. & Tanaka, K. (1983). Histopathology of the brain vascular network in moyamoya disease. *Stroke*, **14**, 50–8.

Yamauchi, T., Houkin, K., Tada, M. & Abe, H. (1997). Familial occurrence of moyamoya disease. *Clinical Neurology and Neurosurgery*, **99**(Suppl. 2), S162–7.

Yang, S.H., Li, B., Wang, C.C. & Zhao, J.Z. (1997). Angiographic study of moyamoya disease and histological study in the external carotid artery system. *Clinical Neurology and Neurosurgery*, **99**(Suppl. 2), S61–3.

Yonekawa, Y., Ogata, N., Kaku, Y., Taub, E. & Imhof, H.G. (1997). Moyamoya disease in Europe, past and present status. *Clinical Neurology and Neurosurgery*, **99**(Suppl. 2), S58–60.

Yoshimoto, T., Houkin, K., Takahashi, A. & Abe, H. (1996). Angiogenic factors in moyamoya disease. *Stroke*, **27**, 2160–5.

Yoshimoto, T., Houkin, K., Takahashi, A. & Abe, H. (1997). Evaluation of cytokines in cerebrospinal fluid from patients with moyamoya disease. *Clinical Neurology and Neurosurgery*, **99**(Suppl. 2), S218–20.

33

Sneddon's syndrome

Jan L. De Bleecker and Jacques L. De Reuck

Department of Neurology, University Hospital, Gent, Belgium

Introduction

Sneddon's syndrome (SS) refers to an infrequent disorder combining skin lesions and ischemic cerebral symptoms in patients without recognizable connective tissue or inflammatory or chronic infectious disease. The skin lesions consist of a purplish mottling of the skin (livedo racemosa, mostly used in synonym with livedo reticularis in English usage), and the central nervous system manifestations range from transient ischemic attacks to multiple confluent infarcts. The first description dates back to Ehrmann in 1906 (Ehrmann, 1906), who described a syphilitic patient with an ischemic stroke and the typical skin lesions. Champion and Rook described a typical patient in 1960 (Champion & Rook, 1960). In 1965, the dermatologist Sneddon was the first to recognize the syndrome as a separate clinical entity (Sneddon, 1965). He was struck by the severe and generalized bluish discoloration of the skin, involving the limbs and often the trunk (Sneddon used the term livedo reticularis), and the multiple strokes 'often leaving little residual disability' in five young females and one young man. All patients had hypertension. Skin biopsies and clinical work-up revealed no known etiology of livedo racemosa such as polyarteritis nodosa, systemic lupus erythematosus, or essential thrombocytopenia. He suggested endarteritis obliterans or an unknown type of arteriopathy causing venous dilatation and stasis of the skin as the underlying pathology.

A similar syndrome combining livedo racemosa and multiple strokes had been reported by Divry and van Bogaert in 1946 as a familial disease leading to dementia, pseudobulbar palsy and epilepsy (Divry & van Bogaert, 1946). Further sporadic and familial cases have been reported under various eponyms: diffuse meningo-cerebral angiomatosis and leukoencephalopathy, cortico-meningeal angiomatosis, venous capillary angiomatosis, Divry-van Bogaert syndrome, etc. (Divry & van Bogaert, 1946; Baro, 1964; Pellat et al., 1976; Bussone et al., 1984; Ellie et al., 1987). This very rare syndrome affects mainly or exclusively men, at least in adults. Meningo-cortical arteriolar proliferation, disseminated cortical infarcts, and white matter gliosis and demyelination were found at autopsy. These patients cannot be distinguished from SS on clinical grounds. Therefore, they can be considered as part of it until the underlying genetic or pathophysiological abnormalities are better defined (Ellie et al., 1987).

Epidemiology

Following Sneddon's description, a number of cases or small series were reported, initially mainly in Europe. Although most reported patients were Caucasians, there is no definite evidence of ethnic differences in incidence. Some authors claim an incidence of four cases per 1 000 000 per year (Zelger et al., 1993). In hospital-based series of stroke patients, the frequency of SS is between 0.25 and 0.50% (De Reuck et al., 1987; Berciano, 1988).

At least in sporadic cases, there is a marked female preponderance. Of 200 literature cases reviewed by us, 80% are females. The average age at onset of the neurological symptoms is around 40 years, with a range of 10–65 years. In more than two-thirds of the patients, the disorder occurs sporadically, while in the others there is familial occurrence (Pettee et al., 1994; Rehany et al., 1998). In apparently familial cases, no single pattern of inheritance is identified, but autosomal dominant inheritance has been most frequently reported (Rebollo et al., 1983; Scott & Boyle, 1986; Berciano, 1988).

Clinical expression

Cutaneous manifestations

The livedo racemosa is usually the first manifestation of the disease, and tends to precede the neurological symptoms by 10 years on average (Sneddon, 1965; Quimby & Perry, 1980; Thomas et al., 1982; Rebollo et al., 1983; Zelger et al., 1993). In some patients, the livedo is firstly detected at the time of stroke occurrence, and rarely it develops years after the first neurological symptoms (Thomas et al., 1982). Livedo racemosa is defined as a dusky erythematous-to-violaceous, irregular, netlike pattern in the skin (Burton, 1988; Daoud et al., 1995). The lesions are typically distributed over the lower trunk, the buttocks and proximal region of the thighs (see colour Fig. 33.1(a)). The lesions occasionally become more generalized and extend to the upper back, the distal extremities (see colour Fig. 33.1(b)), and volar parts of the lower arms. The livedo is increased in the cold, in conjunction with exacerbations of the neurological symptoms, and sometimes during pregnancy (Gibson et al., 1997). In the European literature, the term livedo reticularis refers to a regular, deep-bluish netlike pattern that disappears after the skin is warmed. In the American literature, livedo reticularis is used interchangeably with livedo racemosa, while the reticular changes that disappear after warming are sometimes referred to as 'cutis marmorata'. Livedo reticularis and livedo racemosa have a different pathophysiology (Daoud et al., 1995). Livedo reticularis is caused by temporary vasoconstriction, whereas livedo racemosa results from persistent impairment of peripheral blood flow caused by occlusion of small- or medium-sized arteries. SS patients exhibit the livedo racemosa pattern, and Ehrlich was the first to use the term livedo racemosa apoplectica for the SS (Ehrmann, 1906).

Some patients display acrocyanosis of the distal extremities or typical Raynaud phenomenon (Daoud et al., 1995).

Neurological manifestations

Virtually all syndromes caused by transient or permanent cerebral ischemia have been described. In retrospect, many patients have had vague and transient complaints of dizziness or vertigo, migraine-like headaches (Martinelli et al., 1991), or short-lasting focal neurologic deficits many years before the diagnosis is made. The transient neurological complaints are at that time often not linked to the dermatological manifestations. It is only after the occurrence of multiple minor strokes in young people that the diagnosis of SS is considered by most clinicians.

As a rule, the transient ischemic attacks and strokes are multiple and recurrent in the same or different vascular territories (Stephens & Ferguson, 1982). Both cortical and subcortical areas in the anterior and posterior circulation can be affected. Cortical middle cerebral artery deficits such as aphasia, hemiparesis, hemisensory deficit, and visual field defects are the most common findings. Many strokes are minor, with good recovery. Recurrent transient global amnesia has been the main manifestation in some patients (Rumpl & Rumpl, 1979). Spinal ischemic accidents are rare (Baleva et al., 1995).

In later stages, mild to severe cognitive impairment can occur in many patients, with symptoms varying from inability to concentrate, mild memory loss, frontal lobe type behavioural and emotional disturbances, to severe multi-infarct dementia. Dementia without precedent focal deficits has been the clinical presentation in some patients (Cosnes et al., 1986; Scott and Boyle, 1986; Bruyn et al., 1987; Antoine et al., 1994; Baleva et al., 1995; Devuyst et al., 1996).

Subarachnoid or intracerebral hemorrhage has been reported (Diez-Tejedor et al., 1990; Uitdehaag et al., 1992; Dupont et al., 1996), but an increased incidence of bleeding in SS patients is not supported by larger series.

Focal or secondary generalized seizures are more common than in a general stroke population, probably reflecting the severe cortical involvement. Of 63 randomly selected SS patients from the neurological literature, epilepsy is mentioned in 12 (Sneddon, 1965; Rumpl & Rumpl, 1979; Rebollo et al., 1983; De Reus et al., 1985; Ellie et al., 1987; Stockhammer et al., 1993; Menzel et al., 1994). Population-based prospective incidence studies are not available. Seizures are seldom the presenting manifestation.

Other manifestations

Mild to moderate arterial hypertension occurs in a significant proportion (60–80%) of SS patients. The pathophysiological basis for the hypertension is not well understood. Very few hypertensive SS patients have renal vascular disease (Antoine et al., 1994; Macario et al., 1997).

Valvular heart disease, mostly mitral valve thickening, was found in 36% in one (Lubach et al., 1992) and in up to 61% of patients in another series (Tourbah et al., 1997). The valvular disease was sometimes pre-existent to the neurological symptoms and considered of rheumatic origin in some cases (Vaillant et al., 1990; Antoine et al., 1994; Tourbah et al., 1997). Thrombosis of peripheral arteries and pulmonary embolus can also occur (Alegre et al., 1990).

Ophthalmologic manifestations include transient monocular or binocular blindness, hypertensive vascular changes, retinal artery or vein thrombosis, and microaneurysms (Jonas et al., 1986; Gobert, 1994; Donders et al., 1998), in addition to central nervous system visual symptoms such as homonymous visual field defects, internuclear ophthalmoplegia, diplopia, and pupillary defects (Narbay, 1997; Rehany et al., 1998).

Those patients with antiphospholipid antibodies may present the full clinical spectrum of the primary antiphospholipid antibody syndrome (Levine & Welch, 1987; Hess, 1992; Lockshin, 1992) (see also Chapter 9 in this book).

Pathology

Dermatopathology

For obvious reasons, skin biopsies have been studied more frequently than brain tissue. The most informative skin biopsies are those taken in the central normal areas within the bordering of the livedo (Copeman, 1975; Zelger et al., 1992; Daoud et al., 1995). The main changes involve medium-sized arteries in the deep dermal or subcutaneous tissue and progress over time. The early stage is characterized by arteriolar endothelitis and a mixed inflammatory cellular infiltrate, then followed by occlusion of the arteriolar lumen by a fibrotic plug and dilatation of neighbouring arterioles and venules (Beurey et al., 1984; Marsch & Muckelmann, 1985; Zelger et al., 1992; Stockhammer et al., 1993). Later, subendothelial cell proliferation with collapse of the lamina elastica and recanalization follows. Finally, the arteriole becomes completely involuted and occluded.

Digital artery biopsies have been done by Rebollo (Rebollo et al., 1983). He found segmental intimal hyperplasia, adventitial fibrosis, thrombosis, and narrowing of the lumen. Temporal artery biopsies are usually normal (Rumpl et al., 1985; Pauranik et al., 1987) or show unspecific subintimal hyperplasia and medial fibrosis (De Reus et al., 1985; De Reuck et al., 1987; Kalashnikova et al., 1990). Classical vasculitis with fibrinoid necrosis is not a feature of livedo racemosa.

Neuropathology

Few autopsies or brain biopsies have been reported. Unspecific signs of cortical and subcortical infarction and gliosis, without vascular or perivascular inflammation or fibrinoid necrosis are observed (Rumpl et al., 1985; Scott & Boyle, 1986; Geschwind et al., 1995; Devuyst et al., 1996).

Boortz-Marx et al. found granulomatous inflammation of the leptomeninges without vessel involvement in one patient (Boortz-Marx et al., 1995). Non-inflammatory thrombosis of leptomeningeal arteries has rarely been noted (Pinol-Aguade et al., 1999). As a matter of fact, pathological changes in small- or medium-sized cerebral vessels have often been inferred from observations in skin biopsies, but have rarely been documented in brain biopsy or autopsy tissue.

Pathogenesis

Sneddon's syndrome is unlikely to reflect a single, specific etiology. Two main hypotheses emerge. First, a hypercoagulable state, itself of variable origin, and secondly an intrinsic small-vessel vasculopathy.

Hypercoagulable state

The notion that anticardiolipin antibodies or the lupus anticoagulant are present in about a third of SS patients has greatly supported the theory that the SS is part of the clinical spectrum of the primary antiphospholipid syndrome (Jonas et al., 1986; Levine et al., 1988; Alegre et al., 1990; Kalashnikova et al., 1990; Moral et al., 1991) (see Chapter 9 in this book). The proportion of antiphospholipid antibody positive patients is widely different in various cohorts of SS patients, e.g. 0/17 (Stockhammer et al., 1993), 1/5 (Burton, 1988), 3/13 (Sitzer et al., 1995), 6/17 (Kalashnikova et al., 1990), and 19/33 (Farronay et al., 1992). Natural or treatment-induced fluctuation of antiphospholipid antibody levels, methods for assay determination, and criteria for positive results may partly explain the different incidences (Tanne et al., 1998). Rare familial SS cases with antiphospholipid antibodies have also been documented (Vargas et al., 1989; Pettee et al., 1994).

No major differences in clinical symptoms or outcome have been noted between antiphospholipid antibody positive and negative SS patients (Tourbah et al., 1997), although antiphospholipid antibody positive patients sometimes have a shorter and more disabling disease and may more often present the whole symptom spectrum associated with the antiphospholipid antibody syndrome (Kalashnikova et al., 1990). It is unknown whether skin biopsy data differ between antiphospholipid antibody positive and antibody negative patients (Stockhammer et al., 1993). Cerebral arteriograms in antibody negative SS patients reveal a medium-sized arteriopathy, whereas in the antiphospholipid antibody syndrome, stenosis and occlusion involves larger vessels (Levine & Welch, 1987).

Less frequently, SS occurs in patients with antinuclear antibodies, some of whom turn out to have systemic lupus erythematosus (McHugh et al., 1988; Antoine et al., 1994). Rarely reported coagulation or platelet aggregation deficits include antithrombin-III deficiency (Donnet et al., 1992; Sauter & Rudin, 1992), and essential thrombocythemia (Michel et al., 1996). Up to about 60% of SS patients have a cardiac valvulopathy (Lubach et al., 1992; Antoine et al., 1994; Tourbah et al., 1997). The incidence of valvular disease is unexpectedly high in this young population. It is unclear whether the valvulopathies *per se* are the direct cause of embolic strokes, or become symptomatic because of a coexistent hypercoagulable state (Geschwind et al., 1995).

Primary vasculopathy

In many patients no antiphospholipid antibodies or primary coagulation deficits are detected (Martinez-Menendez et al., 1990; Stockhammer et al., 1993). Mainly based on observations in skin biopsies, it is assumed that a non-vasculitic small- and medium-sized vessel arteriopathy causes both brain and skin symptoms. The common clinical observation of exacerbation of the livedo racemosa at times that new cerebrovascular symptoms develop is indeed suggestive of a common factor causing skin and central nervous system symptoms. The type and origin of the arteriopathy is unknown. In some cases, heritable factors play a role. In others, endothelial dysfunction may be secondary to acquired autoimmune or other factors that circulate in the serum. Circulating proteins, presumably immunoglobulins, could cause both the hypercoagulable state and an endotheliopathy, thus linking both hypothesized mechanisms underlying the SS (Moral et al., 1991). Signalling pathways specific to certain parts of the vascular bed, i.e. brain and skin, may explain why systemic congenital or acquired hypercoagulable states or endotheliopathies produce focal deficits of hemostasis (Rosenberg & Aird, 1999).

Diagnostic work-up

Any patient suspected of SS should undergo extensive blood tests, spinal tap, complete cardiovascular work-up including cardiac monitoring and transoesophageal echo-Doppler, cerebral magnetic resonance imaging (MRI), four-vessel intra-arterial angiography, and skin biopsy. Tests of probable or possible additional value include brain single photon emission computed tomography (SPECT) scan and transcranial echo-Doppler. A meningo-cortical

brain biopsy is only warranted when clinical, angiographic, cerebrospinal fluid, or skin biopsy findings suggest a possible CNS vasculitis or a vasculopathy of other origin.

Blood tests should screen for the lupus anticoagulant, IgG and possibly IgM anticardiolipin antibodies, antinuclear and anti-double stranded DNA autoantibodies, decreased complement factors, thrombocytopenia, leucopenia and other indications for systemic lupus erythematosus, VDRL assay, cryoglobulins, and circulating immune complexes. Heritable causes of hypercoagulable states such as deficiency of antithrombin-III, protein C or protein S should be sought. In many centres, genetic tests for known mutations of these genes and of the factor V Leiden and the prothrombin genes are now available. The current data are too scarce to predict the incidence of such mutations in the SS population.

The cerebrospinal fluid is usually normal. Mild increase of protein content or slight pleocytosis may reflect infarction, but marked lymphocytic pleocytosis suggests other causes of stroke including intracranial vasculitides or chronic CNS infections such as tertiary syphilis or tuberculosis.

MRI scan is more informative than computed tomographic (CT) scan (Ruscalleda et al., 1991). Multiple cortical and subcortical infarcts in various vascular territories are usually present at the time of diagnosis (Fig. 33.2). Mild to moderate cortical and subcortical atrophy with ventricular enlargement are common. Angiography is mandatory to exclude other types of cerebral vasculopathy. Many SS patients have normal angiograms, but a subset of patients have multiple distal arterial occlusions or narrowings, combined with a moya-moya type collateral network in a smaller proportion of the patients (Blom, 1989; Antoine et al., 1994; Pettee et al., 1994). The 'beading type' segmental narrowing and dilatation of large and medium-sized vessels typical of CNS vasculitis is not reported in SS.

Mitral and other cardiac valvulopathies are more commonly observed on transoesophageal echocardiography in SS patients than predicted from observations in age-matched controls (Vaillaint et al., 1990; Donnet et al., 1992). Selection bias alone is unlikely to explain the difference. Some authors claim that the cardiac emboli resulting from these mitral valve abnormalities are the main cause of the brain infarcts (Geschwind et al., 1995). Alternatively, the mitral valve proliferations could be the consequence of a systemic hypercoagulable state. Further study of stroke pathophysiology is needed to sort out the individual contributions of vasculopathy, thrombosis and cardiac embolism in SS.

Cervical Doppler sonography shows no significant atherosclerotic changes in most patients. Clinically silent

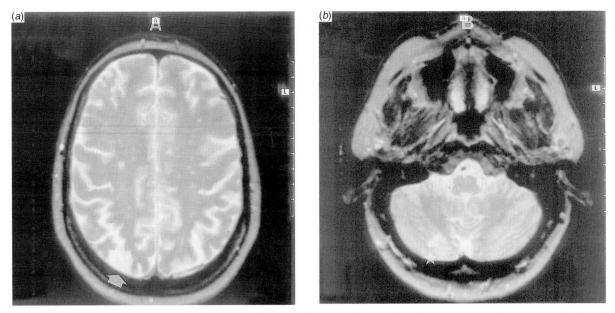

Fig. 33.2. Axial T$_2$-weighted magnetic resonance images show a small cortical infarct in the right occipito-parietal cortex (arrowhead) and a small lacunar infarct in the right centrum semiovale (both in (a)), and a small right hemicerebellar infarct (asterisk in (b)) at the time of diagnosis of Sneddon's syndrome in a 40-year-old female.

cerebral microembolism was detected in one third of the patients by transcranial duplex sonography of the middle cerebral artery in one study. The microemboli may be a marker of disease activity (Sitzer et al., 1995).

Menzel et al. (1994) reported decreased cerebral blood flow as adjudged by Technetium-99m-HMPAO-SPECT scan, even in patients without MRI abnormalities. Transcranial duplex sonography was normal in the same patients. These authors suggested that SPECT scan may allow presymptomatic detection of impaired cerebral blood flow in patients suffering from livedo racemosa. These observations await confirmation by prospective studies.

A skin biopsy including the deep dermis should be taken in the central normal areas within the bordering of the livedo (Zelger et al., 1992; Daoud et al., 1995). The pathologic changes in the various stages of the disease process have been detailed in the dermatopathology paragraph. The differential diagnosis of livedo racemosa should include leukocytoclastic and livedoid vasculitis, polyarteritis nodosa, lupus erythematosus, cryoglobulinemia, macroglobulinemia, polycythemia, thrombotic thrombocytopenic purpura, essential thrombocythemia, atheromatous or cholesterol emboli, disseminated intravascular coagulation, infectious diseases such as syphilis and tuberculosis, and drug toxicity (Daoud et al., 1995; Gibson et al., 1997).

Treatment

No double blind, placebo-controlled or comparative trials of any therapy have been performed. By analogy with the antiphospholipid antibody syndrome and based on the presumed pathogenesis of SS, most clinicians advocate warfarin anticoagulation for the treatment of SS patients. The frequent occurrence of cardiac valvulopathies and the absence of a documented clinical response to aspirin or other platelet inhibitors are additional arguments in favour of anticoagulation. Although some isolated cases of spontaneous or anticoagulation-related intracerebral or subarachnoid hemorrhage have been reported (Diez-Tejedor et al., 1990; Uitdehaag et al., 1992; Dupont et al., 1996), there is no evidence today that intracranial bleeding or hemorrhagic stroke are particularly common in SS (Geschwind et al., 1995). Clinicians should carefully weigh the advantages and disadvantages of anticoagulation therapy in this hypertensive population. In most patients, warfarin can be administered safely. In those in whom anticoagulation is not possible, aspirin combined or not with dipyridamole, or ticlopidine or clopidogrel seem reasonable alternatives for secondary stroke prevention.

Immunosuppressants, such as cyclophosphamide, azathioprine or corticosteroids, have been tried by some authors in individual patients but seemingly did not affect the short- or long-term disease course (Bruyn et al., 1987;

Rautenberg et al., 1988). Large series are not available. Immunosuppressive therapies are therefore not advocated at the present time.

Conclusion

Sneddon's syndrome is a clinically well-delineated syndrome that probably stems from a number of acquired or congenital hemostatic abnormalities that preferentially involve the cerebral and cutaneous vascular beds. Further pathophysiological studies will undoubtedly continue to identify more etiological subgroups. Pending future therapeutic trials that may identify different treatment modalities for different etiological subgroups, the general concept of 'Sneddon's syndrome' is currently still a valid and workable diagnosis in the daily neurological clinical practice.

References

Alegre, V.A., Winkelmann, R.K. & Gastineau, D.A. (1990). Cutaneous thrombosis, cerebrovascular thrombosis, and lupus anticoagulant – the Sneddon syndrome. *International Journal of Dermatology*, **29**, 45–9.

Antoine, J.C., Michel, D., Garnnier, P. et al. (1994). Syndrome de Sneddon: 9 cas. *Revue Neurologique*, **150**, 435–43.

Baleva, M., Chauchev, A., Dikova, C. et al. (1995). Sneddon's syndrome: echocardiographic, neurological, and immunological findings. *Stroke*, **26**, 1303–4.

Baro, F. (1964). Angiomatose méningée non calcifiante, état granulaire de l'écorce, sclérose diffuse axiale et cutis marmorata congenita. Nouvelle observation clinique sporadique du syndrome décrit par Divry et van Bogaert. *Acta Neurologica Psychiatrica Belgica*, **64**, 1042–63.

Berciano, J. (1988). Sneddon syndrome: another Mendelian etiology of stroke. *Annals of Neurology*, **24**, 586–7.

Beurey, J., Weber, M., Edelson, F., Thomas, I. & Eich, D. (1984). Livédo reticularis et accidents vasculaires cérébraux. *Annals of Dermatology and Venereology*, **111**, 25–9.

Blom, R.J. (1989). Sneddon syndrome: CT, arteriography, and MR imaging. *Journal of Computer Assisted Tomography*, **13**, 119–22.

Boortz-Marx, R.L., Clark, H.B., Taylor, S., Wesa, K.M. & Anderson, D.C. (1995). Sneddon's syndrome with granulomatous leptomeningeal infiltration. *Stroke*, **26**, 492–5.

Bruyn, R.P.M., Van Der Veen, J.P.W., Donker, A.J.M., Valk, J. & Wolters, E.C. (1987). Sneddon's syndrome. Case report and review of the literature. *Journal of Neurological Science*, **79**, 243–53.

Burton, J.L. (1988). Livedo reticularis, porcelain-white scars, and cerebral thromboses. *Lancet*, **ii**, 1263–4.

Bussone, G., Parati, E.A., Boiardi, A. et al. (1984). Divry–Van Boogaert syndrome. Clinical and ultrastructural findings. *Archives of Neurology*, **41**, 560–2.

Champion, R.H. & Rook, A.J. (1960). Livedo reticularis. *Proceedings of the Royal Society of Medicine*, **53**, 961–2.

Copeman, P.W.M. (1975.) Livedo reticularis: signs in the skin of disturbance of blood viscosity and of blood flow. *British Journal of Dermatology*, **93**, 519–29.

Cosnes, A., Perroud, A.M., Mathieu, A., Jourdain, C. & Touraine, R. (1986). Livedo reticularis et accidents vasculaires cérébraux. *Annals of Dermatology and Venereology*, **113**, 137–41.

Daoud, M.S., Wilmoth, G.J., Su, W.P.D. & Pittelkow, M.R. (1995). Sneddon syndrome. *Seminars in Dermatology*, **14**, 166–72.

De Reuck, J., De Reus, R. & De Koninck, J. (1987). Sneddon's syndrome. A not unusual cause of stroke in young women. In *Cerebral Vascular Disease 6. Proceedings of the World Federation of Neurology 13th International Salzburg Conference*, ed. J.S. Meyer, H. Lechner, M. Reivich & E.O. Ott, pp. 171–4. Amsterdam: Excerpta Medica.

De Reus, R., De Reuck, J., Vermander, F.D.K.H., Kint, A. & Van de Velde, E. (1985). Livedo racemosa generalisata and stroke. *Clinical Neurology and Neurosurgery*, **87**, 143–8.

Devuyst, G., Sindic, C., Laterre, E-C. & Brucher, J.-M. (1996). Neuropathological findings of a Sneddon's syndrome presenting with dementia not preceded by clinical cerebrovascular events. *Stroke*, **27**, 1008–10.

Diez-Tejedor, E., Lara, M., Frank, A., Gutierrez, M. & Barreiro, P. (1990). Cerebral haemorrhage in Sneddon's syndrome. *Journal of Neurology*, **237**(Suppl.), 78.

Divry, P. & van Bogaert, L. (1946). Une maladie familiale caractérisée par une angiomatose diffuse cortico-meningée non calcifiante et une démyélinisation progressive de la substance blanche. *Journal of Neurology, Neurosurgery and Psychiatry*, **9**, 41–54.

Donders, R.C.J.M., Kappelle, L.J., Derksen, R.H.W.M. et al. (1998). Transient monocular blindness and antiphospholipid antibodies in systemic lupus erythematosus. *Neurology*, **51**, 535–40.

Donnet, A., Khalil, R., Terrier, G., Koeppel, M-C., Njee, B.T. & Aillaud, M.F. (1992). Cerebral infarction, livedo reticularis, and familial deficiency in antithrombine-III. *Stroke*, **23**, 611–12.

Dupont, S., Fénelon, G., Saiag, Ph. & Sirmai, J. (1996). Warfarin in Sneddon's syndrome. *Neurology*, **46**, 1781–2.

Ehrmann, S. (1906). Ein neues Gefassymptom bei Lues. *Wiener Medizinische Wochenschrife*, **16**, 777–82.

Ellie, E., Julien, J., Henry, P., Vital, C. & Ferrer, X. (1987). Angiomatose cortico-méningée de Divry-van Bogaert et syndrome de Sneddon. Etude nosologique. A propos de quatre cas. *Revue Neurologique*, **143**, 798–805.

Farronay, O.W., Kalashnikova, L.A., Vereschaguin, N.V. et al. (1992). Cerebrovascular and immunological studies in Sneddon's syndrome. *Annals of Neurology*, **32**, 266.

Geschwind, D., FitzPatrick, M., Mischel, P. & Cummings, J. (1995). Sneddon's syndrome is a thrombotic vasculopathy: neuropathologic and neuroradiologic evidence. *Neurology*, **45**, 557–60.

Gibson, G.E., Su, W.P. & Pittelkow, M.R. (1997). Antiphospholipid syndrome and the skin. *Journal of the American Academy of Dermatology*, **36**, 970–82.

Gobert, A. (1994). Sneddon's syndrome with bilateral peripheral retinal neovascularization. *Bulletin Société Belge Ophtalmologie*, **255**, 85–90.

Hess, D.C. (1992). Stroke associated with antiphospholipid antibodies. *Stroke*, **23**(Suppl.), 23–8.

Jonas, J., Koelble, K., Voelcker, H.E. & Kalden, J.R. (1986). Central retinal artery occlusion in Sneddon's disease associated with antiphospholipid antibodies. *American Journal of Opthalmology*, **102**, 37–40.

Kalashnikova, L.A., Nasonov, E.L., Kushekbaeva, A.E. & Gracheva, L.A. (1990). Anticardiolipin antibodies in Sneddon's syndrome. *Neurology*, **40**, 464–7.

Levine, S.R. & Welch, K.M.A. (1987). The spectrum of neurologic disease associated with antiphospholipid antibodies. *Archives of Neurology*, **44**, 876–83.

Levine, S.R., Langer, S.L., Albers, J.W. & Welch, K.M.A. (1988). Sneddon's syndrome: an antiphospholipid antibody syndrome? *Neurology*, **38**, 798–800.

Lockshin, M.D. (1992). Antiphospholipid antibody syndrome. *Journal of the American Medical Association*, **268**, 1451–3.

Lubach, D., Schwabe, C., Weissenborn, K., Hartung, K., Creutzig, A. & Drenk, F. (1992). Livedo racemosa generalisata: an evaluation of thirty-four cases. *Stroke*, **23**, 1182–3.

Macario, F., Macario, M.C., Ferro, A., Goncalves, F., Campos, M. & Marques, A. (1997). Sneddon's syndrome: a vascular systemic disease with kidney involvement? *Nephron*, **75**, 94–7.

McHugh, N.J., Mayamo, J., Skinner, R.P., James, I. & Maddison, P.J. (1988). Anticardiolipin antibodies, livedo reticularis and major cerebrovascular and renal disease in systemic lupus erythematosus. *Annals of Rheumatic Diseases*, **47**, 110–15.

Marsch, W.C.L. & Muckelmann, R. (1985). Generalized racemose livedo with cerebrovascular lesions (Sneddon syndrome): an occlusive arteriolopathy due to proliferation and migration of medial smooth muscle cells. *British Journal of Dermatology*, **112**, 703–8.

Martinelli, A., Martinelli, P., Ippoliti, M., Giuliani, S. & Coccagna, G. (1991). Sneddon syndrome presenting with hemicranic attacks: a case report. *Acta Neurologica Scandinavica*, **83**, 201–3.

Martinez-Menendez, B., Perez-Sempere, A., Gonzalez-Rubio, M., Villaverde-Amundarain, F.J. & Bermejo-Pareja, F. (1990). Sneddon's syndrome with negative antiphospholipid antibodies. *Stroke*, **21**, 1510–11.

Menzel, C., Reinhold, U., Grunwald, F. et al. (1994). Cerebral blood flow in Sneddon syndrome. *Journal of Nuclear Medicine*, **35**, 461–4.

Michel, M., Bourquelot, P. & Hermine, O. (1996). Essential thrombocythaemia: a cause of Sneddon's syndrome. *Lancet*, **347**, 395.

Moral, A., Vidal, J.M., Moreau, I., Olhaberriague, L. & Montalban, J. (1991). Sneddon's syndrome with antiphospholipid antibodies and arteriopathy. *Stroke*, **22**, 1327–8.

Narbay, G. (1997). Sneddon's syndrome in a patient with homonymous hemianopia with macular sparing. *Bulletin Société Belge Ophtalmologie*, **263**, 103–7.

Pauranik, A., Parwani, S. & Jain, S. (1987). Simultaneous bilateral central retinal artery occlusion in a patient with Sneddon syndrome: case history. *Journal of Vascular Diseases*, **12**, 158–63.

Pellat, J., Perret, J., Pasquier, B., Bouzet, G., Dubos, G. & Chateau, R. (1976). Etude anatomoclinique et angiographie d'une observation de thromboangiose disséminée à manifestations cérébrales prédominantes. *Revue Neurologique*, **132**, 517–35.

Pettee, A.D., Wasserman, B.A., Adams, N.L. et al. (1994). Familial Sneddon's syndrome. Clinical, hematological, and radiographic findings in two brothers. *Neurology*, **44**, 399–405.

Pinol-Aguade, J., Ferrandiz, C., Ferrer-Roca, O. & Ingelmo, M. (1999). Livedo reticularis y accidentes cerebrovasculares. *Medicina Cutanea Ibero-Latino-Americana*, **3**, 257–65.

Quimby, S.R. & Perry, H.O. (1980). Livedo reticularis and cerebrovascular accidents. *Journal of the American Academy of Dermatology*, **3**, 377–83.

Rautenberg, W., Hennerici, M., Aulich, A., Hoelzle, E. & Lakomek, H.-J. (1988). Immunosuppressive therapy and Sneddon's syndrome. *Lancet*, **ii**, 629–30.

Rebollo, M., Val, J.F., Garijo, F., Quintana, F. & Berg, E.L. (1983). Livedo reticularis and cerebrovascular lesions (Sneddon's syndrome). *Brain*, **106**, 965–79.

Rehany, U., Kassif, Y. & Rumelt, S. (1998). Sneddon's syndrome: neuro-ophthalmologic manifestations in a possible autosomal recessive pattern. *Neurology*, **51**, 1185–7.

Rosenberg, R.D. & Aird, W.C. (1999). Vascular-bed-specific hemostasis and hypercoagulable states. *New England Journal of Medicine*, **340**, 1555–64.

Rumpl, E., Neuhofer, J., Pallua, A. et al. (1985). Cerebrovascular lesions and livedo reticularis (Sneddons's syndrome): a progressive cerebrovascular disorder? *Journal of Neurology*, **231**, 324–30.

Rumpl, E. & Rumpl, H. (1979) Recurrent transient global amnesia in a case with cerebrovascular lesions and livedo reticularis (Sneddon syndrome). *Journal of Neurology*, **221**, 127–31.

Ruscalleda, J., Coscojuela, P., Guardia, E. & De Juan, M. (1991). General case of the day. *Radiographics*, **11**, 929–31.

Scott, I.A. & Boyle, R.S. (1986). Sneddon's syndrome. *Australia and New Zealand Medicine*, **16**, 799–802.

Sitzer, M., Sohngen, D., Siebler, M. et al. (1995). Cerebral microembolism in patients with Sneddon's syndrome. *Archives of Neurology*, **52**, 271–5.

Sneddon, I.B. (1965). Cerebro-vascular lesions and livedo reticularis. *British Journal of Dermatology*, **77**, 777–82.

Stephens, W.P. & Ferguson, I.T. (1982). Livedo reticularis and cerebro-vascular disease. *Postgraduate Medical Journal*, **58**, 70–3.

Stockhammer, G., Felber, S.R., Zelger, B. et al. (1993). Sneddon's syndrome: diagnosis by skin biopsy and MRI in 17 patients. *Stroke*, **24**, 685–90.

Tanne, D., Triplett, D.A. & Levine, S.R. (1998). Antiphospholipid-protein antibodies and ischemic stroke. Not just cardiolipin anymore. *Stroke*, **29**, 1755–8.

Thomas, D.J., Kirby, J.D.T., Britton, K.E. & Galton, D.J. (1982). Livedo reticularis and neurological lesions. *British Journal of Dermatology*, **106**, 711–12.

Tourbah, A., Piette, J., Iba-Zizen, M.T., Lyon-Caen, O., Godeau, P. & Frances, C. (1997). The natural course of cerebral lesions in Sneddon syndrome. *Archives of Neurology*, **54**, 53–60.

Uitdehaag, B.M.J., Scheltens, P., Bertelsmann, F.W. & Bruyn, R.P.M. (1992). Intracerebral hemorrhage and Sneddon's syndrome. *Journal of Neurological Science*, **111**, 227–8.

Vaillant, L., Larmande, P., Arbeille, B., Desveaux, B., Grual, Y. & Lorette, G. (1990). Livedo reticularis, accidents vasculaires cérébraux et maladie mitrale: une nouvelle cause du syndrome de Sneddon. *Annales Dermatologie et Venereologie*, **117**, 925–30.

Vargas, J.A., Yerba, M., Pascual, M.L., Manzano, L. & Durantez, A. (1989). Antiphospholipid antibodies and Sneddon's syndrome. *American Journal of Medicine*, **87**, 597.

Zelger, B., Sepp, N., Schmid, K.W., Hintner, H., Klein, G. & Fritsch, P.O. (1992). Life history of cutaneous vascular lesions in Sneddon's syndrome. *Human Pathology*, **23**, 668–75.

Zelger, B., Sepp, N., Stockhammer, G. et al. (1993). Sneddon's syndrome. A long-term follow-up of 21 patients. *Archives of Neurology*, **129**, 437–47.

34

Cerebral autosomal dominant arteriopathy with subcortical infarcts and leukoencephalopathy

Hugues Chabriat[1], A. Joutel[2], Elisabeth Tournier-Lasserve[2] and Marie-Germaine Bousser[1]

[1]Hôpital Lariboisière and [2]INSERM U25, Paris, France

Introduction

The acronym CADASIL for 'Cerebral Autosomal Dominant Arteriopathy with Subcortical Infarcts and Leuko-encephalopathy' was suggested by us in 1993 (Tournier-Lasserve et al., 1993) for the condition formerly called 'hereditary multi-infarct dementia' (Sourander & Walinder, 1977) and possibly first described in 1955 by Van Bogaert as 'Binswanger's disease with a rapid course in two sisters' (Van Bogaert, 1955). In 1993, the locus of the disease was assigned to chromosome 19 (Tournier-Lasserve et al., 1993). Three years later, mutations of the *notch3* gene were found responsible for the disease (Joutel et al., 1996). The frequency of this autosomal dominant disorder remains unknown. The condition is probably largely underdiagnosed. We are aware of more than 300 affected families in African, Asiatic and Caucasian pedigrees on all continents in 1999.

Clinical presentation

The mean age at onset of symptoms is between 45 and 50 years in the largest series (Chabriat et al., 1995c; Dichgans et al., 1998). It varies among the different pedigrees and within families, and does not significantly differ according to sex.

The first clinical manifestations of CADASIL are attacks of migraine with aura (International Headache Society diagnostic criteria) (Chabriat et al., 1995c, 1997; Dichgans et al., 1998). Migraine with aura is present in about 40% of CADASIL families but its frequency is highly variable within families. It was absent in the family reported by Sabbadini et al. (1995). In contrast, in one family originating from the eastern part of France, 85% of symptomatic members suffered attacks of migraine with aura (Chabriat et al.,

1995b). Globally, 20 to 30% of affected subjects suffer attacks of migraine with aura. The age of onset is 30 years. The first attacks occasionally occur before the age of 20 years (Hutchinson et al., 1995). In a given subject, the frequency of attacks is extremely variable, going from one attack in life to several per month. As usually observed in migraine with aura, the most frequent aura symptoms are visual, sensitive or dysphasic (Vahedi et al., 1996). However, the frequency of attacks with basilar, hemiplegic or prolonged aura is noticeably high. A few patients have been reported with severe attacks including unusual symptoms such as confusion, fever or coma (Chabriat et al., 1995b).

Stroke is the most frequent clinical manifestation of the disease (Dichgans et al., 1998; Chabriat et al., 1995a, b, 1997; Sabbadini et al., 1995; Hutchinson et al., 1995; Vahedi et al., 1996). About 85% of symptomatic subjects suffer TIAs or completed strokes. Ischemic manifestations occur at a mean age of 49 years with a large range from 27 to 65 years. Two-thirds of them are classical lacunar syndromes: pure motor stroke, ataxic hemiparesis, pure sensory stroke, sensory motor stroke. Other focal neurologic deficits of abrupt onset are less frequently observed: dysarthria with or without motor or sensory deficit, isolated ataxia, expressive aphasia, hemianopia. These latters can also be secondary to lacunar infarcts. Ischemic events are isolated in 40% of cases, particularly at onset of the disease. More frequently, they are associated with other symptoms of the disease such as mood disturbances or dementia. In some cases, the onset of the neurologic deficit is progressive within hours (Chabriat et al., 1995a). Some episodes of focal deficits occur in association with headache raising diagnostic difficulties with migraine attacks. The ischemic manifestations of CADASIL most often occur in the absence of vascular risk factors.

Twenty to 30% of CADASIL patients present with severe mood disturbances (Dichgans et al., 1998; Chabriat et al.,

1995a, b, 1997; Sabbadini et al., 1995; Hutchinson et al., 1995; Vahedi et al., 1996). The frequency of such manifestations is widely variable between and within families. Most patients have a severe depression of the melancholic type sometimes alternating with typical manic episodes. The diagnosis of bipolar mood disorder was considered in some subjects until the MRI examination was performed. Thus, the differential diagnosis with a psychiatric disease can be difficult, particularly when such mood disturbances are inaugural and isolated. The late onset of recurrent depressive episodes or of bipolar disorders, their poor response to treatment, their association with a cognitive impairment and even the sole presence of a family history of stroke, migraine with aura or dementia should lead one to perform an MRI of the brain in these subjects. The association of any of these symptoms with WMA at MRI is suggestive of CADASIL and should prompt a genealogical study including all first and second degree relatives as well as the genotypic analysis of the family. The exact cause of mood disturbances in CADASIL remains undetermined. The location of ischemic lesions in basal ganglia or in frontal white matter may play an important role in their occurrence (Aylward et al., 1994; Bhatia & Marsden, 1994).

Dementia is the second most frequent clinical manifestation of CADASIL. It is observed in one third of symptomatic patients. In 90% of cases, dementia aggravates step by step in association with recurrent stroke events. It is a subcortical dementia with predominating frontal symptoms (apragmatism and apathy) and memory impairment. Aphasia, apraxia or agnosia are rare or observed only at the end course of the disease. Dementia is always associated with pyramidal signs, pseudobulbar palsy, gait difficulties and/or urinary incontinence. It is observed at a mean age of 60 years and in 90% of patients before death (Vahedi et al., 1996; Chabriat et al., 1995a). In 10% of cases, dementia is isolated and develops progressively, mimicking the course of Alzheimer's disease. A subtle cognitive deficit only detected with neuropsychological testing has been reported before the occurrence of dementia in some patients (Taillia et al., 1998). The severity and location of lesions are probably determinant for the occurrence of dementia in CADASIL. In a positron emission tomography study of one demented patient and of his asymptomatic cousin, we found a decrease of cortical metabolism only in the demented subject. Both had equally widespread white matter lesions at MRI but the demented subject had far more severe basal ganglia lesions (Chabriat et al., 1995a). In the absence of cortical lesions, these findings suggest the presence of remote metabolic effects of subcortical infarcts (diaschisis) causing dementia.

Other neurologic manifestations have occasionally been reported in CADASIL. Focal or generalized seizures have been observed in 6 to 10% of cases (Dichgans et al., 1998; Chabriat et al., 1995a, b, 1997; Sabbadini et al., 1995; Hutchinson et al., 1995; Vahedi et al., 1996). Deafness of acute or progressive onset has been reported in two cases. The lack of cranial nerve palsy, spinal cord disease [except in one case (Hutchinson et al., 1995)] and of symptoms of muscular origin is noteworthy in CADASIL.

Median age at death is about 65 years. Recently, Dichgans et al. (1998) found that the survival time of men was less than that of women, 64 and 69 years, respectively.

Neuroimaging

MRI is an essential tool for the diagnosis of CADASIL. It is always abnormal in symptomatic subjects. In addition, signal abnormalities can be detected during a presymptomatic period of variable duration. MRI signal abnormalities are observed as early as 20 years of age. After 35, all subjects having the affected gene have an abnormal MRI (Tournier-Lasserve et al., 1993; Sourander et al., 1997; Van Bogaert, 1955; Joutel et al., 1996; Chabriat et al., 1995c).

MRI shows, on T_1-weighted images, punctiform or nodular hyposignals in basal ganglia and in white matter. T_2-weighted images show hypersignals in the same regions associated with widespread areas of increased signal in the white matter. They are observed in the absence of T_1 lesions in one third of affected subjects (Chabriat et al., 1998) (Fig. 34.1). The severity of the lesions dramatically increases with age (Chabriat et al., 1998). In subjects under 40 years, T_2 hypersignals are usually punctuate or nodular with a symmetrical distribution, and predominate in periventricular areas and in the centrum semi-ovale. Later in life, white matter lesions are diffuse and can involve the whole of white matter including the U fibres under the cortex. The severity of the lesions increase with age not only in white matter but also in basal ganglia and brainstem. The frontal and occipital periventricular lesions are constant when MRI is abnormal. The frequency of signal abnormalities in the external capsule (two-thirds of the cases) and in the anterior part of the temporal lobes is noteworthy. Brainstem lesions are mainly observed in the pons. The mesencephalon and medulla are usually spared. Cortical or cerebellar lesions are exceptional. They have been observed in only two cases older than 60 years. Recently, the load of T_1 lesions observed in CADASIL was found related to the clinical severity of the disease (Yousry et al., 1999). CT-scan can

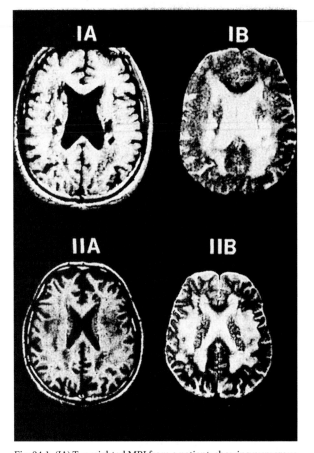

Fig. 34.1. (IA) T$_1$-weighted MRI from a patient, showing numerous low-signal subcortical lesions (left and right thalami, posterior limb of left internal capsule, right external capsule, and left temporo-occipital white matter). (IB) T$_2$-weighted MRI showing corresponding areas of high signal, with a more diffuse increased signal in white matter. (IIA) T$_1$-weighted MRI from an asymptomatic subject, showing that the signal returned from white matter is abnormal, but no focal areas are seen. (IIB) T$_2$-weighted MRI showing diffuse high-signal intensity of the subcortical white matter. (From Tournier-Lasserve et al., 1991, with permission. Copyright American Heart Association.)

also show the white matter and basal ganglia lesions but it is far less sensitive than MRI.

Other investigations

Ultrasound studies and echocardiography are usually normal. Cerebral angiography is normal, showing only in rare cases a narrowing of small arteries. CSF examination is usually normal but oligoclonal bands with pleïocytosis have been reported. A monoclonal immunoglobulin was

detected in two cases of our first family but not in other affected pedigrees (Tournier-Lasserve et al., 1991).

Pathology

Macroscopic examination of the brain shows a diffuse myelin pallor and rarefaction of the hemispheric white matter sparing the U fibres (Baudrimont et al., 1993). Lesions predominate in the periventricular areas and centrum semi-ovale. They are associated with lacunar infarcts located in the white matter and basal ganglia (lentiform nucleus, thalamus, caudate). The most severe hemispheric lesions are the most profound (Ruchoux & Maurage, 1997). In the brainstem, the lesions are more marked in the pons and are similar to the pontine rarefaction of myelin of ischemic origin described by Pullicino et al. (1995). Microscopic investigations show that the wall of cerebral and leptomeningeal arterioles is thickened and that their lumen is significantly reduced (Baudrimont et al., 1993; Ruchoux & Maurage, 1997; Ruchoux et al., 1994, 1995). Such abnormalities can also be detected by leptomeningeal biopsy (Fig. 34.2). The media is thickened with abnormal smooth muscle cells and presence of an eosinophilic non-amyloïd material. Smooth muscle cells are swollen and often degenerated, with multiple nuclei. Sometimes, they are not detectable and are replaced by collagen fibres. By contrast, the endothelium of the vessels is usually spared. On electron microscopy, the eosinophilic material appears dense, granular and osmiophilic. Staining for amyloid substance and elastin are negative. Recently, Ruchoux et al. (1995) made the crucial observation that the vascular abnormalities observed in the brain were also detectable in other organs. The granular material surrounding the smooth muscle cells as seen with electron microscopy is also present in the media of arteries located in the spleen, liver, kidneys, muscle and skin. The presence of this material in the skin, muscle and nerve vessels confirmed the intra vitam diagnosis of CADASIL in several patients (Ruchoux et al., 1994, 1995; Schroder et al., 1995).

Genetics

The defective gene in CADASIL is the *Notch3* gene located on chromosome 19 (Joutel et al., 1996). This gene encodes a large transmembrane receptor. Its exact role in the disease occurence remains so far undetermined. Numerous mis-sense mutations of *Notch3* gene have been detected in CADASIL patients. They are located in

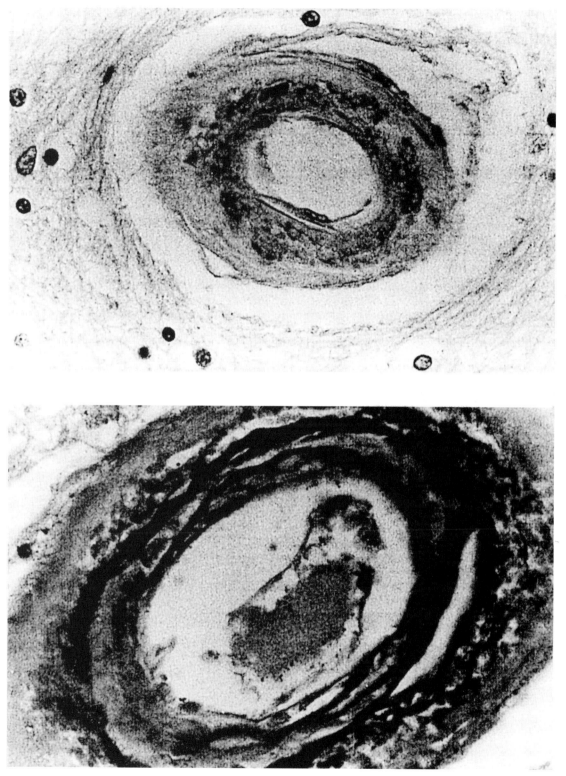

Fig. 34.2. Vascular changes in small arteries of the white matter. Top: Granular eosinophilic material in the media (hematoxylin–eosin stain ×284). Bottom: Thickening and reduplication of the internal elastic lamellae (orcein stain ×284). (From Baudrimont et al., 1993, with permission. Copyright American Heart Association.)

the epidermal-growth-factor-like (EGF-like) repeats in the extracellular domain of the protein (Joutel et al., 1997). Most of the causative mutations are clustered within two exons (3 and 4), which allowed a genetic test to be proposed, which was able to detect 70% of mutations causing the disease (Joutel et al., 1997). The test is now currently used as a diagnostic tool. The testing raises important ethical problems very close to those encounterd in families with Huntington's disease, particularly in asymptomatic members at risk of having the deleterious mutation. In the absence of any effective treatment of the disease, genetic counselling and testing should be performed only in specific and trained centres.

Conclusion

CADASIL is a newly recognized hereditary cause of ischemic strokes associated with white matter lesions. Its characterization is an important step in the dismantling of vascular dementias. Also, the identification of CADASIL will bring new insights in the pathophysiology of leukoaraïosis, subcortical dementia and migraine with aura. The prevalence of the disease remains unknown. In 1999, the disease remains largely undiagnosed.

References

Aylward, E.D., Roberts-Willie, J.V., Barta, P.E. et al. (1994). Basal ganglia volume and white matter hyperintensities in patients with bipolar disorder. *American Journal of Psychiatry*, 5, 687–93.

Baudrimont, M., Dubas, F., Joutel, A. et al. (1993). Autosomal dominant leukoencephalopathy and subcortical ischemic strokes: a clinicopathological study. *Stroke*, 24, 122–5.

Bhatia, K. & Marsden, C. (1994). The behavioural and motor consequences of focal lesions of the basal ganglia in man. *Brain*, 117, 859–76.

Chabriat, H., Bousser, M.G. & Pappata, S. (1995a). Cerebral autosomal dominant arteriopathy with subcortical infarcts and leukoencephalopathy: a positron emission tomography study in two affected family members. *Stroke*, 26(9), 1729–30.

Chabriat, H., Tournier-Lasserve, E., Vahedi, K. et al. (1995b). Autosomal dominant migraine with MRI white-matter abnormalities mapping to the CADASIL locus. *Neurology*, 45(6), 1086–91.

Chabriat, H., Vahedi, K., Iba-Zizen, M.T. et al. (1995c). Clinical spectrum of CADASIL: a study of 7 families. Cerebral autosomal dominant arteriopathy with subcortical infarcts and leukoencephalopathy. *Lancet*, 346(8980), 934–9.

Chabriat, H., Joutel, A., Vahedi, K. et al. (1997). CADASIL. Cerebral Autosomal Dominant Arteriopathy with Subcortical Infarcts and Leukoencephalopathy. *Revue Neurologie (Paris)*, 153(6–7), 376–85.

Chabriat, H., Levy, C., Taillia, H. et al. (1995). Patterns of MRI lesions in CADASIL. *Neurology*, 51(2), 452–7.

Dichgans, M., Mayer, M., Uttner, I. et al. (1998). The phenotypic spectrum of CADASIL: clinical findings in 102 cases. *Annals of Neurology*, 44(5), 731–9.

Hutchinson, M., O'Riordan, J., Javed, M. et al. (1995). Familial hemiplegic migraine and autosomal dominant arteriopathy with leukoencephalopathy (CADASIL). *Annals of Neurology*, 38(5), 817–24.

Joutel, A., Corpechot, C., Ducros, A. et al. (1996). Notch3 mutations in CADASIL, a hereditary adult-onset condition causing stroke and dementia. *Nature*, 383(6602), 707–10.

Joutel, A., Vahedi, K., Corpechot, C. et al. (1997). Strong clustering and stereotyped nature of Notch3 mutations in CADASIL patients. *Lancet*, 350(9090), 1511–15.

Pullicino, P., Ostow, P., Miller, L. et al. (1995). Pontine ischemic rarefaction. *Annals of Neurology*, 37, 460–6.

Ruchoux, M.M. & Maurage, C.A. (1997). CADASIL: Cerebral autosomal dominant arteriopathy with subcortical infarcts and leukoencephalopathy. *Journal of Neuropathology and Experimental Neurology*, 56(9), 947–64.

Ruchoux, M.M., Chabriat, H., Bousser, M.G. et al. (1994). Presence of ultrastructural arterial lesions in muscle and skin vessels of patients with CADASIL. *Stroke*, 25(11), 2291–2.

Ruchoux, M.M., Guerouaou, D., Vandenhaute, B. et al. (1995). Systemic vascular smooth muscle cell impairment in cerebral autosomal dominant arteriopathy with subcortical infarcts and leukoencephalopathy. *Acta Neuropathologica*, 89(6), 500–12.

Sabbadini, G., Francia, A., Calandriello, L. et al. (1995). Cerebral autosomal dominant arteriopathy with subcortical infarcts and leucoencephalopathy (CADASIL). Clinical, neuroimaging, pathological and genetic study of a large Italian family. *Brain*, 118, 207–15.

Schroder, J.M., Sellhaus, B. & Jörg, J. (1995). Identification of the characteristic vascular changes in a sural nerve biopsy of a case with cerebral autosomal dominant arteriopathy with subcortical infarcts and leukoencephalopathy. (CADASIL). *Acta Neuropathologica* (Berlin), 89, 116–121.

Sourander, P. & Walinder, J. (1977). Hereditary multi-infarct dementia. Morphological and clinical studies of a new disease. *Acta Neuropathologica (Berlin)*, 39(3), 247–54.

Taillia, H., Chabriat, H., Kurtz, A. et al. (1998). Cognitive alterations in non-demented CADASIL patients. *Cerebrovascular Diseases*, 8(2), 97–101.

Tournier-Lasserve, E., Iba-Zizen, M.T., Romero, N. & Bousser, M.G. (1991). Autosomal dominant syndrome with stroke-like episodes and leukoencephalopathy. *Stroke*, 22, 1297–302.

Tournier-Lasserve, E., Joutel, A., Melki, J. et al. (1993). Cerebral autosomal dominant arteriopathy with subcortical infarcts and leukoencephalopathy maps to chromosome 19q12. *Natural Genetics*, 3(3), 256–9.

Vahedi, K., Chabriat, H., Ducros, A. et al. (1996). Analysis of

CADASIL clinical natural history in a series of 134 patients belonging to 17 families linked to chromosome 19. *Neurology*, **46**, A211.

Van Bogaert, L. (1955). Encephalopathie sous-corticale progressive (Binswanger) à évolution rapide chez deux soeurs. *Medical Hellenistica*, **24**, 961–72.

Yousry, T.A., Seelos, K., Mayer, M. et al. (1999). Characteristic MR lesion pattern and correlation of T_1 and T_2 lesion volume with neurologic and neuropsychological findings in cerebral autosomal dominant arteriopathy with subcortical infarcts and leukoencephalopathy (CADASIL) [In Process Citation]. *American Journal of Neuroradiology*, **20**(1), 91–100.

35

Cerebrovascular complications of Fabry's disease

Panayiotis Mitsias, Nikolaos I.H. Papamitsakis and Steven R. Levine

Department of Neurology, Henry Ford Hospital, Detroit, MI, USA

Introduction

Fabry's disease (FD), or angiokeratoma corporis diffusum, is a rare X-linked inherited disorder of glycosphingolipid metabolism (Desnick et al., 1995). Deficiency of a lysosomal hydrolase, α-galactosidase, leads to progressive accumulation of glycosphingolipids, mainly ceramide trihexoside, in most visceral tissues, and primarily in the lysosomes of the vascular endothelium. Progressive endothelial glycosphingolipid accumulation results in tissue ischemia and infarction and leads to the major clinical manifestations of the disease (Desnick et al., 1995). The disease is genetically heterogeneous, as it has been linked to multiple mutations in the α-galactosidase gene (Takenaka et al., 1996; Chen et al., 1998; Topaloglou et al., 1999).

Hemizygote males usually have characteristic skin lesions, angiokeratomas, and suffer from unexplained fever, acroparesthesias, episodic crises of excruciating pain, corneal and lenticular opacities, hypohidrosis, and cardiac and renal dysfunction (Desnick et al., 1995). Death usually occurs in adult life from renal, cardiac, and/or cerebral complications of their vascular disease (Desnick et al., 1995).

Heterozygote females are either asymptomatic or exhibit fewer signs and symptoms of the disease, although occasional females have been described with symptoms similar to the males (Bird & Lagunoff, 1978).

The neurological complications of FD include peripheral neuropathy, autonomic neuropathy and cerebrovascular disease (Desnick et al., 1995). Heterozygotes usually present with either no symptoms (Desnick et al., 1995) or with milder manifestations of FD as compared to hemizygotes (Bird & Lagunoff, 1978). However, cerebrovascular manifestations are common in both the hemizygote and the symptomatic heterozygote groups.

In this chapter, we analyse the clinical, radiologic and pathologic features of hemizygote and heterozygote patients FD and cerebrovascular involvement based on our experience and a comprehensive review of the literature (Archer, 1927; Pompen et al., 1947; Brown, 1952; Bass, 1958; Stoughton & Clendenning, 1959; Curry et al., 1961; Bethune et al., 1961; Wise et al., 1962; De Groot, 1964; Wallace & Cooper, 1965; Jensen, 1966; Steward & Hitchcock, 1968; DiLorenzo et al., 1969; Lou & Reske-Nielsen, 1971; Kahn, 1973; Becker et al., 1975; Guin & Saini, 1976; Bird & Lagunoff, 1978; Sher et al., 1978; Zeluff et al., 1978; Schatzki et al., 1979; Ho & Feman, 1981; Cable et al., 1982; Taglianni et al., 1982; Scully et al., 1984; Kaye et al., 1988; Menzies et al., 1988; Petersen et al., 1989; Moumdjian et al., 1989; Roach, 1989; Morgan et al., 1990; Grewal & Barton, 1992; Colley et al., 1958; Maisey & Cosh, 1980; Mutoh et al., 1988; Hasholt et al., 1990; Grewal & McLatchey, 1992; Mitsias & Levine, 1996).

Early diagnostic features

The most consistent early symptoms of FD are episodic crises of pain, lasting for minutes to hours, mostly affecting the feet or the hands, usually precipitated by exercise, fever or hot weather, and prevented by acetophenacetin. The mechanisms responsible for production of the pain crises are not well known, but it is possible that storage of glycophospholipids within the endothelial cells or the vasa nervorum, the perineural cells, or the dorsal root and autonomic ganglia, can cause altered vasomotor reactivity, resulting in a hypoxic state (Desnick et al., 1995).

Anhidrosis, due to infiltration of lipid into the sweat glands and loss of unmyelinated nerve fibres innervating the sweat glands, usually complicates the problem of heat intolerance.

The most often observed sign is the angiokeratoma, appearing in clusters within the superficial layers of the skin. They are usually first noted in the periumbilical area and the extensor surfaces of the elbows and knees, and also the hip and genital areas (Desnick et al., 1995).

Ophthalmological exam typically reveals whirl-like, corneal opacities, dilatation and tortuosity of the conjuctival vessels, and abnormalities of retinal vessels (Desnick et al., 1995). These changes do not usually impair the vision.

Clinical manifestations of cerebrovascular disease

Male hemizygotes develop symptomatic cerebrovascular disease at a young for stroke age, usually in the fourth decade (mean age, 32) (Mitsias & Levine, 1996). Hemiparesis, vertigo, dysarthria, diplopia, ataxia, hemisensory symptoms, nystagmus, and nausea/vomiting are the most common symptoms and signs (Mitsias & Levine, 1996). Headache is rather infrequent, reported by 20% of patients (Mitsias & Levine, 1996). In the majority of patients (58%), the presentation is consistent with vertebrobasilar territory ischemia, while the anterior circulation was definitely symptomatic in approximately 20% of the patients (Mitsias & Levine, 1996).

Vascular dementia from penetrating small vessel disease has also been described in patients with FD and should be a consideration in the evaluation of otherwise unexplained dementia, particularly in males younger than 65 years of age (Mendez et al., 1997).

Heterozygote women develop symptomatic cerebrovascular disease usually a decade later than the hemizygotes (Mitsias & Levine, 1996). Memory loss, vertigo, ataxia, hemiparesis, depressed level of consciousness, hemisensory symptoms and headache are the predominant symptoms and signs (Mitsias & Levine, 1996). In half of the patients the clinical presentation was consistent with involvement within the vertebrobasilar territory, while only in 10% the carotid territory was definitely involved (Mitsias & Levine, 1996). Central retinal artery occlusion (Utsumi et al., 1997) and central retinal vein occlusion (Oto et al., 1998) have also been reported.

Neuroradiologic findings

A multitude of findings on head CT scans has been reported, ranging from completely normal results, to the presence of large superficial territorial infarctions to multiple small deep infarcts, either in the cerebral hemispheres

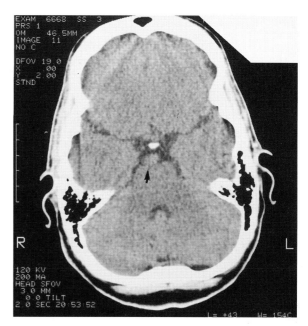

Fig. 35.1. Unenhanced head CT scan from a heterozygote patient, demonstrating basilar artery dilatation and compression of the right side of the anterior pons.

or in the brainstem or cerebellum (Mitsias & Levine, 1996). In addition, dilatation and ectasia of the basilar or vertebral arteries is often seen in both hemizygotes and heterozygotes (Mitsias & Levine, 1996) (Fig. 35.1).

In a large series of patients with FD evaluated with serial head MRI scans it was observed that patients younger than 26 did not have visible lesions, whereas all patients older than 54 had MRI-visible hyperintense lesions, typical for small-vessel disease. Of all patients evaluated, 32% had no lesions (mean age, 36 years), 26% had white matter lesions (mean age, 43 years), and 26% had lesions in both white and grey matter (mean age, 47 years). Approximately one-third of the patients with lesions on MRI had neurological symptoms (Crutchfield et al., 1998). In addition, other MRI reports indicate that prominent, ectatic intracranial basal vessels may be found (Mitsias & Levine, 1996) (Fig. 35.2).

Cerebral angiography could be normal. However, often dolichoectatic intracranial vessels, especially basilar or vertebral arteries, and occasionally internal carotid artery are seen in hemizygotic and heterozygotic patients (Mitsias & Levine, 1996) (Figs. 35.3, 35.4).

In one study (Tedeschi et al., 1999), proton MRS imaging revealed that the ratios of N-acetylaspartate/creatine-phosphocreatine and N-acetylaspartate/choline were significantly decreased compared to controls, while the choline/creatine ratio was not different between FD patients and controls. These findings led to the conclusion

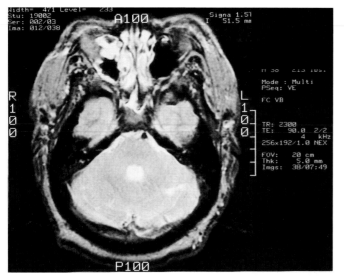

Fig. 35.2. Head MRI scan from a hemizygote patient, revealing ectasia of the basilar artery and a left cerebellar infarction.

that there is decreased *N*-acetylaspartate in FD patients, possibly due to either direct metabolic neuronal dysfunction or to diffuse subclinical ischemia leading to neuronal loss. This neuronal involvement extended beyond the areas of MRI-visible abnormalities. This information could be of help in the assessment of potential therapeutic interventions.

Cerebrovascular pathology

Neuropathologic autopsy findings are consistent with prior events of cerebral ischemia and, rarely, hemorrhage. Large superficial cerebral hemispheric infarcts and multiple small, deep infarcts, and brainstem/cerebellar infarcts are often seen in hemizygotes and symptomatic heterozygotes (Mitsias & Levine, 1996). Intracerebral hemorrhage is rarely observed (Mitsias & Levine, 1996).

The vessels of the circle of Willis often appear thickened. Narrowing of the lumina and intracellular deposits in arteries and arterioles are additional findings. Dolichoectasia of the basilar and vertebral arteries, and less often of the carotid arteries, are frequent findings in both hemizygotes and symptomatic heterozygotes (Mitsias & Levine, 1996).

Ischemic cerebrovascular disease

The majority of patients, male hemizygotes and symptomatic female heterozygotes, present with symptoms and

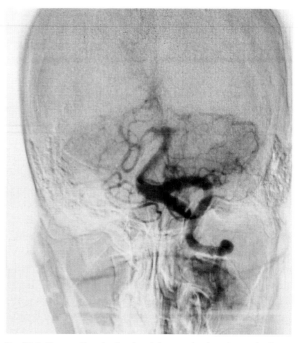

Fig. 35.3. Conventional selective right vertebral angiography from a heterozygote patient, demonstrating an ectatic, tortuous vertebrobasilar system.

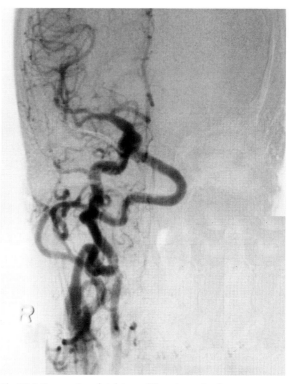

Fig. 35.4. Conventional right carotid angiography from a hemizygote patient, revealing tortuous and ectatic external and internal carotid arteries.

signs related to vertebrobasilar ischemia, while symptoms due to anterior circulation involvement are relatively uncommon. This is in contrast with the general frequency of anterior vs. posterior circulation cerebrovascular disease (Bogousslavsky et al., 1988; Bamford et al., 1958), and suggests a general predilection for involvement of the arteries of the posterior circulation in FD. The combination of large intracranial artery dolichoectasia, especially in the vertebrobasilar system (Wise et al., 1962; Wallace & Cooper, 1965; Petersen et al., 1989; Colley et al., 1958; Mitsias & Levine, 1996), and marked thickening and luminal compromise of the medium- and small-sized arteries (Jensen, 1966; Lou & Reske-Nielsen, 1971; Kahn, 1973; Taglianini et al., 1982; Scully et al., 1984) may cause reduction of blood flow and also stretching, distortion and obstruction of the already stenotic basilar tributaries, thus resulting in brainstem or cerebellar ischemia (Nishizaki et al., 1986). Complete or partial thrombosis resulting in unilateral restricted pontine infarct in the territory of a penetrating artery, large bilateral pontine infarcts from basilar artery occlusion, cerebellar infarcts, or embolic infarction of the occipital lobe or the thalamus have been observed in several patients with FD (Mitsias & Levine, 1996).

Deep small cerebral infarcts, usually multiple, are also a frequent finding (Mitsias & Levine, 1996). The most likely underlying mechanism is progressive occlusion of the small intracranial arteries or arterioles, secondary to deposition of the glycosphingolipid in the vessel wall, as shown pathologically in several patients (Jensen, 1966; Lou & Reske-Nielsen, 1971; Schatzki et al., 1979; Taglianini et al., 1982). Other risk factors (hypertension secondary to renal involvement, diabetes mellitus, etc) may also play a role, but the extent to which each of these factors contributes is unclear.

Cardiac abnormalities are frequently encountered and they can potentially lead to cardiogenic embolism. Coronary artery disease, due to deposition of the glycosphingolipid, resulting in premature myocardial infarction (Wise et al., 1962; Zeluff et al., 1978; Scully et al., 1984), can cause left ventricular wall-motion abnormalities, mural thrombus formation, and subsequent cardiogenic embolism. Valvular heart disease, especially of the mitral valve, is frequently encountered. Mitral valve prolapse is found in 54–56% of the hemizygotes and 39–58% of the heterozygotes (Goldman et al., 1986; Sakuraba et al., 1986). The presence of glycolipid deposits in all the structures of the heart is one of the reasons for the increased incidence of mitral valve prolapse in FD (Becker et al., 1975). Mitral valve prolapse has a role in cerebral ischemia, at least in younger patients (Barnett et al., 1980).

Hypertrophic cardiomyopathy is known to complicate FD (Yokoyama et al., 1987; Cohen et al., 1983), especially in

Table 35.1. *Mechanisms of cerebral ischemia in patients with Fabry's disease*

1. Intracranial arterial dolichoectasia
   a. Complete or partial thrombosis of main arterial trunk
   b. Stretching, distortion and obstruction of tributary vessels
   c. Artery-to-artery embolism
2. Progressive occlusion of small arteries or arterioles secondary to deposition of glucosphingolipid in the vessel wall
3. Cardiogenic embolism
   a. Wall-motion abnormalities secondary to ischemic heart disease
   b. Valvular heart disease, especially mitral valve prolapse
   c. Hypertrophic cardiomyopathy
4. Impaired autonomic function
5. Prothrombotic states
   a. Platelet activation
   b. Activation of endothelial factors

heterozygote women which exhibit a more severe form of cardiac disease (Goldman et al., 1986; Sakuraba et al., 1986). Hypertrophic obstructive cardiomyopathy is associated with increased risk for stroke (Russel et al., 1991), especially when associated with atrial fibrillation (Nishide et al., 1983; Furlan et al., 1984).

Impaired autonomic function in male (Cable et al., 1982) and female (Mutoh et al., 1988) patients with FD, presumably related to glycolipid deposition in the peripheral nervous system and vascular beds, is known to occur. The resulting severe orthostatic hypotension could lead to transient or permanent cerebral ischemia, especially in the presence of cerebral vessel occlusive disease (Dobkin, 1989).

Prothrombotic states are not uncommon in patients with FD. Widespread endothelial abnormalities (Desnick et al., 1995), related to tissue deposits of glucophospholipids, predominantly ceramide trihexoside, and to a lesser extent ceramide digalactoside and the tissue blood type B substance, can lead to platelet activation. This has been demonstrated even in patients without prior history of thrombotic episodes (Igarashi et al., 1986). In addition, analysis of plasma from FD patients for multiple endothelial factors reveals elevated concentrations of soluble intercellular adhesion molecule-1, vascular cell adhesion molecule-1, P-selectin and plasminogen activator inhibitor, lower levels of thrombomodulin, and elevated levels of integrin CDIIb, compared to normal controls (DeGraba et al., 2000). These findings are consistent with a prothrombotic state in FD patients, and could also provide markers of efficacy for therapeutic interventions in the disease (see Table 35.1).

Intracranial arterial dolichoectasia

In FD, in addition to cerebral ischemia, dolichoectatic intracranial arteries may also cause neurovascular compression syndromes. Triventricular hydrocephalus related to dolichoectatic basilar artery has been reported in hemizygote (Kahn, 1973) and heterozygote (Wise et al., 1962; Colley et al., 1958; Maisey & Cosh, 1980) patients. Other presentations, including isolated third nerve palsy (De Groot, 1964), trigeminal neuralgia (Morgan et al., 1990), isolated eighth nerve dysfunction (Wise et al., 1962; De Groot, 1964; Wallace & Cooper, 1965), and dysfunction of the hypoglossal nerve (Maisey & Cosh, 1980) can also be atributed to compression of the individual nerves by dolichoectatic basilar or vertebral arteries. Optic atrophy, observed in three patients (Wise et al., 1962; Wallace & Cooper, 1965; Steward & Hitchcock, 1968) can also be atributed to compression of the optic nerve by a dolichoectatic supraclinoid segment of the internal carotid artery (Schwartz et al., 1993).

The deposition of the glycosphingolipid occurs in all areas of the body, but predominantly in the lysosomes of endothelial, perithelial, and smooth-muscle cells of blood vessels (Desnick et al., 1995), resulting thus in extensive vascular smooth muscle involvement, loss of structural integrity of the arterial wall, eventually leading to the development of the intracranial artery dolichoectasia.

Intracerebral hemorrhage

There are rare reports of intracerebral hemorrhage in hemizygotes (Bass, 1958; Wise et al., 1962) and heterozygotes (Steward & Hitchcock, 1968), and despite incomplete descriptions it appears likely that this was a consequence of malignant hypertension secondary to uremia. It is possible, however, that the degeneration of the cerebral vessels due to deposition of glycosphingolipid in the vessel wall, strongly contributes to the development of this process.

Outcome

The majority (75%) of hemizygote males presenting with cerebral ischemia will eventually develop recurrent cerebrovascular events, and most of them more than one events (Mitsias & Levine, 1996). In three-quarters of patients the recurrence will be in the vertebrobasilar territory (Mitsias & Levine, 1996). Intracerebral hemorrhage is rare as a recurrent event (Mitsias & Levine, 1996). The mean interval

between the first cerebrovascular event and the first recurrence is 6.4 years (range = 0–19) (Mitsias & Levine, 1996). During follow-up time, approximately 50% of patients die, within a mean interval of 8.2 years (± 7.4, range 0–20). In the majority of patients, death is directly linked to the cerebrovascular event, while others die of consequences of renal failure.

The prognosis of symptomatic heterozygotes is also quite poor. One-third die as a direct consequence of the initial cerebrovascular event, usually within one year from presentation with cerebrovascular disease (Mitsias & Levine, 1996). Reported causes of death are progressively deepening coma and pontine hemorrhage. Of the survivors, the vast majority (85%) develop recurrent cerebrovascular disease (Mitsias & Levine, 1996), almost always in the posterior circulation, and usually within 1–4 years (Mitsias & Levine, 1996).

Management

Treatment is far from satisfactory as no specific therapy for the cerebrovascular complications of FD is available. Administration of antiplatelet agents may help to prevent the atherosclerotic and thromboembolic effects of damage to the vascular endothelium, but experience with this approach is limited. In one study, administration of ticlopidine significantly modified platelet aggregation in patients with FD (Sakuraba et al., 1987), but whether this is of value in a clinical setting remains to be shown. Management of underlying cardiac dysfunction, and the use of oral anticoagulant agents, if there are conditions predisposing to cardiogenic embolism, should also be considered.

In addition to correcting renal function, renal transplantation may also prevent the further development of vascular lesions, thus preventing cerebrovascular manifestations, by providing a source of normal enzyme for release in the circulation, although a report of progressive cardiac involvement despite successful renal allotransplantation (Kramer et al., 1985) emphasizes the importance of long-term follow-up studies. Genetic counselling, and prenatal diagnosis based on enzyme assay in amniocytes and chorionic villi (Kleijer et al., 1987) should be offered.

Future directions

Etiologic treatment of FD would be expected to prevent the cerebrovascular complications of the disease. Treatment with infusion of normal human plasma or partially purified preparation of α-galactosidase A has been attempted but the corrective activity of the enzyme was rapidly cleared. A recombinant retroviral vector that delivered the α-galactosidase A cDNA was constructed in 1995, but the recombinant retrovirus was of low titre and no correction of patient cells could be documented (Sugimoto et al., 1995)

A virus-producer cell line, producing high titer recombinant retrovirus constructed to transduce and correct target cells has been developed, skin fibroblasts from FD patients were infected with the recombinant virus, and secreted enzyme was observed to be taken up by uncorrected cells. Similar endogenous enzyme correction and small amount of secretion, as well as uptake by uncorrected cells, was demonstrated in transduced immortalized B cell lines from Fabry patients. These observations lead to the possibility that corrected stem cells (and their progeny) from FD patients, after ex vivo transduction and reimplantation, may become a continuous source of secreted α-galactosidase A activity in vitro. This could be then delivered and taken up by various target cell and tissue types (metabolic co-operativity) (Medin et al., 1996).

In a further move towards clinical utility of a therapeutic approach, cells originating from the bone marrow of FD patients and also healthy volunteers (isolated CD34+-enriched cells and long-term bone marrow culture cells, including non-adherent hematopoietic cells and adherent stromal cells) could be effectively transduced, demonstrating metabolic cooperativity. Increased intracellular α-galactosidase A enzyme activity was demonstrated, as well as functional correction of lipid accumulation. These results demonstrate that a gene transfer approach to bone marrow cells could be of therapeutic benefit for FD patients (Takenaka et al., 1999; Ohsugi et al., 2000). It certainly remains to be shown whether the above mentioned approaches could eventually become of use in the daily practice for etiologic treatment of FD, and therefore primary prevention of cerebrovascular complications.

Acknowledgment

Supported in part by NIH grant NS23393.

References

Archer, B.W.C. (1927). Multiple cavernous angiomata of the sweat glands associated with hemiplegia. *Lancet*, **ii**, 595–6.

Bamford, J., Sandercock, P., Dennis, M. et al. (1991). Classification and natural history of clinically identifiable subtypes of cerebral infarction. *Lancet*, **337**, 1521–6.

Barnett, H.J.M., Boughner, D.R., Taylor, D.W. et al. (1980). Further evidence relating mitral-valve prolapse to cerebral ischemic events. *New England Journal of Medicine*, **302**, 139–44.

Bass, B.H. (1958). Angiokeratoma corporis diffusum. *British Medical Journal*, **1**, 1418.

Becker, A.E., Schoorl, R., Balk, A.G. & van der Heide, R.M. (1975). Cardiac manifestations of Fabry's disease. *American Journal of Cardiology*, **36**, 829–35

Bethune, J.E., Landrigan, P.L. & Chipman, C.D. (1961). Angiokeratoma corporis diffusum universale (Fabry's disease) in two brothers. *New England Journal of Medicine*, **264**, 1280–5.

Bird, T.D. & Lagunoff, D. (1978). Neurological manifestations of Fabry disease in female carriers. *Annals of Neurology*, **4**, 537–40.

Bogousslavsky, J., Van Melle, G. & Regli, F. (1988). The Lausane Stroke Registry: analysis of 1,000 consecutive patients with first stroke. *Stroke*, **19**, 1083–92.

Brown, A. (1952). Diffuse angiokeratoma: report of two cases with diffuse skin changes, one with neurological symptoms and splenomegaly. *Glasgow Medical Journal*, **33**, 361–8.

Cable, W.J.L., Kolodny, E.H. & Adams, R.D. (1982). Fabry disease: impaired autonomic function. *Neurology*, **32**, 498–502.

Chen, C.H., Shyu, P.W., Wu, S.J., Sheu, S.S., Desnick, R.J. & Hsiao, K.J. (1998). Identification of a novel point mutation (S65T) in alpha-galactosidase A gene in Chinese patients with Fabry disease. Mutations in brief no. 169. Online. *Human Mutations*, **11**, 328–30.

Cohen, I.S., Fluri-Lundeen, J. & Wharton, T.P. (1983). Two dimensional echocardiographic similarity of Fabry's disease to cardiac amyloidosis: a function of ultrastructural analogy? *Journal of Clinical Ultrasound*, **11**, 437–41.

Colley, J.R., Miller, D.L., Hutt, M.S.R. & Wallace, H.J. (1958). The renal lesion in angiokeratoma corporis diffusum. *British Medical Journal*, **1**, 1266–8.

Crutchfield, K.E., Patronas, N.J., Dambrosia, J.M. et al. (1998). Quantitative analysis of cerebral vasculopathy in patients with Fabry disease. *Neurology*, **50**, 1746–9.

Curry, H.B., Fleisher, T.L. & Howard, F. (1961). Angiokeratoma corporis diffusum – a case report. *Journal of the American Medical Association*, **175**, 864–8.

DeGraba, T., Azhar, S., Dignat-George, F. et al. (2000). Profile of endothelial and leukocyte activation in Fabry patients. *Annals of Neurology*, **47**, 229–33.

De Groot, W.P. (1964). Angiokeratoma corporis diffusum Fabry. *Dermatologica*, **128**, 321–49.

Desnick, R.S., Ioannou, Y.A. & Eng, C.M. (1995). α-Galactosidase deficiency: Fabry disease. In *The Metabolic Basis of Inherited Disease*, 7th edn, ed. C.R. Scriver, A.L. Beaudet, W.S. Sly & D. Valle, pp. 2741–84. New York: McGraw Hill.

DiLorenzo, P.A., Kleinfeld, J., Tellman, W. & Nay, L. (1969). Angiokeratoma corporis diffusum (Fabry's disese). *Acta Dermatologia Venereologia*, **49**, 319–25.

Dobkin, B.H. (1989). Orthostatic hypotension as a risk factor for symptomatic occlusive cerebrovascular disease. *Neurology*, **39**, 30–4.

Furlan, A.J., Craciun, A.R., Raju, N.R. & Hart, N. (1984). Cerebrovascular complications associated with idiopathic hypertrophic subaortic stenosis. *Stroke*, **15**, 282–4.

Goldman, M.E., Cantor, R., Schwartz, M.F. et al. (1986). Echocardiographic abnormalities and disease severity in Fabry's disease. *Journal of the American College of Cardiology*, **7**, 1157–61.

Grewal, R.P. & Barton, N.W. (1992). Fabry's disease presenting with stroke. *Clinical Neurology and Neurosurgery*, **94**, 177–9.

Grewal, R.P. & McLatchey, SK. (1992). Cerebrovascular manifestations in a female carrier of Fabry's disease. *Acta Neurologica Belgica*, **92**, 36–40.

Guin, G.H. & Saini, N. (1976). Diffuse angiokeratoma (Fabry's disease): case report. *Military Medicine*, **141**, 259–63.

Hasholt, L., Sorensen, S.A., Wandall, A. et al. (1990). A Fabry's disease heterozygote with a new mutation: biochemical, ultra-structural, and clinical investigations. *Journal of Medical Genetics*, **27**, 303–6.

Ho, P.C. & Feman, S.S. (1981). Internuclear ophthalmoplegia in Fabry's disease. *Annals of Ophthalmology*, **13**, 949–51.

Igarashi, T., Sakuraba, H. & Suzuki, Y. (1986). Activation of platelet function in Fabry's disease. *American Journal of Hematology*, **22**, 63–7.

Jensen, E. (1966). On the pathology of angiokeratoma corporis diffusum (Fabry). *Acta Pathologica Microbiologica Scandinavica*, **68**, 313–31.

Kahn, P. (1973). Anderson–Fabry disease: a histopathological study of three cases with observations on the mechanism of production of pain. *Journal of Neurology, Neurosurgery and Psychiatry*, **36**, 1053–62.

Kaye, E.M., Kolodny, E.H., Logigian, E.L. & Ullman, M.D. (1988). Nervous system involvement in Fabry's disease: Clinicopathological and biochemical correlation. *Annals of Neurology*, **23**, 505–9.

Kleijer, W.J., Hussaarts-Odijk, L.M., Sachs, E.S. et al. (1987). Prenatal diagnosis of Fabry's disease by direct analysis of chorionic villi. *Prenatal Diagnosis*, **7**, 283–7.

Kramer, W.J., Thormann, J., Mueller, K. & Frenzel, H. (1985). Progressive cardiac involvement by Fabry's disease despite successful renal allotransplantation. *International Journal of Cardiology*, **7**, 72–5.

Lou, H.O.C. & Reske-Nielsen, E. (1971). The central nervous system in Fabry's disease. *Archives of Neurology*, **25**, 351–9.

Maisey, D.N. & Cosh, J.A. (1980). Basilar artery aneurysm and Anderson–Fabry disease. *Journal of Neurology, Neurosurgery and Psychiatry*, **43**, 85–7.

Medin, J.A., Tudor, M., Simonovitch, R. et al. (1996). Correction in trans for Fabry disease: expression, secretion and uptake of alpha-galactosidase A in patient-derived cells driven by a high-titer recombinant retroviral vector. *Proceedings of the National Academy of Sciences, USA*, **93**, 7917–22.

Mendez, M.F., Stanley, T.M., Medel, N.M., Li, Z. & Tedesco, D.T. (1997). The vascular dementia of Fabry's disease. *Dementia and Geriatric Cognitive Disorders*, **8**, 252–7.

Menzies, D.G., Campbell, I.W. & Kean, D.M. (1988). Magnetic reso-nance imaging in Fabry's disease. *Journal of Neurology, Neurosurgery and Psychiatry*, **51**, 1240–1.

Mitsias, P. & Levine, S.R. (1996). Cerebrovascular complications of Fabry's disease. *Annals of Neurology*, **40**, 8–17.

Morgan, S.H., Rudge, P., Smith, S.J.M. et al. (1990). The neurological complications of Anderson–Fabry Disease (α-galactosidase A deficiency). Investigation of symptomatic and presymptomatic patients. *Quarterly Journal of Medicine*, **75**, 491–504.

Moumdjian, R., Tampieri, D., Melanson, D. & Ethier, R. (1989). Anderson–Fabry disease: a case report with MR, CT, and cerebral angiography. *American Journal of Neuroradiology*, **10**, S69–70

Mutoh, T., Senda, Y., Sugimura, K. et al. (1988). Severe orthostatic hypotension in a female carrier of Fabry's disease. *Archives of Neurology*, **45**, 468–72.

Nishide, M., Irino, T., Gotoh, M. et al. (1983). Cardiac abnormalities in ischemic cerebrovascular disease studied in two-dimensional echocardiography. *Stroke*, **14**, 541–5.

Nishizaki, T., Tamaki, N., Takeda, N. et al. (1986). Dolichoectatic basilar artery: a review of 23 cases. *Stroke*, **17**, 1277–81.

Ohsugi, K., Kobayashi, K., Itoh, K., Sakuraba, H. & Sakuragawa, N. (2000). Enzymatic corrections for cells derived from Fabry disease patients by a recombinant adenovirus vector. *Journal of Human Genetics*, **45**, 1–5.

Oto, S., Kart, H., Kadayifcilar, S., Ozdemir, N. & Aydin, P. (1998). Retinal vein occlusion in a woman with heterozygous Fabry's disease. *European Journal of Ophthalmology*, **8**, 265–7.

Petersen, R.C., Garrity, J.A. & Houser, O.W. (1989). Fabry's disease: an unusual cause of stroke with unique angiographic findings. *Neurology*, **39**(Suppl. 1), 123.

Pompen, A.W.M., Ruiter, M. & Wyers, H.J.G. (1947). Angiokeratoma corporis diffusum (universale) Fabry, as a sign of an unknown internal disease; two autopsy reports. *Acta Medica Scandinavica*, **128**, 234–55.

Roach, E.S. (1989). Congenital cutaneouvascular syndromes. In *Handbook of Clinical Neurology*, vol. II (55): *Vascular Diseases, Part III*, ed. J.F. Toole, pp. 443–62. Amsterdam–New York: Elsevier Science Publishers B.V.

Russel, J.W., Biller, J., Hajduczok, Z.D. et al. (1991). Ischemic cerebrovascular complications and risk factors in idiopathic hypertrophic subaortic stenosis. *Stroke*, **22**, 1143–7.

Sakuraba, H., Yanagawa, Y., Igarashi, T. et al. (1986). Cardiovascular manifestations in Fabry's disease. A high incidence of mitral valve prolapse in hemizygotes and heterozygotes. *Clinical Genetics*, **29**, 276–83.

Sakuraba, H., Igarashi, T., Shibata, T. & Suzuki, Y. (1987). Effect of vitamin E and ticlopidine on platelet aggregation in Fabry's disease. *Clinical Genetics*, **31**, 349–54.

Schatzki, P.F., Kipreos, B. & Payne, J. (1979). Fabry's disease. Primary diagnosis by electron microscopy. *American Journal of Surgical Pathology*, **3**, 211–19.

Schwartz, A., Rautenberg, W. & Hennerici, M. (1993). Dolichoectatic intracranial arteries: Review of selected aspects. *Cerebrovascular Diseases*, **3**, 273–9.

Scully, R.E., Mark, E.J. & McNeely, B.U. (1984). Case records of

Massachusetts General Hospital: Case 2, 1984. *New England Journal of Medicine*, **310**, 106–14.

Sher, N.A., Reiff, W., Letson, R.D. & Desnick, R.J. (1978). Central retinal artery occlusion complicating Fabry's disease. *Archives of Ophthalmology*, **96**, 815–17.

Steward, V.W. & Hitchcock, C. (1968). Fabry's disease (Angiokeratoma corporis diffusum). *Pathology Europe*, **3**, 377–88.

Stoughton, R.B. & Clendenning, W.E. (1959). Angiokeratoma corporis diffusum (Fabry). *Archives of Dermatology*, **79**, 601–2.

Sugimoto, Y., Aksentijevich, I., Murray, G.J., Brady, R.O., Pastan, I. & Gottesman, M.M. (1995). Retroviral coexpression of a multidrug resistance gene (MDR1) and human alpha-galactosidase A for gene therapy of Fabry disease. *Human Gene Therapy*, **6**, 905–15.

Taglianini, F., Pietrini, V., Gemignani, F. et al. (1982). Anderson–Fabry's disease: neuropathological and neurochemical investigation. *Acta Neuropathologica (Berlin)*, **56**, 93–8.

Takenaka, T., Sakuraba, H., Hashimoto, K. et al. (1996). Coexistence of gene mutations causing Fabry disease and Duchenne muscular dystrophy in a Japanese boy. *Clinical Genetics*, **49**, 255–60.

Takenaka, T., Hendrickson, C.S., Tworeck, D.M. et al. (1999). Enzymatic and functional correction along with long-term enzyme secretion from transduced bone marrow hematopoietic stem/progenitor and stromal cells derived from patients with Fabry disease. *Experimental Hematology*, **27**, 1149–59.

Tedeschi, G., Bonavita, S., Banerjee, T.K., Virta, A. & Schiffmann, R. (1999). Diffuse central neuronal involvement in Fabry disease. A proton MRS imaging study. *Neurology*, **52**, 1663–7.

Topaloglou, A.K., Ashley, G.A., Tong, B. et al. (1999). Twenty novel mutations in the alpha-galactosidase A gene causing Fabry disease. *Molecular Medicine*, **5**, 806–11

Utsumi, K., Yamamoto, N., Kase, R. et al. (1997). High incidence of thrombosis in Fabry's disease. *Internal Medicine*, **36**, 327–9.

Wallace, R.D. & Cooper, W.J. (1965). Angiokeratoma corporis diffusum universale (Fabry's disease). *American Journal of Medicine*, **39**, 656–61.

Wise, D., Wallace, H.J. & Jellinek, E.H. (1962). Angiokeratoma corporis diffusum. *Quarterly Journal of Medicine*, **122**, 177–206.

Yokoyama, A., Yamazoe, M. & Shibata, A. (1987). A case of heterozygous Fabry's disease with a short PR interval and giant T waves. *British Heart Journal*, **57**, 296–9.

Zeluff, G.W., Caskey, C.T. & Jackson, D. (1978). Heart attack or stroke in a young man? Think Fabry's disease. *Heart and Lung*, **7**, 1056–61.

36

Metabolic causes of stroke

Engin Y. Yilmaz, Betsy B. Love and José Biller

Department of Neurology, Indiana University School of Medicine, Indianapolis, IN, USA

It is extremely challenging to assess the frequency and mortality of 'metabolic strokes' in the general population, because reports are often biased towards the rare causes of strokes that are seen in tertiary care centres.

Mitochondrial disorders

Historical background

The concept of mitochondrial disease was first described by Luft et al. in a young Swedish woman with severe hypermetabolism (Luft et al., 1962). Engel and Cunningham (1963) defined abnormal deposits of mitochondria as 'ragged-red fibers' in 1963. Defects of respiratory chain complexes were described during the 1970s (Spiro et al., 1970; Willems et al., 1977). The acronym MELAS to describe a clinical syndrome with mitochondrial encephalomyopathy, lactic acidosis and stroke-like episodes, was introduced by Pavlakis et al. in 1984. In 1988, Holt et al. described pathogenic mutation of mitochondrial DNA (mtDNA) in a patient with mitochondrial myopathy. Since that time, disorders with pathogenic mtDNA and related diseases have emerged as major clinical entities (Johns, 1995).

MELAS (Mitochondrial encephalomyopathy, lactic acidosis, and stroke-like episodes)

Genetics

MELAS results from extrachromosomal, abnormal mtDNA causing mitochondrial respiratory chain dysfunction (Ciafaloni et al., 1992). The defects of mtDNA include inherited heteroplasmic (coexistance of normal and mutant mtDNA in the same cell) point mutations or rarely, sporadic deletions. MtDNA is inherited maternally and therefore, MELAS can demonstrate a maternal pattern of inheritance. However, sporadic cases are also common. Four point mutations have been found in association with MELAS, three mutations at nucleotide pairs 3243, 3250, 3271 and one at the coding region for subunit 4 of complex 1 (Lyon et al., 1996). Eighty to ninety percent of cases are associated with a point mutation of the leucine transfer RNA gene of mtDNA at nucleotide 3243 (Goto et al., 1990). Subsequent studies have identified additional point mutations establishing that MELAS is a genetically heterogeneous disorder (Goto et al., 1991). Maternal relatives of patients with MELAS may be normal or may have hearing loss, migraines, myopathy, or cardiomyopathy. Rarely, an mtDNA mutation of subunit 4 of complex (ND4) of the respiratory chain can cause MELAS (Lertrit et al., 1992).

Prevalence /incidence

Among patients younger than 45 years of age, the frequency of mitochondrial disease as a cause of stroke ranges between 2 and 10% (Bogousslavsky et al., 1993; Majamaa et al., 1997).

Clinical manifestations (early diagnostic features)

MELAS is a multisystem disease characterized by recurrent migraine-like headaches in the setting of stroke-like episodes, and prolonged focal or generalized seizures (Montagna et al., 1988). Most patients with MELAS are asymptomatic in infancy and have normal early development. However, in early childhood, parents may seek care for less well-known clinical features such as short stature, muscle fatigability, exercise intolerance, and myalgias. Migraine-like headaches, nausea, or vomiting are present in more than 90% of patients (Hirano et al, 1992). The episodes may be precipitated by febrile illnesses. In a study of 40 patients, 80% were aged 5–15 years, and the most frequent symptom was episodic headache with vomiting and convulsions (Goto et al., 1992). Stroke-like episodes manifest as transient hemiparesis, alternating hemiparesis, homonymous hemianopia, cortical blindness, ataxia or aphasia (Pavlakis et al., 1984). Strokes generally do not follow vascular arterial territories but occur predominantly in the posterior half of the brain. As a result, many patients develop cortical visual field deficits that may be reversible. Other features include; sensorineural hearing loss (Sue et al., 1998a), cataracts, optic nerve atrophy (Hanna et al., 1998) migraine complicated by stroke (Ohno et al., 1997), occipital strokes (Pavlakis et al., 1984), chronic asthma (Shanske et al., 1993), purpura as a manifestation of mitochondrial angiopathy (Horiguchi et al., 1991), myoclonic seizures, and hypogonadism (Topaloglu et al., 1998). Recurrent episodes of cortical infarction may lead to a gradual decline in cognitive and motor function. Multisystem involvement may cause ocular signs such as bilateral eyelid ptosis, chronic external ophthalmoplegia, posterior subcapsular cataracts, atypical pigmentary retinopathy and optic nerve atrophy (Rummelt et al., 1993). Cardiac involvement may cause mitral regurgitation (Suzuki et al., 1993), hypertrophic or dilated cardiomyopathy (Inui et al., 1992), and cardiac conduction defects. Endocrine manifestations include diabetes mellitus and hypothyroidism (Inui et al., 1992). Full expression of the disease may result in dementia and death before age 20.

Increased blood and CSF concentrations of lactate and pyruvate are often seen, but are not always present (Hammans et al., 1995). Serum creatine kinase is often normal. EMG may show active myopathic changes. EEG may show features suggestive of occipital lobe seizures.

MR imaging may demonstrate asymmetrically distributed cortical and subcortical infarcts. Infarcts often do not correspond to vascular territories (Valanne et al., 1998). Focal lesions may preferentially (Kuriyama, 1984) affect the parietal and occipital lobes (Kuriyama et al., 1984; Yamamoto et al., 1984). Infarcts predominantly affect grey matter. Symmetric basal ganglia calcification occurring most commonly in the globus pallidus can be seen. An additional early neuroimaging feature may be fourth ventricular enlargement (Sue et al., 1998b) (Fig. 36.1).

SPECT findings include focal hypoperfusion in the parietal and occipital lobes and decreased cerebral perfusion reserve (Morita et al., 1989; Watanabe et al., 1998). Proton MR spectroscopy may show increased concentrations of lactate (Barkovich et al., 1993).

The diagnosis of possible MELAS requires incorporating

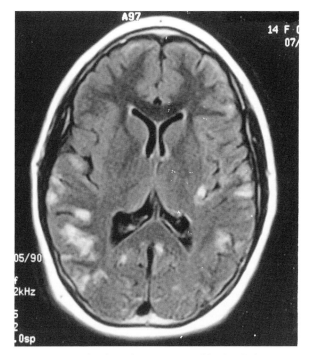

Fig. 36.1. T_1-weighted MRI from a 14-year-old girl with short stature and proximal muscle weakness, showing multiple bilateral hemispheric infarcts.

clinical, neuroimaging, histochemical and molecular biological investigations. Hirano et al. (1992) proposed clinical criteria for establishing a diagnosis of MELAS. Main criteria were: (i) stroke-like episodes before the age of 40 years, (ii) encephalopathy characterized by seizures, dementia, or both, (iii) lactic acidosis, ragged red fibres, or both. Additional criteria were (i) normal early development, (ii) recurrent headaches, and (iii) recurrent vomiting. However, in the presence of consistent clinical and neuroimaging features, the clinician should keep a high index of suspicion to prompt a search for the diagnosis of 'mitochondrial strokes'. Genetic mutation analysis may be performed on peripheral blood leukocytes, skeletal muscle or both.

Neuropathology

Skeletal muscle biopsy using histochemical techniques to document ragged red fibres and Cytochrome–C oxidase deficient muscle fibres may be very valuable. Since one study found that ragged red fibres were absent in 3 of 22 patients, their absence does not exclude the diagnosis of MELAS (Zeviani et al., 1996). Spongy degeneration of the brain may be seen. Extracellular, and pericapillary calcification may also be seen (Sue et al., 1998a).

Treatment

The current management of MELAS is unsatisfactory and involves the use of drugs that inhibit mitochondrial metabolism. Coenzyme Q, vitamin K3 (menadiol sodium diphosphate), C, B2 (riboflavin), B6 (pyridoxine) and sodium dichloroacetate have been used (Matthews et al., 1993b; Argov et al., 1986). Although the results of open studies are controversial, coenzyme Q is the most widely used drug. A trial of Coenzyme Q is recommended, as it may be beneficial in some cases (Goda et al., 1987; Chan et al., 1998; Nishikawa et al., 1989). Intravenous treatment with sodium dichloroacetate has been shown to decrease arterial and brain lactate levels. However, its efficacy and safety needs to be investigated (Pavlakis et al., 1998; Kimura et al., 1997).

Leigh disease

Necrotizing encephalomyelopathy and lactic acidosis, or Leigh disease is an uncommon condition with clinical, biochemical and pathological features similar to the mitochondrial encephalomyopathies.

Historical background

This condition was first described in a 7-month-old infant boy. Focal, symmetric neuropathological abnormalities resembling Wernicke encephalopathy were described and were referred to as subacute necrotizing encephalomyelopathy (Leigh, 1951).

Biochemistry

All of the defects described in Leigh disease affect oxidative metabolism and impair energy production. MtDNA dysfunction (Holt et al., 1990), and deficiencies of pyruvate dehydrogenase complex (Matthews et al., 1993a), cytochrome C oxidase (Willems et al., 1977; DiMauro et al., 1987), Complex IV, Complex I (Morris et al., 1996) have been described.

Genetics

Leigh disease is genetically heterogenic, transmitted by X-linked recessive, autosomal recessive, or mitochondrial modes of inheritance.

Clinical manifestations

Clinical presentation may vary according to age of onset; Neonatal, classic infantile and juvenile forms have been described. The neonatal form presents with sucking, swallowing, and respiratory difficulties. Death occurs rapidly.

The infantile form begins within the first year of life, usually in infants less than four months of age. Motor and intellectual retardation, feeding and swallowing difficulties, episodic hyperventilation, hypotonia, weakness, blindness, ataxia, seizures and signs of brainstem dysfunction; including ophthalmoparesis, nystagmus, facial weakness, and deafness can occur. The infantile form progresses very rapidly and results in death within 2 years. (Montpetit et al., 1971; Pincus, 1972). A rare juvenile form presents with a slowly progressive course in the first decade of life and leads to mild spastic paraparesis, visual impairment, and movement disorders (dystonia, choreoathetosis, and parkinsonism). In the second decade of life, the juvenile form has a subacute or acute course resulting in marked respiratory depression and coma (Grunnet et al., 1991). Neuropathy, ataxia and retinitis pigmentosa (NARP) can occur with Leigh disease in the maternally inherited mitochondrial form. Retinitis pigmentosa may represent a useful diagnostic clue in the mitochondrially inherited form, as it is not seen with patients pyruvate dehydrogenase complex and cytochrome C oxidase deficiency (Holt et al., 1990).

Elevated plasma and CSF pyruvate and lactate levels are frequent during episodic metabolic acidosis. Muscle and skin biopsies can be helpful. Neuroimaging studies provide strong diagnostic support. The characteristic findings on magnetic resonance imaging include symmetric high signal intensity T_2-weighted lesions in the putamen, globus pallidus, substantia nigra, periaqueductal grey matter, lower medulla, and periventricular white matter (Valanne et al., 1998).

Neuropathology

The main pathology is grey matter degeneration with symmetric foci of partial necrosis and capillary proliferation involving the thalami, brain stem and posterior columns of the spinal cord. The mammillary bodies and hypothalamus are relatively spared (Swaiman, 1994). Microscopically, these spongiform lesions show cystic cavitation, vascular proliferation, with relative preservation of neurons and associated demyelination and gliosis (Richter, 1957).

Treatment

Treatment is palliative and symptomatic. Dichloroacetate administration has a mild benefit in some cases of Leigh disease due to pyruvate dehydrogenase deficiency. (Kimura et al., 1997).

Hyperhomocyst(e)inemia and homocystinuria

Hyperhomocyst(e)inemia is a clinical syndrome caused by several enzyme deficiencies in methionine metabolism.

Biochemistry

Homocysteine is a sulfur-containing amino acid produced during the metabolism of methionine. Its intracellular metabolism is controlled by two pathways, transsulfuration to cysteine and remethylation to methionine. The majority of homocysteine is catabolized via pyridoxine (B6)-dependent condensation with serine to form cystathionine. This step is catalysed by cystathionine beta synthetase. A second pathway is remethylation of homocysteine back to methionine by methionine synthase. Methionine synthase requires methylenetetrahydrofolate and methylcobalamine as cofactors.

Different enzyme defects, nutritional deficiencies, toxins and drugs can cause hyperhomocyst(e)inemia. Deficiency of three enzymes; cystathionine beta synthetase, methylenetetrahydrofolate reductase (MTHFR), and methionine synthase, lead to hyperhomocyst(e)inemia (Mudd et al., 1995). In addition, nutritional deficiencies in vitamin B12(cobalamine), pyridoxine (vitamin B6), or folic acid can cause hyperhomocyst(e)inemia.

The most common enzyme deficiency is cystathionine beta synthetase deficiency (Mudd et al., 1964). The genetic defect in cystathionine beta synthetase is located on chromosome 21 (Kraus et al., 1993). The homozygous trait; congenital homocystinuria, is rare. Heterozygosity for cystathionine beta synthetase is more common and at least 24 mutations have been identified. Plasma homocysteine concentrations are mildly elevated (two to four times more than normal) in heterozygotes. MTHFR mutation is an autosomal recessive disorder affecting folate metabolism. The gene is localized to chromosome 1p.

Many toxins and drugs increase plasma homocyst(e)ine concentrations. Smoking may lower pyridoxal phosphate concentrations and may cause accelerated atherogenesis (Vermaak et al., 1990). Phenytoin and theophylline, may cause homocyst(e)inemia (Ueland & Refsum, 1989; Ubbink et al., 1996).

Incidence

The estimated incidence of homocystinuria is approximately 1 in 332 000 live births. Approximately 0.3% to 1.5% of the population is heterozygous for cystathionine beta synthetase deficiency. Methylenetetrahydrofolate reductase (MTHFR) mutation is also prevalent in the population; about 50% of North Americans are heterozygous, and 11% are homozygous for a thermolabile mutation of MTHFR (Rozen, 1996). In the Framingham study, 40% of elderly subjects had a vitamin deficiency that can raise plasma homocyst(e)ine levels (Lindenbaum, et al. 1994). Plasma homocyst(e)ine levels are greater than 14 μmol/l in 20% of North Americans (Rozen, 1996).

Pathology

Homocystinuria promotes premature atherosclerosis. Fibrous intimal plaques, medial fibrosis, and disruption of the internal elastic lamina are typical features (McCully, 1969). Homocyst(e)ine may damage vascular endothelial cells and interfere with the regulatory functions of endothelial cells in coagulation and nitric oxide generation (Harpel et al., 1996). Furthermore, homocyst(e)ine may induce proliferation of smooth muscle cells (Tsai et al., 1996). Homocyst(e)ine suppresses expression of thrombomodulin and heparan sulfate, resulting in a prothrombotic state (Lentz & Sadler, 1991). Neuropathologic changes are widespread and include microgyria and perivascular changes such as demyelination, macrophage infiltration, and gliosis.

Clinical features

There is widespread vascular involvement including the cerebrovascular and cardiovascular systems. Most patients present with peripheral venous thrombosis, including pulmonary embolism. However, stroke, arterial occlusion, or myocardial infarction can be the initial presentation. Other manifestations include dystonia, or osteoporosis (Kempster et al., 1988) Hyperhomocyst(e)inemia is accepted as an independent risk factor for cardiovascular disease and stroke (Graham et al., 1997). In the Framingham Heart Study, there was a graded, strong relationship between elevated homocyst(e)ine levels and carotid artery stenosis (Selhub et al., 1995). Homocyst(e)ine levels more than 10.5 μmol/l, increase the risk of carotid artery thickening by three times (Malinow et al., 1993). Mild hyperhomocyst(e)inemia is also an independent risk factor for venous thromboembolism (den Heijer et al., 1996).

The classic early childhood homocystinuria is associated with early atherosclerosis, marfanoid features, mental retardation, and ectopia lentis (Mudd et al., 1985). The increased tendency for thrombosis usually presents as an ischemic stroke. Malar flush, livedo reticularis, myopia, glaucoma and rarely optic atrophy may be present. The multiple clinical presentations that are

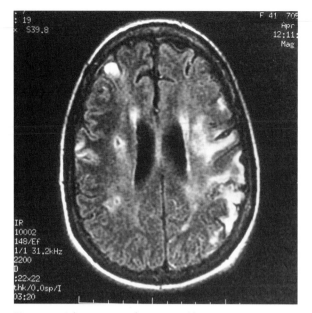

Fig. 36.2. Axial FLAIR MRI of a 41-year-old woman with heterozygous mutation of MTHFR, demonstrates extensive ischemic changes involving the left middle cerebral artery, the right middle cerebral artery, and the right anterior cerebral artery watershed distribution. There were also extensive ischemic changes involving the left posterior cerebral artery distribution.

possible relate to the genetic heterogeneity involved with this deficiency state. Approximately 50% of these patients will have a thromboembolic event before age 30 (Mudd et al., 1985).

MTHFR deficiency is the most common inherited disorder of folate metabolism. A typical presentation is infantile global delay and failure to thrive, with associated seizures and progressive neurological deterioriation. With infantile onset, cerebrovascular manifestations tend to be more striking than in cystathionine beta synthetase deficiency. MTHFR deficiency is associated with a possible increase in myocardial infarctions (Kluijtmans et al., 1996). Adult-onset cerebrovascular disease is also possible, but currently data are lacking for support of this mutation as a risk factor in stroke (Fig. 36.2).

Diagnosis

All young patients and adults with unexplained stroke should be considered for plasma homocyst(e)ine testing. The range of normal plasma homocyst(e)ine levels is still debatable. Plasma homocyst(e)ine levels 10.2 μmol/l or higher, were associated with an increase in vascular disease (Graham et al., 1997). The Vitamin Intervention in Stroke Prevention trial is currently following patients with

atherosclerotic cerebral infarctions and homocyst(e)ine levels greater than 9.5 μmol/l.

Infants with cystathionine beta synthetase deficiency may be identified with neonatal screening for methionine. The cyanide nitroprusside test may be utilized for neonatal screening of infants with cystathionine beta synthetase. Prenatal diagnosis can be possible by amniocentesis and enzymatic essay of cultured amniocytes (Fowler et al., 1982).

MTHFR deficiency is also characterized by low cerebro-spinal fluid folate levels, and low plasma methionine without megaloblastic anemia. Prenatal diagnosis is possible.

Treatment

Vitamin supplementation with folic acid, pyridoxine and vitamin B12 is generally effective. Minimal doses of folate 1–5 mg per day alone or combined with B6 and B12 have been shown to reduce homocyst(e)ine concentrations within four to six weeks (Brattstrom et al., 1988). Treatment with a combination of folic acid, pyridoxine and vitamin B12, in patients with plasma homocyst(e)ine levels more than 14 μmol/l, may prevent progression of carotid athero-sclerosis (Peterson & Spence, 1998).

Fabry's disease (Fig. 36.3)

Fabry's disease (angiokeratoma corporis diffusum) is an X-linked recessive disorder of glycosphingolipid metabolism due to deficiency of the lysosomal enzyme alpha galactosi-dase A. Patients present with multifocal thromboembolic vascular disease secondary to progressive accumulation of ceramide trihexoside within the vessel walls. Major mani-festations are corneal opacifications, episodic acropares-thesias, heat intolerance, postprandial abdominal cramping, hypohydrosis and other manifestations of auto-nomic dysfunction. A hallmark of Fabry's disease is angioke-ratomas which are especially prominent between the umbilicus and knees (Fig. 36.3). Cardiac ischemia in combi-nation with renovascular failure increases the likelihood of cerebrovascular complications, such as strokes. Management includes antiplatelet agents, antipyretics, and analgesics. (Fabry's disease is discussed in Chapter 35 in detail.)

Menkes disease

Menkes disease (Kinky hair disease, Steely hair disease) is a multifocal disorder associated with a defect in the intes-

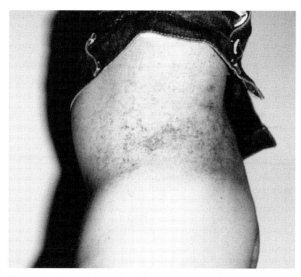

Fig. 36.3. Fabry's disease. Angiokeratoma corporis diffusum.

tinal absorption of copper. Serum copper and ceruloplas-min are very low. The brain and liver copper content are reduced, while the copper content in the intestinal mucosa is increased. The disease is inherited as an X-linked trait; the mutant gene has been located on the X chromosome in the q13.3 region. Affected individuals have abnormal, col-ourless, twisted and friable hair and eyebrows. Focal and generalized seizures, hypotonia, and hypothermia are often present. Menkes disease can also present with sub-dural hematomas. Multiple intracranial occlusions can occur. Thalamic degeneration can be seen (Martin & Leroy, 1985; Williams et al., 1978). Cerebral angiography and mag-netic resonance angiography usually reveal tortous, irreg-ular, and elongated intracranial vessels (Takahashi et al., 1993).

Tangier disease

Tangier disease causes premature atherosclerosis. It is an autosomal recessive disorder characterized by deficiency or absence of HDL in plasma. Serum cholesterol and low density lipoproteins are low, and triglycerides are normal or mildly elevated. Homozygotes can develop cholesterol ester deposition in the tonsils (orange tonsils), liver, spleen, lymph nodes, gastrointestinal tract, and Schwann cells. Cerebral infarcts can be seen (Serfaty-Lacrosniere et al., 1994).

Cardiovascular involvement is thought to be related to the deposition of cholesterol esters (Schaefer et al., 1980).

Organic acid disorders

Propionic acidemia, methylmalonic acidemia, and isovaleric acidemia

Recurrent episodes of vomiting, dehydration leading to metabolic acidosis and coma are the common features of organic acid disorders. Cerebrovascular complications such as infarctions may be seen probably secondary to dehydration, metabolic acidosis, anemia, and thrombocy-topenia.

Propionic acidemia is a disorder of propionyl-CoA car-boxylase activity. This enzyme converts propionyl CoA to methylmalonyl CoA. Osteoporosis, and mental retardation may occur. Basal ganglia infarction may cause chorea and dystonia (Haas et al., 1995). Diagnosis is made by organic acid analysis of the urine.

In methylmalonic acidemia the defective enzyme is methylmalonyl CoA mutase. Most patients have a monilial erythematous eruption and failure to thrive. Renal tubular acidosis may be seen. Basal ganglionic strokes leading to an extrapyramidal syndrome or death may occur (Heidenreich et al., 1988). In a subgroup of patients, meth-ylmalonic acidemia and homocystinuria may coexist. This subgroup may respond to large doses of vitamin B12.

Isovaleric acidemia, or 'sweaty foot syndrome', is a disor-der of isovaleryl CoA dehydrogenase in the catabolism of leucine. Infants usually present in the first week of life with recurrent attacks of vomiting, acidosis, tremors and sei-zures. If they survive, consistent clinical features include mental retardation, persistent ataxia, and involuntary movements. Infants may have leukopenia causing recur-rent infections or thrombocytopenia. The gene for this enzyme is localized to chromosome 15q12–15 (Nyhan & Hass, 1996). Rarely, cerebellar hemorrhages have been described (Fischer et al., 1981).

Diagnosis of the organic acidemias includes prenatal enzyme assay in cultured amniocytes, and organic acid analysis of the urine. Therapy includes dietary restriction of proteins to less than 1 g/kg per day, vitamin B12, biotin, vigorous use of parenteral fluids, and hemodialysis. In iso-valeric acidemia restriction of leucine, and supplementa-tion with glycine may be tried (Cohn et al., 1978).

Glutaric aciduria (types I and II)

Glutaric aciduria is a neurodegenerative disorder charac-terized by macrocephaly, seizures, spasticity and extrapy-ramidal dysfunction. Frontotemporal atrophy, basal ganglia infarctions and bilateral subdural accumulations may be seen in neuroimaging studies (Kohler & Hoffmann, 1998; Osaka et al., 1993; Hoffmann et al., 1994).

Glutaric aciduria type I (GA I)

Typical features are macrocephaly and attacks of fever of unknown origin and sweating. Following acute cerebral infarctions, seizures and coma may occur (Hoffmann et al., 1991). Additionally, spasticity, dystonia, intellectual impairment, and choreoathetosis may be seen (Goodman et al., 1975). This condition may resemble Leigh disease or the 'shaken baby syndrome' with retinal hemorrhages and intracranial bleeding (Stutchfield et al., 1985). Neuroimaging studies may show frontotemporal atrophy, and signal changes in putamen and caudate nuclei (Altman et al., 1991). Glutaryl-CoA dehydrogenase is the deficient enzyme in this disorder. The gene is located on the short arm of chromosome 19. Organic acid analysis of urine or culture of fibroblasts and leukocytes are useful in the diagnosis of this enzyme deficiency (Goodman & Kohlof, 1975).

Treatment includes low protein diet, and a combination of riboflavin and carnitine (Lipkin et al., 1988). Baclofen may be also be useful (Brandt et al., 1979).

Glutaric aciduria type II (GA II)

In glutaric aciduria type II (GA II), there is impairment of various acyl-CoA dehydrogenases. This condition is also referred to as multiple acyl-CoA dehydrogenase deficiency (MAD). There are three different forms; neonatal, infantile and later onset. All forms are characterized by vomiting, hypoglycemia, metabolic acidosis, a strong 'sweaty-feet' odour, and early death (Vallee et al., 1994). Cardiomyopathy and renal cysts may also present. Pathologically there is fatty degeneration of multiple organs. Diagnosis is made by detection of large amounts of urinary organic acids.

Sulfite oxidase deficiency

Sulfite oxidase deficiency is a rare autosomal recessive disorder of sulfur metabolism. Main clinical features are hemiplegia, seizures, progressive choreoathetoid movements, and dislocated lenses. Presence of sulfide in fresh urine is diagnostic. Prenatal diagnosis is also possible (Shih et al., 1977).

Ornithine transcarbamylase (OTC) deficiency

The most common urea cycle deficiency is ornithine transcarbamylase. The X-linked recessive inheritance results in hyperammonemia and neonatal death of affected males. In females, symptoms are variable, with onset of symptoms in early childhood. The initial presentation of OTC deficiency may be hemiparesis, encephalopathy, or intracranial hemorrhage (Amir et al., 1982; Gilchrist & Coleman, 1987; de Grauw et al., 1990; Christodoulou et al., 1993). Therapy includes protein restriction, ketoacid derivative administration to provide a substrate for ammonia fixation and intravenous fluids for dehydration (Rowe et al., 1986).

References

Altman, N.R., Rovira, M. & Bauer, M. (1991). Glutaric aciduria type I: MR findings in two cases. *American Journal of Neuroradiology*, **12**(5), 966–8.

Amir, J., Albert, G., Slatter, M. et al. (1982). Intracranial haemorrhage in siblings and ornithine transcarbamylase deficiency. *Acta Paediatrica Scandinavica*, **71**(4), 671–3.

Argov, Z., Bank, W.J., Maris, J. et al. (1986). Treatment of mitochondrial myopathy due to complex III deficiency with vitamins K3 and C: A ^{31}P-NMR follow-up study. *Annals of Neurology*, **19**(6), 598–602.

Barkovich, A.J., Good, W.V., Koch, T.K. et al. (1993). Mitochondrial disorders: analysis of their clinical and imaging characteristics. *American Journal of Neuroradiology*, **14**(5), 1119–37.

Bogousslavsky, J., Regli, F., Maeder, P. et al. (1993). The etiology of posterior circulation infarcts: a prospective study using magnetic resonance imaging and magnetic resonance angiography. *Neurology*, **43**(8), 1528–33.

Brandt, N.J., Gregersen, N., Christensen, E. et al. (1979). Treatment of glutaryl-CoA dehydrogenase deficiency (glutaric aciduria). Experience with diet, riboflavin, and GABA analogue. *Journal of Pediatrics*, **94**(4), 669–73.

Brattstrom, L.E., Israelsson, B., Jeppsson, J. et al. (1988). Folic acid—an innocuous means to reduce plasma homocysteine. *Scandinavian Journal of Clinical Laboratory Investigation*, **48**(3), 215–21.

Chan, A., Reichmann, H., Kogel, A. et al. (1998). Metabolic changes in patients with mitochondrial myopathies and effects of coenzyme Q10 therapy. *Journal of Neurology*, **1245**(10), 681–5.

Christodoulou, J., Qureshi, I., McInnes, R. et al. (1993). Ornithine transcarbamylase deficiency presenting with stroke-like episodes. *Journal of Pediatrics*, **122**(3), 423–5.

Ciafaloni, E., Ricci, E., Shanske, S. et al. (1992). MELAS: clinical features, biochemistry, and molecular genetics. *Annals of Neurology*, **31**(4), 391–8.

Cohn, R.M., Yudkoff, M., Rothman, R. et al. (1978). Isovaleric acidemia:use of glycine therapy in neonates. *New England Journal of Medicine*, **299**(18), 996–9.

de Grauw, T.J., Smit, L.M., Brockstedt, M. et al. (1990). Acute hemiparesis as the presenting sign in a heterozygote for ornithine transcarbamylase deficiency. *Neuropediatrics*, **21**(3), 133–5.

den Heijer M., Koster, T., Blorn, H.J. et al. (1986). Hyperhomocysteinemia as a risk factor for deep-vein thrombosis. *New England Journal of Medicine*, **334**(12), 759–62.

DiMauro, S., Servidei, S., Zeviani, M. et al. (1987). Cytochrome c oxidase deficiency in Leigh syndrome. *Annals of Neurology*, **22**(4), 498–506.

Engel, W.K. & Cunningham, G. (1963). Rapid examination of muscle tissue. *Neurology*, **13**(11), 919–23.

Fischer, A.Q., Chall, V., Burton, B. et al. (1981). Cerebellar hemorrhage complicating isovaleric acidemia. A case report. *Neurology*, **31**(6), 746–8.

Fowler, B., Bressen, A. & Boman, N. (1982). Prenatal diagnosis of homocystinuria. *Lancet*, **ii**(8303), 875.

Gilchrist, J.M. & Coleman, R. (1987). Ornithine transcarbamylase deficiency: adult onset of severe symptoms. *Annals of Internal Medicine*, **106**(4), 556–8.

Goda, S., Hamada, T., Ishimoto, S. et al. (1987). Clinical improvement after administration of coenzyme Q10 in a patient with mitochondrial encephalomyopathy. *Journal of Neurology*, **234**(1), 63–9.

Goodman, S.I., Markey, S.P., Moe, P.G. et al. (1975). Glutaric aciduria: a 'new' disorder of amino acid metabolism. *Biochemical Medicine*, **12**(1), 12–21.

Goodman, S.I. & Kohlof, J.G. (1975). Glutaric aciduria: inherited deficiency of glutaryl-CoA dehydrogenase activity. *Biochemical Medicine*, **13**(2), 138–40.

Goto, Y., Nonaka, I. & Horai, S. (1990). A mutation in the tRNA(Leu)(UUR) gene associated with the MELAS subgroup of mitochondrial encephalomyopathies. *Nature*, **348**(6302), 651–3.

Goto, Y., Nonaka, I. & Horai, S. (1991). A new mtDNA mutation associated with mitochondrial myopathy, encephalopathy, lactic acidosis and stroke-like episodes (MELAS). *Biochimica et Biophysica Acta*, **1097**(3), 238–40.

Goto, Y., Horai, S., Matsuoka, T. et al. (1992). Mitochondrial myopathy, encephalopathy, lactic acidosis, and stroke-like episodes (MELAS): a correlative study of the clinical features and mitochondrial DNA mutation. *Neurology*, **42**(3, 1), 545–50.

Graham, I.M., Daly, L.E., Refsum, H.M. et al. (1997). Plasma homocysteine as a risk factor for vascular disease: the European Concerted Action Project. *Journal of the American Medical Association*, **277**(22), 1775–81.

Grunnet, M.L., Zalneraitis, E.L., Russman, B.S. et al. (1991). Juvenile Leigh's encephalomyelopathy with peripheral neuropathy, myopathy, and cardiomyopathy. *Journal of Child Neurology*, **6**(2), 159–63.

Haas, R.H., Marsden, D.L., Capistrano-Estrada, S. et al. (1995). Acute basal ganglia infarction in propionic acidemia. *Journal of Child Neurology*, 1995. **10**(1), 18–22.

Hammans, S.R., Sweeney, M.E., Hanna, M.G. et al. (1995). The mitochondrial DNA transfer RNALeu(UUR) A→G(3243) mutation. A clinical and genetic study. *Brain*, **118**(3), 721–34.

Hanna, M.G., Nelson, I., Morgan-Hughes, J. et al. (1998). Melas: a new disease associated with mitochondrial DNA mutation and evidence for further genetic heterogenity. *Journal of Neurology, Neurosurgery and Psychiatry*, **65**, 512–17.

Harpel, P., Zhang, X. & Borth, W. (1996). Homocysteine and hemostasis: pathogenic mechanisms predisposing to thrombosis. *Journal of Nutrition*, **126**(Suppl. 4), 1285S–9S.

Heidenreich, R., Natowicz, M., Hainline, B.E. et al. (1988). Acute extrapyramidal syndrome in methylmalonic acidemia: 'metabolic stroke' involving the globus pallidus. *Journal of Pediatrics*, **113**(6), 1022–7.

Hirano, M., Ricci, E., Koenigsberger, M.R. et al. (1992). Melas: an original case and clinical criteria for diagnosis. *Neuromuscular Disorder*, **2**(2), 125–35.

Hoffmann, G.F., Trefz, F.K., Barth, P.G. et al. (1991). Glutaryl-CoA dehydrogenase deficiency: a distinct encephalopathy. *Pediatrics*, **88**(6), 1194–203.

Hoffmann, G.F., Gibson, K.M., Trefz, F.K. et al. (1994). Neurological manifestations of organic acid disorders. *European Journal of Pediatrics*, **153**(7 Suppl. 1), S94–100.

Holt, I., Harding, A. & Morgan-Hughes, J. (1988). Deletions of muscle mitochondrial DNA in patients with mitochondrial myopathies. *Nature*, **331**(6158), 717–19.

Holt, I.J., Harding, A.E., Petty, R.K. et al. (1990). A new mitochondrial disease associated with mitochondrial DNA heteroplasmy. *American Journal of Human Genetics*, (46), 428–33.

Horiguchi, Y., Fujii, T. & Imamura, S. (1991). Purpuric cutaneous manifestations in mitochondrial encephalomyopathy. *Journal of Dermatology*, **18**(5), 295–301.

Inui, K., Fukushima, H., Tsukamoto, H. et al. (1992). Mitochondrial encephalomyopathies with the mutation of the mitochondrial tRNA(Leu(UUR)) gene. *Journal of Pediatrics*, **120**(1), 62–6.

Johns, D. (1995). Seminars in medicine of Beth Israel Hospital, Boston; Mitochondrial DNA and disease. *New England Journal of Medicine*, **333**(10), 638–44.

Kempster, P.A., Brenton, D.P., Gale, A.N. et al. (1988). Dystonia in homocystinuria. *Journal of Neurology, Neurosurgery and Psychiatry*, **51**(6), 859–62.

Kimura, S., Ohtuke, N., Nezu, A. et al. (1997). Clinical and radiologic improvements in mitochondrial encephalomyelopathy following sodium dichloroacetate therapy. *Brain and Development*, **19**(8), 535–40.

Kluijtmans, L.A., van den Heuvel, L.P., Boers, G.H. et al. (1996). Molecular genetic analysis of mild hyperhomocysteinemia: a common manifestation in the methylenetetrahydrofolate reductase gene is a genetic risk factor for cerebrovascular disease. *American Journal of Human Genetics*, **58**(581), 35–41.

Kohler, M. & Hoffmann, G. (1998). Subdural haematoma in a child with glutaric aciduria type I. *Pediatric Radiology*, **28**(8), 582.

Kraus, J.P., Le, K., Swaroop, M. et al. (1993). Human cystathionine beta synthetase c DNA: sequence, alternative splicing and expression in cultured cells. *Human Molecular Genetics*, **2**(10), 1633–8.

Kuriyama, M., Umezaki, H., Fukuda, Y. et al. (1984). Mitochondrial encephalomyopathy with lactate-pyruvate elevation and brain infarctions. *Neurology*, **34**(1), 72–7.

Leigh, D. (1951). Subacute necrotizing encephalomyelopathy in an infant. *Journal of Neurology, Neurosurgery and Psychiatry*, **14**, 216–21.

Lentz, S.R. & Sadler, J. (1991). Inhibition of thrombomodulin surface expression and protein C activation by the thrombogenic agent homocysteine. *Journal of Clinical Investigation*, **88**(6), 1906–14.

Lertrit, P., Noer, A.S., Jean-Francois, M.J. et al. (1992). A new disease-related mutation for mitochondrial encephalopathy lactic acidosis and strokelike episodes (MELAS) syndrome affects the ND4 subunit of the respiratory complex I. *American Journal of Human Genetics*, **51**(3), 457–68.

Lindenbaum, J., Rosenberg, I.H., Wilson, P.W. et al. (1994). Prevalence of cobalamine deficiency in the Framingham elderly population. *American Journal of Clinical Nutrition*, **60**(1), 2–11.

Lipkin, P.H., Roe, C.R., Goodman, S.I. et al. (1988). A case of glutaric acidemia type I; effect of riboflavin and carnitine. *Journal of Pediatrics*, **112**(1), 62–5.

Luft, R., Ikkos, D., Palmieri, G. et al. (1962). A case of severe hypermetabolism of nonthyroid origin with a defect in the maintenance of mitochondrial respiratory control: a correlated clinical, biochemical and morphological study. *Journal of Clinical Investment*, **41**(9), 1776–804.

Lyon, G., Adams, R.D. & Kolodny, E.H. (1996). *Neurology of Hereditary Metabolic Diseases of Children*, pp. 256–7. New York: McGraw Hill.

McCully, K. (1969). Vascular pathology of homocyst(e)inemia: implications for pathogenesis for atherosclerosis. *American Journal of Pathology*, **56**(1), 111–28.

Majamaa, K., Turrka, J., Karppa, M. et al. (1997). The common MELAS mutation A3243G in mitochondrial DNA among young patients with an occipital brain infarct. *Neurology*, **49**(5), 1331–4.

Malinow, M.R., Nieto, F.J., Szklo, M. et al. (1993). Carotid artery intimal-medial wall thickening and plasma homocyst(e)ine in asymptomatic adults. The Atherosclerosis Risk in Communities Study. *Circulation*, **87**(4), 1107–13.

Martin, J.J. & Leroy, J.G. (1985). Thalamic lesions in a patient with Menkes kinky-hair disease. *Clinical Neuropathology*, **4**(5), 206–9.

Matthews, P.M., Marchington, D.R., Squier, M. et al. (1993a). Molecular genetic characterization of an X-linked form of Leigh's syndrome. *Annals of Neurology*, **33**, 652–5.

Matthews, P.M., Ford, B., Dandurand, R.J. et al. (1993b). Coenzyme Q10 with multiple vitamins is generally ineffective in treatment of mitochondrial disease. *Neurology*, **43**(5), 884–90.

Montagna, P., Gallassi, R., Medori, R. et al. (1988). MELAS syndrome: characteristic migrainous and epileptic features and maternal transmission. *Neurology*, **38**(5), 751–4.

Montpetit, V.J., Andermann, F., Carpenter, S. et al. (1971). Subacute necrotizing encephalomyelopathy; a review and a study of two families. *Brain*, **94**, 1–30.

Morita, K., Ono, S., Fukunaga, M. et al. (1989). Increased accumulation of N-isopropyl-p-(123I)-iodoamphetamine in two cases with mitochondrial encephalomyopathy with lactic acidosis and strokelike episodes (MELAS). *Neuroradiology*, **31**(4), 358–61.

Morris, A.A., Leonard, J.V., Brown, G.K. et al. (1996). Deficiency of respiratory chain complex I is a common cause of Leigh disease. *Annals of Neurology*, **40**, 25–30.

Mudd, S.H., Finkelstein, J., Irrevere, F. et al. (1964). Homocystinuria; an enzymatic defect. *Science*, **143**, 1443.

Mudd, S.H., Skorby, F., Levy, H.L. et al. (1985). The natural history of homocystinuria due to cystathione beta-synthetase deficiency. *American Journal of Human Genetics*, **37**(1), 1–31.

Mudd, S., Levy, H. & Skovby, F. (1995). Disorders of transsulfuration. In *The Metabolic and Molecular Basis of Inherited Disease*, ed. C. Scriver, pp. 1279–323. New York: McGraw Hill.

Nishikawa, Y., Takahashi, M., Yorifuji, S. et al. (1989). Long-term coenzyme Q10 therapy for a mitochondrial encephalomyopathy with cytochrome c oxidase deficiency: a ^{31}P-NMR study. *Neurology*, **39**(3), 399–403.

Nyhan, W.L. & Hass, R. (1996). Inborn errors of amino acid metabolism and transport. In *The Molecular and Genetic Basis of Neurological Disease*, ed. P.S. Rosenberg, S. Dimauro & R.L. Barchi, pp. 1129–50. Boston, Oxford, Johannesburg, Melbourne, New Delhi, Singapore: Butterworth-Heinemann.

Ohno, K., Isotani, E. & Hirakawa, K. (1997). MELAS presenting as migraine complicated by stroke: case report. *Neuroradiology*, **39**(11), 781–4.

Osaka, H., Kimura, S., Nezu, A. et al. (1993). Chronic subdural hematoma, as an initial manifestation of glutaric aciduria type-1. *Brain Development*, **15**(2), 125–7.

Pavlakis, S.G., Phillips, P., DiMauro, S. et al. (1984). Mitochondrial myopathy, encephalopathy, lactic acidosis, and stroke-like episodes: a distinctive clinical syndrome. *Annals of Neurology*, **16**, 481–8.

Pavlakis, S.G., Kingsley, P.B., Kaplan, G.P. et al. (1998). Magnetic resonance spectroscopy: use in monitoring MELAS treatment. *Archives of Neurology*, **55**(6), 849–52.

Peterson, J.C. & Spence, J. (1998). Vitamins and progression of atherosclerosis in patients with hyper-homocyst(e)inemia. *Lancet*, **351**(9098), 263.

Pincus, J. (1972). Subacute necrotizing encephalomyelopathy (Leigh's disease): A consideration of clinical features and etiology. *Developmental Medicine and Child Neurology*, **14**, 87–101.

Richter, R. (1957). Infantile subacute necrotizing encephalopathy with predilection for the brain stem. *Journal of Neuropathology and Experimental Neurology*, **16**(3), 281–307.

Rowe, P.C., Newman, S.L. & Brusilow, S.W. (1986). Natural history of symptomatic partial ornithine transcarbamylase deficiency. *New England Journal of Medicine*, **314**(9), 541–7.

Rozen, R. (1996). Molecular genetic aspects of hyperhomocyst(e)inemia and its relation to folic acid. *Clinical Investigative Medicine*, **19**(3), 171–8.

Rummelt, V., Folberg, R., Ionasescu, V. et al. (1993). Ocular pathology of MELAS syndrome with mitochondrial DNA nucleotide 3243 point mutation. *Ophthalmology*, **100**(12), 1757–66.

Schaefer, E.J., Zech, L.A., Schwartz, D.E. et al. (1980). Coronary heart disease prevalence and other clinical features in familial high-density lipoprotein deficiency (Tangier disease). *Annals of Internal Medicine*, **93**(2), 261–6.

Selhub, J., Jacques, P.F., Bostom, A.G. et al. (1995). Association between plasma homocysteine concentrations and extracranial carotid-artery stenosis. *New England Journal of Medicine*, **332**(5), 286–91.

Serfaty-Lacrosniere, C., Civeira, F., Lanzberg, A. et al. (1994). Homozygous Tangier disease and cardiovascular disease. *Atherosclerosis*, **107**(1), 85–98.

Shanske, A.L., Silvestri, G., Tanji, K., Wertheim, D. & Lipper, S. (1993). MELAS point mutation with unusual clinical presentation. *Neuromuscular Disorders*, **3**(3), 191–3.

Shih, V.E., Abroms, I.F., Johnson, J.L. et al. (1977). Sulfite oxidase deficiency. Biochemical and clinical investigations of a hereditary metabolic disorder in sulfur metabolism. *New England Journal of Medicine*, **297**(19), 1022–8.

Spiro, A.J., Moore, C.L., Prineas, J.W. et al. (1970). A cytochrome-related inherited disorder of the nervous system and muscle. *Archives of Neurology*, **23**, 103–12.

Stutchfield, P., Edwards, M.A., Gray, R.G. et al. (1985). Glutaric aciduria type I misdiagnosed as Leigh's encephalopathy and cerebral palsy. *Developmental Medicine and Child Neurology*, **27**(4), 514–18.

Sue, C.M., Lipsett, L.J., Crimmins, D.S. et al. (1998a). Cochlear origin of hearing loss in MELAS syndrome. *Annals of Neurology.*, **43**(3), 350–9.

Sue, C.M., Crimmins, D.S., Soo, Y.S. et al. (1998b). Neuroradiological features of six kindreds with MELAS tRNA(Leu) A2343G point mutation: implications for pathogenesis. *Journal of Neurology, Neurosurgery and Psychiatry*, **65**(2), 233–40.

Suzuki, Y., Harada, K., Miura, Y. et al. (1993). Mitochondrial myopathy, encephalopathy, lactic acidosis, and stroke-like episodes (MELAS) decrease in diastolic left ventricular function assessed by echocardiography. *Pediatric Cardiology*, **14**(3), 162–6.

Swaiman, K. (1994). Aminoacidopathies and organic acidemias resulting from deficiency of enzyme activity. In *Neurology Principles and Practice*, ed. K. Swaiman, pp. 1220–1. St Louis, MO: Mosby.

Takahashi, S., Ishii, K., Matsumoto, K. et al. (1993). Cranial MRI and MR angiography in Menkes' syndrome. *Neuroradiology*, **35**(7), 556–8.

Topaloglu, H., Seyrantepe, V., Kandemir, N. et al. (1998). mtDNA nt3243 mutation, external ophthalmoplegia, and hypogonadism in an adolescent girl. *Pediatric Neurology*, **18**(5), 429–31.

Tsai, J.C., Wang, H., Perrella, M.A. et al. (1996). Induction of cyclin A gene expression by homocysteine in vascular smooth muscle cells. *Journal of Clinical Investigation*, **97**(1), 146–53.

Ubbink, J.B., van der Merwe, A., Delport, R. et al. (1996). The effect of a subnormal vitamin B6 status on homocysteine metabolism. *Journal of Clinical Investigation*, **98**(1), 177–84.

Ueland, P.M. & Refsum, H. (1989). Plasma homocysteine, a risk factor for vascular disease: plasma levels in health, disease, and drug therapy. *Journal of Laboratory Clinical Medicine*, **114**, 473–501.

Valanne, L., Ketonen, L., Majander, A. et al. (1998). Neuroradiologic findings in children with mitochondrial disorders. *American Journal of Neuroradiology*, **19**(2), 369–77.

Vallee, L., Fontaine, M., Nuyts, J.P. et al. (1994). Stroke, hemiparesis and deficient mitochondrial beta-oxidation. *European Journal of Pediatrics*, **153**(8), 598–603.

Vermaak, W.J., Ubbink, J., Barnard, H. et al. (1990). Vitamin B6 nutrition status and cigarette smoking. *American Journal of Clinical Nutrition*, **51**, 1058–61.

Watanabe, Y., Hashikawa, K., Moriwaki, H. et al. (1998). SPECT findings in mitochondrial encephalomyopathy. *Journal of Nuclear Medicine*, **39**(6), 961–4.

Willems, J.L., Monnens, L.A., Trijbels, J.M. et al. (1977). Leigh's encephalomyelopathy in a patient with a cytochrome c oxidase deficiency in muscle tissue. *Pediatrics*, **60**, 850–7.

Williams, R.S., Marshall, P.C., Lott, I.T. et al. (1978). The cellular pathology of Menkes steely hair syndrome. *Neurology*, **28**(6), 575–83.

Yamamoto, T., Beppu, H. & Tsubaki, T. (1984). Mitochondrial encephalomyopathy: fluctuating symptoms and CT. *Neurology*, **34**(11), 1456–60.

Zeviani, M., Bertagnolio, B. & Uziel, G. (1996). Neurological presentations of mitochondrial diseases. *Journal of Inheritable Metabolic Diseases*, **19**(4), 504–20.

37

Marfan's syndrome

Luís Cunha and V. Barbosa

Servizio de Neurologia, Hospital Universidade Coimbra, Portugal

Bernard Marfan described the disease, that still bears his name, at a meeting of the Medical Society of Paris in 1896. He presented the case of a 5-year-old girl called Gabrielle, pointing out what is still considered to be one of the hallmarks of the disease, her disproportionately long limbs. Further elucidation on the clinical features of the disease and its causes still continues today.

Marfan's syndrome is a connective tissue disorder responsible for an extensive and generalized malformation of organs and systems. The skeleton is disproportionate and unstable, the eyes often have lens dislocations and are myopic, a cystic disease of the lungs can be present. . . . All the organic departments can be affected in different degrees, leading to multiple medical problems. Nevertheless, defective formation of cardiac valves and blood vessels are the origin of the more serious occurrences in Marfan's syndrome.

Marfan's syndrome is an inherited disorder, transmitted as a dominant trait, being sporadic in less than one-quarter of the cases. The condition is present in 1:5000–10 000 people, and both men and women of any ethnic group can be affected. In 1990–91, the gene defect was definitively located to chromosome 15, opening a new era in the management of Marfan's syndrome.

The clinical spectrum of Marfan's syndrome is large and unpredictable. Moreover, its complete extent was only progressively made clear. That was the origin of distinct denominations during the last century (dolichosestenomelia, arachnodactyly . . .) and, almost certainly, of the inclusion in clinical series of patients suffering from different diseases. Genetic definition of the Marfan's entity allows a more precise identification of the cases, but the spreading use of the Marfan's syndrome designation still persists, and diagnosis remains based on a careful clinical assessment of the patients.

So, a methodical exploration of the organic depart-ments, and the hierarchic organization of the findings in major and minor criteria were proposed and adopted by The American Academy of Pediatrics.

Skeletal system

The skeletal peculiarities, particularly the long and thin extremities, were first recognized by Marfan and were the core of his original description. Actually, an excessive length of the long bones – usually, but not always, resulting in tall stature – pes planus, pectus carinatum, pectus excavatum requiring surgery – the consequence of an excessive growth of ribs – wrist and thumb signs, scoliosis . . ., are the most striking features of a Marfan's patient and are some of the major signals.

Ocular system

The eye abnormalities were described by Boerger only two decades after the Marfan communication. Ectopia lentis, provoked by the lassitude or rupture of the suspensory ligaments of the lens, is one of the cardinal manifestations of the syndrome, present in nearly half of the cases and the single major ocular criterion. Increased axial length of globe with myopia and a tendency to detachment of the retina are also common.

Cardiovascular system

Cardiovascular abnormalities, the other major component of Marfan's syndrome, are the cause of the most damaging or even fatal complications of the disease. It is remarkable that those abnormalities were first described only in 1943,

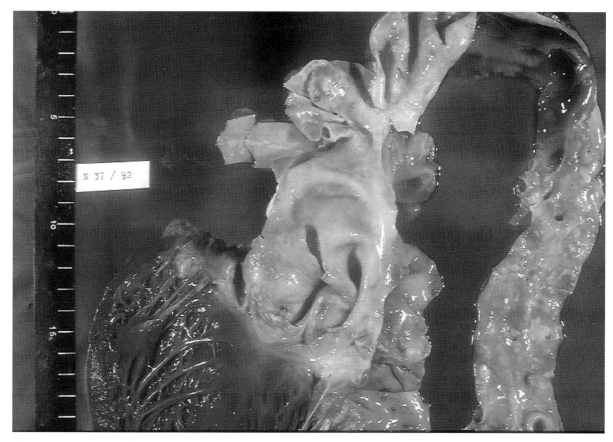

Fig. 37.1. Aorta rupture and dissection in a Marfan's patient.

in spite of the fact that a dissecting aneurysm of the aorta was reported in association with a left recurrent nerve palsy as early as 1909.

Dilatation of the ascending aorta with or without aortic regurgitation, and involving at least the sinuses of valsalva or dissection of the ascending aorta, is the major criterion. Aortic root dilatation is present in 80% of cases. The first identifiable enlargement can be as early as 10 years of age or as late as the sixth decade. Aorta and large arteries are unusually wide and fragile, even in very young patients, and can rapidly progress to aneurysms and aneurysm dissection. The main histologic abnormality affects the aortic media, which presents a severe loss of elastic fibres in advanced forms (Figs. 37.1 and 37.2).

Mitral valve prolapse affects two-thirds of the patients, and mitral leakage or rhythm disturbances are very often associated. The mitral valve modifications, as well the more rare dilatation of pulmonary artery and dilatation or dissection of the descending aorta, are minor criteria of the disease.

Other major criteria are a positive family and genetic history and lumbosacral dural ectasia in CT or MR imaging. Minor alterations were also documented in the pulmonary system and the skin.

The final diagnosis of a Marfan's syndrome needs a minimal cluster of the signals mentioned. No cerebrovascular manifestation was reported to be contributive for that diagnosis.

Nevertheless, the occurrence of a cerebrovascular event along the natural course of a Marfan syndrome is possible. Secondary placement of neurological manifestations relates to their lesser frequency, probably because the most dramatic consequences of cardiovascular anomalies are not expressed primarily by neurological syndromes.

Two main causes underlie the neurological complications of Marfan's syndrome.

Dissection of ascending aorta, carotids and vertebral arteries

It was said earlier that the first reference to a neurological complication in a Marfan's patient, in 1909, described a recurrent paralysis. It was not a stroke or other vascular ocurrence but its cause was a dissecting aneurysm of the

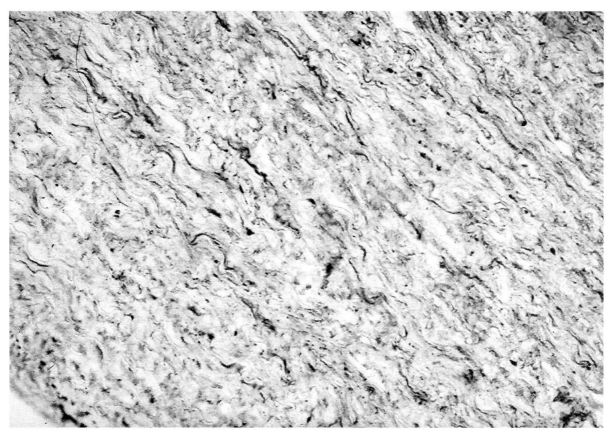

Fig. 37.2. Shortened and thickened elastic fibres (Elastin & Alcian Blue 200 × 2.5).

aorta. Since then, most of the references to cerebrovascular events underline the existence of an arterial malformation: dilatation, aneurysm, dissection, extending from the aorta or occurring independently in the internal carotid or vertebral arteries.

Embolic mechanisms

Valvular dysfunction and disturbances of cardiac rhythm can produce embolic strokes basically no different from any other embolic stroke.

Intracerebral aneurysms and aneurysmatic rupture have for a long time been considered a frequent complication of Marfan's disease. The controversy has not been resolved but has come closer to a conclusion: there is an excess of aneurysms in Marfan's syndrome but not an excess of subarachnoid haemorrhages.

Other neurological complications have been described in Marfan's syndrome. Particular attention must to be given to spinal defects, particularly at the cranio-spinal junction. As many as 54% of patients with Marfan's syndrome have increased atlantoaxial translation and a radio-

graphic prevalence of 36% for basilar impression was described in the same population. Distinct varieties of headaches and other cranio-facial manifestations have been related to spinal and vascular anomalies.

An estimate of the risk of developing a cerebrovascular event in Marfan's syndrome is entirely elusive, both in general and for a particular patient. Severity of the vascular malformations differs from patient to patient and, in the worst cases, the chance of a disastrous event is largely related to causes other than neurological.

In spite of the advances in the genetics of Marfan's syndrome, a simple diagnostic test does not exist. Diagnosis of Marfan's syndrome is difficult and remains based on clinical criteria. Unfortunately, clinical appearance varies greatly among affected people and, in the absence of familial history (15–20% of the cases) and congenital ectopia lentis (perhaps the most specific trait of the syndrome), considerable risk of misdiagnosis exists.

Homocystinuria is the main condition to be distinguished from Marfan's syndrome. Both diseases can present with skeletal deformities, eye defects and vascular disease. However, homocystinuria presents a high frequency of mental retardation, is transmitted as a recessive trait, and can be identified by specific tests.

Congenital contractural arachnodactyly, like Marfan's syndrome, is a dominant inherited disorder. The habitus is marfanoid and cardiovascular defects, although somewhat different, may be also present. Ocular anomalies may be present or not but, if present, are not so serious.

A complete physical examination, focusing on the systems affected by the disorder, is crucial for diagnosis, but equally is the most effective way to follow the progress of the malformations. There is no treatment for the basic defect of the Marfan's syndrome, and the malformations tend to progress continuously. So, the principal concerns in the management of those patients are the precocious identification of functional and structural defects and implementation of corrective measures. Some basic protective procedures and a careful medical management, which can greatly improve the prognosis and lengthen the lifespan, are listed below:

(i) lifestyle adaptations, such as the avoidance of strenuous exercise;

(ii) monitoring of the skeletal system, specially during childhood and adolescence;

(iii) annual echocardiogram to monitor the size and function of the heart and aorta;

(iv) regular ophthalmologic evaluation, including slit-lamp eye examination.

Beta-blockers to reduce aortic stress, and cardiovascular surgery, are specifically directed to patients with aortic dilatation, which means a potential indication for most of the patients. An aortic diameter greater than 50–60 mm (or, in children, doubling its normal dimension) is critical and makes a decision on the surgical repair of the vessel urgent.

Valvular dysfunctions have an approach basically analogous to similar conditions in non-Marfan patients, including reconstructive surgery and valvular replacement.

Anticoagulation is indicated for patients submitted to graft surgery.

Antibiotics are recommended prior to dental or genitourinary treatment in patients who have mitral valve prolapse, artificial heart valves or in those who have had aortic surgery.

The defective component of connective tissue, the fibrillin, and the functional and structural modifications with which it operates, have been investigated for the last decade. More than 150 mutations in the critical gene for fibrillin have been discovered, prenatal diagnosis was made in certain cases, and an experimental model is available.

Progress in understanding genetics and biochemical defects, and in the elucidation of the ultimate mechanisms related to malformations in Marfan's syndrome makes it conceivable that in the future diagnosis will be easier and there will be a more effective management of the disease. Future perspectives are no different from usual: an easy and effective test for prenatal and presymptomatic diagnosis, and a treatment effective in the prevention, and eradication, of the disease by acting on the genes responsible.

Prenatal diagnosis is now available for some families with this condition, at least for those families where a mutation in the fibrillin gene has been demonstrated.

Bibliography

American Academy of Pediatrics Committee on Genetics. (1996). Health supervision for children with Marfan syndrome. *Pediatrics*, **98**(5), 978–82.

De Paepe, A., Devereux, R.B., Dietz, H.C., Hennekam, R.C. & Pyeritz, R.E. (1996). Revised diagnostic criteria for the Marfan syndrome. *American Journal of Medical Genetics*, **62**(4), 417–26.

Fukutake, T., Sakakibara, R., Mori, M., Araki, M. & Hattori, T. (1997). Chronic intractable headache in a patient with Marfan's syndrome. *Headache*, **37**(5), 291–5.

Gott, V.L. (1998). Antoine Marfan and his syndrome: one hundred years later. *Maryland Medical Journal*, **47**(5), 247–52.

Hobbs, W.R., Sponseller, P.D., Weiss, A.P. & Pyeritz, R.E. (1997). The cervical spine in Marfan syndrome. *Spine*, **22**(9), 983–9.

Huggon, I.C., Burke, J.P. & Talbot, J.F. (1990). Contractural arachnodactyly with mitral regurgitation and iridodonesis. *Archives of Diseases in Children*, **65**(3), 317–19.

Hwa, J., Richards, J.G., Huang, H. et al. (1993). The natural history of aortic dilatation in Marfan syndrome. *Medical Journal of Australia*, **158**(8), 558–62.

Kainulainen, K., Pulkkinen, L., Savolainen, A., Kaitila, I. & Peltonen, L. (1990). Location on chromosome 15 of the gene defect causing Marfan syndrome. *New England Journal of Medicine*, **323**(14), 935–9.

Kainulainen, K., Steinmann, B., Collins, F. et al. (1991). Marfan syndrome: no evidence for heterogeneity in different populations, and more precise mapping of the gene. *American Journal of Human Genetics*, **49**(3), 662–7.

Magenis, R.E., Maslen, C.L., Smith, L., Allen, L. & Sakai, L.Y. (1991). Localization of the fibrillin (FBN) gene to chromosome 15, band q21.1. *Genomics*, **11**(2), 346–51.

Nagatani, T., Inao, S. & Yoshida, J. (1998). Hemifacial spasm associated with Marfan's syndrome: a case report. *Neurosurgical Review*, **21**(2–3), 152–4.

Pereira, L., Andrikopoulos, K., Tian, J. et al. (1997). Targetting of the gene encoding fibrillin-1 recapitulates the vascular aspect of Marfan syndrome. *Nature Genetics*, **17**(2), 218–22.

Ramos Arroyo, M.A., Weaver, D.D. & Beals, R.K. (1985). Congenital contractural arachnodactyly. Report of four additional families and review of literature. *Clinical Genetics*, **27**(6), 570–81.

Schievink, W.I., Björnsson, J. & Piepgras, D.G. (1994). Coexistence of fibromuscular dysplasia and cystic medial necrosis in a patient with Marfan's syndrome and bilateral carotid artery dissections. *Stroke*, **25**(12), 2492–6.

Schievink, W.I., Michels, V.V. & Piepgras, D.G. (1994). Neurovascular manifestations of heritable connective tissue disorders. A review. *Stroke*, **25**(4), 889–903.

Schievink, W.I., Parisi, J.E., Piepgras, D.G. & Michels, V.V. (1997). Intracranial aneurysms in Marfan's syndrome: an autopsy study. *Neurosurgery*, **41**(4), 866–70.

Van den Berg, J.S., Limburg, M. & Hennekam, R.C. (1996). Is Marfan syndrome associated with symptomatic intracranial aneurysms? *Stroke*, **27**(1), 10–12.

Youl, B.D., Coutellier, A., Dubois, B., Leger, J.M. & Bousser, M.G. (1990). Three cases of spontaneous extracranial vertebral artery dissection. *Stroke*, **21**(4), 618–25.

Zambrino, C.A., Berardinelli, A., Martelli, A., Vercelli, P., Termine, C. & Lanzi, G. (1999). Dolicho-vertebrobasilar abnormality and migraine-like attacks. *European Neurology*, **41**(1), 10–14.

38

Pseudoxanthoma elasticum

Louis R. Caplan[1] and Chin-Sang Chung [2]

[1]Beth Israel Deaconess Medical Center, Boston, MA, USA
[2]Department of Neurology, Samsung Medical Center, Sungkyunkwan University School of Medicine, Seoul, S. Korea

Introduction

Pseudoxanthoma elasticum (PXE) is an inherited connective tissue disorder, characterized predominantly by skin, eye, cardiac, and vascular abnormalities. Hypertension is common and the elevated blood pressure and vascular lesions often lead to strokes and damage to many body organs.

The skin manifestations were first described by the French dermatologist Rigal in 1881. Two Swedish physicians: Gronblad, an ophthalmologist, and Strandberg, a dermatologist, in 1929 recognized that the skin findings were accompanied by angioid streaks in the retina. PXE is often referred to as Gronblad–Strandberg disease after these two physicians.

Clinical findings and organ involvement

Skin

The characteristic skin lesions are linear, round, and oval-shaped yellow–orange elevated skin lesions that resemble xanthomas (Viljoen, 1993). The flexoral surfaces are most often involved. The face, neck, axilla, and the antecubital, inguinal, and periumbilical regions contain the most frequent skin lesions (Neldner, 1988, 1993; Strole & Margolis, 1983). The skin in affected regions can become thickened and grooved resembling course-grained leather. Later the skin becomes quite lax and redundant (Lebwohl, 1993). Fig. 38.1 shows an example of very abnormal redundant lax skin within the upper arm of a patient with PXE (Mayer et al., 1994). The lips show similar lesions. The mucosa of the palate, buccal region, vagina, and rectum may also show typical xanthomas. In some patients the skin abnormalities are very subtle, and abnormalities can only be definitively shown by biopsy (Lebwohl et al., 1993). The same process that affects mucocutaneous surfaces can also affect other regions that contain elastic fibres. Endoscopy sometimes shows similar lesions in the gastric mucosa and within the gastrointestinal tract (Strole & Margolis, 1983); the process also may involve the endocardium and the heart valves (Lebwohl et al., 1982).

The skin and mucosal abnormality consists of very abnormal elastic tissue. Biopsy early in the course of illness shows irregularity, fragmentation, and clumping of elastic fibres in the skin. Calcification of the abnormal mucocutaneous regions develops later.

Eye

The most characteristic and diagnostic feature of PXE is the angioid streaks found in the retina. The streaks are red–brown or grey, are usually wider than veins, and radiate from the optic disc (Stroke & Margolis, 1983). The retinal streaks are thought to be the result of cracks or ruptures in Bruch's membrane which has been weakened by disruption of elastic fibers. Fig. 38.2 shows two examples of angioid streaks. Chorioretinal scarring, hemorrhages, pigmentary deposits and macular degeneration also occur and many patients with PXE have very diminished visual acuity. About 85% of patients with PXE have angioid streaks (Pessin & Chung, 1995).

Angioid streaks also occur in other conditions. Patients with sickle cell anemia and Paget's disease of bone often have angioid streaks when ophthalmoscopy is thoroughly performed (Clarkson & Altman, 1982; Neldner, 1988; Lebwohl et al., 1993). Angioid streaks have occasionally been described in patients with hyperphosphatemia, Ehlers–Danlos syndrome, lead poisoning, trauma, idiopathic thrombocytopenic purpura, and pituitary diseases (Lebwohl et al., 1993).

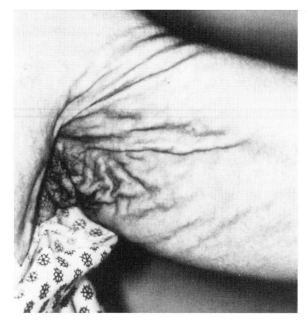

Fig. 38.1. Very abnormal wrinkled, lax, redundant skin with a cobblestone appearance in the upper arm of a patient with PXE. (From Mayer et al., 1994 with permission.)

Heart

Cardiac abnormalities are very common and may dominate the clinical presentation. Cardiac manifestations relate to premature coronary artery disease, and endocardial abnormalities. Coronary artery disease with resulting angina pectoris, myocardial infarction, and sudden death are common and may occur at quite a young age (Lebwohl et al., 1993). Some patients have an ischemic cardiomyopathy.

Abnormalities in the elastic tissue of the endocardium can produce dramatic cardiac findings. Huang et al. (1967) described thickened mitral valves, mitral annular calcification, and mitral stenosis in patients with PXE. The abnormal mitral valve can show fragmentation, coiling, and disruption of collagen bundles (Davies et al., 1978). Lebwohl et al. (1982) reported a high frequency of mitral valve prolapse in patients with PXE who had echocardiography. The elastic tissue abnormalities can cause dramatic calcification of the endocardium and a restrictive cardiomyopathy (Navarro-Lopez et al., 1980; Rosenzweig et al., 1993). Rosenzweig et al. (1993) described a woman with PXE, who had extensive mitral annulus calcification. The calcification extended from the mitral valve into the left ventricular endocardium. The entire left atrium was encircled with calcific endocardial plaques. A 5 mm mobile calcific lesion was attached to the junction of the left atrial appendage and the left atrium (Rosenzweig et al., 1993).

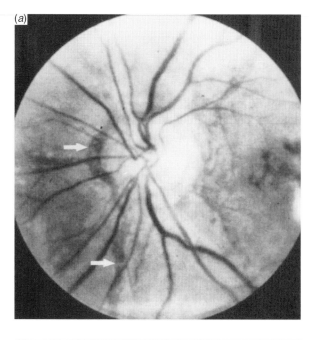

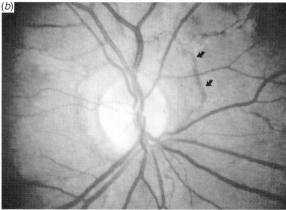

Fig. 38.2. Fundus photographs of angioid streaks in patients with PXE. (a) Large angioid streak (white arrows) in the patient whose skin is shown in Fig. 38.1. A macular scar is also present. (From Mayer et al., 1994 with permission.) (b) Large tortuous angioid streak (curved black arrows) in a patient with PXE.

Gastrointestinal tract

Gastrointestinal hemorrhages are quite common in patients with PXE, and are often the presenting symptom. Superficial mucosal and intestinal erosions, and a diffuse gastritis are the result of vascular lesions. Gastroscopic examination may show yellow cobblestone-like changes in the gastric mucosa. Examination of gastric tissue removed at surgery and necropsy show mucosal and submucosal capillaries, and veins may be dilated. Small and medium-sized arteries can show degenerative abnormalities that predominantly involve the internal elastic lamina (Kaplan & Hartman, 1954; Strole & Margolis, 1983). Angiography of abdominal arteries may show tortuosity with narrowing and occlusions. Microaneurysms and angiomatous malformations also occur (Strole & Margolis, 1983). Abdominal angina and ischemic bowel disease occasionally develop.

Aorta and peripheral vessels

The aorta may be involved and show aneurysmal dilatation. Peripheral limb arteries are often calcified. Intermittent claudication is relatively common. Extremity arteries may become firm on palpation and plain X-rays may show calcification. Hypertension is also very common in patients with PXE and often contributes to the cardiac and cerebrovascular pathology.

Prevalence and inheritance

About 1 in a 100 000 individuals have PXE (Viljoen, 1993; Neldner, 1993; Schievink et al., 1994). The genetics are complex: two autosomal recessive and two autosomal dominant forms have been described (Schievink et al., 1994). The majority of patients probably have the autosomal recessive form (Neldner, 1993). Patients with the autosomal dominant form may have more severe vascular disease. The basic molecular defect is not known. Preliminary studies of the elastin and fibrillin genes have been undertaken with negative results (Alberts, 1999). Curiously, patients with B-thalassemia seem to have an unexpectedly high frequency of PXE (Aessopos et al., 1989, 1997).

Cerebrovascular disease

Premature occlusive cervico-cranial disease and aneurysmal subarachnoid hemorrhage are the two cerebrovascular problems directly attributable to PXE. Some patients with PXE show the common complications of hypertension – intracerebral hemorrhages, multiple lacunar infarcts, and microvascular disease of the Binswanger type (Mayer et al., 1994).

Rios-Montenegro et al. (1972) described a patient with PXE, who had a moya-moya like syndrome of bilateral internal carotid artery occlusion at the skull base associated with a 'rete-mirabile' of abnormal small vessels. Their patient also had a carotid-cavernous fistula. Koo and Newton (1972) also reported a patient with PXE and a carotid 'rete mirabile'. Internal carotid artery, and basilar artery occlusive disease has also been reported (Tay, 1970;

Goto, 1975; Sharma et al., 1974; Iqbal et al., 1978). The occlusive lesions can be extracranial or intracranial (Schievink et al., 1994). Brain ischemic symptoms most often develop in the fifth or sixth decade of life, but occasional patients develop cervico-cranial occlusive disease in their twenties. Some patients with PXE show tortuosity and ectasia of the neck arteries on angiography (Schievink et al., 1994).

Mayer et al. (1994) reported two women with PXE who had multiple strokes and extensive white matter abnormalities on MRI. Both of these patients had long-standing hypertension. We have cared for a patient with angioid retinal streaks, blindness, pseudobulbar palsy, gait abnormalities, dementia and Binswanger changes on MRI who had PXE and hypertension. Hypertension is common in patients with PXE. It is difficult in patients with Binswanger-like abnormalities, PXE, and hypertension to know how much of the abnormalities, if any, relate directly to PXE and how much are attributable to the hypertension.

Aneurysm formation and subarachnoid hemorrhage (SAH) have also been reported in patients with PXE. Some of the aneurysms are located within the cavernous sinus and patients have presented with cranial nerve palsies rather than SAH. Kito et al. (1983) reported a 37-year-old woman with PXE who ruptured an aneurysm that arose from the thoracic portion of the anterior spinal artery.

Dissections have occasionally been reported in patients with PXE but it is not certain if the association is a chance one. The frequency of dissection in patients with PXE does not approach that known for Ehlers–Danlos syndrome and Marfan's disease. Josien (1992) described a 17-year-old boy who had PXE and a cervical vertebral artery dissection. One patient of Mokri et al. (1979), with a spontaneous cervical ICA dissection, had an angioid retinal streak.

References

Aessopos, A., Stamatelos, G., Savvides, P. et al. (1989). Angioid streaks in homozygous B thalassemia. *American Journal of Opthalmology*, **108**, 356–9.

Aessopos, A., Farmakis, D., Karagiorga, M., Rombos, I. & Loucopoulos, D. (1997). Pseudoxanthoma elasticum lesions and cardiac complications as contributing factors for strokes in B-thalassemia patients. *Stroke*, **28**, 2421–4.

Alberts, M.J. (1999). *Genetics of Cerebrovascular disease*. Armonk, NY: Futura Publ Co. Inc.

Clarkson, J.G. & Altman, R.D. (1982). Angioid streaks. *Survey of Ophthalmology*, **26**, 235–46.

Davies, M.J., Moore, B.P. & Brainbridge, M.V. (1978). The floppy mitral valve: study of incidence, pathology, and complications in surgical, necropsy, and forensic material. *British Heart Journal,* **40**, 468–81.

Goto, K. (1975). Involvement of central nervous system in pseudoxanthoma elasticum. *Folia Psychiatrica et Neurologica Japonica,* **29**, 263–77.

Gronblad, E. (1929). Angioid streaks: pseudoxanthoma elasticum. *Acta Opthalmologica,* **7**, 329–33.

Huang, S., Kumar, G., Steele, H.D. & Parker, J.O. (1967). Cardiac involvement in pseudoxanthoma elasticum: report of a case. *American Heart Journal,* **74**, 680–6.

Iqbal, A., Alter, M. & Lee, S.H. (1978). Pseudoxanthoma elasticum: a review of neurological complication. *Annals of Neurology,* **4**, 18–20.

Josien, E. (1992). Extracranial vertebral artery dissection: nine cases. *Journal of Neurology,* **239**, 327–30

Kaplan, L. & Hartman, S.W. (1954). Elastica disease: case of Gronblad–Strandberg syndrome with gastrointestinal hemorrhage. *Archives of Internal Medicine,* **94**, 489–92.

Kito, K., Kobayashi, N., Mori, N. & Kohno, H. (1983). Ruptured aneurysm of the anterior spinal artery associated with pseudoxanthoma elasticum: case report. *Journal of Neurosurgery,* **58**, 126–8.

Koo, A.H. & Newton, T.H. (1972). Pseudoxanthoma elasticum associated with carotid rete mirabile: a case report. *American Journal of Roentgenology,* **116**, 16–22.

Lebwohl, M. (1993). Pseudoxanthoma elasticum. *New England Journal of Medicine,* **329**, 1240.

Lebwohl, M.G., Distefano, D., Prioleau, P.G., Uram, M., Yannuzzi, L.A. & Fleischmajer, R. (1982). Pseudoxanthoma elasticum and mitral-valve prolapse. *New England Journal of Medicine,* **307**, 228–31.

Lebwohl, M., Halperin, J. & Phelps, R.G. (1993). Brief report: occult pseudoxanthoma elasticum in patients with premature cardiovascular disease. *New England Journal of Medicine,* **329**, 1237–9.

Mayer, S., Tatemichi, T.K., Spitz, J. et al. (1994). Recurrent ischemic events and diffuse white matter disease in patients with pseudoxanthoma elasticum. *Cerebrovascular Diseases,* **4**, 294–7.

Mokri, B., Sundt, T.M. Jr & Houser, O.W. (1979). Spontaneous internal carotid artery dissection, hemicrania, and Horner's syndrome. *Archives of Neurology,* **36**, 677–80.

Navarro-Lopez, F., Liorian, A., Ferrer-Roca, O., Betriu, A. & Sans, G. (1980). Restrictive cardiomyopathy in pseudoxanthoma elasticum. *Chest,* **78**, 113–15.

Neldner, K.H. (1988). Pseudoxanthoma elasticum. *Clinical Dermatology,* **6**, 1–159.

Neldner, K.H. (1993). Pseudoxanthoma elasticum. In *Connective Tissue and its Heritable Disorders: Molecular, Genetic, and Medical Aspects,* ed. P.M. Royce & B. Steinman, pp. 425–36. New York: Wiley-Liss.

Pessin, M.S. & Chung, C.S. (1995). Eales's disease and Gronenblad–Strandberg disease (pseudoxanthoma elasticum). In *Stroke Syndromes,* 1st edn, ed. J. Bogousslavsky & L.R. Caplan, pp. 443–7. Cambridge, UK: Cambridge University Press.

Rigal, D. (1881). Observation pour servir a l'histoire de la cheloide diffuse xanthelasmique. *Annals of Dermatology and Syphilology,* **2**, 491–501.

Rios-Montenegro, E.N., Behrens, M.M. & Hoyt, W.F. (1972). Pseudoxanthoma elasticum. Association with bilateral carotid rete mirabile and unilateral carotid-cavernous sinus fistula. *Archives of Neurology,* **26**, 151–5.

Rosenzweig, B.P., Guarneri, E. & Kronzon, I. (1993). Echocardiographic manifestations in a patient with pseudoxanthoma elasticum. *Annals of Internal Medicine,* **119**, 487–90.

Schievink, W.I., Michels, V.V. & Piepgras, D.G. (1994). Neurovascular manifestations of heritable connective tissue disorders: a review. *Stroke,* **25**, 889–903.

Sharma, N.G.K., Beohar, P.C., Ghosh, S.K. & Gupta, P.S. (1974). Subarachnoid hemorrhage in pseudoxanthoma elasticum. *Postgraduate Medical Journal,* **50**, 774–6.

Strandberg, J.V. (1929). Pseudoxanthoma elasticum. *Zentralblatt Haut- und Geschlechtskrankenheiten,* **31**, 689–93.

Strole, W.E. & Margolis, R. (1983). Case records of the Massachusetts General Hospital: case 10–1983. *New England Journal of Medicine,* **308**, 579–85.

Tay, C.H. (1970). Pseudoxanthoma elasticum. *Postgraduate Medical Journal,* **46**, 97–108.

Viljoen, D. (1993). Pseudoxanthoma elasticum. In *McKusick's Heritable Disorders of Connective Tissue,* 5th edn, ed. P. Beighton. pp. 335–365. St Louis, CV: Mosby Co.

39

Ehlers–Danlos syndrome

Carol F. Zimmerman and E. Steve Roach

Department of Ophthalmology, Southwestern Medical School, Dallas, TX, USA

The Ehlers–Danlos syndromes (EDS) are a group of connective tissue diseases, classically characterized by fragile or hyperelastic skin, hyperextensible joints, vascular lesions, easy bruising and excessive scarring after an injury (Beighton, 1993). Based on the clinical manifestations, inheritance pattern, and (in some cases) specific collagen defects, there are at least ten subtypes of the Ehlers–Danlos syndrome (Byers, 1994). Exact categorization is not always possible because of overlapping clinical features and because there is substantial phenotypic variability even among patients with the same subtype (Byers et al., 1979). Over 80% of the patients have types I, II, or III, and the other subtypes are much less common.

Most of the patients with cerebrovascular complications have type IV EDS, the most lethal of the EDS subtypes. Fortunately, the prevalence of EDS type IV is only 1 in 50 000 to 500 000 individuals (Byers, 1995). All cases of type IV EDS confirmed by biochemical and molecular methods have shown autosomal dominance (Beighton, 1993). Earlier reports of autosomal recessive transmission may be due to parental mosaicism (Byers, 1994). All confirmed patients have abnormal production of type III collagen, the major collagen type in blood vessels, bowel, and uterus (North et al., 1995). Numerous mutations in the COL3A1 gene on chromosome 2, including point mutations, exon skipping mutations and multi-exon deletions, have been described. All result in abnormal type III procollagen that causes tissue to be thin and friable (Byers, 1994). Characteristic facial features and/or easy bruising are described in some individuals (Schievink, 1997), but neither hyperelastic skin (Fig. 39.1) nor hyperextensible joints are prominent features of type IV EDS, and diagnosis is often delayed in these patients until major vascular complications occur.

Intracranial aneurysm, carotid-cavernous fistula, and arterial dissection are the most serious cerebrovascular complications of EDS. North and colleagues identified 20 cerebrovascular complications in 19 of 202 individuals with type IV EDS from 121 families in which the diagnosis was confirmed by molecular or biochemical studies (North et al., 1995). Outside the central nervous system, spontaneous hemorrhage, aneurysms, arterial dissection, bowel perforation and uterine rupture are major causes of morbidity and mortality in patients with type IV EDS (Freeman et al., 1996; Bergqvist, 1996; Peaceman & Cruikshank, 1987).

Diagnosis depends on recognition of the typical clinical findings and, for type IV, demonstration of defective synthesis of type III collagen. Careful family history of sudden unexplained death (especially during childbirth) or family or personal history of spontaneous hemorrhage, major hemorrhage from relatively minor trauma, hemorrhagic complications during surgery, and bowel rupture may be important clues to the diagnosis in individuals with subtle findings.

Aneurysm

Rubinstein and Cohen (1964) first reported the occurrence of intracranial aneurysms with EDS in a 47-year-old woman with aneurysms of both the internal carotid and vertebral arteries. Numerous patients with extracranial and intracranial aneurysms have since been reported, including several individuals with multiple intracranial aneurysms (Mirza et al., 1979; Krog et al., 1983; Schievink et al., 1990; North et al., 1995). The most common intracranial vessel to develop an aneurysm is the internal carotid artery, typically in the cavernous sinus or just as it emerges from the sinus (Figs. 39.2 and 39.3). Aneurysms have been found in most of the other intracranial arteries as well (Imahori et al., 1969). Rupture of an intracavernous carotid

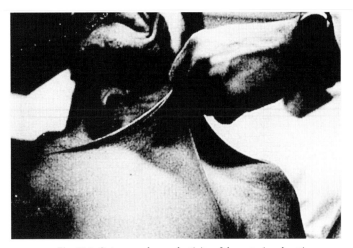

Fig. 39.1. Cutaneous hyperelasticity of the anterior chest in a patient with Ehlers–Danlos syndrome. (Reproduced from Roach, 1989 with permission.)

aneurysm to create a carotid-cavernous fistula or rupture with subarachnoid hemorrhage are the most common means of presentation. Rupture of the aneurysm can occur spontaneously or during vigorous activity (North et al., 1995; McKusick, 1972; Rubinstein & Cohen, 1964; Schievink et al., 1990).

While aneurysms are common in EDS IV, few patients with intracranial aneurysms have hereditary connective tissue disorders. Aneurysms occasionally occur with EDS type I (Krog et al., 1983) and Marfan syndrome (Stehbens et al., 1989; Hainsworth & Mendelow, 1991). Several giant aneurysms have been reported in Marfan patients (Hainsworth & Mendelow, 1991; Matsuda et al., 1979; Finney et al., 1976), and, as with EDS type IV, these lesions tend to affect the intracranial carotid artery. Occasional reports of berry aneurysms in Marfan patients (Stehbens et al., 1989) could be coincidental. Marfan patients have defective fibrillin synthesis; the abnormal gene is located on the long arm of chromosome 15 (Godfrey, 1993). Other heritable connective tissue diseases associated with intracranial aneurysms include neurofibromatosis type I, autosomal dominant polycystic kidney disease, pseudoxanthoma elasticum, osteogenesis imperfecta and α-antitrypsin deficiency (Schievink, 1997).

Mutations of the COL3A1 gene are rare in unselected patients with cerebral aneurysms (Kuivaniemi et al., 1993; Hamano et al., 1998). However, abnormal production of type III collagen has been demonstrated in some families with familial intracranial aneurysms (Pope et al., 1990) as well as occasional people with berry aneurysms (Pope et al., 1981; Schievink, 1997) even though these individuals have no other features of EDS.

Carotid-cavernous fistula

Graf (1965) described two EDS patients with a spontaneous carotid-cavernous fistula, and numerous patients have subsequently been reported (Schievink et al., 1991; Halbach et al., 1990; Debrun et al., 1996; Zimmerman et al., 1994; Pollock et al., 1997). Symptoms sometimes follow minor head trauma (Krog et al., 1983) but most occur spontaneously. The patient may complain of periorbital swelling, blurred or double vision, pain, and pulsatile tinnitus. Clinical findings include proptosis, chemosis, abnormal ocular motility, tortuous episcleral vessels (from arterialized blood flow), elevated intraocular pressure, and retinal venous engorgement. Vision may be lost if the fistula is not treated.

Occasionally, arteriovenous fistulae occur in other sites as well. The authors have observed one patient who developed posterior fossa ischemia from vertebral artery steal due to bilateral vertebral artery fistulae.

Intracavernous aneurysms sometimes occur in the same patient (Farley et al., 1983; Lach et al., 1987). Most carotid-cavernous fistulae in EDS patients result from rupture of an internal carotid artery aneurysm within the cavernous sinus (direct fistula) (Schievink et al., 1991; Graf, 1965; Fox et al., 1988). Schoolman and Kepes (1967) describe bilateral carotid-cavernous fistulae in a 39-year-old woman with EDS. At autopsy she had fragmentation of the internal elastic membrane and fibrosis of portions of the carotid wall. Similar fragmentation of the internal elastic membrane was recorded by Krog and colleagues along with several arteries with microscopic ruptures between the media and adventitia (Krog et al., 1983).

The fistula is best demonstrated by angiography (Fig. 39.4). However, the vascular fragility of type IV EDS makes both standard angiography and intravascular occlusion of the fistula difficult (Beighton & Thomas, 1969). Driscoll and colleagues reported the perforation of the superior vena cava during intravenous digital angiography, and other patients have developed localized hematomas or cutaneous tears at the site of catheter insertion (Driscoll et al., 1984). Complications of diagnostic angiography may be as high as 67%, and 6 to 17% of patients die from the procedure (Freeman et al., 1996; Schievink et al., 1991; Cikrit et al., 1987).

Endovascular embolization (Fig. 39.4) is the procedure of choice for treating carotid-cavernous fistulae, and this procedure has also been successful in some EDS patients (Fox et al., 1988; Halbach et al., 1990; Schievink et al., 1991; Kashiwagi et al., 1993; Zimmerman et al., 1994; Foulodou et al., 1996; Debrun et al., 1996). Lach and colleagues attempted to occlude their patient's fistula with a

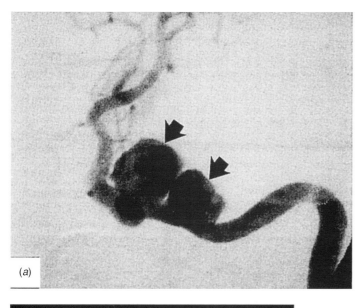

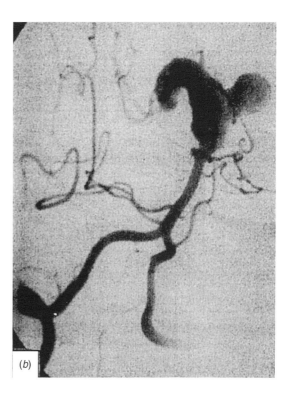

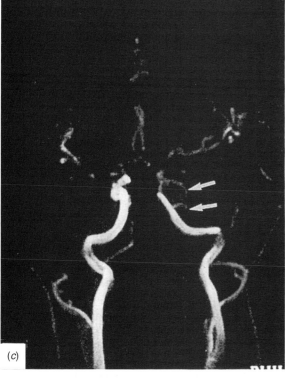

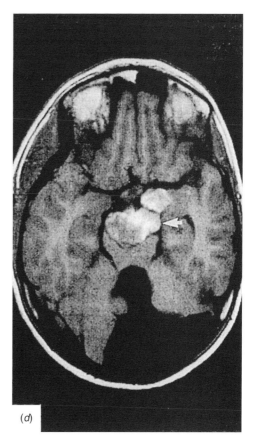

Fig. 39.2. A 13-year-old boy with type IV Ehlers–Danlos syndrome and multiple intracranial aneurysms. (*a*) Left internal carotid angiogram demonstrates two adjacent aneurysms (arrows). (*b*) Right vertebral angiogram demonstrates another large fusiform aneurysm with saccular component at the tip of the basilar artery. (*c*) Magnetic resonance angiogram, frontal projection, reveals two aneurysms (arrows) of the left internal carotid artery. (*d*) The T_1-weighted magnetic resonance scan with gadolinium showed the vertebral artery aneurysm (arrows) plus incidental cerebellar hypoplasia.

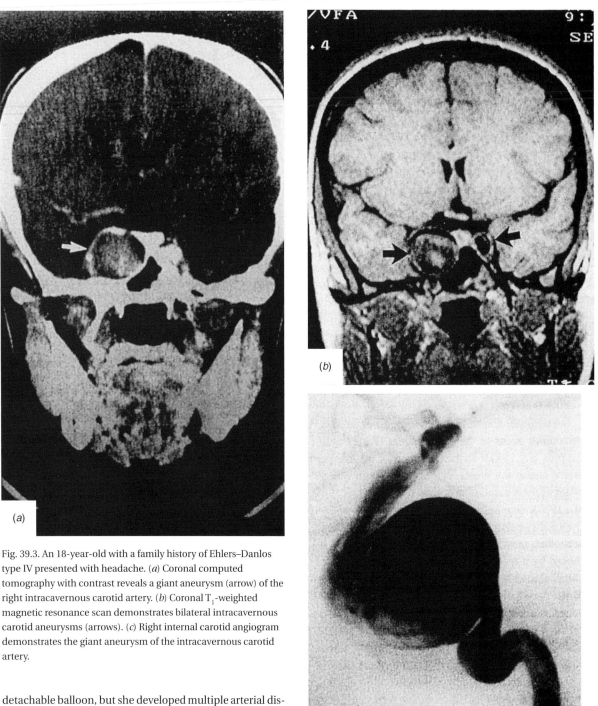

Fig. 39.3. An 18-year-old with a family history of Ehlers–Danlos type IV presented with headache. (*a*) Coronal computed tomography with contrast reveals a giant aneurysm (arrow) of the right intracavernous carotid artery. (*b*) Coronal T$_1$-weighted magnetic resonance scan demonstrates bilateral intracavernous carotid aneurysms (arrows). (*c*) Right internal carotid angiogram demonstrates the giant aneurysm of the intracavernous carotid artery.

detachable balloon, but she developed multiple arterial dissections which caused massive retroperitoneal hemorrhage and death (Lach et al., 1987). Others have reported death as a direct complication of the embolization procedure or occurring in the days to months following a successful procedure, due to complications of the disease (Farley et al., 1983; Schievink et al., 1991; Halbach et al., 1990; Debrun et al., 1996; Pollock et al., 1997). Careful insertion and

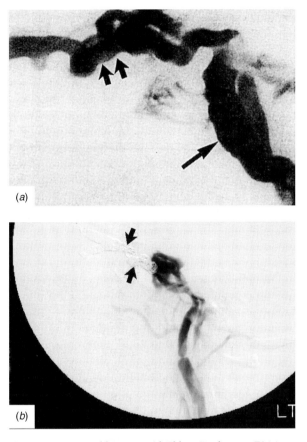

Fig. 39.4. A 28-year-old woman with Ehlers–Danlos type IV. (*a*) Her left internal carotid angiogram revealed a carotid-cavernous fistula and an enlarged, tortuous internal carotid artery (single arrow). The superior orbital vein (double arrows) is markedly dilated. (*b*) The fistula has been occluded with platinum coils.

manipulation of small angiographic catheters may reduce the risk from arteriography (Mirza et al., 1979). If possible, transvenous access to occlude the cavernous sinus and superior ophthalmic vein may be safer than transarterial balloon occlusion (Zimmerman et al., 1994). Still others may require 'trapping' of the fistula by occlusion of the carotid artery proximal and distal to the fistula.

Arterial dissection

It is not surprising that EDS patients develop arterial dissections. Surgeons have likened the tissue of these patients to 'wet blotting paper' or 'porridge' (Schievink et al., 1990). During surgery the arteries fail to hold sutures, and handling the tissue leads to tears of the artery or separation of the arterial layers (Sheiner et al., 1985). Dissection has been

documented in most of the intracranial and extracranial arteries, and the clinical presentation depends primarily on which artery is affected. Carotid dissection may cause ipsilateral oculosympathetic paresis and headache (Pope et al., 1991). One patient with a vertebral dissection developed a painful, pulsatile mass of the neck (Edwards & Taylor, 1969). Dissection of an intrathoracic artery can secondarily occlude cervical vessels (Hunter et al., 1982), and cerebral infarction distal to a carotid dissection has been reported (Pope et al., 1988).

Carotid dissection could cause a carotid-cavernous fistula in some patients. One of Graf's (Graf, 1965) patients had a very tortuous, dilated internal carotid artery ipsilateral to the carotid-cavernous fistula. Several years later at autopsy she had multiple arterial aneurysms but no evidence of an intracavernous carotid aneurysm (Imahori et al., 1969). Another patient with a carotid-cavernous fistula died from a dissection of the abdominal aorta; an autopsy revealed multiple smaller dissections in the abdomen, but the carotid-cavernous fistula was clearly caused by a true aneurysm with an interruption of the internal elastic lamina (Lach et al., 1987). Dissection of intra-abdominal, pelvic, intrathoracic, cervical and intracranial carotid arteries often follows diagnostic or therapeutic angiography and is, indeed, a major cause of morbidity and mortality with these procedures.

Infantile polycystic kidney disease was described (Mauseth et al., 1977) in one child with EDS. At autopsy, this youngster's carotid and basilar arteries were thin-walled, enlarged and tortuous. A dissecting aortic aneurysm was also found.

Segmental narrowing of the lumen is the classic angiographic sign of arterial dissection (Schievink et al., 1990), but subtle narrowing may be difficult to demonstrate in patients with tortuous vessels (Graf, 1965). Distinguishing an arterial dissection from a true aneurysm can be difficult (Edwards & Taylor, 1969).

Because of the risk of angiography in EDS patients, the need for an arteriogram must be weighed carefully. Magnetic resonance angiography may be less accurate but is undoubtedly safer.

Despite justifiable concern about the risk of arterial manipulation and angiography in these patients, balloon occlusion has been successful in some patients (Kashiwagi et al., 1993; Fox et al., 1988). Surgery is also difficult because the arteries are friable and difficult to suture (Krog et al., 1983; Edwards & Taylor, 1969).

References

Beighton, P. (1993). The Ehlers–Danlos syndromes. In *Heritable Disorders of Connective Tissue*, ed. P Beighton, pp. 189–251. St Louis: Mosby-Year Book, Inc.

Beighton, P. & Thomas, M.L. (1969). The radiology of the Ehlers–Danlos syndrome. *Clinical Radiolology*, **20**, 354–61.

Bergqvist, D. (1996). Ehlers–Danlos type IV syndrome. A review from a vascular surgical point of view. *European Journal of Surgery*, **162**, 163–70.

Byers, P.H. (1994). Ehlers–Danlos Syndrome: recent advances and current understanding of the clinical and genetic heterogeneity. *Journal of Investigative Dermatology*, **103S**, 47S–52S.

Byers, P.H. (1995). Ehlers–Danlos syndrome type IV: a genetic disorder in many guises. *Journal of Investigative Dermatology*, **105**, 311–13.

Byers, P.H., Holbrook, K.A., McGillivray, B., MaCleod, P.M. & Lowry, R.B. (1979). Clinical and ultrastructural heterogeneity of Type IV Ehlers–Danlos syndrome. *Human Genetics*, **47**, 141–50.

Cikrit, D.F., Miles, J.H. & Silver, D. (1987). Spontaneous arterial perforation: the Ehlers–Danlos specter. *Journal of Vascular Surgery*, **5**, 248–55.

Debrun, G.M., Aletich, V.A., Miller, N.R. & Dekeiser, R.J.W. (1996). Three cases of spontaneous direct carotid cavernous fistulas associated with Ehlers–Danlos syndrome type IV. *Surgical Neurology*, **46**, 247–52.

Driscoll, S.H.M., Gomes, A.S. & Machleder, H.I. (1984). Perforation of the superior vena cava: a complication of digital angiography in Ehlers–Danlos syndrome. *American Journal of Radiology*, **142**, 1021–2.

Edwards, A. & Taylor, G.W. (1969). Ehlers–Danlos syndrome with vertebral artery aneurysm. *Proceedings of the Royal Society of Medicine*, **62**, 734–5.

Farley, M.K., Clark, R.D., Fallor, M.K., Geggel, H.S. & Heckenlively, J.R. (1983). Spontaneous carotid-cavernous fistula and the Ehlers–Danlos syndromes. *Ophthalmology*, **90**, 1337–42.

Finney, L.H., Roberts, T.S. & Anderson, R.E. (1976). Giant intracranial aneurysm associated with Marfan's syndrome. Case report. *Journal of Neurosurgery*, **45**, 342–7.

Foulodou, P., De Kersaint-Gilly, A., Pizzanelli, J., Viarouge, M.P. & Auffray-Calvier, E. (1996). Ehlers–Danlos syndrome with a spontaneous caroticocavernous fistula occluded by detachable balloon: case report and review of literature. *Neuroradiology*, **38**, 595–7.

Fox, R., Pope, F.M., Narcisi, P. et al. (1988). Spontaneous carotid cavernous fistula in Ehlers–Danlos syndrome. *Journal of Neurology, Neurosurgery and Psychiatry*, **51**, 984–6.

Freeman, R.K., Swegle, J. & Sise, M.J. (1996). The surgical complications of Ehlers–Danlos syndrome. *American Surgeon*, **62**, 869–73.

Godfrey, M. (1993). The Marfan syndrome. In *McKusick's Heritable Disorders of Connective Tissue*, ed. P. Beighton, pp. 51–135. St Louis: Mosby-Year Book, Inc.

Graf, C.J. (1965). Spontaneous carotid-cavernous fistula. *Archives of Neurology*, **13**, 662–72.

Hainsworth, P.J. & Mendelow, A.D. (1991). Giant intracranial aneurysm associated with Marfan's syndrome: a case report. *Journal of Neurology, Neurosurgery and Psychiatry*, **54**, 471–2.

Halbach, V.V., Higashida, R.T., Dowd, C.F., Barnwell, S.L. & Hieshima, G.B. (1990). Treatment of carotid-cavernous fistulas associated with Ehlers–Danlos syndrome. *Neurosurgery*, **26**, 1021–7.

Hamano, K., Kuga, T., Takahashi, M. et al. (1998). The lack of type III collagen in a patient with aneurysms and an aortic dissection. *Journal of Vascular Surgery*, **28**, 1104–6.

Hunter, G.C., Malone, J.M., Moore, W.S., Misiorowski, D.L. & Chvapil, M. (1982). Vascular manifestations in patients with Ehlers–Danlos syndrome. *Archives of Surgery*, **117**, 495–8.

Imahori, S., Bannerman, R.M., Graf, C.J. & Brennan, J.C. (1969). Ehlers–Danlos syndrome with multiple arterial lesions. *American Journal of Medicine*, **47**, 967–77.

Kashiwagi, S., Tsuchida, E., Goto, K. et al. (1993). Balloon occlusion of a spontaneous carotid-cavernous fistula in Ehlers–Danlos syndrome type IV. *Surgical Neurology*, **39**, 187–90.

Krog, M., Almgren, B., Eriksson, I. & Nordstrom, S. (1983). Vascular complications in the Ehlers–Danlos syndrome. *Acta Chirugica Scandinavica*, **149**, 279–82.

Kuivaniemi, H., Prockop, D.J., Wu, Y. et al. (1993). Exclusion of mutations in the gene for type III collagen (COL3A1) as a common cause of intracranial aneurysms or cervical artery dissections: results from sequence analysis of the coding sequences of type III collagen from 55 unrelated patients. *Neurology*, **43**, 2652–8.

Lach, B., Nair, S.G., Russell, N.A. & Benoit, B.G. (1987). Spontaneous carotid-cavernous fistula and multiple arterial dissections in type IV Ehlers–Danlos syndrome. *Journal of Neurosurgery*, **66**, 462–7.

McKusick, V.A. (1972). *Heritable Disorders of Connective Tissue*. St. Louis: C.V. Mosby Company.

Matsuda, M., Matsuda, I., Handa, H. & Okamoto, K. (1979). Intracavernous giant aneurysm associated with Marfan's syndrome. *Surgical Neurology*, **12**, 119–21.

Mauseth, R., Lieberman, E. & Heuser, E.T. (1977). Infantile polycystic disease of the kidneys and Ehlers–Danlos syndrome in an 11-year-old patient. *Journal of Pediatrics*, **90**, 81–3.

Mirza, F.H., Smith, P.L. & Lim, W.N. (1979). Multiple aneurysms in a patient with Ehlers–Danlos syndrome: Angiography without sequelae. *American Journal of Radiology*, **132**, 993–5.

North, K.N., Whiteman, D.A.H., Pepin, M.G. & Byers, P.H. (1995). Cerebrovascular complications in Ehlers–Danlos syndrome type IV. *Annals of Neurology*, **38**, 960–4.

Peaceman, A.M. & Cruikshank, D.P. (1987). Ehlers–Danlos syndrome and pregnancy: association of type IV disease with maternal death. *Obstetrics and Gynecology*, **69**, 428–31.

Pollock, J.S., Custer, P.L., Hart, W.M., Smith, M.E. & Fitzpatrick, M.M. (1997). Ocular complications in Ehlers–Danlos syndrome type IV. *Archives of Ophthalmology*, **115**, 416–19.

Pope, F.M., Narcisi, P., Dwyer, N.G., Nicholls, A.C., Bartlett, J. & Doshi, B. (1981). Some patients with cerebral aneurysms are deficient in type III collagen. *Lancet*, **i**, 973–5.

Pope, F.M., Narcisi, P., Nicholls, A.C., Liberman, M. & Oorthuys, J.W. (1988). Clinical presentations of Ehlers–Danlos syndrome type IV. *Archives of Diseases in Childhood*, **63**, 1016–25.

Pope, F.M., Limburg, M. & Schievink, W.I. (1990). Familial cerebral aneurysms and type III collagen deficiency. *Journal of Neurosurgery*, **72**, 156–7.

Pope, F.M., Kendall, B.E., Slapak, G.I. et al. (1991). Type III collagen mutations cause fragile cerebral arteries. *British Journal of Neurosurgery*, **5**, 551–74.

Roach, E.S. (1989). Congenital cutaneovascular syndromes. In *Handbook of Clinical Neurology: Vascular Diseases*, vol 11, ed. P.J. Vinken, G.W. Bruyn, H.L. Klawans & J.F. Toole, pp. 443–62. Amsterdam: Elsevier.

Rubinstein, M.K. & Cohen, N.H. (1964). Ehlers–Danlos syndrome associated with multiple intracranial aneurysms. *Neurology*, **14**, 125–32.

Schievink, W.I. (1997). Genetics of intracranial aneurysms. *Neurosurgery*, **40**, 651–63.

Schievink, W.I., Limburg, M., Oorthuys, J.W., Fleury, P. & Pope, F.M. (1990). Cerebrovascular disease in Ehlers–Danlos syndrome type IV. *Stroke*, **21**, 626–32.

Schievink, W.I., Piepgras, D.G., Earnest, I.V.F. & Gordon, H. (1991). Spontaneous carotid-cavernous fistulae in Ehlers–Danlos syndrome type IV. *Journal of Neurosurgery*, **74**, 991–8.

Schoolman, A. & Kepes, J.J. (1967). Bilateral spontaneous carotid-cavernous fistulae in Ehlers–Danlos syndrome. *Journal of Neurosurgery*, **26**, 82–6.

Sheiner, N.M., Miller, N. & Lachance, C. (1985). Arterial complications of Ehlers–Danlos syndrome. *Journal of Cardiovascular Surgery*, **26**, 291–6.

Stehbens, W.E., Delahunt, B. & Hilless, A.D. (1989). Early berry aneurysm formation in Marfan's syndrome. *Surgical Neurology*, **31**, 200–2.

Zimmerman, C.F., Batjer, H.H., Purdy, P., Samson, D., Kopitnik, T. & Carstens, G.J. (1994). Ehlers–Danlos syndrome type IV: neuro-ophthalmic manifestations and management (abstract). *Ophthalmology*, **101S**, 133.

40

Progeria

E. Steve Roach[1], Irena Anselm[2], N. Paul Rosman[3] and Louis R. Caplan[4]

[1]Department of Neurology, University of Texas, Southwestern Medical School, Dallas, TX, USA
[2]Department of Neurology, Children's Hospital, Boston, MA, USA
[3]Department of Neurology, Floating Hospital, New England Medical Center, Boston, MA, USA
[4]Beth Israel Deaconess Medical Center, Boston, MA, USA

Introduction

Progeria is a rare condition characterized by premature ageing beginning in very early life and invariably ending in premature death. The term progeria is derived from *pro* meaning before and *geras* – old age. The aging involves the skin and appendages, the joints, and blood vessels causing coronary and cerebrovascular disease in boys and girls still in their youth. The original report of this condition was by Jonathan Hutchinson (1886). In 1895, Hutchinson reported a second similar patient (DeBusk, 1972). Hastings Gilford (1904) later studied these same two patients and dubbed the disorder progeria. Progeria has often been called the Hutchinson–Gilford syndrome after these early observations. DeBusk (1972) later summarized the findings in 60 patients with this disorder. Only about 100 patients with progeria have been reported.

Frequency and genetic and pathogenetic aspects

Progeria is a very rare disorder. The estimated incidence is 1 in 4–8 million births (DeBusk, 1972). The genetic defect is as yet unknown. Most instances are attributed to a sporadic autosomal dominant mutation, a hypothesis supported by an increase in paternal age of patients. Boys and girls are affected equally. Although siblings are usually not affected, the presence of affected siblings in some families suggests an autosomal recessive form of inheritance (Franklyn, 1976; Parkash et al., 1991; Viegas et al., 1974). The occasional involvement of siblings has also been explained by somatic mosaicism or stem cell mutations of the ovary or testes (Rosman & Anselm, in press).

In one study, cultured skin fibroblasts derived from a patient with progeria had reduced levels of mRNA coding for the macromolecules of the extracellular matrix (Colige et al., 1991). In another study, skin fibroblast cultures showed 76% of the DNA regenerative capacity of normals (Matsuo et al., 1994). Progeria could also result from an abnormality of telomerase, a substance recently shown to determine the number of cell replications before cellular senescence develops.

General findings and course

The signs of progeria are often first noted during the first two years of life. At birth some babies show scleroderma-like skin especially over the abdomen. By the end of the first year of life, decreased weight gain and retarded growth become evident. The head and facial appearance is characteristic – the head looks relatively large for the face. The scalp veins are prominent. The head is usually bald or has scant hair (Fig. 40.1). Alopecia is always present by adolescence. Eyebrows and eyelashes are often sparse. The nose is narrow and beaked. The ears and mandible are small and the teeth are crowded together. The ears often protrude laterally. The voice is usually high-pitched (Feingold, 1980; DeBusk, 1972).

Children with progeria are short and their growth is severely retarded. Growth hormone is often present in a form that has reduced bioavailability. Sexual maturation does not occur. Subcutaneous fat is scanty and the skin is lax. Superficial veins are prominent. The nails are small and dystrophic. Bone and joint abnormalities are always present. The bones are thinner than normal and fractures are common. The distal clavicles show thinning and resorption of bone. The ribs are thin. There is progressive loss of bone from the distal phalanges. The joints are

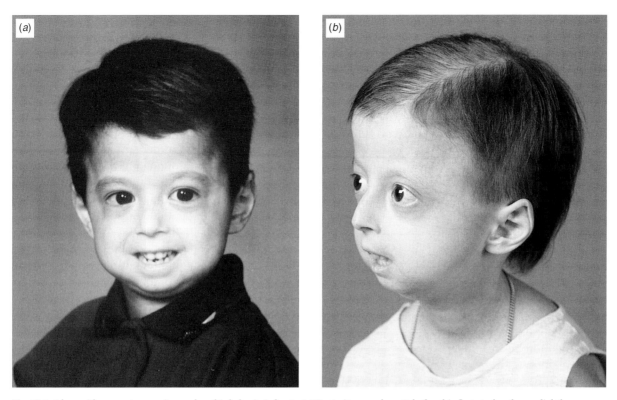

Fig. 40.1. A boy with premature ageing and multiple brain infarcts. (*a*) Portrait around age 3, before his first stroke, shows slightly dysmorphic facial features but normal subcutaneous tissue and full scalp hair. (*b*) By age 8 years, his thin hair, stooped posture, thinned skin, and loss of subcutaneous fat make him appear prematurely aged. (Reproduced with permission from Miller & Roach, 1999.)

enlarged and have limited mobility. Coxa valga is common. The bow-legged appearance gives the patients a characteristic 'horse riding stance'.

Most children with progeria develop premature severe vascular disease. Heart disease is the leading cause of death (DeBusk, 1972). Coronary artery disease and myocardial infarction are very common (Dyck et al., 1987). Congestive heart failure can result from myocardial fibrosis (Gabr et al., 1960). The median age at death is 13.4 years (McKusick, 1988). Although most patients with progeria die during the second decade, some less severely affected individuals do survive until middle age (Ogihara et al., 1986).

Strokes and cerebrovascular disease (Fig. 40.2)

Cerebrovascular disease plays an important role in the morbidity of progeria. Green (1981) reported a patient with progeria who had cerebral aneurysms. Progeria was diagnosed at age 6 years because of the characteristic features. At age 22, she developed pain in the right eye, headache, and right ophthalmoplegia. Angiography showed a very

large (2.5 × 1.5 cm) aneurysm of the right internal carotid artery within the cavernous sinus. She also had a left internal carotid artery aneurysm on the extracranial portion of the artery just before penetration into the skull base.

Dyck et al. (1987) reported a girl with progeria who had episodes of right sided limb paralysis at ages 7 and 9. She also had recurrent vertigo. Angiography showed occlusion of the left internal carotid artery and severe vertebrobasilar arterial disease. The authors did not report or show images that localize the occlusions to the extracranial or intracranial circulations. She developed angina pectoris at age 9 and had a myocardial infarct at age 11. Coronary angiography showed severe premature coronary artery occlusive disease (Dyck et al., 1987).

Naganuma et al. (1990) described a boy who, at age 7 years, had transient ischemic attacks and developed a right hemiplegia. Cranial CT showed multiple cerebral infarcts. Angiography showed occlusion of the left internal carotid artery and occlusive vertebral artery disease. Wagle et al. (1992) reported an 8-year-old girl who had a stroke with left hemiplegia. She had been diagnosed as having progeria at age 14 months because of her characteristic body habitus

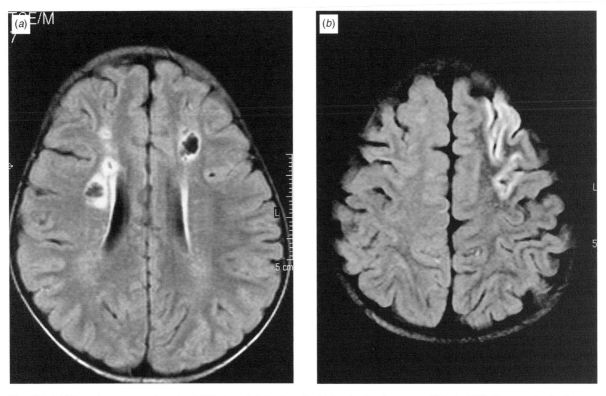

Fig. 40.2. (*a*) Magnetic resonance imaging (MRI) shows bilateral cerebral infarcts of various ages. (*b*) Later MRI after an episode of hemiplegia with aphasia shows a new infarct in the left frontal lobe. (Fig. 40.2(*a*) reproduced with permission from Miller & Roach, 1999.)

and features. Brain MRI showed an infarct in the distribution of the superior division of the right middle cerebral artery. Neither echocardiography nor MRA nor extracranial Duplex ultrasonography revealed a cardiac or cervicocranial vascular cause of the embolic stroke.

Smith et al. (1993) reported a boy who, at age 4 years, developed headaches, drooling and right arm weakness. One month later he had a right-sided seizure followed by a right hemiparesis. Brain MRI showed an acute left posterior parietal infarct, bilateral subdural fluid collections, and diffuse abnormalities involving the white matter and basal ganglia, and a right posterior parietal infarct. The proximal portions of the internal carotid arteries and the origins of the vertebral arteries were all occluded in the neck, and there was extensive collateral circulation. He later had transient left limb weakness and biparietal and right frontal lobe infarcts (Smith et al., 1993). Matsuo et al. (1994) reported a 7-year-old boy who had a right putaminal infarct shown on brain MRI. This patient later developed coronary artery disease. No vascular studies were reported.

Two of the authors cared for an African–American boy in whom the diagnosis of progeria was made very early in life because of severe growth failure, absence of subcutaneous

fat, and premature ageing. He had the characteristic facial features and habitus of progeria. Hypertension develped by age 5 and was treated with atenolol. At age 5 he had three left-sided seizures followed by paralysis of the left arm and weakness of the left face. MRI showed bilateral parietal lobe infarcts and MRA showed severe stenosis of the petrous portion of the left internal carotid artery and stenosis of the cavernous portion of the right internal carotid artery. Cardiac echo showed a protrusion under the aortic valve that could have represented a vegetation or a thrombus. There was a small patent foramen ovale. He was anticoagulated with heparin then coumadin. Three months later he had multiple focal seizures of the right arm followed by temporary right hemiparesis. Two months later a recurrence of right-sided seizures prompted repeat MRA which then showed occlusion of the right internal carotid artery within the siphon. The valve lesion was unchanged on echocardiography.

The occlusive vascular disease in progeria probably most often involves the cervical carotid and vertebral arteries but the intracranial large arteries may also be involved. The chronic basal ganglia and white matter changes found on brain imaging raise the possibility of concurrent penetrating artery disease. There is almost no pathological data about the histopathological nature of the occlusive vascular lesions.

Differential diagnosis and other causes of premature ageing

Several other conditions cause premature ageing and arterial occlusions and stroke. Werner's syndrome is an autosomal recessive disorder characterized by cataract formation, scleroderma and subcutaneous calcifications, a beak-like nose, and the features of premature aging such as greying of hair, senile macular degeneration, osteoporosis and atherosclerosis.

In 1904, Otto Werner in his doctoral thesis described the findings in four siblings who had premature ageing (Herrero, 1980; Werner, 1904). Little has been added since Werner's original description of the findings in this disorder. His patients were short and had a senile appearance. Their hair started to become grey during their 20s. Cataracts appeared during their third decade of life. They developed atrophic hyperkeratotic ulcerated skin, mostly over the hands and feet, and their skeletal limb muscles showed marked atrophy. With time, physicians have learned that diabetes, hypogonadism and retinitis pigmentosa are also usually pesent. Cataracts are posterior cortical and subcapsular and always bilateral (Herrero, 1980). Liver dysfunction, hyperuricemia, and hyperlipidemia are usually present. Some patients have subnormal intelligence. Seizures and hyperreflexia are common.

The facies are characteristic. Affected individuals look 20 to 30 years older than their actual age. The face is thin and the sharp angle of the bridge of the nose gives it a beaked appearance. Most patients have a high-pitched voice due to a variety of vocal cord abnormalities. The muscles of the extremities are usually severely atrophied. Electromyographic studies show a myopathic pattern of abnormality. Patients with Werner's syndrome have a striking predilection for developing non-carcinomatous tumours. Meningiomas and neural sheath sarcomas are found within the central nervous system. Age at death averages about 48 years (range 30–63) (Herrero, 1980). Death is often from malignancies, diabetic coma, or liver failure.

Patients with Werner's syndrome develop accelerated atherosclerosis. The aorta and great vessels are often calcified. Atherosclerosis also involves the coronary and craniocervical arteries. Myocardial infarcts are common. Often there is heavy calcification of the mitral and/or the aortic valves (Tokunaga et al., 1976). Although Werner's syndrome has been called adult progeria, the age of onset, clinical features and length of survival are quite different from progeria (Perloff & Phelps, 1958). Individuals with Werner's syndrome live until their 40s or 50s while progeria patients are usually dead by age 15 years. As with progeria, death from cardiac disease is more common than stroke-related death, but patients with Werner's syndrome have a much higher frequency of malignancies than patients with progeria.

The Werner syndrome gene on the short arm of chromosome 8 encodes a 1432 amino acid DNA helicase (Gray et al., 1997; Goddard et al., 1996). The DNA helicase family unwinds double stranded DNA and so plays a role in DNA replication and repair, recombination and transcription (Gray et al., 1996; Huang et al., 1998). Dysfunction of the Werner syndrome gene leads to genomic instability, accounting for the frequency of neoplasia in this condition. In one study, Werner's syndrome gene was not found among any of seven patients with progeria (Oshima et al., 1996).

Mandibulocranial dysplasia is another autosomal recessive disorder that features alopecia and short stature, along with clavicular and mandibular hypoplasia, stiff joints, and persistently open cranial sutures (Palotta & Morgese, 1984; Zina et al., 1981). It is not clear if this is an entirely separate syndrome.

References

Baker, P.B., Baba, N. & Boesel, C.P. (1981). Cardiovascular abnormalities in progeria: case report and review of the literature. *Archives of Pathology and Laboratory Medicine*, **105**, 384–6.

Colige, A., Roujeau, J.C., De la Roque, F. & Lapiere, C.M. (1991). Abnormal gene expression in skin fibroblasts from a Hutchinson–Gilford patient. *Laboratory Investigations*, **64**, 799–806.

DeBusk, F.L. (1972). The Hutchinson–Gilford progeria syndrome. *Journal of Pediatrics*, **80**, 697–724.

Dyck, J.D., David, T.E., Burke, B., Webb, G.D., Henderson, M.A. & Fowler, R.S. (1987). Management of coronary artery disease in Hutchinson–Gilford syndrome. *Journal of Pediatrics*, **111**, 407–10.

Feingold, M. (1980). Progeria (Hutchinson–Gilford syndrome). In *Neurogenetic Directory Part ll. Handbook of Clinical Neurology*, vol. 43, ed. P.J. Vinken, G.W. Bruyn & H. Klawans, pp. 465–6. Amsterdam: North Holland Publishing Company,

Franklyn, P.P. (1976). Progeria in siblings. *Clinical Radiology*, **27**, 327–33.

Gabr, M., Hashem, N., Hashem, M., Fahmi, A. & Safouh, M. (1960). Progeria: a pathological study. *Journal of Pediatrics*, **57**, 70–7.

Gilford, H. (1904). Progeria: a form of senilism. *The Practitioner*, **73**, 188–217.

Gray, M.D., Shen, J-C., Kamath-Loeb, A.S. et al. (1997). The Werner syndrome protein is a DNA helicase. *Nature Genetics*, **17**, 100–3.

Goddard, K.A.B., Yu, C-E., Oshima, J. et al. (1996). Toward localization of the Werner syndrome gene by linkage dysequilibrium and ancestral haplotyping: lessons learned from analysis of 35 chromosome 8p11.1–21.1 markers. *American Journal of Human Genetics*, **58**, 1286–302.

Green, L.N. (1981). Progeria with carotid artery aneurysms. Report of a case. *Archives of Neurology*, **38**, 659–61.

Herrero, F.A. (1980). Neurological manifestations of hereditable connective tissue disorders. In *Neurological Manifestations of Systemic Diseases Part II. Handbook of Clinical Neurology*, vol. 39, ed. P.J. Vinken, G.W. Bruyn & H.L. Klawans, pp. 379–418. Amsterdam: North Holland Publishing Company.

Huang, S., Baomin, L., Gray, M.D., Oshima, J., Saira, M. & Campisi, J. (1998). The premature ageing syndrome protein WRN, is a 3′→5′ exonuclease. *Nature Genetics*, **20**, 114–16.

Hutchinson, J. (1886). Congenital absence of hair and mammary glands with an atrophic condition of the skin and its appendages in a boy whose mother had been almost wholly bald from alopecia areata from the age of 6. *Transactions of the Medical and Chirurgical Society of Edinburgh*, **69**, 473–7.

McKusick, V. (1988). *Mendelian Inheritance in Man*, 8th edn, p. 630. Baltimore: Johns Hopkins University Press.

Matsuo, S., Takeuchi, Y., Hayashi, S., Kinugasa, A. & Sawada, T. (1994). Patients with unusual Hutchinson–Gilford syndrome (progeria) *Pediatric Neurology*, **8**, 476–7.

Miller, V.S. & Roach, E.S. (1999). Neurocutaneous syndromes. In *Neurology in Clinical Practice*, 3rd edn, ed. W.G. Bradley et al. Boston, MS: Butterworth-Heinemann.

Naganuma, Y., Konishi, T. & Hongou, K. (1990). A case of progeria syndrome with cerebral infarction. *No To Hattatsu*, **22**, 71–6.

Ogihara, T., Hata, T., Tanaka, K., Fukuchi, K., Tabuchi, Y. & Kamahara, Y. (1986). Hutchinson–Gilford progeria syndrome in a 45-year-old man. *American Journal of Medicine*, **81**, 135–8.

Oshima, J., Brown, W.T. & Martin, G.M. (1996). No detectable mutations at Werner helicase locus in progeria. *Lancet*, **348**, 1106–???.

Palotta, R. & Morgese, G. (1984). Mandibular dysplasia: a rare progeroid syndrome. Two brothers confirm autosomal recessive inheritance. *Clinical Genetics*, **26**, 133–8.

Parkash, H., Sidhu, S.S., Raghavan, R. & Deshmukh, R.N. (1990). Hutchinson–Gilford progeria: familial occurrence. *American Journal of Medical Genetics*, **36**, 431–3.

Perloff, J.K. & Phelps, E.T. (1958). A review of Werner's syndrome with a report of the second autopsied case. *Annals of Internal Medicine*, **48**, 1205–20.

Smith, A.S., Wiznitzer, M. & Karaman, B.A. (1993). MRA detection of vascular occlusion in a child with progeria. *American Journal of Neuroradiology*, **14**, 441–3.

Tokunaga, M., Mori, S., Sato, K., Nakamura, K. & Wakamatsu, E. (1976). Postmortem study of a case of Werner's syndrome. *Journal of the American Geriatric Society*, **24**, 407–11.

Viegas, J., Souza, L.R. & Salzano, F.M. (1974). Progeria in twins. *Journal of Medical Genetics*, **11**, 384–6.

Wagle, W.A., Haller, J.S. & Cousins, J.P. (1992). Cerebral infarction in progeria. *Pediatric Neurology*, **8**, 476–7.

Werner, O. (1904). Uber Kataraki in Verbindung mit Sklerodermis. Thesis. Kiel, Germany, Kiel, Schmidt und Klaunig.

Zina, A.M., Cravaior, A. & Bundino, S. (1981), Familial mandibulo-cranial dysplasia. *British Journal of Dermatology*, **105**, 719–23.

41

Microangiopathy of the retina, inner ear and brain: Susac's syndrome, 'SICRET' syndrome, RED-M syndrome or retinocochleocerebral arteriolopathy

Isabel Henriques[1], Julien Bogousslavsky[2] and Louis R. Caplan[3]

[1]Neurologia, Hospital do Espírito Santo, Evora, Portugal
[2]Department of Neurology, University of Lausanne, Switzerland
[3]Beth Israel Deaconess Medical Center, Boston, MA, USA

History

First reports, designations and eponyms

A clinical triad of encephalopathy, deafness and branch retinal artery occlusions was first reported in 1979 by Susac, a neurologist from Florida, USA (Susac et al., 1979). This first description included one case observed by Susac in 1975 and presented in a previous conference, and another patient from Dr John Selhorst. With the contribution of a neuropathologist John Hardiman, they reported these patients as having a microangiopathy of the brain and retina (Susac et al., 1979).

A previous description of a multifocal non-embolic occlusion of the retinal arteries, with similar brain involvement in two young female patients, classified as probable disseminated lupus erythematosus was already published in 1973 by Pfaffenbach and Hollenhorst (Pfaffenbach & Hollenhorst, 1973). Other partial forms of what is nowadays supposed to be the same syndrome were also described in patients with retinal vascular occlusions and bilateral sensorioneural hearing loss, but with no brain involvement (Delaney & Torrisi, 1976). During the 1980s, a total of 13 new patients were reported with similar descriptions (Coppeto et al., 1984; Monteiro et al., 1985; MacFadyen et al., 1987; Mass et al., 1988; Heiskala et al., 1988; Bogousslavsky et al., 1989). All these patients were women of childbearing age. In 1996, the first case of a 29-year-old man was published by Ballard (Ballard et al., 1996).

Different designations of what is supposed to be the same clinical entity have been used. After being called microangiopathy of the brain and retina, Coppeto referred to it as an arterial-occlusive retinopathy and encephalopathy (Coppeto et al., 1984). Mass designated it as RED-M syndrome (Retinopathy, Encephalopathy, Deafness associated Microangiopathy) (Mass et al., 1988) and

Bogousslavsky as retinocochleocerebral arteriolopathy (Bogousslavsky et al., 1989). Schwitter et al. refer to to it as 'SICRET' syndrome (Small Infarction of Cochlear, Retinal and Encephalic Tissue) (Schwitter et al., 1992).

Since 1994, after the review of the syndrome by Susac in *Neurology* (Susac, 1994), the eponym Susac's syndrome is generally used in publications.

Clinical features

Prototypal case

A young caucasian woman with no significant previous history, who develops a subacute neurological syndrome with a triad of diffuse encephalopathy, neurosensory auditory dysfunction and retinal involvement, without evidence of systemic disease can be considered the typical case of this clinical entity (Susac et al., 1979; Coppeto et al., 1984; Monteiro et al., 1985; Schwitter et al., 1992; MacFadyen et al., 1987; Mass et al., 1988; Heiskala et al., 1988; Bogousslavsky et al., 1989; Gordon et al., 1991). All first reported cases were women of childbearing age, except one with a partial form of the syndrome who presented in an 8-year-old girl (Delaney & Torrisi, 1976). The first description of a male patient appeared in 1996 referring to a 29-year-old man, who presented with the triad and an outcome comparable concerning clinical and laboratorial evaluation (Ballard et al., 1996).

Early reports of similar syndromes, confined only to two systems (inner ear and retina or retina and nervous system), were published, but it is not sure if they represent the same entity with atypical (incomplete) presentation or a different disease (McCabe, 1979; Pfaffenbach & Hollenhorst, 1973; Susac et al., 1979; Delaney & Torrisi, 1976).

Table 41.1. *Common clinical signs*

Eye involvement
  Retinal arteriolar occlusions
Hearing loss
  Neurosensory, bilateral
Encephalopathy
  Personality/behavioural changes
  Corticospinal tract

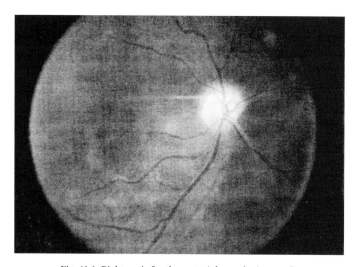

Fig. 41.1. Right optic fundus: arteriolar occlusions and submacular edema.

Clinical presentation

The triad of encephalopathy, hearing loss and retinopathy, usually develops in patients without any remarkable previous medical history. However, it is frequent to find behavioral disturbances and personality changes a few weeks or months prior to onset of symptoms. Signs of diffuse encephalopathy with difficulties in auditory and visual perception are common (Bogousslavsky et al., 1989). A smoother onset was also observed and the involvement of the brain, inner ear and retina is not always simultaneous. Table 41.1 summarizes the main clinical features.

Encephalopathy

Prodomal symptoms of encephalopathy included headache and psychiatric features. Slowly progressive personality changes, with indifference, mood changes, eating disorders, bizarre behaviour or hallucinations were described (MacFadyen et al., 1987). In one-fourth of the patients the first attack was preceded by slowly progressive personality and mental changes (Susac, 1994). Cognitive

dysfunction is characterized by short-term memory loss, and periods of apathy or disorientation. Recently, a male case was described in which neuropsychological testing were suggestive of diffuse cerebral dysfunction, with presumed prominent involvement of reciprocal diencephalic–cortical projections (Ballard et al., 1996).

Primitive reflexes may also be present as well as long tract signs. Ataxic gait, pseudobulbar speech, dysmetria, hyperactive tendon reflexes, Babinski's sign and nystagmus of vestibular or nonvestibular origin were the most commonly referred motor signs. Cranial nerve palsies (III, VI, VII), hemidysesthesia, urinary incontinence, and hemiparesis were less frequent. Generalized tonic-clonic seizures and myoclonus may also occur.

Retinopathy and hearing loss

Auditory and visual involvement may not occur at the same time in the course of the disease, and may be delayed in relation to motor dysfunction. Auditory dysfunction consists of a progressive difficulty in perceiving low to medium frequency sounds, with uni- or bilateral involvement, or it might be asymptomatic and only found in the audiogram. Vertigo, nausea and tinnitus may also occur, vertigo probably associated with microinfarction in the vestibular labyrinth (Ballard et al., 1996). The loss of low-and-moderate-frequency tones is thought to result from microinfarction of the apical portions of the cochlea, which are supplied by end arterioles of the inner ear (Monteiro et al., 1985). Concerning eye involvement, scotomas that may lead to total visual loss are due to multiple bilateral retinal branch occlusions. Fundoscopic examination shows arteriolar occlusions with narrowing of arterioles, as well as signs of other ischemic changes in the affected vascular area, such as edema and increased vascular permeability (Fig. 41.1 and Fig. 41.2). The macula may show a cherry-red appearance (Coppeto et al., 1984). When the occlusions are limited to the peripheral branches of the retinal artery, vision symptomatology may not occur and fundoscopy may be normal.

A suggestion for diagnostic criteria is given in Table 41.2.

Course of disease: evolution of the symptoms, bursts and 'end stage'

The initial symptoms generally improve with or without treatment. Weeks or months later, a second burst may occur leading to further deterioration. After each burst, there is a tendency towards remission, but the degree of recovery is variable. On fundoscopy it is occasionally possible to observe a partial reopening of previously occluded artery branches (Wildemann et al., 1996); on MRI, one case

Table 41.2. *Diagnostic criteria*

Neurosensory hearing loss[a]
Retinal branch arteriolar occlusion[b]
Encephalopathy

Notes:
[a] Neurosensory bilateral non-symmetrical auditory loss, more evident for low and medium frequencies.
[b] Retinal branch arteriolar occlusions frequently bilateral and with arterial narrowing, and microvascular lesions showing increased vascular permeability.

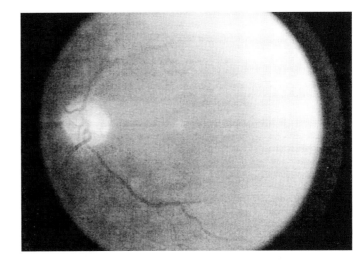

Fig. 41.2. Left optic fundus: perimacular whitish edema and arteriolar occlusion.

showed disappearance of hypersignal images on T_2 after two years of onset (Mala et al., 1998). The reported number of bursts was between 1 and 8, appearing with an interval of 1 to 34 months between attacks. A 'final stage' is commonly achieved after a period varying from 1 to 5 years. Most patients spontaneously improve but it is common that they remain with some degree of disturbances, commonly gait difficulties, auditory and visual deficits. Patients are left with a more or less severe deficit that may remain stable for the rest of their lives. These deficits vary from slight pyramidal signs to complete dependency upon others.

Although the natural history of the disease is unknown, the disease seems to have a self-limited course of action in most instances. In most of the cases patients were given some treatment, but the effect of treatment on the natural evolution of the disease is unknown.

Pathology and pathogenesis

Pathology

Pathological specimens were obtained from biopsies from the frontal cortical white matter and from autopsies (Petty et al., 1998). Pathological material showed the presence of microinfarcts in the territories of the end arterioles of the brain (both in white and grey matter), the retina and inner ear (Bogousslavsky et al., 1989; Gordon et al., 1991; Heiskala et al., 1988; Monteiro et al., 1985). The most significant findings include multiple foci of necrosis in the cerebral cortex and white matter, with loss of neurons, axons and myelin, as well as diffuse proliferation of hypertrophied astrocytes in the white matter, especially around the small vessels. The walls of small arterioles were thickened and surrounded by abnormal reticulin network. The

normal capillary network was destroyed and replaced by fragmented material that was extremely reactive to antibodies for laminin and fibronectin. Electronic microscopy showed very thick basal lamina in the capillary walls. There was no evidence of amyloid angiopathy.

We should explain that some of these biopsies were performed after different treatments, including steroids, so the interpretation of the minimal perivascular inflammation changes may have been influenced.

Pathological findings suggest a specific vascular disease of small arterial vessels. Retinal fluorescence angiography is also consistent with the hypothesis of microvascular lesions that cause increased vascular permeability and the mechanism of arterial occlusion is more consistent with thrombosis rather than embolism.

Pathology of the other organs showed no associated disease except for the case of microangiopathy in the muscles in one case (Ballard et al., 1996); in all other cases, the arteriopathy was circumscribed to a cephalic localization. Cerebral biopsies are described in Table 41.3.

Mechanism of arteriolar occlusion

Although all pathological evidence converges to the presence of the typical lesion, the arteriolar occlusion, the exact mechanism of occlusion is unknown. There is no evidence of vasculitis, although the clinical evolution with fluctuations could suggest it. In no case was any evidence for a coagulopathy observed except for one female, heterozygotic for the factor V Leiden mutation, and another one with a protein S deficiency (Cafferty et al., 1994). The Leiden mutation occurs in 5% of the population and,

Table 41.3. *Cerebral biopsies*

Case 1: Sclerosis of the media and adventitia of small pial and cortical vessels, consistent with a 'healed' angiitis.

Case 2: Numerous microinfarcts (500 μm maximum diameter) in the grey matter. No evidence for inflammation. Small vessels with muscular walls present within most of the infarcts, possibly precapillary arterioles. Reactive astrocytic gliosis associated with the infarcts. No infarct in white matter. Leptomeninges without abnormality.

Case 3: Microinfarcts in the white and grey matter (500 μm maximum diameter) with loss of neurons, axons and myelin and proliferation of hypertrophic astrocytes. Walls of several arterioles were thick and surrounded by an abnormal reticulin network and occasional lymphocytes. Normal capillary network was destroyed and replaced by fragmented material that was extremely reactive to antibodies for laminin and fibronectin. Electron microscopy showed a thick basal lamina.

Case 4: Moderate gliosis with neuronal loss, suggesting chronic hypoxic changes. Slightly thickened blood vessels, possibly only cortical tissue involved. No amyloid deposits nor fibrosis nor hyalinosis were present.

Case 5: Foci of necrosis and minimal perivascular infiltration of small blood vessels by mononuclear cells.

Case 6: Mild arteriolar wall sclerosis without vasculitis in leptomeningeal and small arterioles.

Case 7: Chronic organizing multifocal microinfarcts in the white matter, associated with focal acute ischemic neuronal necrosis in the grey matter.[a]

Case 8: Microinfarcts of varying ages with tiny foci of eosinophilic ischemic neurons in the cerebral cortex and perivascular rarefaction, breakdown of axons and accumulation of foamy macrophages in the white matter.

Note:
[a] Muscle biopsy showed inflammatory and occlusive microangiopathy.

although associated with venous thrombosis, was never associated with microangiopathy.

The localization of the infarcts limited to the brain, eye and ear, may be related to the common embriologic origin of these tissues (Monteiro et al., 1985), with a common endothelium and barriers similar to blood–brain barrier, where antigens might act and cause delayed arteriolar occlusion. Most arguments seem to favour a disease of the vascular wall as an etiology for this syndrome (Mala et al., 1998).

Pathogenesis

Although the etiopathogenesis of this entity remains obscure, several hypotheses have been considered. The first authors found some clinical similarities with CNS vasculitis and a diagnosis of cerebral systemic lupus erythematosus (SLE) was proposed (Pfaffenbach & Hollenhorst 1973; MacFadyen et al., 1987), but no reported case fulfilled the criteria for SLE.

Another hypothesis was that of an immune-mediated process. Increase in CSF protein content, erythrocyte sediment rate, and in the Leu 3a/Leu 2a ratio (with a decrease in Leu 7) in the first patient of Bogousslavsky et al. suggested an immunological dysfunction, despite the negativity of all other immunological markers. Intra-arterial thrombosis and occlusion could be induced by circulating immune complexes. A process directed primarily against the small vessels through antibodies against the endothelial antigens seems less plausible because antibodies directed against endothelial antigens are not observed in human models of vasculitic syndromes (Coppeto et al., 1984; Moore & Cupps, 1983).

The hypothesis of an atypical viral infection, triggering subsequent pathological or immunological changes has also been proposed. This theory was favoured by the case of an anencephalic fetus from a mother who became pregnant 2 months after the first burst of the disease. She had a sore throat and skin rash with fever before the development of the first signs (Coppeto et al., 1984).

An iatrogenic origin linked to fenfluramine has also been suggested. Fenfluramine is an anoretic drug that can injure serotoninergic neurons and cause a transient decrease in dopamine turnover in the rat brain (Zaczek et al., 1990). This drug was taken by both patients of Schwitter et al., before the onset of the disease (Schwitter et al., 1992).

Pregnancy in this age group can be just coincidental, but was also thought to be a possible contributing factor. Puerperium is known as a period where an increased tendency for thrombosis exists (Davidson et al., 1963). No laboratory test supported this theory. On the other hand, the reactivation of symptoms in the postpartum period (patient 2 of Coppeto et al., 1984), is another argument favouring an immune-modulated disease.

Whatever the true pathogenesis, the reversibility of some of the lesions is an indirect argument in favour of a nondestructive process (Coppeto et al., 1984). Despite extensive investigation including autopsies, there has never been strong evidence for systemic disease and pathogenesis remains unclear.

Differential diagnosis

Differential diagnosis is the key for the diagnosis of Susac's syndrome. Probably, one very common misdiagnosis is multiple sclerosis, but differential diagnosis must include all causes of multifocal neurologic symptoms with hearing and or visual loss.

Multiple sclerosis
Age of onset and sex predominance are similar as are MRI lesions in the subacute phase, but liquor hyperproteinemia does not show typical oligoclonal bands, the number of burst and the deterioration was always limited, and chronic lesions on MRI differ from multiple sclerosis, as well as lesion size (smaller and in higher number) and location (lesions located in both white and grey matter). Concerning eye abnormalities, a diagnosis of demyelinating multifocal sclerosis could be sought, but visual fields showed no retrobulbar optic neuropathy or retinal periphlebitis. Hearing loss and arteriolar occlusive retinal disease are unlikely in multiple sclerosis.

Cerebral infarction
The typical lesions are small infarcts in large artery territories. They can resemble lacunar infarcts but patients have no classic risk factors for lacunar infarction.

Systemic lupus erythematosus
Seronegative cerebral type of systemic lupus erythematosus (SLE) was one of the first diagnoses proposed for this syndrome (Pfaffenbach & Hollenhorst, 1973; MacFadyen et al., 1987). There were previous reports of multiple retinal artery occlusions in SLE patients (Wong et al., 1981; Gold et al., 1977; Coppetto & Lessell, 1977; Bishko, 1972; DuBois, 1974; Estes & Christian, 1971; Johnson & Richardson, 1968; Kayazawa & Honda, 1981). Although SLE can cause cerebral and retinal ischemia, retinal involvement is a rare complication of SLE, although less rare when there is CNS involvement. None of these patients had positive antinuclear antibody determinations or LE cells.

Polyarteritis nodosa
Classic polyarteritis nodosa (PAN) is a multisystem disease involving all the organs except the lung and spleen (Travers et al., 1979; Cupps & Fauci, 1981; Blau et al., 1977). Ocular and auditory deficits may be present (Peitersen & Carlson, 1966; Moore & Sevel, 1966; Dick et al., 1972). CNS abnormalities occur in 20–40% of patients. Common CNS presentations are diffuse encephalopathy with focal or multifocal brain or spinal cord involvement caused by vasculitis. Symptoms may resolve spontaneously over weeks, and reoccurrence is unusual. Blurred vision and visual loss are common symptoms of affected choroid or retinal vessels, but more often choroidal.

Untreated patients with PAN have only 13% survival rate over 5 years.

Wegener granulomatosis
Wegener granulomatosis is a systemic necrotizing vasculitis with granulomatous vasculitis of the respiratory tract with or without glomerulonephritis (Wolff et al., 1974; Fauci & Wolff, 1973). Neurologic symptoms occur in 20–50% of untreated patients (Drachman, 1963; Anderson et al., 1975). Involvement of II and VIII cranial nerves is possible by a compressing granuloma or by ischemia. There is no evidence that hearing loss in Susac's syndrome is due to VIII nerve involvement. Slight alterations in cognitive function may occur. Seizures, stroke and encephalopathy are late complications in untreated patients.

Hypersensitivity vasculitis
Hypersensitivity vasculitis, including allergic vasculitis and drug-induced vasculitis, should also be considered. Neurological, as well as inner ear and retinal, involvement is rare. Commonly, skin and small veins are involved. Concerning iatrogenic cases, CNS arteritis has been described in patients with history of drug abuse; this includes anorectic drugs, particularly amphetamines. Angiography shows that the typical beaded artery appearance is common.

Isolated angiitis of the CNS
This can have the same early manifestations and CSF changes. Visual loss is possible but by a mechanism of decompensated papilledema (Susac et al., 1979). Retinal arteriography can be normal. Nevertheless, it is usually a fatal disease, with small artery and vein involvement and a necrotizing vasculitis on brain biopsy. Retinal occlusions are uncommon and brain biopsy is required for the diagnosis (Cogan, 1969).

CNS infections
Several infections can cause multifocal signs. Posterior fossa meningitis may appear with cranial nerve signs. CSF may help the diagnosis. Syphilis can occasionally cause retinal periphlebitis and neurological involvement (Delaney & Torrisi, 1976). Labyrinthitis has been reported and is accompanied by hearing loss over months or years.

Migraine
Headache is a prodromal symptom of Susac's syndrome and migraine can cause cerebral and retinal ischemia, but cerebral infarction usually involves large artery territories. Scotomas may also occur.

Temporal arteritis

Temporal arteritis may also cause retinal and cerebral infarction, although ocular signs in temporal arteritis are due to posterior ciliary artery occlusion.

Cerebral autosomal dominant arteriopathy with subcortical infarcts and leukoencephalopathy

Cerebral autosomal dominant arteriopathy with subcortical infarcts and leukoencephalopathy (CADASIL) has an hereditary nature and can show retinal changes, but on fundoscopy juxtafoveal telangiectasis does occur.

Other

Other differential diagnoses for patients with microangiopathy of the retina, inner ear and brain, include (although not having any clinical or laboratorial evidence) diseases like Cogan's syndrome (rarely involving CNS), Usher's syndrome (retinopathia pigmentosa and labyrinthitis with deafness, transmitted as a recessive trait), Vogt–Koyanagi–Harada's syndrome (deafness with blindness that results from diffuse exudative choroiditis and retinal detachment), Rocky Mountain spotted fever (that can lead to necrosis of retinal vascular walls), Norrie's disease or Takayasu's disease (Heynes et al., 1980; Bruyn & Went, 1964; Delaney & Torrisi, 1976; Vernon, 1979; Wilson et al., 1979).

Investigation

Patients have been extensively investigated in order to exclude diseases which may mimic some aspects of this syndrome. Apart from routine examinations (biochemistry, hemoleucogram, urine analysis, chest X-ray, EKG) some other investigation is recommended including CSF studies (elevated protein and minimal cell content), cerebral MRI (normal or showing multiple areas of increased signal on T_2-weighted images, both in white and grey matter), neuropsychological examination, audiogram (neurosensorial bilateral asymmetrical hearing loss, more intense for low and medium frequencies), brainstem auditory evoked potentials, fundoscopy (peripheral ophthalmoscopy), and retinal angiography (retinal branch arteriolar occlusions frequently bilateral, with artery narrowing and microvascular lesions showing increased vascular permeability). Other laboratory tests, including immunology, exclude a vasculitic or infectious process. CT scan shows no lesions or only discrete to mild generalized atrophy. CT is considered not necessary when MRI is also available. Neither CT nor cerebral angiography or angioMRI detected lesions that explain the neuropsychiatric disturbances. Small size of lesions

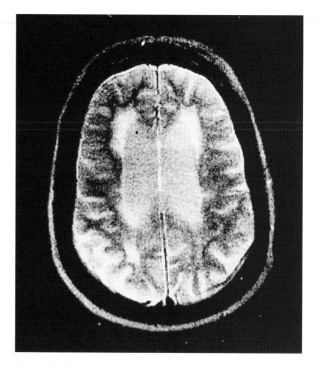

Fig. 41.3. MRI: spots of increased signal in subcortical white matter.

may be responsible (Coppeto et al., 1984) (Fig. 41.3) The predominance of microinfarcts in white matter may contribute to the difficulty in the differential diagnosis with multiple sclerosis. On MRI, lesions are enhanced by gadolinium in the subacute phase, and brain atrophy is common in the chronic stage. EEG performed in the encephalopathic phase is diffusely slow (Susac, 1994). Indication for brain biopsy is individual, considering both the lack of knowledge on etiopathogenic mechanisms and on effective treatment. Peripheral ophthalmoscopy is obligatory (Coppeto et al., 1984).

Management

As all rare diseases, treatment trials are neither available nor expected and so therapy remains empirical, symptomatic and based on anecdotal case reports and 'personal experience'. It would also be difficult to establish the benefit of any single therapy, as the natural history of the disease is unknown.

Corticotherapy and immunossuppressive therapy have been used as an immune dysfunction was presumed. Steroid therapy seems to achieve clinical improvement, at least temporarily, in most patients. Some authors advise corticosteroids as first line treatment (Petty et al., 1998). Immunosuppressive therapy was used alone or in association with steroids, also with some positive results reported. However, the benefit of prolonged immunosuppressive therapy is not established. Plasmapheresis was used in one patient together with oral cyclophosphamide but the patient continued to deteriorate.

Five patients were treated with anticoagulants, with only one report describing clinical improvement. Recently, Wildemann reported improvement of clinical signs in a patient with combined therapy using an antiplatelet drug (ASA) and the calcium antagonist agent nimodipine (Wildemann et al., 1996). A possible mechanism for the effect of nimodipine includes increased cerebral blood flow related to vasodilatation. In another case, improvement of visual symptoms was obtained after hyperbaric oxygen therapy (Li et al., 1996).

Neither the number of cases described, nor the severity of individual symptoms, would let us expect randomization of therapy. As spontaneous recovery and remission were reported (Susac, 1994), treatment efficacy is even more difficult to evaluate, but might include comparison to placebo. The only consensus therapy is rehabilitation, including vestibular rehabilitation or hearing aids, when required. It seems difficult to establish new effective therapeutical approaches while further knowledge in pathogenesis is not available.

Research trends

The unique clinical features of this syndrome suggest that it is a clinically distinct disease. One reason for the rarity of case reports of this syndrome is the difficulty of recognizing it. It would be desirable to include this syndrome routinely in the differential diagnoses mentioned above. As knowledge of the pathogenesis and the natural history of this entity accumulates, treatment possibilities may go beyond an empirical approach.

References

Anderson, J.M., Jamieson, D.G. & Jefferson, J.M. (1975). Non-healing granuloma and the nervous system. *Quarterly Journal of Medicine*, **44**, 309–11.

Ballard, E., Butzer, J.F. & Donders, J. (1996). Susac's syndrome: neuropsychological characteristics in a young man. *Neurology*, **47**, 266–8.

Bishko, F. (1972). Retinopathy in systemic lupus erythematosus. A case report and review of the literature. *Arthritis and Rheumatism*, **15**, 57.

Blau, E.B., Morris, R.F. & Yunis, E.J. (1977). Polyarteritis in older children. *Pediatrics*, **60**, 227–34.

Bogousslavsky, J., Gaio, J.M., Caplan, L.R., et al. (1989). Encephalopathy, deafness and blindness in young women: a distinct retinocochleocerebral arteriolopathy? *Journal of Neurology, Neurosurgery and Psychiatry*, **52**, 43.

Bruyn, G.W. & Went, L.N. (1964). A sex-linked heredodegenerative neurological disorder associated with Leber's optic atrophy: I. Clinical studies. *Journal of the Neurological Sciences*, 159.

Cafferty, M.S., Notis, C. & Kitei, R. (1994). Retinal artery occlusions, hearing loss and stroke in a 19-year old (abstract). *Neurology*, **44**, A267.

Cogan, D.G. (1969). Retinal and papillary vasculitis. In *The William MacKenzie Centenary Symposium on the Ocular Circulation in Health and Disease*, ed. J. Cant, p. 249. St Louis: CV Mosby.

Coppeto, J.R. & Lessell, S. (1977). Retinopathy in systemic lupus erythematosus. *Archives of Ophthalmology*, **95**, 1580.

Coppeto, J.R., Currie, J.N., Monteiro, M.L.R. & Lessell, S. (1984). A syndrome of arterial-occlusive retinopathy and encephalopathy. *American Journal of Ophthalmology*, **98**, 189–202.

Cupps, T.R. & Fauci, A.S. (1981). The vascilitides. In *Major Problems in Internal Medicine*, ed. L. Smith Jr, vol. 21, p. 18. Philadelphia: WB Saunders.

Davidson, E., Tomlin, S., Hoffman, G.S. & Epstein, W.V. (1963). The levels of plasma coagulation factors after trauma and childbirth. *Journal of Clinical Pathology*, **16**, 112.

Delaney, W.V. & Torrisi, P.F. (1976). Occlusive retinal vascular disease and deafness. *American Journal of Ophthalmology*, **82**(2), 232–6.

Dick, P., Conn, D.L. & Okazaki, H. (1972). Necrotizing angiopathic neuropathy: three dimensional morphology of fiber degeneration related to sites of occluded vessels. *Mayo Clinic Proceedings*, **47**, 461.

Drachman, D.A. (1963). Neurological complications of Wegener's granulomatosis. *Archives of Neurology*, **8**, 145.

DuBois, E.L. (ed.). (1974). *Lupus Erythematosus*, 2nd edn, p. 323. Los Angeles: University of Southern California Press.

Estes, D. & Christian, C.L. (1971). The natural history of systemic lupus erythematosus by prospective analysis. *Medicine*, **50**, 85.

Fauci, A.S. & Wolff, S.M. (1973). Wegener's granulomatosis: studies in eighteen patients and a review of the literature. *Medicine*, **52**, 535.

Gold, D., Feiner, L. & Henkind, P. (1977). Retinal arterial occlusive disease in systemic lupus erythematosus. *Archives of Ophthalmology*, **95**, 1580.

Gordon, D.L., Hayreh, S.S. & Adams, H.P. Jr. (1991). Microangiopathy of the brain, retina, and ear: Improvement without immunosuppressive therapy. *Stroke*, **22**, 993–7.

Heynes, B.F., Kaiser-Kupfer, M.I., Mason, P. & Fauci, A.S. (1980). Cogan syndrome. *Medicine*, **59**(6), 426–41.

Heiskala, H., Somer, H., Kovanen, J., Poutiainen, E., Karli, H. & Haltia, M. (1988). Microangiopathy with encephalopathy, hearing loss and retinal arteriolar occlusions: two new cases. *Journal of the Neurological Sciences*, **86**, 239–50.

Johnson, R.T. & Richardson, E.P. (1968). The neurological manifestations of systemic lupus erythematosus. *Medicine*, **47**, 337.

Kayazawa, F. & Honda, A. (1981). Severe retinal vascular lesions in systemic lupus erythematous. *Annals of Ophthalmology*, **13**, 1291.

Li, H.K., Dejean, B.J. & Tang, R.A. (1996). Reversal of visual loss with hyperbaric oxygen treatment in a patient with Susac syndrome. *Ophthalmology*, **103**, 2091–8.

McCabe, B.F. (1979). Autoimmune sensorineural hearing loss. *Annals of Otology, Rhinology and Laryngology*, **88**, 585–9.

MacFadyen, D.J., Schneider, R.J. & Chisholm, I.A. (1987). A syndrome of brain, inner ear and retinal microangiopathy. *Canadian Journal of Neurological Sciences*, **14**, 315–18.

Mala, L., Bazard, M.C., Berrod, J.P., Wahl, D. & Raspiller, A. (1998). Petits infarctus rétiniens, cochléaires et cérébraux du sujet jeune, ou 'SICRET' syndrome ou syndrome de Susac. *Journal Français Ophtalmologie*, **21**(5), 375–80.

Mass, M., Bourdette, D., Bernstein, W. & Hammerstad, J. (1988). Retinopathy, encephalopathy, deafness associated microangiopathy (the RED M syndrome): three new cases. *Neurology*, **38**(Suppl.), 215.

Monteiro, M.L.R., Swanson, R.A., Coppeto, J.R., Cuneo, R.A., DeArmond, S.J. & Prusiner, S.B. (1985). A microangiopathic syndrome of encephalopathy, hearing loss, and retinal arteriolar occlusions. *Neurology*, **35**, 1113–21.

Moore, J. & Sevel, D. (1966). Corneoscleral ulceration in periarteritis nodosa. *British Journal of Ophthalmology*, **50**, 651.

Moore, P.M. & Cupps, T.R. (1983). Neurological complications of vasculitis. *Annals of Neurology*, **14**, 155–67.

Peitersen, E. & Carlson, B.H. (1966). Hearing impairment as the initial sign of polyarteritis nodosa. *Acta Otolaryngologica*, **61**, 189.

Petty, G., Engel, A., Vounge, B.R. et al. (1998). Retinocochleocerebral vasculopathy. *Medicine*, **77**, 122–40.

Pfaffenbach, D.D. & Hollenhorst, R.W. (1973). Microangiopathy of the retinal arterioles. *Journal of American Medical Association*, **225**(5), 480–3.

Schwitter, J., Agosti, R., Ott, P., Kalman, A. & Waespe, W. (1992). Small infarctions of cochlear, retinal, and encephalic tissue in young women. *Stroke*, **23**, 903–7.

Susac, J.O. (1994). Susac's syndrome: the triad of microangiopathy of the brain and retina with hearing loss in young women. *Neurology*, **44**, 591–3.

Susac, J.O., Hardman, J.M. & Selhorst, J.B. (1979). Microangiopathy of the brain and retina. *Neurology*, **29**, 313–16.

Travers, R.L., Allison, D.J., Brettle, R.P. & Hughes, G.R.V. (1979). Polyarteritis nodosa: a clinical and angiographic analysis of 17 cases. *Seminars in Arthritis and Rheumatism*, **8**, 184–9.

Vernon, N. (1979). Usher's syndrome. *Journal of Chronic Diseases*, **22**, 133.

Wilson, L.A., Warlow, C.P. & Ross Russell, R.W. (1979). Cardiovascular disease in patients with retinal artery occlusion. *Lancet*, 292–4.

Wildemann, B., Schulin, C., Stroch-Hagenlocher, B. et al. (1996). Susac's syndrome: improvement with combined antiplatelet and calcium antagonist therapy. *Stroke*, **1**, 149–50 (Letter).

Wolff, S.M., Fauci, A.S., Horn, R.G. & Dale, D.C. (1974). Wegener's granulomatosis. *Annals of Internal Medicine*, **81**, 513–25.

Wong, K., Ai, E., Jones, J.V. & Young, D. (1981). Visual loss as the initial symptom of lupus erythematosus. *American Journal of Ophthalmology*, **92**, 238.

Zaczek, R., Battaglia, G., Culp, S., Appel, N., Contrera, J. & De Souza, E. (1990). Effects of repeated fenfluramine administration on indices of monoamine function in the rat brain: Pharmacokinetic, dose response, regional specificity and time course data. *Journal of Pharmacology and Experimental Therapeutics*, **253**, 104–12.

42

Hereditary endotheliopathy with retinopathy, nephropathy and stroke (HERNS)

Joanna C. Jen and Robert W. Baloh

Department of Neurology, UCLA Medical Center, Los Angeles, CA, USA

Background

There have been few reports of familial multi-infarct syndromes. In 1977, Sourender and Wålinder reported a family with hereditary progressive leukoencephalopathy in middle-aged adults without hypertension (Sourander & Wålinder, 1977). That family is probably the first reported case of cerebral autosomal dominant arteriopathy with subcortical infarcts and leukoencephalopathy (CADASIL) (Tournier-Lasserve et al., 1993). In 1988, Grand et al. reported a family with clinical features similar to CADASIL; in addition, family members develop visual loss due to characteristic retinal capillary abnormalities (Grand et al., 1988). Gutmann et al. described another family with a similar syndrome of progressive visual loss and leukoencephalopathy without any renal or other organ involvement (Gutmann et al., 1989). In 1997, we reported a large Chinese family who manifested a hereditary vasculopathy similar to cerebral retinal vasculopathy with subcortical leukoencephalopathy and retinopathy but, in addition, manifested renal dysfunction (Jen et al., 1997). Ultrastructural studies identified characteristic alterations of vascular basement membranes not previously described. CADASIL, hereditary cerebral retinal vasculopathy and HERNS all present with progressive neuropsychiatric deterioration typically beginning in the third to fourth decade (Table 42.1). There are clear diagnostic and vasculopathic features that separate CADASIL from hereditary cerebral retinal vasculopathy and HERNS (Baudrimont et al., 1993; Jen et al., 1997), but it is unclear whether hereditary cerebral retinal vasculopathy and HERNS are distinct entities or the same systemic disorder.

Clinical characteristics

HERNS typically begins with progressive visual loss in the third or fourth decades of life followed by focal neurologi-cal deficits within 4 to 10 years. The visual loss begins in the central vision with decreased visual acuity. Blind spots in the visual field are also common. Many affected individuals will report long-standing psychiatric symptoms such as depression, anxiety and paranoia with onset as early as the second decade of life. Stroke-like episodes occur in most and in some are the presenting symptom. Often the stroke will progress over several days before reaching its completed stage. Later in the disease, signs of multifocal cortical and subcortical involvement such as dysarthria, hemiparesis, apraxia, ataxia, and dementia are common. More than half of patients report migraine headaches. About half of the patients exhibited evidence of renal dysfunction including azotemia, proteinuria, and hematuria.

Diagnosis

Ophthalmologic examination

There is a characteristic retinal vasculopathy which is most prominent in the macular region. Drop-out of macular capillaries may be associated with macular edema. One can typically identify dilated tortuous telangiectatic vessels and capillary shunts. Fluorescein angiograms show juxtafoveolar capillary obliteration with tortuous telangiectatic microaneurysms (Fig. 42.1).

Neuroimaging

On MRI, multifocal T_2 high signal intensity lesions in the deep white matter can often be identified with the initial onset of retinal involvement before neurologic symptoms and signs develop. With the onset of focal neurologic deficits, the patients will have contrast-enhancing lesions with surrounding vasogenic edema most commonly in the deep frontoparietal regions (Fig. 42.2(*a*)). Larger lesions can act

Table 42.1. *Comparison of dominantly inherited leukoencephalopathic syndromes*

Syndrome	Clinical features	Radiographic features	Vasculopathic features
CADASIL	Strokes, migraine, mood disorders, dementia	Non-contrast-enhancing white matter high T_2 signal lesions	Systemic non-atheromatous, non-amyloid arteriopathy with destruction of the vascular smooth muscle cells and the formation of granular, electron-dense, eosinophilic material
Hereditary cerebroretinal vasculopathy	Strokes, retinopathy, dementia	Contrast-enhancing white matter lesions with vasogenic edema	Fibrinoid necrosis without inflammation[a]
Hereditary endotheliopathy with retinopathy, nephropathy, and stroke (HERNS)	Strokes, retinopathy, nephropathy, migraine, mood disorders, dementia	Contrast-enhancing white lesions with vasogenic edema	Systemic vasculopathic changes with multilaminated basement membrane

Note:
[a] Light microscopy only.
Source: From Jen et al. (1997), with permission from Lippincott, Williams & Wilkins.

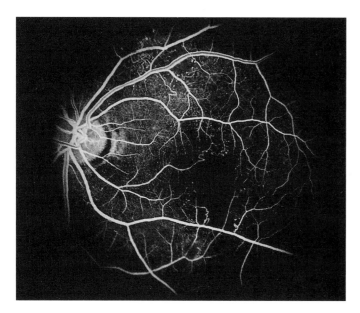

Fig. 42.1. Mid-venous phase fluorescein angiogram from a patient demonstrating areas of macular capillary dropout as well as dilated tortuous telangiectatic vessels and capillary shunts. (Jen et al., 1997, with permission from Lippincott, Williams & Wilkins.)

as a space-occupying mass causing herniation of brain structures (Fig. 42.2(*b*)).

Pathology

On light microscopy, the brain lesions with HERNS appear to be cerebral infarcts with extensive nuclear fragmentation and spongy change, often centered on small blood vessels occluded by fibrin thrombi. Ultrastructural studies show distinctive multilaminated vascular basement membranes in the brain and other tissues including the kidney, stomach, appendix, omentum and skin. The original (sub-epithelial) basement membranes are normal but basement membranes are multilaminated with alternating medium, dense and loosened zones (Fig. 42.3). Endothelial cell cytoplasm is normal or slightly swollen. There was no evidence of either abnormal mitochondria or accumulation of mitochondria in any tissue examined by electron microscopy.

Genetics

The hereditary pattern of HERNS is most consistent with autosomal dominant inheritance. Shared clinical symptoms between HERNS and CADASIL prompted us to examine whether the disease locus in HERNS would map to the same chromosomal region as CADASIL. We typed a series of microsatellite markers near the *Notch3* locus on

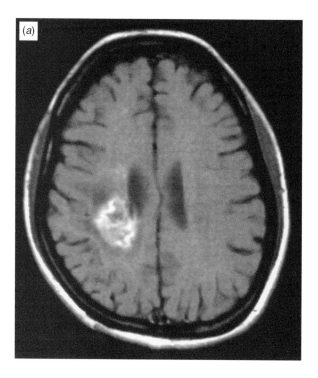

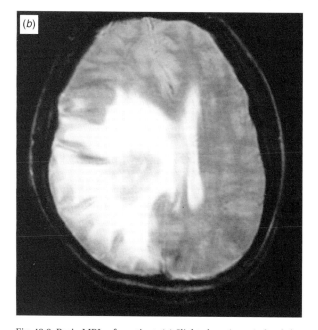

Fig. 42.2. Brain MRIs of a patient. (*a*) Slight clumsiness in her left hand and left leg, contrast-enhancing lesions with surrounding edema in the right frontoparietal subcortical region on T_1-weighted images. (*b*) Persistent headache with one episode of projectile vomiting but no other neurologic changes, increased size of the lesions with marked edema on proton-weighted images. (Jen et al., 1997, with permission from Lippincott, Williams & Wilkins.)

chromosome 19 (Ducros et al., 1996). Linkage data in the HERNS pedigree yielded negative lod scores, thus making it unlikely that *Notch3* mutations causing CADASIL are involved in the pathogenesis of HERNS.

Pathophysiology

The underlying mechanism of HERNS appears to be a generalized vasculopathy with disruption of the integrity of capillaries and arterioles. Fluorescein angiograms clearly demonstrate retinal vasculopathic changes. That the intracerebral lesions show contrast enhancement on MRI indicates breakdown in the blood–brain barrier. The surrounding edema in a vasogenic pattern also suggests increased capillary permeability. Since the basement membrane is synthesized by endothelial cells, the basement membrane abnormalities seen on EM probably reflect a primary endothelial injury.

Why should a generalized vasculopathy preferentially affect the brain, the retina and the kidney? One explanation may be that these organs rely heavily on an intact endothelial barrier to maintain proper function and are particularly 'eloquent' when injured. Furthermore, the basis for the regional vulnerability in the brain is intriguing in that the intracranial mass lesions tend to involve the frontoparietal region in both HERNS and cerebral retinal vasculopathy.

Treatment

At the present time there is no known treatment that is effective in patients with HERNS. Most patients have been maintained on aspirin for its antiplatelet action but there is no indication that this altered the course of the disease. Resection of a 'pseudotumour' has not helped in those who have undergone surgery. Laser treatments have been of little benefit in controlling the retinal vasculopathy but may be indicated to prevent retinal hemorrhages. Corticosteroids have been useful to decrease cerebral edema and may even be life-saving in patients with large edematous lesions. Often patients must be kept on a maintenance dose of corticosteroids since the edema returns if they are discontinued. Grand et al. noted the histologic similarities between hereditary cerebral retinal vasculopathy and delayed radiation-induced cerebral necrosis. Delayed cerebral radiation necrosis appears to result from damage of endothelial cells in small vessels (Rottenberg et al., 1977; Glantz et al., 1994). The observation of similarities between hereditary cerebral retinal vasculopathy and delayed radiation-induced cerebral

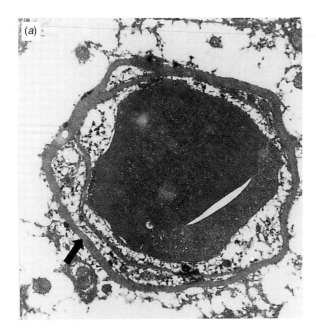

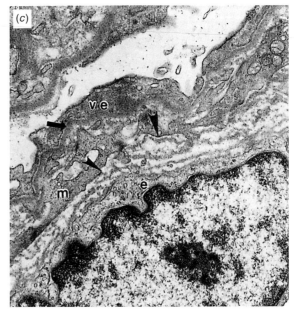

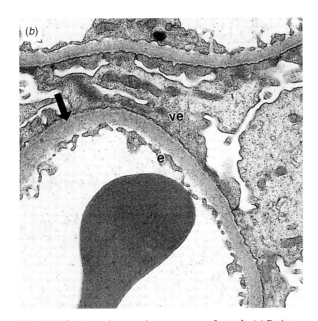

Fig. 42.3. Electron microscopic appearance of vessels. (*a*) Brain. Reprocessed specimen with several layers of basement membrane (arrow) in cerebral capillary (×11000). (*b*) Normal glomerular capillary wall from age-matched control. Note uniform appearance and thickness of basement membrane (arrow) (ve: visceral epithelial cell, e: endothelial cell) (×11000). (*c*) Glomerular capillary wall, patient. The original basement membrane (arrow) beneath visceral epithelial cell (ve) appears normal, while the basement membrane (arrowheads) beneath endothelial cell (e) is multilayered. A mesangial cell (m) separates the two basement membranes (×12800). (Jen et al., 1997, with permission from Lippincott, Williams & Wilkins.)

necrosis may have important therapeutic implications since anticoagulation may arrest and even reverse endothelial injury due to radiation. However, a trial of anticoagulation in a single patient with HERNS was not beneficial and bleeding complications developed.

References

Baudrimont, M., Dubas, F., Joutel, A., Tournier-Lasserve, E. & Bousser, M.G. (1993). Autosomal dominant leukoencephalopathy and subcortical ischemic stroke. A clinicopathological study. *Stroke*, **24**, 122–5.

Ducros, A., Nagy, T., Alamowitch, S. et al (1996). Cerebral autosomal dominant arteriopathy with subcortical infarcts and leukoencephalopathy, genetic homogeneity, and mapping of the locus within a 2-cM interval. *American Journal of Human Genetics*, **58**, 171–81.

Glantz, M.J., Burger, P.C., Friedman, A.H., Radtke, R.A., Massey, E.W. & Schold, S.C., Jr. (1994). Treatment of radiation-induced nervous system injury with heparin and warfarin. *Neurology*, **44**, 2020–7.

Grand, M.G., Kaine, J., Fulling, K. et al. (1988). Cerebroretinal vasculopathy. A new hereditary syndrome. *Ophthalmology*, **95**, 649–59.

Gutmann, D.H., Fischbeck, K.H. & Sergott, R.C. (1989). Hereditary retinal vasculopathy with cerebral white matter lesions. *American Journal of Medical Genetics*, **34**, 217–20.

Jen, J., Cohen, A.H., Yue, Q. et al. (1997). Hereditary endotheliopathy with retinopathy, nephropathy, and stroke (HERNS). *Neurology*, **49**, 1322–30.

Rottenberg, D.A., Chernik, N.L., Deck, M.D., Ellis, F. & Posner, J.B. (1977). Cerebral necrosis following radiotherapy of extracranial neoplasms. *Annals of Neurology*, **1**, 339–57.

Sourander, P. & Wålinder, J. (1977). Hereditary multi-infarct dementia. Morphological and clinical studies of a new disease. *Acta Neuropathalogica (Berlin)*, **39**, 247–54.

Tournier-Lasserve, E., Joutel, A., Melki, J. et al. (1993). Cerebral autosomal dominant arteriopathy with subcortical infarcts and leukoencephalopathy maps to chromosome 19q12. *Natural Genetics*, **3**, 256–9.

43

MELAS and stroke in mitochondrial diseases

Lorenz Hirt[1] and Julien Bogousslavsky[2]

[1]Massachusetts General Hospital, Charlestown, MA, USA
[2]Department of Neurology, University of Lausanne, Switzerland

Introduction

MELAS is one of the multisystemic syndromes associated with mutations of mitochondrial DNA. The mitochondrial genome consists of a 16.5 kilobase circular DNA molecule located within the mitochondrion, and present in a large copy number, which is tissue dependent. Mitochondrial DNA (mtDNA) is maternally transmitted and encodes mitochondrial tRNAs and rRNAs and 13 proteins out of approximately 80 proteins that are required for the respiratory chain (Anderson et al., 1981; DiMauro et Moraes, 1993; Mitomap, 1999; DiMauro, 1999). The remaining of these respiratory chain proteins are encoded by nuclear DNA, synthesized in the cytoplasm and transported to the mitochondria, as are most proteins found in the mitochondria (e.g. mitochondrial DNA polymerase, mitochondrial superoxide dismutase). MtDNA mutations may therefore cause respiratory chain dysfunction and ATP depletion and tissues with high energy expenditure like brain and muscle are more at risk of not being able to meet their energy demands. Since 1988, numerous mtDNA mutations have been identified in association with human diseases. Mutations have been found in tRNA, rRNA and protein encoding genes. More recently several mutations in nuclear genes encoding proteins involved in the respiratory chain have been identified in patients with mitochondrial dysfunction (Bourgeron et al., 1995; Triepels et al., 1999), but not so far in MELAS syndrome. An interesting feature of mtDNA mutations is heteroplasmy. As mentioned above, the mtDNA is present in a large copy number within the mitochondrion, wild type and mutated DNA commonly coexist within one cell. The proportions of mutated and wild type mtDNA vary between cells and between tissues. If the proportion of mutated mtDNA exceeds a certain threshold, the normal functioning of the cell is disturbed.

The threshold above which a function impairment becomes apparent depends on the tissue. For instance, in a symptomatic mitochondrial myopathy, the ratio typically exceeds 50% of total mtDNA in affected muscle. The degree of heteroplasmy varies from one tissue to another within one individual, and the distribution of the mutation throughout this organism plays a part in determining the phenotype, and there is poor correlation between abundance of mutant mtDNA in peripheral tissues and neurological phenotype. The distribution of the mutation varies between individuals and participates in the wide phenotypic variability encountered in mtDNA mutations associated diseases, but other unknown factors (e.g. genetic, environmental) are likely to contribute to the phenotypic expression of a mutation. With time, the degree of heteroplasmy may vary, due to a better survival of cells with a low degree of heteroplasmy, or due to an altered replication speed of the mutated mtDNA molecules. MtDNA is exposed to free radicals generated by the respiratory chain, and DNA repair mechanisms are less efficient in the mitochondrion than in the nucleus. MtDNA is therefore more prone to mutations than nuclear DNA. During the normal aging process, spontaneous mtDNA mutations accumulate and slowly impair mitochondrial function. The age-related phenomenon may contribute to the appearance of a phenotype. Following early reports of the association of stroke with mitochondrial myopathy (Bogousslavsky et al., 1982; Kuriyama et al., 1984), the acronym MELAS, for Mitochondrial Encephalomyopathy, Lactic Acidosis and Stroke-like episodes was introduced in 1984 (Pavlakis et al., 1984), defining a multisystemic syndrome most commonly associated with a maternally inherited mtDNA point mutation (A to G transition) at position 3243 within the tRNA$^{Leu(UUR)}$ encoding gene (Goto et al., 1990).

Clinical presentation

The MELAS syndrome affects young patients, and its most striking feature is stroke or stroke-like episodes, occurring as early as teenage, with transient or permanent hemianopia, cortical blindness, aphasia or hemiparesis. Fever and infections have been reported as possible triggering factors for stroke like episodes (Sue et al., 1998). Episodic vomiting, sudden episodes of headache and seizures are common in MELAS patients. Blood lactate levels are increased, which is attributable to a dysfunction of the respiratory chain, with resulting inhibition of the citric acid cycle and accumulation of pyruvate and lactate. Most commonly, MELAS is associated with a mtDNA point mutation at position 3243 within the tRNA$^{Leu(UUR)}$ encoding gene. This mutation is transmitted in a maternal mode of inheritance. It always is heteroplasmic, suggesting that the presence of wild type DNA is required for survival. Other mutations reported in association with the MELAS syndrome are listed in Table 43.2 and are discussed below. Since mitochondrial diseases are remarkable by their phenotypic and genotypic heterogeneity, siblings of MELAS patients carrying the 3243 mutation may not present MELAS syndrome but a different phenotype.

Many different phenotypes, alone or in various combinations, have been reported with this mutation (Table 43.1). A recent population survey (Majamaa et al., 1998) in a Finnish province with 245 201 inhabitants has, for the first time, established the prevalence of the mitochondrial 3243 A to G mutation in an adult population to 16.3/100 000. This mutation therefore classes as a frequent genetic anomaly. While 2 in 35 probands with occipital stroke carry the mutation, the most frequent phenotype in this survey is not MELAS syndrome, but short stature, hearing impairment and cognitive decline.

A list of other clinical features and syndromes reported with the mtDNA 3243 A to G transition is provided in Table 43.1 and includes muscle involvement with ophthalmoparesis and palpebral ptosis due to myopathy of the extrinsic eye muscles. Muscle biopsy shows a mitochondrial myopathy with ragged-red fibres (trichrome gomorrhi staining) and cytochrome c oxidase negative with reduced respiratory chain activity (complexes I, III and/or IV). Overlaps between different mitochondrial syndromes are common.

Brain imaging

Neuroradiological features of six kindreds carrying the MELAS tRNALeu$^{(UUR)}$ 3243 A to G mutation have been reported recently (Sue et al., 1998). The most common

Table 43.1. *Clinical features associated with the mtDNA A3243G mutation*

MELAS syndrome	Goto et al. (1990)
Diabetes mellitus	Reardon et al. (1992); Gerbitz et al. (1995)
Hearing impairment	Morgan-Hughes et al. (1995); Majamaa et al. (1998)
Epilepsy	Majamaa et al. (1998)
Short stature	Majamaa et al. (1998)
Progressive external ophthalmoplegia	Majamaa et al. (1998)
Pigmentary retinopathy	Sue et al. (1997)
Ataxia	Damian et al. (1995); Majamaa et al. (1998)
Basal ganglia calcification	Morgan-Hughes et al. (1995); Majamaa et al. (1998)
Hypertrophic cardiomyopathy	Morgan-Hughes et al. (1995); Majamaa et al. (1998)
Cognitive decline	Majamaa et al. (1998)
MERRF	Folgero et al. (1995)
Ischemic colitis	Hess et al. (1995)
Nephropathy	Damian et al. (1995)
Leigh syndrome	Sue et al. (1999)

feature visible on computerized axial tomography (CT) and by magnetic resonance imaging (MRI) was symmetrical calcifications of the basal ganglia (in 14 out of 22 patients). These calcifications always involved the globus pallidus, and were also seen in the caudate, putamen and thalamus. None of the patients with such calcifications had clinical features suggesting basal ganglia dysfunction. Histopathology obtained from two patients showed neuronal sparing between the calcifications. Serum calcium levels were normal in all patients, and parathyroid hormone was also normal in all tested patients.

Other findings included focal lesions, and cerebellar and cerebral atrophy. Focal hypodensities by CT were seen in nine patients, mainly in the occipital and parietal lobes, and in both cerebellar hemispheres in one patient. In four patients, lesions were not confined to the vascular territory of one large artery. By CT, lesions involved grey and white matter. In the acute stage, there was enhancement with intravenous contrast, and mass effect was also seen. By MRI, there was an increase in T$_2$ signal, mainly within the cortex. All patients with focal hypodensities had a history of stroke-like episodes. Enlargement of the fourth ventricle

Table 43.2. *Mutations associated with stroke in mitochondrial encephalomyopathy*

Mutation	affected gene	Phenotype	
mtDNA A3243G	tRNA[Leu(UUR)]	MELAS	Goto et al. (1990)
mtDNA deletion			Zupanc et al. (1991)
mtDNA T3271C	tRNA[Leu(UUR)]	MELAS	Goto et al. (1991)
mtDNA A11084G	ND4		Lertrit et al. (1992)
mtDNA A8356C	tRNA[Lys]	MERRF MELAS overlap	Zeviani et al. (1993)
mtDNA T7512C	tRNA[Ser(UCN)]	MERRF MELAS overlap	Nakamura et al. (1995)
mtDNA T9957C	COX III	MELAS	Manfredi et al. (1995)
mtDNA T8993G	ATPase 6	NARP, Leigh syndrome	Uziel et al. (1997)
mtDNA 3260	tRNA[Leu(UUR)]	MELAS	Nishino et al. (1996)
mtDNA G13513A	ND5	MELAS	Santorelli, et al. (1997)
mtDNA T3308C	ND1	MELAS and bilateral striatal necrosis	Campos et al. (1997)

or/and cerebellar atrophy was seen in nine patients. Four patients had generalized atrophy of the cerebellum which correlated with wide-based gait and mild limb ataxia. Cerebral atrophy was seen in six patients.

Stroke in other mitochondrial syndromes

Stroke has been reported in association with other mtDNA mutations (Table 43.2). These mutations are point mutations lying within tRNA encoding genes, within protein encoding genes, or deletions encompassing several genes, demonstrating that all these different genetic anomalies can cause a similar dysfunction of the mitochondrion resulting in stroke. In many instances a patient's clinical presentation is a combination of features of two or more syndromes (Table 43.2). A MELAS-MERRF (Myoclonic epilepsy with ragged-red fibres) has been reported with point mutations at positions 8356 and 7512. Stroke has been reported in association with a mitochondrial DNA deletion in two siblings in an overlap between MELAS and Kearns–Sayre Syndrome (Zupanc et al., 1991). Both showed a pigmentary retinopathy, progressive external ophthalmoplegia, neurosensorial hearing loss and lactic acidosis and there was diabetes in one individual and hypoparathyroidism in the other.

Diagnostic evaluation

The clinical evaluation includes a careful family history, searching for other phenotypes of the mitochondrial 3243 A to G mutation (e.g. diabetes and deafness). Brain imaging is important and can reveal calcifications of the basal ganglia and focal lesions in the occipital and parietal lobes. Blood lactate measurement (resting, or after exercise) is useful, as is a muscle biopsy (modified trichrome-gomorrhi staining, cytochrome c oxidase and succinate-, NADH-reductase histochemistry) with measurement of the respiratory chain activity. The diagnosis can be confirmed by mtDNA analysis (muscle biopsy, blood or buccal-epithelial sample).

Treatment

Various approaches have been tried including dietary measures, administration of redox compounds, vitamins and coenzymes, but due to the rarity of the MELAS syndrome, reports of treatment are anecdotal and sometimes controversial. Recently published therapies include coenzyme Q10 (Abe et al., 1999), sodium dichloroacetate (Pavlakis et al., 1998; Saitoh et al., 1998), nicotinamide (Majamaa et al., 1997), coadministration of cytochrome c, vitamin B1 and B2 (Tanaka et al., 1997).

Discussion

Mitochondrial cytopathies have been studied in an in vitro model, in a cell culture system (King & Attardi, 1989) leading to interesting observations on the relative role of the nuclear and the mitochondrial genome in given pathologies, and demonstrating that cells carrying mitochondrial DNA mutations are more susceptible to oxydants, in a calcium-dependent way (Wong & Cortopassi, 1997). However, to understand cerebral injury and stroke in MELAS syndrome, an animal model would be very important and none is currently available. The mechanisms leading to stroke episodes in the MELAS syndrome are not known at present.

The function of the mtDNA is to encode proteins participating in the respiratory chain, and mtDNA mutations affect the respiratory chain activity. The most likely origin of stroke-like episodes is a sudden metabolic failure, in neuronal tissue with a high proportion of mutant mitochondrial DNA, with loss of function and transient or permanent cellular damage, perhaps triggered by fever or infection. This would be consistent with the observation that lesions in some cases are not confined to a single vascular territory (Sue et al., 1998).

Alternatively, there are reports of involvement of smooth muscle cells within the arterial wall, with a high rate of mutated DNA in a case of ischemic colitis associated with the 3243 mutation (Hess et al., 1995). Lesions of the arterial wall cause narrowing or occlusion of the arterial lumen with resulting mesenteric ischemia. A similar mechanism may occur in cerebral arteries and induce cerebral ischemia, but cerebral angiograms have not shown narrowing or irregularities of intracranial arteries, the lesion is in some cases not confined to the territory of a large intracranial vessel and does not evoke an arteriolopathy (Sue et al., 1998). Anomalies of blood clotting have not been reported in MELAS patients.

Recent evidence links mitochondria to neuronal death: mitochondria participate in intracellular calcium buffering, and in calcium signalling processes, and early steps of apoptosis involve the mitochondria (Miller, 1998; Green & Reed, 1998). Apoptotic pathways are complex and incompletely characterized. Fas mediated apoptosis in so-called type I cells is an example of mitochondrial involvement. Fas receptor stimulation activates caspase 8, which cleaves BID, a pro-apoptotic Bcl2 family member; truncated BID migrates to mitochondria and triggers cytochrome c release from the mitochondrial intermembrane space into the cytoplasm (Li et al., 1998; Luo et al., 1998). Cytochrome c with APAF-1 activates caspase 9, which cleaves and activates caspase 3, currently believed to be the major effector protease of apoptosis (Li et al., 1997). Several members of the Bcl2 family of proteins regulating apoptosis are located in the mitochondrion (Adams & Cory, 1998). AIF (apoptosis inducing factor) is also a protein that, like cytochrome c, is released from the mitochondria and promotes apoptosis. These apoptotic pathways are of interest in stroke (Barinaga 1998), since caspase 3 activation has been demonstrated in rodent cerebral ischemia models (Namura et al., 1998),

since caspase inhibitors reduce the infarct size and neurological deficits after cerebral ischemia in mice (Endres et al., 1998), and since cytochrome c release has been demonstrated in rat and mouse cerebral ischemia (Fujimura et al., 1998; Perez-Pinzon et al., 1999). A dysfunction of the mitochondrial respiratory chain may affect calcium signalling, free radical production or apoptosis regulation in the mitochondrion and thereby promote cell death.

It remains very puzzling why the mtDNA A3243G mutation leads to stroke-like episodes more often than other mitochondrial mutations.

References

Abe, K., Matsuo, Y., Kadekawa, J., Inoue, S. & Yanagihara, T. (1999). Effect of coenzyme Q10 in patients with mitochondrial myopathy, encephalopathy, lactic acidosis, and stroke-like episodes (MELAS): evaluation by noninvasive tissue oximetry. *Journal of Neurological Science*, **162**(1), 65–8.

Adams, J.M. & Cory, S. (1998). The Bcl-2 protein family: arbiters of cell survival. *Science*, **281**(5381), 1322–6.

Anderson, S., Bankier, A.T., Barrell, B.G. et al. (1981). Sequence and organization of the human mitochondrial genome. *Nature*, **290**, 457–65.

Barinaga, M. (1998). Stroke-damaged neurons may commit cellular suicide. *Science*, **281**(5381), 1302–3.

Bogousslavsky, J., Perentes, E., Deruaz, J.P. & Regli, F. (1982). Mitochondrial myopathy and cardiomyopathy with neurodegenerative features and multiple brain infarcts. *Journal of Neurological Science*, **55**(3), 351–7.

Bourgeron, T., Rustin, P., Chretien, D. et al. (1995). Mutation of a nuclear succinate dehydrogenase gene results in mitochondrial respiratory chain deficiency. *Nature Genetics*, **11**(2), 144–9.

Campos, Y., Martin, M.A., Rubio, J.C., Gutierrez Del Olmo, M.C., Cabello, A. & Arenas, J. (1997). Bilateral striatal necrosis and MELAS associated with a new T3308C mutation in the mitochondrial ND1 gene. *Biochemical and Biophysical Research Communications*, **238**(2), 323–5.

Damian, M.S., Seibel, P., Reichmann, H. et al. (1995). Clinical spectrum of the MELAS mutation in a large pedigree. *Acta Neurologica Scandinavica*, **92**(5), 409–15.

DiMauro, S. (1999). Mitochondrial encephalomyopathies: Back to mendelian genetics. *Annals of Neurology*, **45**, 693–4.

DiMauro, S. & Moraes, C.T. (1993). Mitochondrial encephalomyopathies. *Archives of Neurology*, **50**(11), 1197–208.

Endres, M., Namura, S., Shimizu-Sasamata, M. et al. (1998) Attenuation of delayed neuronal death after mild focal ischemia by inhibitors of the caspase family. *Journal of Cerebral Blood Flow Metabolism*, **18**, 238–47.

Folgero, T., Torbergsen, T. & Oian, P. (1995). The 3243 MELAS mutation in a pedigree with MERRF. *European Neurology*, **35**(3), 168–71.

Fujimura, M., Morita-Fujimura, Y., Murakami, K., Kawase, M. & Chan, P.K. (1998). Cytosolic redistribution of cytochrome c after transient focal cerebral ischemia in rats. *Journal of Cerebral Blood Flow Metabolism*, **18**, 1239–47.

Gerbitz, K.D., van den Ouweland, J.M.W., Maassen, J.A. & Jaksch, M. (1995). Mitochondrial diabetes mellitus: a review. *Biochimica et Biophysica Acta*, **1271**, 253–60.

Goto, Y., Nonaka, I. & Horai, S. (1990). A mutation in the tRNALeu(UUR) gene associated with the MELAS subgroup of mitochondrial encephalomyopathies. *Nature*, **348**, 651–3.

Goto, Y., Nonaka, I. & Horai, S. (1991). A new mtDNA mutation associated with mitochondrial myopathy, encephalopathy, lactic acidosis and stroke-like episodes (MELAS). *Biochimica et Biophysica Acta*, **1097**, 238–40.

Green, D.R. & Reed, J.C. (1998). Mitochondria and apoptosis. *Science*, **281**(5381), 1309–12.

Hess, J., Burkhard, P., Morris, M., Lalioti, M., Myers, P. & Hadengue, A. (1995). Ischaemic colitis due to mitochondrial cytopathy. *Lancet*, **346**(8968), 189–90.

King, M. P. & Attardi, G. (1989). Human cells lacking mtDNA: repopulation with exogenous mitochondria by complementation. *Science*, **246**(4929), 500–3.

Kuriyama, M., Umezaki, H., Fukuda, Y. et al. (1984). Mitochondrial encephalomyopathy with lactate-pyruvate elevation and brain infarctions. *Neurology*, **34**, 72–7.

Lertrit, P., Noer, A.S., Jean-Francois, M.J. et al. (1992). A new disease-related mutation for mitochondrial encephalopathy lactic acidosis and strokelike episodes (MELAS) syndrome affects the ND4 subunit of the respiratory complex I. *American Journal of Human Genetics*, **51**(3), 457–68.

Li, P., Nijhawan, D., Budihardjo, I. et al. (1997). Cytochrome c and dATP-dependent formation of Apaf-1/caspase-9. *Cell*, **91**(4), 479–89.

Li, H., Zhu, H., Xu, C.J. & Yuan, J. (1998). Cleavage of BID by caspase 8 mediates the mitochondrial damage in the Fas pathway of apoptosis. *Cell*, **94**(4), 491–501.

Majamaa, K., Rusanen, H., Remes, A. & Hassinen, I.E. (1997). Metabolic interventions against complex I deficiency in MELAS syndrome. *Molecular and Cellular Biochemistry*, **174**(1–2), 291–6.

Majamaa, K., Moilanen, J.S., Uimonen, S. et al. (1998). Epidemiology of A3243G, the mutation for mitochondrial encephalomyopathy, lactic acidosis, and strokelike episodes: prevalence of the mutation in an adult population. *American Journal of Human Genetics*, **63**(2), 447–54.

Manfredi, G., Schon, E.A., Moraes, C.T. et al. (1995). A new mutation associated with MELAS is located in a mitochondrial DNA polypeptide-coding gene. *Neuromusculular Disorders*, **5**(5), 391–8.

Miller, R.J. (1998). Mitochondria – the Kraken wakes! *Trends in Neuroscience*, **21**(3), 95–7.

MITOMAP: A Human Mitochondrial Genome Database. Center for Molecular Medicine, Emory University, Atlanta, GA, USA, http://www.gen.emory.edu/mitomap.html, 1999.

Morgan-Hughes, J.A., Sweeney, M.G., Cooper, J.M. et al. (1995).

Mitochondrial DNA (mtDNA) diseases: correlation of genotype to phenotype. *Biochimica et Biophysica Acta*, **1271**(1), 135–40.

Nakamura, M., Nakano, S., Goto, Y. et al. (1995). A novel point mutation in the mitochondrial tRNA(Ser(UCN)) gene detected in a family with MERRF/MELAS overlap syndrome. *Biochemical and Biophysical Research Communications*, **214**(1), 86–93.

Namura, S., Zhu, J., Fink, K. et al. (1998). Activation and cleavage of caspase-3 in experimental cerebral ischemia in mice. *Journal of Neuroscience*, **18**, 3659–68.

Nishino, I., Komatsu, M., Kodama, S., Horai, S., Nonaka, I. & Goto, Y. (1996). The 3260 mutation in mitochondrial DNA can cause mitochondrial myopathy, encephalopathy,lactic acidosis, and strokelike episodes (MELAS). *Muscle Nerve*, **19**(12), 1603–4.

Pavlakis, S.G., Phillips, P.C., DiMauro, S., de Vivo, D.C. & Rowland, L.P. (1984). Mitochondrial myopathy, encephalopathy, lactic acidosis, and strokelike episodes: a distinctive clinical syndrome. *Annals of Neurology*, **16**(4), 481–8.

Pavlakis, S.G., Kingsley, P.B., Kaplan, G.P., Stacpoole, P.W., O'Shea, M. & Lustbader, D. (1998). Magnetic resonance spectroscopy: use in monitoring MELAS treatment. *Archives of Neurology*, **55**(6), 849–52.

Perez-Pinzon, M.A., Xu, G.P., Born, J. et al. (1999). Cytochrome C is released from mitochondria into the cytosol after cerebral anoxia or ischemia. *Journal of Cerebral Blood Flow Metabolism*, **19**(1), 39–43.

Reardon, W., Ross, R.J., Sweeney, M.G. et al. (1992). Diabetes mellitus associated with a pathogenic point mutation in mitochondrial DNA. *Lancet*, **340**(8832), 1376–9.

Saitoh, S., Momoi, M.Y., Yamagata, T., Mori, Y. & Imai, M. (1998). Effects of dichloroacetate in three patients with MELAS. *Neurology*, **50**(2), 531–4.

Santorelli, F.M., Tanji, K., Kulikova, R. et al. (1997). Identification of a novel mutation in the mtDNA ND5 gene associated with MELAS. *Biochemical and Biophysical Research Communications*, **238**(2), 326–8.

Sue, C.M., Mitchell, P., Grimmins, D.S., Moshegov, C., Byrne, E. & Morris, J.G.L. (1997). Pigmentary retinopathy associated with the mitochondrial DNA 3243 point mutation. *Neurology*, **49**, 1013–17.

Sue, C.M., Crimmins, D.S., Soo, Y.S. et al. (1998). Neuroradiological features of six kindreds with MELAS tRNA(Leu) A2343G point mutation: implications for pathogenesis. *Journal of Neurology, Neurosurgery and Psychiatry*, **65**, 233–40.

Sue, C.M., Bruno, C., Andreu, A.L. et al. (1999). Infantile encephalopathy associated with the MELAS A3243G mutation. *Journal of Pediatrics*, **134**(6), 696–700.

Tanaka, J., Nagai, T., Arai, H. et al. (1997). Treatment of mitochondrial encephalomyopathy with a combination of cytochrome C and vitamins B1 and B2. *Brain Development*, **19**(4), 262–7.

Triepels, R.H., van den Heuvel, L.P., Loeffen, J.L. et al. (1999). Leigh syndrome associated with a mutation in the NDUFS7 (PSST) nuclear encoded subunit of complex I. *Annals of Neurology*, **45**(6), 787–90.

Uziel, G., Moroni, I., Lamantea, E. et al. (1997). Mitochondrial disease associated with the T8993G mutation of the mitochondrial ATPase 6 gene: a clinical, biochemical, and molecular study in six families. *Journal of Neurology, Neurosurgery and Psychiatry*, **63**, 16–22.

Wong, A. & Cortopassi, G. (1997). MtDNA mutations confer cellular sensitivity to oxidant stress that is partially rescued by calcium depletion and cyclosporin A. *Biochemical and Biophysical Research Communications*, **239**(1), 139–45.

Zeviani, M., Muntoni, F., Savarese, N. et al. (1993). MERRF/MELAS overlap syndrome associated with a new point mutation in the mitochondrial DNA tRNA(Lys) gene. *European Journal of Human Genetics*, **1**(1), 80–7.

Zupanc, M.L., Moraes, C.T., Shanske, S., Langman, C.B., Ciafaloni, E. & DiMauro, S. (1991). Deletion of mitochondrial DNA in patients with combined features of Kearns–Sayre and MELAS syndromes. *Annals of Neurology*, **29**(6), 680–3.

44

Sturge–Weber syndrome

E. Steve Roach

Department of Neurology, The University of Texas, Southwestern Medical School, Dallas, TX, USA

Introduction

Sturge–Weber syndrome is characterized by a facial cutaneous nevus (port-wine stain) and a leptomeningeal angioma, often found ipsilateral to the facial lesion. Frequent additional findings include mental retardation, epileptic seizures, contralateral hemiparesis and hemiatrophy, homonymous hemianopia, and glaucoma. However, the clinical features and their severity are quite variable, and patients with the cutaneous nevus and seizures but with normal intelligence and no focal neurologic deficit are common (Uram & Zubillaga, 1982).

The syndrome occurs sporadically in all races and has no predilection for either sex. Sturge–Weber syndrome (encephalofacial angiomatosis) remains an enigmatic disorder that is rarely difficult to diagnose, but frequently hard to predict or treat effectively. This difficulty is due to the highly variable nature of the clinical manifestations and to the lack of effective treatment for some of its more devastating features.

Cutaneous manifestations

The nevus characteristically involves the forehead and upper eyelid, but it commonly affects both sides of the face and may extend onto the trunk and extremities (Fig. 44.1). Patients whose nevus involves only the trunk, or the maxillary or mandibular area but not the upper face, have little risk of an intracranial angioma (Tallman et al., 1991; Enjolras et al., 1985; Uram & Zubillaga, 1982). Although the facial angioma is obvious in most children from birth, occasional patients have the characteristic neurologic and radiographic features of Sturge–Weber syndrome without the skin lesion (Ambrosetto et al., 1983; Crosley & Binet, 1978). More often, the typical cutaneous angioma is present without any evidence of an intracranial lesion (Morelli, 1999). Even the children with classic Sturge–Weber syndrome usually have normal neurologic function at first, and it is not always easy to identify which neonates have an intracranial angioma.

The leptomeningeal angioma is typically ipsilateral to a unilateral facial nevus, but bilateral brain lesions occur in at least 15% of patients, including some with a unilateral cutaneous nevus (Boltshauser et al., 1976). The extent of the cutaneous lesion correlates poorly with the severity of neurologic impairment (Uram & Zubillaga, 1982), although children with an extensive cutaneous lesion are more likely to have bilateral brain angiomas. Children with bilateral brain lesions have a greater risk of neurologic impairment and tend to have an earlier onset of seizures (Bebin & Gomez, 1988).

The location of the port-wine nevus of Sturge–Weber syndrome has traditionally been linked to the distribution of the trigeminal nerve branches, but the occurrence of facial and leptomeningeal angiomas can be better explained by the common embryological derivation of these two regions.

Occasionally the port-wine nevus is extensive, involving parts of the trunk and extremities in addition to the face. Patients with extensive cutaneous lesions and limb hypertrophy have been separately classified as Klippel–Trenaunay–Weber syndrome (Meyer, 1979), but if their cutaneous lesion involves the upper face, their neurological picture may be identical to that of Sturge–Weber syndrome.

Ophthalmologic findings

Glaucoma is a common problem in patients with a port-wine nevus near the eye, whether or not they manifest the intracranial disease characteristic of Sturge–Weber syn-

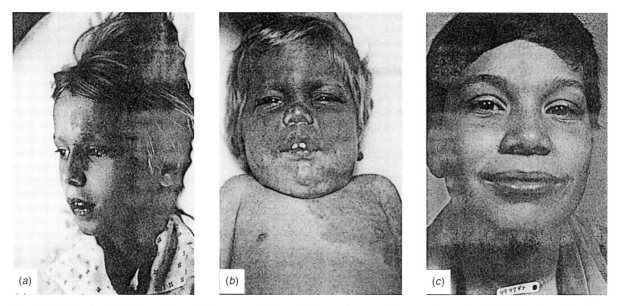

Fig. 44.1. (*a*) Classic distribution of the port-wine nevus of Sturge-Weber syndrome on the upper face and eyelid. (*b*) Another patient's nevus involved both sides of his face and extends onto the trunk and arm. (*c*) This boy had epilepsy and the typical radiographic features of Sturge–Weber syndrome, but only a subtle skin lesion. (From Roach, 1989, and Roach & Riela, 1995, with permission.)

drome (Stevenson et al., 1974). Sullivan and colleagues found glaucoma in 36 of 51 patients (71%); 26 of these developed glaucoma by age 2 years (Sullivan et al., 1992). Buphthalmos and amblyopia are present in some newborns, evidently due to an anomalous anterior chamber angle (Cibis et al., 1984). In other patients, the glaucoma becomes symptomatic later and untreated leads to progressive blindness (Sujansky & Conradi, 1995). Therefore, periodic measurement of the intraocular pressure is mandatory regardless of the patient's age, particularly when the nevus is near the eye. The intracranial angioma is frequently in the occipital region and, not surprisingly, visual field defects are common.

Neurologic manifestations

Epileptic seizures, mental retardation, and focal neurological deficits are the primary neurologic abnormalities of Sturge–Weber syndrome (Roach & Bodensteiner, 1999). Seizures and hemiparesis typically develop acutely during the first or second year of life, often during a febrile illness. The age when symptoms begin and the overall clinical severity are highly variable, but onset of seizures prior to age two tends to increase the likelihood of future mental retardation and refractory epilepsy (Sujansky & Conradi, 1995). Patients with refractory seizures are much more likely to be mentally retarded, while patients who have

never had seizures are typically normal (Roach & Bodensteiner, 1999).

Seizures occur in 72–80% of Sturge–Weber patients with unilateral lesions and in 93% of patients with bihemispheric involvement (Bebin & Gomez, 1988; Oakes, 1992). Focal motor seizures or generalized tonic-clonic seizures are most typical of Sturge–Weber syndrome initially, but infantile spasms, myoclonic seizures and atonic seizures occur (Chevrie et al., 1988). The first few seizures are often focal even in patients who later develop generalized tonic-clonic seizures or infantile spasms. Older children and adults are more likely to have complex partial seizures or focal motor seizures. Some patients continue to have daily seizures after the initial deterioration in spite of various daily anticonvulsant medications, while others have long seizure-free intervals, sometimes even without medication, punctuated by clusters of seizures (Chevrie et al., 1988; Roach & Bodensteiner, 1999).

Hemiparesis often develops acutely in conjunction with the initial flurry of seizure activity. Although often attributed to postictal weakness, hemiparesis may be permanent or persist much longer than the few hours typical of a postictal deficit. Other patients suddenly develop weakness without seizures, either as repeated episodes of weakness similar to transient ischemic attacks or as a single stroke-like episode with persistent deficit (Garcia et al., 1981). Children who develop hemiparesis early in life often have arrested growth in the weak extremities.

Other focal neurologic deficits depend on the anatomic site and the extent of the intracranial vascular lesion. Because the occipital region is frequently involved, visual field deficits are common (Aicardi & Arzimanoglou, 1991). Patients with glaucoma are doubly at risk, because they may become amblyopic in one or both eyes from the glaucoma plus they have a superimposed visual field loss from the cortical lesion (Cheng, 1999).

Early development is usually normal, but mental deficiency eventually develops in about half of Sturge–Weber patients (Uram & Zubillaga, 1982; Aicardi & Arzimanoglou, 1991). Only 8% of the patients with bilateral brain involvement are intellectually normal (Bebin & Gomez, 1988). The degree of intellectual impairment ranges from mild to profound. Behavioural abnormalities are often a problem even in patients who are not mentally retarded.

Intracranial hemorrhage rarely occurs in Sturge–Weber patients. Cushing in 1906 described three patients that he assumed had spontaneous hemorrhage, but all three had acutely developed seizures and weakness, fairly typical of the pattern seen during the initial neurologic deterioration in children without hemorrhage. Even with operative or postmortem examination of the brain in two of these patients, no direct evidence of hemorrhage was found (Cushing, 1906). Anderson and Duncan presented one adult with subarachnoid hemorrhage attributed to Sturge–Weber syndrome (Anderson & Duncan, 1974). Microscopic hemorrhages are mentioned in autopsy series but probably have limited clinical significance.

Mechanisms of neurologic deterioration

Neurologic function at birth is typically normal, but most children with Sturge–Weber syndrome eventually develop seizures which are often difficult to control especially during the acute illness (Roach & Bodensteiner, 1999). Some children undergo saltatory deterioration via a series of discrete episodes of neurologic dysfunction (Garcia et al., 1981), and episodic neurologic deficits can occur even without overt seizure activity (Alexander & Norman, 1960). Although the mechanism of neurologic deterioration in Sturge–Weber patients is debated, several different factors probably contribute.

Chronic hypoxia of the cerebral cortex adjacent to the angioma resulting from reduced blood flow has been postulated, and increased metabolic requirements during seizures could potentiate the oxygen deficit (Aicardi & Arzimanoglou, 1991). Frequent epileptic seizures, no doubt, cause additional impairment in some children, because children with refractory seizures from a variety of other causes also deteriorate. Also important is the extent and location of the vascular lesion in the brain: children with an extensive lesion often have more difficult to control seizures and more intellectual impairment.

Hemiparesis is often attributed to postictal weakness, but in some patients the hemiparesis clearly begins before the onset of seizures. In patients with both hemiparesis and seizures, it is often difficult to be certain which came first. Some patients undergo saltatory deterioration of neurologic function and others display episodic neurologic dysfunction without obvious seizures, and it has been suggested that both of these phenomena result from repeated venous thromboses (Garcia et al., 1981). Venous thrombosis could also explain the typical first episode of neurologic dysfunction: the clinical picture at the time of the initial deterioration resembles the pattern seen with venous thromboses from other causes. However, a similar pattern of episodic dysfunction without seizures could result from elevated venous pressure without actual thrombosis of the veins.

Diagnostic evaluation

Most of the children with facial port-wine nevi do not have an intracranial angioma (Enjolras et al., 1985), and neuroimaging studies and other tests help to distinguish the children with Sturge–Weber syndrome from those with an isolated cutaneous lesion. Neuroimaging, electroencephalography, and functional testing with positron emission tomography (PET) and single photon emission computed tomography (SPECT) may also help to define the extent of the intracranial lesion for possible epilepsy surgery (Chugani et al., 1989; Chiron et al., 1989).

Although gyral calcification is a classic feature of Sturge–Weber syndrome, this 'trolley track' appearance is not always present. Bilateral calcification is common (Boltshauser et al., 1976). Calcification often becomes more apparent as the patient becomes older but is sometimes already present at birth (McCaughan et al., 1975; Yeakley et al., 1992). Intracranial calcification can be demonstrated much earlier with computed cranial tomography (Fig. 44.2) than with standard skull films.

Cerebral atrophy is more apparent with magnetic resonance imaging than with computed tomography (Chamberlain et al., 1989). In addition to cortical atrophy, magnetic resonance imaging sometimes demonstrates accelerated myelination in very young Sturge–Weber patients (Jacoby et al., 1987; Maria et al., 1999a). The addition of gadolinium contrast (Fig. 44.3) allows magnetic resonance imaging to effectively demonstrate the abnormal intracranial vessels in Sturge–Weber patients (Benedikt et

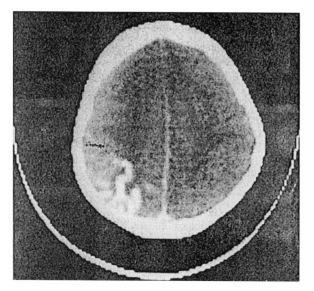

Fig. 44.2. Cranial CT from a patient with Sturge–Weber syndrome shows a gyriform pattern of calcification in the parieto-occipital region. (From Garcia et al., 1981, with permission.)

al., 1993); currently this is the best test to determine intracranial involvement. Magnetic resonance angiography has recently been used to directly image the larger abnormal vessels.

Functional imaging with PET indicates reduced brain glucose utilization adjacent to the leptomeningeal lesion, but often extending beyond the area of abnormality depicted by computed tomography or magnetic resonance imaging (Chugani et al., 1989; Maria et al., 1999a). Glucose utilization tends to be reduced after the first year of life (Chugani et al., 1989), although PET activation studies suggest that these abnormal areas retain some functional responsiveness (Muller et al., 1997). SPECT typically shows reduced cerebral perfusion even in regions of the brain with normal glucose uptake (Chiron et al., 1989; Maria et al., 1999b). As with PET, the area with abnormal perfusion shown with SPECT is often more extensive than the abnormality seen with computed tomography or magnetic resonance imaging (Chiron et al., 1989; Griffiths et al., 1997; Maria et al., 1999b).

Cerebral arteriography is no longer routinely required for the evaluation of Sturge–Weber syndrome, but it may be helpful in atypical patients or prior to surgery for epilepsy (Maria et al., 1999a). The veins are typically more abnormal than the arteries (Probst, 1980). Occasional patients have evidence of arterial occlusion, and the homogeneous blush of the intracranial angioma is sometimes present (Poser & Taveras, 1957). The superficial cortical veins are reduced in number (Fig. 44.4) and the deep draining veins are dilated and tortuous (Farrell et al., 1992).

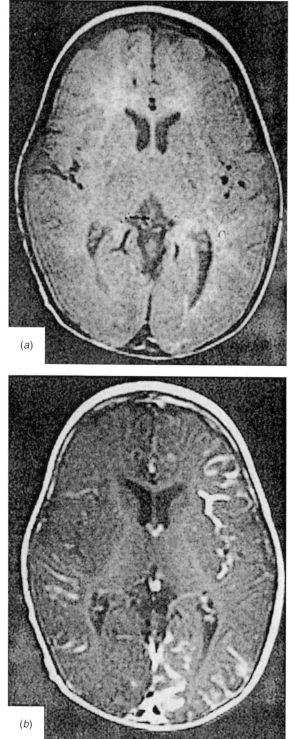

Fig. 44.3. (a) Normal cranial MRI without contrast from a patient with Sturge–Weber syndrome. (b) Addition of gadolinium contrast in this patient revealed a left leptomeningeal vascular lesion plus extensive intraparenchymal vascular abnormalities. (From Roach, 1992, with permission.)

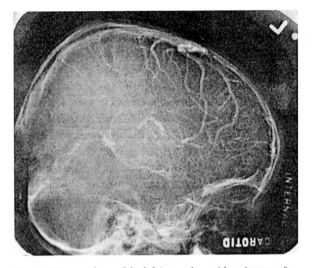

Fig. 44.4. Venous phase of the left internal carotid angiogram of a patient with Sturge–Weber syndrome. Note the paucity of superficial cortical veins posteriorly and the prominent deep venous system. (From Garcia et al., 1981, with permission.)

Failure of the sagittal sinus to opacify after ipsilateral carotid injection may be secondary to thrombosis of the superficial cortical veins (Bentson et al., 1971), and the abnormal deep venous channels probably have a similar origin as they form collateral conduits for nonfunctioning cortical veins (Probst, 1980).

Pathology

The parietal and occipital lobes are affected more often than the frontal lobes (Hatfield et al., 1988). The leptomeninges are thickened and discolored by increased vascularity. Angiomatous vessels may obliterate the subarachnoid space, and the tortuous deep-draining veins that are seen radiographically can also be seen in pathologic specimens (Wohlwill & Yakovlev, 1957). Microscopically these vessels are primarily thin-walled veins of variable size (Di Trapani et al., 1982; Wohlwill & Yakovlev, 1957). Angiomatous vessels sometimes extend into the superficial brain parenchyma and the ipsilateral choroid plexus is often involved. Microscopic abnormalities are frequently found in normal looking areas adjacent to the visible malformation, and some vessels are narrowed or occluded by progressive hyalinization and subendothelial proliferation (Wohlwill & Yakovlev, 1957; Norman & Schoene, 1977).

Cerebral atrophy adjacent to the angioma is typical. In some patients the atrophy becomes progressively more severe in early childhood before eventually stabilizing. Other children, particularly those with mild clinical features, may not develop visible atrophy at all. Microscopic features include neuronal loss and gliosis which, like the angioma itself, usually extend beyond the area of obvious abnormality.

The typical gyriform calcification results from deposition of calcium within the outer cortical layers (Wohlwill & Yakovlev, 1957; Di Trapani et al., 1982). Norman and Schoene (1977) found that the foci of calcium typically lie adjacent to a blood vessel, and Di Trapani et al., (1982) believe the calcium is deposited in an intravascular mucopolysaccharide substance before shifting into the brain parenchyma adjacent to the vessel. Chronic venous stasis with anoxic damage of the nearby cortex has been postulated as the mechanism for inducing cortical calcifications.

Treatment

Treatment of Sturge–Weber syndrome is problematic. The syndrome is rare and its manifestations so variable that controlled trials to evaluate therapy are difficult. The majority of patients with Sturge–Weber syndrome at some point develop seizures, and seizure control can markedly improve their quality of life. Careful attention to dosing schedules and periodic monitoring of serum anticonvulsant levels help to assure the best possible control of seizures. Complete seizure control with medication is possible in some patients.

Hemispherectomy sometimes improves seizure control and may promote more normal intellectual development (Ogunmekan et al., 1989). Early hemispherectomy has been recommended for patients whose seizures begin in infancy (Hoffman et al., 1979). More recently, resection of the area predominantly affected has achieved good results (Aicardi & Arzimanoglou, 1991; Bye et al., 1989), and corpus callosum section may be a useful alternative for some patients (Rappaport, 1988). Despite the general agreement that surgical resection is effective, there remains some debate about patient selection and about the timing of surgery. Almost one patient in five has bilateral cerebral lesions, limiting the surgical options unless one hemisphere is clearly causing most of the seizures. Most physicians do not feel comfortable recommending surgery in a patient who has not yet developed seizures or one whose seizures are fully controlled with medication, and there is also understandable reluctance to resect a still functional portion of the brain and cause a deficit (Arzimanoglou & Aicardi, 1992; Bruce, 1999). Thus, surgery is often reserved for individuals with severe refractory seizures who already have clinical dysfunction of the area to be removed (e.g. hemiparesis or hemianopia).

Surgical guidelines for Sturge–Weber patients have been published (Roach et al., 1994). Hemispherectomy should be undertaken for patients with clinically significant seizures who fail to respond to an adequate trial of anticonvulsants. Surgery should not be done automatically just because the diagnosis of Sturge–Weber syndrome is made. Surgery should only be done in a centre with an ongoing program in pediatric epilepsy surgery and age-appropriate facilities for preoperative and postoperative care. Patients with less extensive lesions should have a limited resection rather than a complete hemispherectomy that preserves as much normal brain as possible, even at the risk of having to do another operation later. Corpus callosotomy should be reserved for patients with refractory tonic or atonic seizures. In effect, much the same approach should be used in children with Sturge–Weber syndrome as with other epileptic patients (Roach et al., 1994).

Daily aspirin has been tried in an effort to prevent recurrent vascular thrombosis that may cause neurologic deterioration (Garcia et al., 1981; McCaughan et al., 1975). Controlled studies with aspirin present the same difficulties as with hemispherectomy, and until more information is available, routine use of aspirin can not be enthusiastically endorsed. It does seem reasonable to use aspirin for patients with repeated clinical episodes suggesting transient ischemic attacks (Garcia et al., 1981; Cambon et al., 1987) and for patients with bihemispheric disease for whom surgery is not a reasonable option. Low-dose daily aspirin seems to be well tolerated in children, although the optimum dose has not been established.

Periodic monitoring of the intraocular pressure is an important aspect of management that is easily overlooked in patients who have no initial ocular findings. Glaucoma may be present at birth or symptoms may arise later. Occasional patients develop glaucoma only after several years, so yearly ophthalmologic examination with intraocular pressure measurement is recommended. Patients who develop ocular pain or visual symptoms should be promptly reevaluated.

The patient's appearance can be dramatically improved by pulsed dye laser treatment, although it is not often possible to completely obliterate the lesion (Nguyen et al., 1998). Early treatment is preferable because the skin lesions tend to hypertrophy with time and thereafter require more extensive treatment (Morelli, 1999). Pulsed dye laser treatment of port-wine lesions has been reviewed in detail (Morelli, 1999). Some physicians reserve cosmetic procedures for those patients with reasonably good neurologic function.

References

Aicardi, J. & Arzimanoglou A. (1991). Sturge–Weber syndrome. *International Pediatrics*, **6**, 129–34.

Alexander, G.L. & Norman, R.M. (1960). *Sturge–Weber Syndrome*. Bristol: John Wright & Sons Ltd.

Ambrosetto, P., Ambrosetto, G., Michelucci, R. & Bacci, A. (1983). Sturge–Weber syndrome without port-wine facial nevus – report of 2 cases studied by CT. *Child's Brain*, **10**, 387–92.

Anderson, F.H., & Duncan, G.W. (1974). Sturge–Weber disease with subarachnoid hemorrhage. *Stroke*, **5**, 509–11.

Arzimanoglou, A. & Aicardi, J. (1992). The epilepsy of Sturge–Weber syndrome: clinical features and treatment in 23 patients. *Acta Neurologica Scandinavica (Suppl.)*, **140**, 18–22.

Bebin, E.M. & Gomez, M.R. (1988). Prognosis in Sturge–Weber disease: comparison of unihemispheric and bihemispheric involvement. *Journal of Child Neurology*, **3**, 181–4.

Benedikt, R.A., Brown, D.C., Walker, R., Ghaed, V.N., Mitchell, M. & Geyer, C.A. (1993). Sturge–Weber syndrome: cranial MR imaging with Gd-DTPA. *American Journal of Neuroradiology*, **14**, 409–15.

Bentson, J.R., Wilson, G.H. & Newton, T.H. (1971). Cerebral venous drainage pattern of the Sturge–Weber syndrome. *Radiology*, **101**, 111–18.

Boltshauser, E., Wilson, J. & Hoare, R.D. (1976). Sturge–Weber syndrome with bilateral intracranial calcification. *Journal of Neurology, Neurosurgery and Psychiatry*, **39**, 429–35.

Bruce, D.A. (1999). Neurosurgical aspects of Sturge–Weber syndrome. In *Sturge–Weber Syndrome*, ed. J.B. Bodensteiner & E.S. Roach, pp. 39–42. Mt Freedom, NJ: Sturge–Weber Foundation.

Bye, A.M., Matheson, J.M. & MacKenzie, R.A. (1989). Epilepsy surgery in Sturge–Weber syndrome. *Australian and New Zealand Journal of Ophthalmology*, **25**, 103–5.

Cambon, H., Truelle, J.L., Baron, J.C., Chiras, J., Tran Dinh, S. & Chatel, M. (1987). Focal chronic ischemia and concomitant migraine: an atypical form of Sturge–Weber angiomatosis? *Review Neurologie*, **143**, 588–94.

Chamberlain, M.C., Press, G.A. & Hesselink, J.R. (1989). MR imaging and CT in three cases of Sturge–Weber syndrome: prospective comparison. *American Journal of Neuroradiology*, **10**, 491–6.

Cheng, K.P. (1999). Ophthalmologic manifestations of Sturge–Weber syndrome. In *Sturge–Weber Syndrome*, ed. J.B. Bodensteiner & E.S. Roach, pp. 17–26. Mt Freedom, NJ: Sturge–Weber Foundation.

Chevrie, J.J., Specola, N. & Aicardi, J. (1988). Secondary bilateral synchrony in unilateral pial angiomatosis: successful surgical management. *Journal of Neurology, Neurosurgery and Psychiatry*, **15**, 95–8.

Chiron, C., Raynaud, C., Tzourio, N. et al. (1989). Regional cerebral blood flow by SPECT imaging in Sturge–Weber disease: an aid for diagnosis. *Journal of Neurology, Neurosurgery and Psychiatry*, **52**, 1402–9.

Chugani, H.T., Mazziotta, J.C. & Phelps, M.E. (1989). Sturge–Weber syndrome: a study of cerebral glucose utilization with positron emission tomography. *Journal of Pediatrics*, **114**, 244–53.

Cibis, G.W., Tripathi, R.C. & Tripathi, B.J. (1984). Glaucoma in Sturge–Weber syndrome. *Ophthalmology*, **91**, 1061–71.

Crosley, C.J. & Binet, E.F. (1978). Sturge–Weber Syndrome presentation as a focal seizure disorder without nevus flammeus. *Clinical Pediatrics*, **17**, 606–9.

Cushing, H. (1906). Cases of spontaneous intracranial hemorrhage associated with trigeminal nevi. *Journal of the American Medical Association*, **47**, 178–83.

Di Trapani, G., Di Rocco, C., Abbamondi, A.L. et al. (1982). Light microscopy and ultrastructural studies of Sturge–Weber disease. *Brain*, **9**, 23–36.

Enjolras, O., Riche, M.C. & Merland, J.J. (1985). Facial port-wine stains and Sturge–Weber syndrome. *Pediatrics*, **76**, 48–51.

Farrell, M.A., Derosa, M.J., Curran, J.G. et al. (1992). Neuropathologic findings in cortical resections (including hemispherectomies) performed for the treatment of intractable childhood epilepsy. *Acta Neuropathology*, **83**, 246–59.

Garcia, J.C., Roach, E.S. & McLean, W.T. (1981). Recurrent thrombotic deterioration in the Sturge–Weber syndrome. *Child's Brain*, **8**, 427–33.

Griffiths, P.D., Boodram, M.B., Blaser, S., Armstrong, D., Gilday, D.L. & Harwood-Nash, D. (1997). ^{99m}Technetium HMPAO imaging in children with the Sturge–Weber syndrome: a study of nine cases with CT and MRI correlation. *Neuroradiology*, **39**, 219–24.

Hatfield, M., Muraki, A., Wollman, R., Hekmatpanah, J., Mojtahedi, S. & Duda, E.E. (1988). Isolated frontal lobe calcification in Sturge–Weber syndrome. *American Journal of Neuroradiology*, **9**, 203–4.

Hoffman, H.J., Hendrick, E.B., Dennis, M. & Armstrong, D. (1979). Hemispherectomy for Sturge–Weber syndrome. *Child's Brain*, **5**, 233–48.

Jacoby, C.G., Yuh, W.T., Afifi, A.K., Bell, W.E., Schelper, R.L. & Sato, Y. (1987). Accelerated myelination in early Sturge–Weber syndrome demonstrated by MR imaging. *Journal of Computer Assisted Tomography*, **11**, 226–31.

McCaughan, R.A., Ouvrier, R.A., De Silva, K. & McLaughlin, A. (1975). The value of the brain scan and cerebral arteriogram in the Sturge–Weber syndrome. *Proceedings of the Australian Association of Neurology*, **12**, 185–90.

Maria, B.L., Hoang, K.N., Robertson, R.L. et al. (1999a). Imaging brain structure and function in Sturge–Weber syndrome. In *Sturge–Weber Syndrome*, ed. J.B. Bodensteiner & E.S. Roach, pp. 43–69. Mt Freedom, NJ: Sturge–Weber Foundation.

Maria, B.L., Neufeld, J.A., Rosainz, L.C. et al. (1999b). Bihemispheric brain disease is common in Sturge–Weber syndrome. *Journal of Child Neurology*, (In press).

Meyer, E. (1979). Neurocutaneous syndrome with excessive macrohydrocephalus (Sturge–Weber/Klippel–Trenaunay syndrome). *Neuropediatrie*, **10**, 67–75.

Morelli, J.G. (1999). Port-wine stains and the Sturge–Weber syndrome. In *Sturge–Weber Syndrome*, ed. J.B. Bodensteiner & E.S. Roach, pp. 11–16. Mt Freedom, NJ: Sturge–Weber Foundation.

Muller, R.A., Chugani, H.T., Muzik, O., Rothermel, R.D. & Chakraborty, P.K. (1997).Language and motor functions activate calcified hemisphere in patients with Sturge–Weber syndrome: a positron emission tomography study. *Journal of Child Neurology*, **12**, 431–7.

Nguyen, C.M., Yohn, J.J., Huff, C., Weston, W.L. & Morelli, J.G. (1998). Facial port wine stains in childhood: prediction of the rate of improvement as a function of the age of the patient, size and location of the port wine stain and the number of treatments with the pulsed dye (585 nm) laser. *British Journal of Dermatology*, **138**, 821–5.

Norman, M.G. & Schoene, W.C. (1977). The ultrastructure of Sturge–Weber disease. *Acta Neuropathology*, **37**, 199–205.

Oakes, W.J. (1992). The natural history of patients with the Sturge–Weber syndrome. *Pediatric Neurosurgery*, **18**, 287–90.

Ogunmekan, A.O., Hwang, P.A. & Hoffman, H.J. (1989). Sturge–Weber–Dimitri disease: role of hemispherectomy in prognosis. *Canadian Journal of Neurological Science*, **16**, 78–80.

Poser, C.M. & Taveras, J.M. (1957). Cerebral angiography in encephalo-trigeminal angiomatosis. *Radiology*, **68**, 327–36.

Probst, F.P. (1980). Vascular morphology and angiographic flow patterns in Sturge–Weber angiomatosis. *Neuroradiology*, **20**, 73–8.

Rappaport, Z.H. (1988). Corpus callosum section in the treatment of intractable seizures in the Sturge–Weber syndrome. *Child's Nervous System*, **4**, 231–2.

Roach, E.S. (1989). Congenital cutaneovascular syndromes. In *Handbook of Clinical Neurology: Vascular Diseases, Volume 11*, ed. P.J. Vinken, G.W. Bruyn, H.L. Klawans & J.F. Toole, pp. 443–62. Amsterdam: Elsevier.

Roach, E.S. (1992). Neurocutaneous syndromes. *Pediatric Clinics of North America*, **39**, 591–620.

Roach, E.S., Riela, A.R., Chugani, H.T., Shinnar, S., Bodensteiner, J.B. & Freeman, J. (1994). Sturge–Weber syndrome: recommendations for surgery. *Journal of Child Neurology*, **9**, 190–3.

Roach, E.S. & Bodensteiner, J.B. (1999). Neurologic manifestations of Sturge–Weber syndrome. In *Sturge–Weber Syndrome*, ed. J.B. Bodensteiner & E.S. Roach, pp. 27–38. Mt Freedom, NJ: Sturge–Weber Foundation.

Roach, E.S. & Riela, A.R. (1995). *Pediatric Cerebrovascular Disorders*. New York: Futura.

Stevenson, R.F., Thomson, H.G. & Morin, L.D. (1974). Unrecognized ocular problems associated with port-wine stain of the face in children. *Canadian Medical Association Journal*, **111**, 953–4.

Sujansky, E. & Conradi, S. (1995). Sturge–Weber syndrome: age of onset of seizures and glaucoma and the prognosis for affected children. *Journal of Child Neurology*, **10**, 49–58.

Sullivan, J., Clarke, M.P. & Morin, J.D. (1992). The ocular manifestations of the Sturge–Weber syndrome. *Journal of Pediatric Ophthalmology and Strabismus*, **29**, 349–56.

Tallman, B., Tan, O.T., Morelli, J.G. et al. (1991). Location of port-wine stains and the likelihood of ophthalmic and/or central nervous system complications. *Pediatrics*, **87**, 323–7.

Uram, M. & Zubillaga, C. (1982). The cutaneous manifestations of

Sturge–Weber syndrome. *Journal of Clinical Neuro-Ophthalmology*, **2**, 245–8.

Wohlwill, F.J. & Yakovlev, P.I. (1957). Histopathology of meningo-facial angiomatosis (Sturge–Weber's disease). *Journal of Neuropathology and Experimental Neurology*, **16**, 341–64.

Yeakley, J.W., Woodside, M. & Fenstermacher, M.J. (1992). Bilateral neonatal Sturge–Weber–Dimitri disease: CT and MR findings. *American Journal of Neuroradiology*, **13**, 1179–82.

45

Von Hippel–Lindau disease

John M. Duff[1] and Luca Regli[2]

[1]Department of Neurosurgery, Tufts New England Medical Center, Boston, MA, USA
[2]Department of Neurology, University of Lausanne, Switzerland

Introduction

Von Hippel–Lindau (VHL) disease is an inherited tumour susceptibility syndrome manifesting a variety of benign and malignant tumours. It has an autosomal dominant inheritance with incomplete but high penetrance whose most characteristic central nervous system lesion is the hemangioblastoma. The hemangioblastoma is a capillary-rich neoplasm containing variably lipid laden interstitial or stromal cells, and is histologically identical at all sites (including the retina) in VHL patients. Its exact histogenesis is unknown (Burger & Scheithauer, 1994). These neoplasms account for 2–3% of all central nervous system tumours and familial forms comprise anywhere from 5.3 to 11.8% of cases according to the literature (Resche et al., 1993). As Resche et al. point out, genetic inquiry in many cases is lacking implying that the real familial incidence is in fact higher (Resche et al., 1993). Stroke as a mode of presentation of a hemangioblastoma is rare, with hemorrhage being described in only 2% of cases in a large series of hemangioblastomas (Resche et al., 1985). By extrapolation, we can say that intracerebral hemorrhage as a clinical presentation of VHL disease would be proportionally less common again and is confined to small series and case reports. However, it forms an integral part of the subject matter of this chapter. We did not find any reported cases or series of acute cerebral ischemia as a direct complication of VHL disease.

Historically, the first case of hemangioblastoma was described at autopsy in 1872 by Hughlings Jackson. Von Hippel first described a retinal hemangioblastoma in 1904 and subsequently the association of visceral and cerebral lesions with retinal hemangioblastomas was observed in 1926 by Lindau (Rengachary, 1985). The term hemangioblastoma was coined by Bailey and Cushing in 1928 to delineate all vascular tumours of the central nervous

system and to differentiate these lesions from primary vascular malformations.

Contentious issues regarding hemangioblastomas are uncertain histogenesis, factors predictive of tumour recurrence, factors predictive of multifocal disease, and the cumulative morbidity of central and retinal lesions.

Genetics

VHL is due to a defect on the short arm of chromosome 3 (Hosoe et al., 1990). The VHL tumour suppressor gene was cloned in 1993 and localized at 3p25–26 (Decker et al., 1994), and a large number of different mutations have thus far been identified (Shuin et al., 1994). Recent genetic mutation studies show that the VHL tumour suppressor gene is mutated not only in hereditary tumours in VHL patients but also in sporadic cases of the same tumours. For example, the VHL gene is the most frequently mutated cancer related gene identified to date in sporadic renal cell carcinoma (Shuin et al., 1994). Tumour development is due to inactivation or loss of the remaining wild-type allele in a susceptible cell. The highly vascular nature of the VHL associated tumours may be explained by the fact that under normal conditions, the VHL gene product (p VHL) negatively regulates the hypoxia-inducible mRNA encoding vascular endothelial growth factor (VEGF) under normoxic conditions (Kaelin et al., 1998). Thus with VHL disease, loss of this p VHL leads to an inappropriate accumulation of this m RNA and results in a dramatic upregulation of VEGF in stromal cells and of its corresponding receptors VEGFR-1 and VEGFR-2 in tumour endothelial cells. It is thought that this signalling pathway may play a role in angiogenesis and cyst formation of these lesions (Wizigmann-Voos et al., 1995). In addition to its role in angiogenesis regulation, the p VHL is a tumour suppressor protein also known to play a role in regulating extracellular matrix formation and regulating the ability of cells to exit the cell cycle (Ohh et al., 1999).

Diagnostic criteria

Clinical diagnosis of VHL disease is based on the presence of (a) multiple hemangioblastomas of the central nervous system or (b) one hemangioblastoma in association with a known associated visceral manifestation (as described below) or (c) one visceral or central nervous system manifestation in a patient with an affected first-order family member (Filling-Katz et al., 1989).

The constellation of visceral lesions associated with VHL disease include two neoplasms and various cysts. Associated neoplasms are renal clear cell carcinoma (25–40% cases of VHL) which is bilateral in 15% of VHL cases and in only 1.8% of sporadic cases (Vermillion et al., 1972), and pheochromocytoma (10% cases of VHL). Solid organ cysts (50–70% cases of VHL) may be seen in the kidney, pancreas, adrenals, and epididymis and more rarely in liver, skin, ovary, lungs and spleen.

Central nervous system hemangioblastomas are seen in over 60% of cases of VHL which may be multiple in up to half of these (Neumann et al., 1992). Sites of predilection for hemangioblastoma within the central nervous system include the cerebellum, the brainstem (particularly the medulla) and the spinal cord parenchyma although they can occur anywhere along the neuraxis. Cerebellar hemangiomas are by far the most common central nervous system manifestation of the disease, followed by metastases from renal cell carcinoma while supratentorial hemangioblastomas (Neumann et al., 1992; Levine et al., 1982; Ho et al., 1992; Huson et al., 1986), optic nerve hemangioblastomas (Raila et al., 1997; Kerr et al., 1995) and endolymphatic sac tumours (Kempermann et al., 1996; Ouallet et al., 1997) have all been rarely described in the context of VHL disease. Other characteristic features of the typical central nervous system hemangioblastoma in VHL disease include a high frequency of multiplicity (so-called 'hemangioblastomatosis'), and occasional production and release of erythropoiesis-stimulating factor with resultant secondary polycythemia. This hematological manifestation is, strictly speaking, an erythrocythemia without leukocytosis, thrombocytosis or splenomegaly, with increased values of hematocrit, hemoglobin, blood mass and an erythroblastosis on bone marrow examination (Resche et al., 1993). Erythropoetic activity has been described in the aspirated cyst fluid (Skultety et al., 1970). Erythrocytosis is most often seen with solid hemangioblastomas producing erythropoiesis-stimulating factor (Cramer & Kimsey, 1952; Resche, 1971), and may resolve upon tumour resection. It is often more prominent with recurrent hemangioblastoma than with initial presentation and regresses with complete tumour resection. Such findings were observed in 18% of surgical cases on initial presentation and in 63.6% of recurrences in one series (Cramer & Kimsey, 1952). Thus, its appearance may be a harbinger for tumor recurrence. The precise nature of the erythropoiesis-stimulating factor of hemangioblastoma origin is uncertain, and it may be either ectopic erythropoetin or a form of precursor (Resche et al., 1993).

Retinal hemangioblastomas (von Hippel's disease) are seen in 40–50% of cases of VHL and are histologically identical to the central nervous system lesions. Retinal lesions are multiple in one-third and bilateral in one-half of cases (Braffman et al., 1990) and can be readily seen on fundoscopic examination in the absence of hemorrhage and subretinal exudate.

Clinical presentation

In general, hemangioblastomas present earlier in patients with VHL disease than in sporadic cases, the mean age at diagnosis being 5.6 years earlier than in sporadic cases. In one series, the mean age for males with familial disease at presentation was $31(+/-11.6)$ years and for females $28.7(+/-11)$ years (Resche et al., 1993). Clinical presentation of central nervous system hemangioblastoma before puberty is very uncommon. Retinal hemangioblastomas typically manifest clinically in the third decade, hemangioblastomas of the brain and spinal cord in the fourth decade and renal cell carcinoma in the fifth decade.

Overall, males are more commonly affected with hemangioblastoma with a ratio of 1.5:1 male to female. From a series of VHL patients with retinal and cerebellar hemangiomas, the initial presenting lesion was retinal in 62 cases, and was followed by cerebellar manifestations in 31 of these patients within 10 years and in a further 16 patients more than 10 years after initial presentation (Resche et al., 1985). Retinal hemangioblastomas may present with progressive visual loss or with ocular pain (Resche et al., 1993). With posterior fossa hemangioblastoma, headache is the most common presenting symptom. Associated vomiting when present suggests raised intracranial pressure. Other presenting symptoms are ataxia and gait disturbance. Rare symptoms include abnormal head attitudes and the so-called cerebellar 'fits' (Resche et al., 1993). An abnormal neurological examination was found in 87.7% of cases in a series, with the remaining

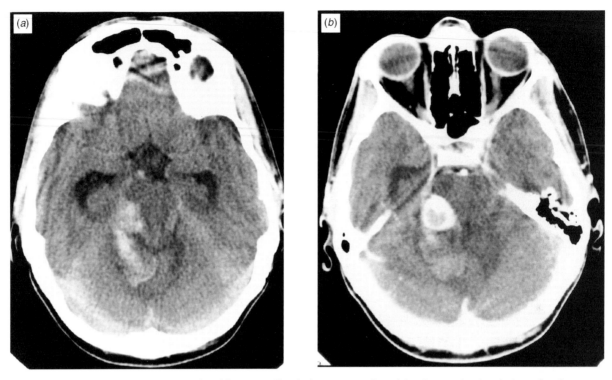

Fig. 45.1. 35-year-old woman presenting with sudden onset of headache, nausea and vomiting. On examination she is confused, somnolent, showing mesenecephalic as well as cerebellar signs. Non-enhanced CT-scan (*a*) shows a superior vermian hemorrhage with mass effect and compression of the IV ventricle and secondary obstructive hydrocephalus. Note also the presence of subarachnoid blood. The enhanced CT-scan (*b*) reveals a markedly enhancing lesion in the right superior cerebellar peduncle. Surgical resection confirmed the diagnosis of hemangioblastoma. (By courtesy of Dr P. Maeder, Department of Radiology, Centre Hospitalier Universitaire Vaudois, Lausanne.)

12.3% being normal (Resche et al., 1993). Clinical presentation of supratentorial hemangioblastomas depends on location, and these present similarly to other supratentorial mass lesions.

Most familial cases exhibit multiple CNS hemangiomas associated with visceral lesions, however there is interfamily variability. For example, pheochromocytoma may be prominent in certain predisposed VHL families whilst in others, renal cell carcinoma appears to predominate, and in others still, there may be a predilection for spinal hemangioblastomas (Resche et al., 1993).

Presentation of hemangioblastomas with a stroke syndrome is rare despite their highly vascular nature. Spontaneous hemorrhage due to any underlying tumour accounts for only 3.0–7.5% of all spontaneous intracerebral hemorrhages (Zimmerman & Balaniuk, 1980). Most of these occur in glial and metastatic lesions, meningiomas and tumours of reticuloendothelial origin. They infrequently occur in ependymomas, choroid plexus papillomas, and hemangioblastomas (Agegbite et al., 1983).

Although the occurrence of microscopic subclinical hemorrhages in hemangioblastomas is known (Russell & Rubenstein, 1977; Rubenstein, 1970), presentation in the form of clinically apparent intracranial subarachnoid or parenchymal hemorrhage (Figs. 45.1, 45.2) is decidedly uncommon and accounted for only 2% of the 262 cases in the French Society of Neurosurgery series (Resche et al., 1985). There are several reports of gross hemorrhage with posterior fossa hemangioblastomas (Skultety et al., 1970; Resche, 1971; Wakai et al., 1984; Wagenvoort et al., 1962; Raynor & Kingman, 1965; Mondkar et al., 1967; Meredith & Hennigar, 1954; Matsumara et al., 1985; Ismail & Cole, 1984; Green & Vaughan, 1972; Chapman et al., 1959) and also with supratentorial lesions (Agegbite et al., 1983; Wakai et al., 1984). Case fatalities following acute hemorrhage have also been described (Agegbite et al., 1983; Meredith & Hennigar, 1954; Ismail & Cole, 1984; Boker et al., 1984)

Precise clinical presentation depends on the localization and extent of the spontaneous hemorrhage in each case. In

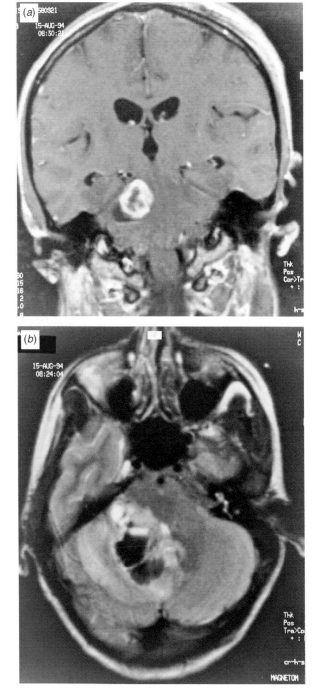

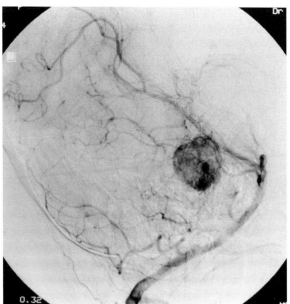

Fig. 45.3. Selective lateral vertebral angiography showing a highly vascular mass typical of hemangioblastoma. (By courtesy from Dr P. Maeder, Department of Radiology, Centre Hospitalier Universitaire Vaudois, Lausanne.)

Fig. 45.2. T_1-weighted coronal MRI (*a*) showing a markedly enhancing lesion in the right superior cerebellar peduncle that presented with vermian and subarachnoid hemorrhage. Note also the associated cyst suggestive of hemangioblastoma. T_2-weighted axial MRI (*b*) showing the typical finding of an acute hemorrhage. Same case as Fig. 45.1, after emergent external ventricular drainage. (By courtesy of Dr P. Maeder, Department of Radiology, Centre Hospitalier Universitaire Vaudois, Lausanne.

a series of six cases of spontaneous hemorrhage secondary to hemangioblastoma, the patients were between 2 and 74 years at presentation (mean 44 years), whose initial clinical presentation was decreased level of consciousness, generalized seizures, nausea, vomiting and focal neurological deficits. Four of these six cases were supratentorial lesions. In each case, a typical contrasting enhancing mass was masked by acute hemorrhage, and angiography (Fig. 45.3) revealed abnormal vessels or blush in only two cases. However, at surgery, a highly vascular mass was identified within the hematoma wall in each case (Wakai et al., 1984). In a separate reported case, no obvious source of hemorrhage was found at surgical exploration (Matsumara et al., 1985).

Spontaneous intracranial hemorrhage in the context of known VHL disease also provokes the question of the presence of intracranial metastatic renal clear cell carcinoma which is susceptible to intratumoural hemorrhage. According to Horton et al. (1976), renal cell carcinoma has already metastasized in more than 50% of cases at the time of diagnosis.

An unusual phenomenon associated with intracranial hemangioblastoma and probably of vascular etiology is the occurrence of pulsatile tinnitus (Williamson, 1892; Sargent & Greenfield, 1929; Daum & LeBeau, 1963).

Investigations

Detailed investigation starts with a thorough physical examination bearing in mind all the potential manifestations of VHL disease. In addition to a neurological examination, fundoscopy, abdominal and genital examinations are most pertinent. Laboratory investigations should include red cell count, hemoglobin, hematocrit, serum epinephrine and norepinephrine, a 24-hour urinary analysis for vanillylmandelic acid and catecholamine levels. Total neuraxis MRI scan is conducted with and without gadolinium. Selective cerebral angiography depending on the tumour location is often also necessary. Finally, use abdominal CT scanning with intravenous contrast to detect visceral lesions (Vernet & de Tribolet, 1999).

Cerebral CT scanning typically reveals a hypodense cerebellar cyst with an isodense non-calcified mural nodule on the part of the cyst closest to a pial surface which enhances brightly with administration of intravenous contrast. Cyst wall contains gliotic tissue which is typically non-enhancing. Occasionally, prominent feeding vessels of the tumour can be seen with IV contrast injection.

MRI of the entire neuraxis is indispensable for delineating single or multiple hemangiomas. Cystic lesions appear hypointense on T_1-weighted and hyperintense on T_2-weighted images with minimal edema and an isointense mural nodule which enhances intensely with intravenous gadolinium. Solid hemangioblastomas typically enhance intensely and uniformly with gadolinium. Vascular flow voids of prominent vessels may also be seen. Cerebral CT and MRI (Figs. 45.1, 45.2) will also confirm the presence of hydrocephalus in such affected cases. Differential diagnosis of the typical single lesion on MRI are pilocytic astrocytoma (more common in children), pleomorphic xanthoastrocytoma (uncommon in the cerebellum) or metastasis (common in the posterior fossa but rarely cystic).

Conventional angiography should be used selectively for the purposes of surgical planning for larger posterior fossa lesions (Fig. 45.3). It shows in detail the vascular pedicle, which may be of mixed pial-dural origin, and often an early draining vein indicating AV shunting. The solid mass/mural nodule shows up as a dense prolonged vascular stain. If indicated for a posterior fossa lesion, bilateral vertebral injections are necessary and should include posterior inferior cerebellar arteries. Large solid hemangioblastomas with high flow on angiography may occasionally mimic an arteriovenous malformation.

It should be noted that radiological absence of a typical cystic component raises the real possibility of a metastatic renal cell carcinoma in view of the known association of these lesions, however the two can be readily differentiated histologically.

Treatment

A patient presenting with a hemorrhage in the posterior fossa warrants an emergency neurosurgical consultation. Urgent surgical evacuation of the hematoma with the underlying hemangioblastoma may be life saving, and is particularly indicated in these rare instances of acute hemorrhagic presentation of a hemangioblastoma. These patients with VHL tend to present at a younger age than most with spontaneous intracerebral hemorrhage, most have a reasonable overall prognosis (in the absence of renal cell carcinoma) and some may be known VHL patients. Acute hydrocephalus induced by a posterior fossa hematoma may be treated initially with external ventricular drainage with smaller hematomas (Figs. 45.1, 45.2).

With regard to cerebral lesions, surgical resection is the treatment of choice for symptomatic hemangioblastomas as a complete resection is possible in most cases. At surgery, it usually appears as a highly vascular nodule and usually abuts the leptomeninges. Surgical attack of cystic lesions should be targeted only at the enhancing mural nodule and cyst wall should only be resected in those rare 'purely' cystic lesions without a mural nodule evident radiologically or at the time of surgery. Further details of surgical technique are beyond the scope of this chapter but may be found elsewhere (Vernet & de Tribolet, 1999). Postoperative mortality for cerebellar hemangioblastomas has been reported as high as 16%, being higher for solid tumours (Resche et al., 1985). This may be explained in part by the multisystem nature of the disease and the multitude of potential complications. Of particular surgical relevance is difficulty with control of systemic blood pressure as a previously unsuspected pheochromocytoma is unmasked under general anesthesia. Some of the above surgical results date from the premicrosurgical era and may not extrapolate to modern standards. It is also known that in patients with hemangioblastomatosis, resection of one tumour may lead to the development of other previously quiescent tumours (Resche et al., 1993). The mechanism of this remains unknown, but lends credence to a policy of observing and not operating on asymptomatic lesions. However, patients with incidentally discovered asymptomatic lesions should also be subjected to a full investigation as previously discussed.

Radiation treatment reduces tumour size and vascularity but may not prevent regrowth. Size reduction has been measured on pre- and postirradiation angiograms to be in the order of 15–55% in various studies (Helle et al., 1980; Vinci and Lostia, 1972), whilst in others, no size reduction was noted (Lamont et al., 1984). The role of radiation is limited and it has been recommended for non resectable or recurrent tumours of the high cervical cord or medulla

(Smalley et al., 1990). Currently, the role of radiosurgery remains to be fully elucidated and may prove to be useful particularly for brainstem lesions not abutting a pial surface.

Management of spinal, retinal and visceral lesions is beyond the scope of this chapter and will not discussed.

Prognosis/outcome

Survival depends largely on the presence or otherwise of visceral lesions particularly renal cell carcinoma (25–40% of VHL cases). The main factors at the time of diagnosis predicting a poor prognosis in affected patients are the presence of multiple CNS hemangioblastomas, the association of CNS and retinal hemangioblastomas, and onset of disease before the age of 30 years (Resche et al., 1993). The development of an adjacent primary lesion must be considered in cases of 'recurrence' after total resection.

Conclusions

With younger patients who present with spontaneous intracerebral hemorrhage, particularly in the posterior fossa, one may add hemangioblastoma as part of a differential diagnosis. The possibility of the VHL syndrome should be entertained in the context of (i) multiple cerebral lesions, particularly cystic masses in the posterior fossa of a young patient, or (ii) progressive visual loss with retinal lesions or (iii) suggestive family history. Such patients should be examined with this possibility in mind and other 'stigmata' of the VHL complex should be sought.

Screening for VHL disease following the diagnosis of a cerebral hemangioblastoma is warranted given the high risk of associated lesions with hereditary forms. The most commonly associated lesions are cerebellar and retinal hemangioblastomas, a pattern which occurs in 25% of VHL cases (Resche et al., 1993), so the diagnosis of VHL disease can occasionally be made on fundoscopy following the discovery of a typical posterior fossa hemangioblastoma. Direct genetic testing is available for patients affected with VHL disease where the majority of germline mutations can be detected. This mutational analysis has proved to be of important prognostic significance and gene testing has become an important tool in the management of VHL patients. Further understanding of the function of the VHL gene product will inevitably lead to treatment strategies targeted at a molecular level. Thus the importance of early detection and long-term follow-up cannot be over-emphasized to recognize affected individuals and at-risk relatives. In this way, one can avoid complications and treat lesions at an earlier presymptomatic stage, thus leading to improved quality of life and better long -term prognosis (Levine et al., 1982; Green, 1986; Lamiell et al., 1989).

References

Agegbite, A.B., Rozdilsky, B. & Varughese, G. (1983). Supratentorial capillary hemangioblastoma presenting with fatal spontaneous intracerebral hemorrhage. *Neurosurgery*, **12**, 327–30.

Boker, D.K., Wasserman, H. & Solymosi, L. (1984). Multiple spinal hemangioblastomas in a case of Lindau's disease. *Surgical Neurology*, **22**, 439–43.

Braffman, B.H., Bilanuik, C.T. & Zimmermann, R.A. (1990). MR of central nervous system neoplasia of the phakomatoses. *Seminars in Roentgenology*, **25**, 198–217.

Burger, P.C. & Scheithauer, B.W. (1994). *Tumors of the Central Nervous System*. Washington DC: Armed Forces Institute of Pathology.

Chapman, R.C., Kemp, V.E. & Taliaferro, I. (1959). Pheochromocytoma associated with multiple neurofibromatosis and intracranial hemangioma. *American Journal of Medicine*, **26**, 883–90.

Cramer, F. & Kimsey, W. (1952). The cerebellar hemangioblastomas: review of fifty-three cases, with special reference to cerebellar cysts and association of polycythemia. *Archives of Neurology and Psychiatry*, **67**, 237–52.

Daum, S. & Le Beau, J. (1963). Hemangioblastome du cervelet opere au même age chez la mère et le fils (maladie de von Hippel-Lindau). *Revue Neurologique (Paris)*, **108**, 50–4.

Decker, H.J., Klauck, S.M., Lawrence, J.B. et al. (1994). Cytogenetic and fluorescence in situ hybridization studies on sporadic and hereditary tumors associated with von Hippel–Lindau syndrome(VHL). *Cancer Genetics and Cytogenetics*, **7**(1), 1–13.

Filling-Katz, M.R., Choyke, P.L., Patronas, N.J. et al. (1989). Radiologic screening for von Hippel–Lindau Disease: the role of Gd-DTPA enhanced MR imaging of the CNS. *Journal of Computer Assisted Tomography*, **13**, 743–55.

Green, J.R. & Vaughan, R.J. (1972). Blood vessel tumours and hematomas of the posterior fossa in adolescence. *Angiology*, **23**, 475–87.

Green, J.S. (1986). Von Hippel–Lindau disease in a Newfoundland kindred. *Canadian Medical Association Journal*, **134**, 133–46.

Helle, T.L., Conley, F.K. & Britt, R.H. (1980). Effect of radiation therapy on hemangioblastoma: a case report and review of the literature. *Neurosurgery*, **6**, 82–6.

Ho, V.B., Smirniotopoulos, J.G., Murphy, F.M. et al. (1992). Radiologic–pathologic correlation: hemangioblastoma. *American Journal of Neuroradiology*, **13**, 1343–52.

Horton, W.A., Wong, V. & Eldridge, R. (1976). Von Hippel–Lindau disease. Clinical and pathological manifestations in nine families with 50 affected members. *Archives of Internal Medicine*, **136**, 769–77.

Hosoe, S., Brauch, H., Latif, F. et al. (1990). Localization of the von

Hippel–Lindau disease to a small region of chromosome 3. *Genomics*, **8**, 634–40.

Huson, S.M., Harper, P.S., Hourihan, M.D. et al. (1986). Cerebellar hemangioblastoma and von Hippel–Lindau disease. *Brain*, **109**, 1297–310.

Ismail, S.M. & Cole, G. (1984). Von Hippel–Lindau syndrome with microscopic hemangioblastomas of the spinal nerve roots. *Journal of Neurosurgery*, **60**, 1279–81.

Kaelin, W.G., Illopoulos, O., Lonergan, K.M. et al. (1998). Functions of the von Hippel–Lindau tumour suppressor protein. *Journal of Internal Medicine*, **243**(6), 535–9.

Kempermann, G., Neumann, H.P., Scheremet, R. et al. (1996). Deafness due to bilateral endolymphatic sac tumours in a case of von Hippel–Lindau syndrome. *Journal of Neurology, Neurosurgery and Psychiatry*, **61**(3), 318–20.

Kerr, D.J., Scheithauer, B.W., Miller, G.M. et al. (1995). Hemangioblastoma of the optic nerve: case report. *Neurosurgery*, **36**(3), 573–80.

Lamiell, J.M., Salazar, F.G. & Hsia, Y.E. (1989). Von Hippel–Lindau disease affecting 43 members of a single kindred. *Medicine*, **68**, 1–29.

Lamont, P.M., Jacobson, I., Gunn, A. et al. (1984). Lindau's disease and familial hyperparathyroidism. *Surgical Neurology*, **22**, 36–8.

Levine, E., Collins, D.L., Horton, W.A. et al. (1982). CT screening of the abdomen in von Hippel–Lindau disease. *American Journal of Radiology*, **139**, 505–10.

Matsumura, A., Maki, Y., Munekata, K. et al. (1985). Intracerebellar hemorrhage due to cerebellar hemangioblastoma. *Surgical Neurology*, **24**, 227–30.

Meredith, J.M. & Hennigar, G.R. (1954). Cerebellar hemangiomas; a clinico-pathologic study of fourteen cases. *American Surgery*, **20**, 410–23.

Mondkar, V.P., McKissock, W. & Russell, R.W.R. (1967). Cerebellar hemangioblastomas. *British Journal of Surgery*, **54**, 45–9.

Neumann, H.P.H., Eggert, H.R., Scheremet, R. et al. (1992). Central Nervous System Lesions in von Hippel–Lindau Syndrome. *Journal of Neurology, Neurosurgery and Psychiatry*, **55**, 898–901.

Ohh, M. & Kaelin, W.G. Jr. (1999). The von Hippel–Lindau tumour supressor protein: new perspectives. *Molecular Medicine Today*, **5**(6), 257–63.

Ouallet, J.C., Marsot-Dupuch, K., Van Effenterre, R. et al. (1997). Papillary adenoma of endolymphatic sac origin: a temporal bone tumor in von Hippel–Lindau disease. Case report. *Journal of Neurosurgery*, **87**(3), 445–9.

Raila, F.A., Zimmermann, J., Azordegan, P. et al. (1997). Successful surgical removal of an asymptomatic optic nerve hemangioblastoma in von Hippel–Lindau disease. *Journal of Neuroimaging*, **7**(1), 48–50.

Raynor, R.B. & Kingman, A.F. Jr. (1965).Hemangioblastoma and vascular malformations as one lesion. *Archives of Neurology*, **12**, 39–48.

Rengachary, S.S. (1985). Hemangioblastoma. In *Neurosurgery*, ed. R.H. Wilkins & S.S. Rengachary. New York: McGraw-Hill.

Resche, F. (1971). Les angioreticulomes-hemangioblastomes-du nevraxe. *Thesis Nantes*, No. 875:1–147.

Resche, F., Chabannes, J., Combelles, G. et al. (1985). Les hemangioblastome infra-tentoriels. *Neurochirurgie*, **31**, 91–149.

Resche, F., Moisan, J.P., Mantoura, J. et al. (1993). Haemangioblastoma, Haemangioblastosis, and von Hippel–Lindau Disease. In *Advances and Technical Standards in Neurosurgery*, ed. L. Symon, L. Calliauw, F. Cohadon et al., pp. 197–303. Wien, New York: Springer-Verlag.

Rubenstein, L.J. (1970). Tumors of the central nervous system. *Atlas of Tumors*, pp. 235–40. Washington DC: Armed Forces Institute of Nervous Pathology.

Russell, D.S. & Rubenstein, L.J., eds. (1977). *Pathology of Tumors of the Nervous System* 4th edn, pp. 116–27. London: E. Arnold.

Sargent, P. & Greenfield, J.G. (1929). Haemangeiomatous cysts of the cerebellum. *British Journal of Surgery*, **17**, 84–101.

Shuin, T., Kondo, K., Torigoe, S. et al. (1994). Frequent somatic mutations and loss of heterozygosity of the von Hippel–Lindau tumor suppressor gene in primary human renal cell carcinomas. *Cancer Research*, **54**(11), 2852–5.

Skultety, F.M., Sorrell, M.F. & Burcklund, C.W. (1970). Hemangioblastoma of the cerebellum associated with erythrocytosis and an unusual blood supply. Case report. *Journal of Neurosurgery*, **32**, 700–5.

Smalley, S.R., Schomberg, P.J., Earle, J.D. et al. (1990). Radiotherapeutic considerations in the treatment of hemangioblastomas of the central nervous system. *International Journal of Radiation, Oncology and Biological Physics*, **18**, 1165–71.

Vermillion, C.D., Skinner, D.G. & Pfister, R.C. (1972). Bilateral renal cell carcinoma. *Journal of Urology*, **108**, 219–22.

Vernet, O. & de Tribolet, N. (1999). Posterior fossa hemangioblastoma. In *Operative Neurosurgery*, 1st edn, ed. A. Kaye & P.M. Black, pp. 635–40. W.B. Saunders.

Vinci, A. & Lostia, G. (1972). Angioreticulomi cerebellari: modificazioni regressive indotte dalla radioterapia in un caso documentato mediante l'indagine neuroradiologica. *Bulletin Science Medicale*, **144**, 131–40.

Wagenvoort, C.A., Baggenstoss, A.H. & Love, J.G. (1962). Subarachnoid hemorrhage due to cerebellar hemangioma associated with congenital hepatic fibrosis and polycystic kidneys: report of case. *Proceedings of the Mayo Clinics*, **37**, 301–6.

Wakai, S., Inoh, S., Ueda, Y. et al. (1984). Hemangioblastoma presenting with intraparenchymatous hemorrhage. *Journal of Neurosurgery*, **61**, 956–60.

Williamson, R.T. (1892). Serous cysts in the cerebellum. *American Journal of Medical Science*, **104**, 151–7.

Wizigmann-Voos, S., Breier, G., Risau, W. et al. (1995). Up-regulation of vascular endothelial growth factor and its receptors in von Hippel–Lindau disease-associated and sporadic hemangioblastomas. *Cancer Research*, **55**(6), 1358–64.

Zimmerman, R.A. & Bilaniuk, L.T. (1980). Computed tomography of acute intratumoral hemorrhage. *Radiology*, **135**, 355–9.

46

Cerebrovascular manifestations in neurofibromatosis

Alain Carruzzo and Julien Bogousslavsky

Department of Neurology, University of Lausanne, Switzerland

General considerations

Neurofibromatosis (NF), first described in 1882 by Friedrich von Recklinghausen, is an autosomal dominant disorder occurring in one in 3000 or 3200 individuals (Crow et al., 1956). The genes for the two main types, NF 1 and NF 2, have been located on chromosomes 17 and 22, respectively. About 50% of cases of NF 1 are due to spontaneous mutation and family history is negative. Main clinical features include café-au-lait spots, neurofibroma and axillary or inguinal freckling. The phenotype is quite variable, so that a thorough clinical examination is sometimes needed to detect cutaneous or ocular stigmata (for diagnostic criteria, see Riccardi 1992). When present, hamartoma of the iris (so-called Lisch spots) are considered to be specific of NF 1.

Since the first observation of Reubi (1944), vascular pathologies in NF have been observed in cases of NF 1 only. The best-known vascular manifestation is renal hypertension, which occurs in about 1% of patients with neurofibromatosis. In NF patients, though, most cerebrovascular events result from NF 1-specific focal arterial disease, and not from hypertensive microangiopathy. In older patients, the prevalence of cardiovascular and cerebrovascular disease does not differ from the general population. Although anecdotal association has been reported (Hilal et al., 1971), there is no conclusive evidence that radiotherapy for optic gliomas is a significant cause of cerebral arteriopathy in NF 1 patients (Rudoltz et al., 1998).

Pathological findings

In his 1944 autoptic study, Reubi described two main types of arterial lesions in thymic and renal arteries of a patient in NF 1: an occlusive intimal form affecting small arteries and an aneurysmal form with replacement of the muscular wall with fibrohyaline thickening in arterioles of 0.1–1 mm. Subsequent microscopic examination of specimens of diseased intracranial or carotid arteries mostly revealed hyperplasia of the intima and fragmentation or reduplication of the internal elastica. Thinning of the media was also described in one case of aneurysma of an intracranial vessel (Greene et al., 1974).

Reubi originally proposed the proliferating intimal cells to be of neural origin (i.e. derived from Schwann cells). Aided with immunohistochemistry and ultrastructural studies, later investigators concluded that these cells probably are of muscular origin in both cerebral and renal vessels (Greene et al., 1974; Malecha & Rubin, 1992). Although NF 1 is caused by a mutation of the gene encoding neurofibromin, we have no clear picture yet of the role that this protein might play in the vascular pathology of NF 1 (Schievink, 1997; Shen et al., 1996). Intimal cell proliferation can be found in stenosed, dilated or grossly normal arteries, suggesting that it may be a general mechanism for vascular involvement in NF (Malecha & Rubin, 1992).

Clinical manifestations (Fig. 46.1)

In NF 1, both occlusive and dilatative arterial disorder are encountered. As for neural or cutaneous stigmata, there is a great variation of number and severity of the vascular lesions from one patient to the other. Familial occurrence of arterial occlusive disease is anecdotal (Erickson et al., 1980). Ischemic symptoms may occur at any age, but more than half of the reported cases concerned children or young adults. Vascular anomalies may be present in intra- or extracranial arteries. Carotid or vertebral arteries are commonly involved, but also other neck arteries (a. pharyngea ascendens or truncus thyreo-cervicalis) (Anegawa

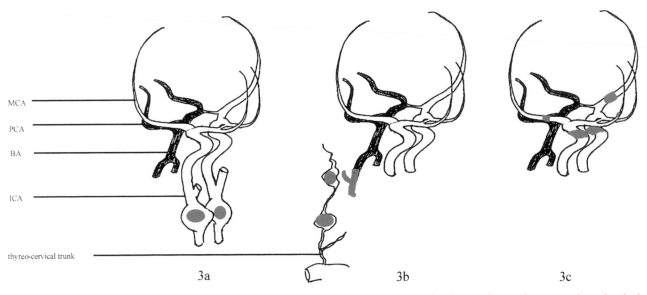

Fig. 46.1. Schematic representation of various types of vascular abnormalities associated with NF 1 (abnormal segments shown hatched). (*a*) Bilateral aneurysms of common carotid arteries (modified from Malecha et al., 1992). (*b*) Occlusion of distal vertebral artery associated with a pseudo-aneurysm of the thyreo-cervical trunk (own patient, see Fig. 46.2. (*c*) Multiple stenoses/occlusions of major intracranial arteries. MCA = middle cerebral artery, PCA = posterior cerebral artery, BA = basilar artery, ICA = internal carotid artery.

et al., 1997; Latchaw et al., 1980; Smith & White, 1974; Wada et al., 1989). Sometimes, many other major arteries are affected as well (Debure et al., 1984).

Stroke, intracranial hematoma and subarachnoidal bleeding are the most common clinical manifestations in NF 1. Stroke or transient ischemic attacks can be unique, recurrent in the same or in different territories. Ocular involvement has been reported, including both occlusive disorder (retinal arteries) (Tholen et al., 1998) and global ocular ischemia (Barral & Summers, 1996). In NF 1, whole regions may show dysplastic vessels, a feature which gives the disease peculiar features. A classical clinical manifestation is laterocervical hematoma, due to aneurysm of the vertebral artery or another neck artery, quite often combined with arterio-venous fistulae (Schievink & Piepgras, 1991). In case of a large vertebral aneurysm, plexus palsy or even medullary compression with paraparesis may result (Anegawa et al., 1997; Schubiger & Yasargil, 1978; Wada et al., 1989). Fusiform aneurysma of the intrapetrosal part of the carotid artery may result in abducens palsy.

Occlusive disorder

Stenoses in NF 1 differ from those in atherosclerotic lesions in that they generally do not occur at sites of maximal flow turbulence, like the origin of vertebral artery or the carotid bifurcation. The vertebral artery, for instance, may be narrowed in the V3 or V4 portion rather than at the origin. When affected, the internal carotid artery is almost always narrowed in the supraclinoidal portion, not infrequently on both sides (Malecha & Rubin, 1992; Momose & New, 1973; Gebarski et al., 1983; Götze & Kühne, 1976; Klatte et al., 1976; Lamas et al., 1978; Levisohn et al., 1978; Vignes et al., 1973). Every artery of large or medium calibre can be affected, and some patients have multiple stenoses of intracranial vessels combined with stenoses or occlusion of carotid arteries (Gebarski et al., 1983; Pellock et al, 1980; Taboada et al., 1979). Voigt reported one case with multiple intracranial stenoses in only one hemisphere, with stealing mechanisms from one hemisphere to the other (Voigt & Beck, 1971). The majority of reported cases concern hemispheric territorial infarction, often in the superficial territory of the middle cerebral artery (de Kersaint-Gilly et al., 1980; Gilly et al., 1982; Levisohn et al., 1978; Pellock et al., 1980; Rossi Lopez et al., 1985).

Many cases found in the literature were probably partly published because of spectacular angiographic findings (including moya-moya), so that there might be a bias towards lesions of large or middle-sized vessels. We have personally seen one case of laterobulbar infarction and two cases of hemispheric lacunar infarction in which, in the absence of other cerebrovascular risk factors, the ischemic lesion was most probably due to neurofibromatosis (A. Carruzzo & J. Bogousslavsky, unpublished data).

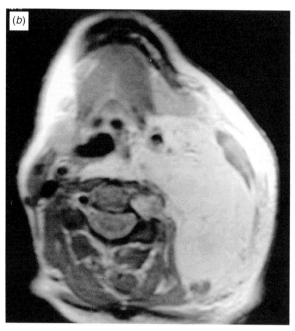

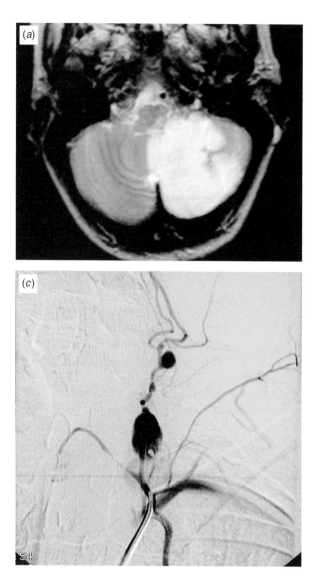

Fig. 46.2. (*a*) T$_2$-weighted MR showing an acute ischemic infarction in the territory of the posterior inferior cerebellar artery (PICA). (*b*) Two days later, T$_2$-weighted MR showing a voluminous left lateral cervical soft tissue bleeding consecutive to the rupture of a pseudoaneurysm of the thyreo-cervical trunk. (*c*) Conventional angiography showing a displasic left thyreo-cervical trunk with two pseudoaneurysms; coiling was attempted without success and surgical ligation of the subclavian artery had to be performed in emergency. (Courtesy of Dr Maeder, Radiology, Lausanne, CHUV.)

Aneurysms

Intracranial aneurysms may be saccular or fusiform. They may be found on the circle of Willis, but also more distally or on other vessels like the posterior choroid artery (Leone et al., 1982). Intracranial aneurysms commonly present as subarachnoidal hemorrhage (Bergouignan & Arne, 1951). Aneurysms of the vertebral artery, especially when combined with arteriovenous fistulae, may cause laterocervical hematoma, or even compression of brachial plexus or the spinal cord (Anegawa et al., 1997; Schubiger & Yasargil, 1978; Wada et al., 1989). Fusiform aneurysma of the intracranial portion of the carotid artery may be associated with sphenoid wing dysplasy and cranial nerve palsies (VI) (Steel et al., 1994). It is not clear though if patients with NF 1 have

a significantly increased risk of developing an aneurysm and should benefit from a screening when asymptomatic. Rupture of cervical aneurysma shortly after chiropractic manipulations has been reported (Lennington et al., 1980).

Radiological findings (Fig. 46.2)

Various angiographic patterns can be found. When intimal hyperplasia spreads over long distances, the arteries appear hypoplastic without luminal stenosis (Leone et al., 1982). Focal concentric stenosis or irregular narrowing over a long distance, remembering fibromuscular dysplasia, is also encountered. Other typical findings include bilateral fusiform aneurysm of the carotid siphon.

Vertebral arteries are particularly prone to develop arterio-venous fistulae. In this latter case, the fistula can be combined with stenoses and pseudoaneurysmal dilatation of the feeding arterial vessel.

Probably because occlusive disorder progresses in a slow fashion, extensive collateral pathways may develop. In case of bilateral carotid stenosis or/and occlusion, moyamoya staining is almost invariably found at angiography; in many cases of proximal stenoses of intracranial arteries, collateralization through leptomeningeal anastomoses, i.e. anastomosis from the external carotid artery, and through the circle of Willis, can be observed.

Diagnosis and treatment

Because they may have multiple stenoses of major intracranial vessels or asymptomatic aneurysms, patients with NF1 and stroke should benefit from extensive neuroradiological work-up including conventional angiography or angio-MRI.

Surgery or angioplasty can be performed to minimize the natural risk of hemorrhage in case of aneurysms or arterio-venous malformations, especially in extracranial malformations originating from the vertebral artery (Negoro et al., 1990). Because many of these malformations are tortuous or have several feeding arteries, embolization may be difficult to realize or allow only partial occlusion of feeding vessels; in some cases, surgery is still necessary after endovascular treatment (Latchaw et al., 1980). In NF 1, diseased vessels are often fragile; massive hemorrhage is thus a feared complication of both surgery and endovascular treatment. Stroke management and prophylactic drug treatment do not differ from those in stroke of atheromatous origin.

References

Anegawa, S., Hayashi, T., Torigoe, R. et al. (1997). Symptomatic arteriovenous fistula in a patient with neurofibromatosis type 1. *No Shinkei Geka*, **25**, 373–8.

Barral, J.L. & Summers, C.G. (1996). Ocular ischemic syndrome in a child with moyamoya disease and neurofibromatosis. *Survey of Ophthalmology*, **40**, 500–4.

Bergouignan, M. & Arne, L. (1951). A propos des anévrysmes des artères cérébrales associés à d'autres malformations. *Acta Neurologica et Psychiatrica Belgica*, **51**, 529–35.

Crow, F.W., Schull, J. & Neel, J.V. (1956). A Clinical, *Pathological and Genetical Study of Multiple Neurofibromatosis*. Illinois: Charles C. Thomas Springfield.

Debure, C., Fiessinger, J.N., Bruneval, P., Vuong, N.P., Cormier, J.M. & Housset, E. (1984). Lésions artérielles multiples au cours de la maladie de von Recklinghausen: une observation. *Presse Medicin*, **13**, 1776–8.

de Kersaint-Gilly, A., Zenthe, L., Dabouis, G. et al. (1980). Anomalies de modelage des vaisseaux intra-cérébraux dans une observation de neurofibromatose de Recklinghausen. *Journal of Neuroradiology*, **7**, 193–8.

Erickson, R.P., Woolliscroft, J. & Allen, R.J. (1980). Familial occurrence of intracranial arterial occlusive disease (Moyamoya) in neurofibromatosis. *Clinical Genetics*, **18**, 191–6.

Gebarski, S.S., Gabrielsern, T.O., Knake, J.E. & Latack, J.T. (1983). Posterior circulation intracranial arterial occlusive disease in neurofibromatosis. *American Journal of Neuroradiology*, **4**, 1245–6.

Gilly, R., Elbaz, N., Langue, J. & Raveau, J. (1982). Sténoses artérielles cérébrales multiples et progressives, sténose d l'artère rénale et maladie de Recklinghausen. *Pédiatrie*, **38**, 523–30.

Götze, P. & Kühne, D. (1976). Moyamoya-Syndrome (hämangiomartiges Gefässnetz an der Schädelbasis) verbunden mit einer Neurofibromatose von Recklinghausen. *Nervenarzt*, **47**, 34–9.

Greene, J.F., Fitzwater, J.E. & Burgess, J. (1974). Arterial lesions associated with neurofibromatosis. *American Journal of Clinical Pathology*, **62**, 481–7.

Hilal, S.K., Solomon, G.E., Gold, A.P. & Carter, S. (1971). Primary cerebral arterial occlusive disease in children. *Radiology*, **99**, 87–93.

Klatte, E.C., Franken, E.A. & Smith, J.A. (1976). The radiographic spectrum in neurofibromatosis. *Seminars in Roentgenology*, **11**, 17–33.

Lamas, E., Diez Lobato, R., Cabello, A. & Abad, J.M. (1978). Multiple intracranial arterial occlusions (Moyamoya disease) in patients with neurofibromatosis. One case report with autopsy. *Acta Neurochirurgica*, **45**, 133–45.

Latchaw, R.E., Harris, R.D., Chou, S.N. & Gold, L.H.A. (1980). Combined embolization and operation in the treatment of cervical arteriovenous malformations. *Neurosurgery*, **6**, 131–7.

Lennington, B.R., Laster, D.W., Moody, D.M. & Ball, M.R. (1980). Traumatic pseudoaneurysm of ascending cervical artery in neurofibromatosis: complication of chiropractic manipulation. *American Journal of Neuroradiology*, **1**, 269–70.

Leone, R.G., Schatzki S.C., Wolpow, E.R. (1982). Neurofibromatosis with extensive intracranial arterial occlusive disease. *American Journal of Neuroradiology*, **3**, 572–6.

Levisohn, P.M., Mikhael, M.A. & Rothman, S.M. (1978). Cerebrovascular changes in neurofibromatosis. *Developmental Medicine and Child Neurology*, **20**, 789–93.

Malecha, M.J. & Rubin, R. (1992). Aneurysms of the carotid arteries associated with von Recklinghausen's neurofibromatosis. *Pathology, Research and Practice*, **188**, 145–7.

Momose, K.J. & New, P.F. (1973). Non-atheromatous stenosis and occlusion of the internal carotid artery and its main branches. *American Journal of Roentgenology*, **118**, 550–6.

Negoro, M., Nakaya, T., Terashima, K. & Sugita, K. (1990).

Extracranial vertebral artery aneurysm with neurofibromatosis. Endovascular treatment by detachable ballon. *Neuroradiology*, **31**, 533–6.

Pellock, J.M., Kleinman, P.K., McDonald, B.M. & Wixson, D. (1980). Hypertensive stroke with neurofibromatosis. *Neurology*, **30**, 656–9.

Reubi, F. (1994). Les vaisseaux et les glandes endocrines dans la neurofibromatose. *Z. Path. u. Bakt.*, **7**, 168.

Riccardi, V.M. (1992). *Neurofibromatosis: Phenotype, Natural History and Pathogenesis.* Baltimore: John Hopkins University Press.

Rossi Lopez, R.E., Romero, J., Gracia, R., Rallo, B. & Gonzalez-Elipe, J. (1985). Neurofibromatosis de von Recklinghausen con afeccion vascular cerebral. *Revue Clinica España*, **176**, 94–7.

Rudoltz, M.S., Regine, W.F., Langston, J.W., Sanford, R.A., Kovnar, E.H., Kun, L.E. (1998). Multiple causes of cerebrovascular events in children with tumors of the parasellar region. *Journal of Neuro-Oncology*, **37**, 251–61.

Schievink, W.I. (1997). Genetics of intracranial aneurysms. *Neurosurgery*, **40**, 651–63.

Schievink, W.I. & Piepgras, D.G. (1991). Cervical vertebral artery aneurysms and arteriovenous fistulae in neurofibromatosis type 1: case reports. *Neurosurgery*, **29**, 760–5.

Schubiger, O. & Yasargil, M.G. (1978). Extracranial vertebral aneurysm with neurofibromatosis. *Neuroradiology*, **15**, 171–3.

Shen, M.H., Harper, P.H. & Upadhyaya, M. (1996). Molecular genetics of neurofibromatosis type 1. *Journal of Medical Genetics*, **33**, 2–17.

Smith, M.A.P. & White, J.A.M. (1974). Ruptured cervical aneurysm with neurofibromatosis. *South African Medical Journal*, **48**, 945.

Steel, T.R., Bentivoglio, P.B. & Garrick, R. (1994). Vascular neurofibromatosis affecting the internal carotid artery: a case report. *British Journal of Neurosurgery*, **8**, 233–7.

Taboada, D., Alonso, A., Moreno, J., Muro, D. & Mulas, F. (1979). Occlusion of the cerebral arteries in Recklinghausen's disease. *Neuroradiology*, **18**, 281–4.

Tholen, A., Messmer, A.P. & Landau, K. (1998). Peripheral retinal vascular occlusive disorder in a young patient with neurofibromatosis 1. *Retina*, **18**, 184–6.

Vignes, B., Guvert, J-P., Martin, G. & Labrune, B. (1973). Maladie de Moyamoya et maladie de Recklinghausen. A propos d'une observation. *Seminars Hôpital Paris*, **20**, 469–76.

Voigt, K. & Beck, U. (1971). Arterial developmental anomalies of one hemisphere with inter- and intrahemispheric steal effects in neurofibromatosis (Recklinghausen's disease). *Radiological and Clinical Biology*, **43**, 483–93.

Wada, K., Ohtsuka, K., Terayama, K., Maruyama, M., Kumaki, S. & Murata, S. (1989). Neurofibromatosis with spinal paralysis due to arteriovenous fistula. *Archives of Orthopedics and Trauma Surgery*, **108**, 322–4.

47

Bone disorders and cerebrovascular disease

Natan M. Bornstein and Vadim G. Karepov

Department of Neurology, Tel Aviv Sourasky Medical Center, Israel

This chapter reviews rare and unusual cases of cerebrovascular disease related to bone abnormalities or caused by various kinds of bone disorders. The main mechanism by which bone disorders cause ischemic vascular events are: embolism to the brain, mechanical compression of the brain vessels, and the formation of the different cerebral vascular abnormalities, such as the moya-moya phenomenon, or in association with premature arteriosclerosis.

Embolic mechanism

Fibrocartilaginous emboli

The phenomenon of fibrocartilaginous embolism (FE) is well documented in the veterinary literature (Ryan et al., 1981; Uhthoff & Rahn, 1981; Kon & de Visser, 1981; Cook, 1988; Johnson et al., 1988; Schubert, 1980; Bischel et al., 1984; Neer, 1992; Fuentealba et al., 1991; Jeffrey & Weels, 1986). However, FE is a rare cause of brain ischemia and its pathogenesis remains poorly understood. Only one case of FE was reported in humans (Toro-Gonzales et al., 1993). A previously healthy 17-year-old girl fell while playing basketball. Left hemiparesis and unresponsiveness developed, followed by signs of right uncal herniation over a period of 3 days and then by death. She had no evidence of neck, head, or spine trauma, and the cardiac evaluation was normal. The neuropathologic examination showed an extensive ischemic infarction of the right middle cerebral artery territory due to complete embolic occlusion by fibrocartilaginous material, consistent with nucleus pulposus. Small, terminal coronary artery branches also showed embolism by the same material in addition to limited areas of myocardial infarction.

FE from the ruptured nucleus pulposus was described in the spinal cord in only 17 cases as of 1981 (Bots et al., 1981).

In 1994, Toro et al. (1994) reported another 32 cases of nucleus pulposus embolism. Women were more frequently affected (69%) and age distribution was bimodal, with peaks at ages 22 and 60 years (median 38.5). Embolization was either arterial and venous (50%) or purely arterial (50%). Ischemic myelopathy occurred more commonly in the cervical (69%) and lumbosacral (22%) regions. Shmorl's nodes, larger volume, and vascularization of the nucleus pulposus in younger patients, and spinal arteriovenous communications, trauma, and degenerative changes in older patients, are potentially important pathogenetic factors.

Multifocal ischemic encephalomyelopathy associated with fibrocartilaginous emboli was first described in a lamb in 1986 (Jeffrey & Weels, 1986). The emboli contained mucosubstances that were identified by the Alcian blue critical electrolyte concentration method as mainly keratin sulphate. This composition indicates that the probable origin of the emboli was the nucleus pulposus of intervertebral disks.

Mechanical compression

Paget's disease

Paget's disease, a common pathology of the bony structure, is a chronic osteodystrophy of unknown etiology that usually occurs in adults (≥50 years of age) (Farre & Delcambre, 1989). This disorder is characterized by the progressive and extensive replacement of normal bone tissue by tissue with a rough and irregular structure which produces hyperdensity and hypertrophy of the affected bones (Renier, 1989). The condition results from the action of abnormal and overactive osteoclasts containing 3 virus-like intranuclear and intracytoplasmic inclusions. It profoundly alters the physiology of the bones. The viral-appearing inclusions that enter the osteoclasts seem to induce a loss of control of bone renewal and remodelling. The resorption-formation mechanism continues but it is irregular, first facilitating bone resorption for two to five years and then inducing bone formation. In that way, patients with Paget's disease, who have reached the age of physiological osteopenia, often display a significant increase in bone density and mass. Paget's disease of bone is a condition grafted on the skeleton, thus it is partly dependent on the skeletal status of the host. The activity of this disease is evaluated by measuring the ratio of plasma alkaline phosphatase levels to the volumes of normal and pagetic bones (Renier, 1989). Some authors prefer the term 'osteitis deformans' for this condition. Pains and bone deformations are the main functional symptoms. Bone fractures are frequent and are sometimes the first signs of the disease (Farre & Delcambre, 1989). Patients with Paget's disease have no hypercalcemia unless they are bedridden (Fournie et al., 1989). Radiographic patterns of this disease include homogeneous sclerosis, trabecular coarsening, cortical thickening, and lysis (Friedman et al., 1982). Cardiovascular complications are rare except for arterial hypertension which seems to be closely related to the skeletal dystrophy (Farre & Delcambre, 1989).

Neurologic manifestations are diverse and are caused by anatomic alterations and vascular steal syndromes (Farre & Delcambre, 1989). Because of its temporal bone involvement, Paget's disease can produce loss of hearing, tinnitus and vertigo (Ginsberg et al., 1992; Marcos-Perez et al., 1992). An association between this disease and syringomyelia was also reported (Pryce & Wiener, 1990). The main mechanism of these neurological disorders is the compression of neural structures (Ginsberg et al., 1992).

Cerebrovascular disorders in these patients have a mainly mechanical origin (Fournie et al., 1989). There were 14 patients (nine males and five females) who had Paget's disease and were admitted to the Tel Aviv Medical Center because of cerebrovascular events from January 1988 to June 1999. Two of them had intracerebral hemorrhage, seven had first-ever ischemic stroke, two had recurrent ischemic stroke, and three had recurrent TISs. However, only three patients had no other vascular risk factors. We suggest that Paget's disease might be associated with cerebrovascular events but is not their main cause.

Osteopetrosis

The osteopetroses are a group of conditions which are characterized by varying combinations of bony sclerosis and modelling defects (Beighton et al., 1977).

Osteopetrosis (OP) is an extremely rare hereditary metabolic disease of unknown etiology. The incidence of OP varies from 1:500000 in the North American population as a whole (Colonia et al., 1993) to 1:20000 in the Caucasian population (Dahl et al., 1992; Bollerslev, 1987) This hereditary disorder is characterized by an abnormal accumulation of bone mass (Bollerslev et al., 1987) resulting in a pathologic alteration of osteoclast resorption of bone which leads to thickening of cortical and lammellar bone. OP is characterized by increased skeletal density and fractures. The relentless bone growth may progressively obliterate the various craniofacial skeletal foramina because of skeletal thickening, leading to vessels and nerve compression and a diversity of neurological disorders. Symptoms directly and indirectly stem from the increased amount of bone. Clinically, three types can be distinguished: the infantile malignant autosomal recessive form, the benign form of the adult patient and the intermediate 5 type (Colonia et al., 1993; Ohlsson et al., 1980; Shapiro, 1993). Recessive OP with renal tubular acidosis and cerebral calcification is also known as 'marble brain disease' or 'marble bone' disease. (Al Rajeh et al., 1988; Whyte et al., 1980; Eddy et al., 1992; Scwartz et al., 1992). The adult form of OP is known as Albers–Schonberg disease. In the study which was conducted by Bollerslev (1987), 39% of the OP patients were asymptomatic. The age of first appearance of symptoms also varied widely (8–76 years), with a tendency to increasing symptoms with aging. Neurologic sequelae include cranial nerve compression (optic nerve, deafness; facial nerve, paresis), hydrocephalus, convulsions, mental retardation, and compressive myelopathy (Shapiro, 1993; McCleary et al., 1987).

Facial nerve paralysis or symptoms of audiovestibular nerve dysfunction may be the first indication of one of the group of the OP bone diseases. Radiographs show uniform bone density without corticomedullary demarcation, broadened metaphases, 'bone within a bone' or endobone phenomena (tarsals, carpals, phalanges, vertebra, ilium), and thickened growth plates if there is superimposed rickets. Transverse pathologic fractures are likely to occur, often followed by massive periosteal bone formation. Petrous carotid canal and internal carotid artery stenoses occur frequently in patients with malignant osteopetrosis (Cure et al., 1996). Makin et al. (1986) described one patient with severe stenosis of the internal carotid artery, a posterior fossa aneurysm and abnormal intracranial hemodynamics. Another patient was reported to have probable occlusion of one internal jugular vein and retrograde thrombosis of the contributing dural venous sinuses was demonstrated. Computed tomographic scans and magnetic resonance imaging scans provide specific diagnostic information (Shapiro, 1993). While some neurologic complications have been described in patients with OP (McCleary et al., 1987; Lerman-Sagie et al., 1987; Szappanos & Thomazy, 1987; Allen et al., 1982; Chinidia et al., 1991; Miyamoto et al., 1980; Benecke, 1993), cerebrovascular involvement is very rare. Wilms et al. (1990) reported a 16-year-old patient with OP who had transient sensory and motor disturbances in the left upper limb and dizziness upon changing the position of his head. Selective angiography of the cerebral vessels showed severe narrowing of the internal carotid artery within the petrous carotid canal and in its supraclinoid portion. The cervical vertebral arteries showed multiple stenosis within the vertebral canal. These findings are explained by a mechanical narrowing of the basal foramina by the osteopetrotic bone. Stroke associated with OP is rare and probably due to compression of the arteries by osteoporotic bones.

Craniosynostosis

Premature fusion of multiple cranial sutures has been associated with increased intracranial pressure and the potential for mental impairment. Isolated craniosynostosis, however, has been thought to be a benign condition (David et al., 1996). Craniosynostosis may be associated with decreased cerebral blood flow as a result of the constriction of the brain because of the prematurely fused suture. Single positron emission computed tomography (SPECT) was used to assess differences in cerebral perfusion in the areas that were compressed secondary to the fused cranial suture before and after cranial reconstructive surgery in patients with simple craniostenosis (David et al., 1996). These authors prospectively studied seven children with craniostenosis, six boys and one girl (3–28 months age). Six of the seven had cranial asymmetry on preoperative cranial computed tomographic scans, and one had a symmetric defect and served as a control. Each patient had a preoperative SPECT scan approximately 3 to 5 days before the cranial reconstructive procedure and a follow-up scan 6 to 10 weeks postoperatively. Preoperative asymmetries in cerebral perfusion ranged from 0 to 30% (mean, 13%) and were found in the areas that were compressed secondary to the premature suture fusion. In five patients, cerebral blood flow, which was asymmetric before surgery, became symmetric after craniofacial reconstruction, and no new perfusion defects were documented. The control patient and one other patient had symmetric perfusion both pre- and postoperatively. This difference in blood flow supports a policy of early surgical intervention to prevent any potential central nervous system compromise secondary to abnormal blood flow in these patients.

Association with moya-moya or arteriosclerosis

Spondyloepiphyseal dysplasia

Immuno-osseous dysplasia is an autosomal recessive spondyloepiphyseal dysplasia (SD) that was first described by Schimke et al. (1971). It is associated with premature arteriosclerosis and cerebral ischemia. Boerkoel et al. (1998) described two girls with immunoosseous dysplasia and cerebral ischemia associated with the moyamoya phenomenon. This was the first presentation of the cerebral vascular abnormality found in SD and it was based on magnetic resonance angiography and magnetic resonance venography. Three other children who had a transient ischemic attack associated with focal segmental glomerulosclerosis, nephrotic syndrome, chronic renal failure, spondyloepiphyseal dysplasia, growth failure and lymphopenia were reported (1995). Positron emission tomography revealed perfusion defects of both cerebral and cerebellar arteries. Two boys and one girl developed the full syndrome at age 5, 6 and 10 years.

In summary, we consider that these rare cases of stroke with bone diseases are infrequently accidental in character and that their association with these diseases is indirect. Bone-related disorders and their association with stroke are rare and should be considered only in cases in which the osteopathy is well defined.

References

Allen, H.A., Haney, P. & Rao, K.C. (1982). Vascular involvement in cranial hyperostosis. *American Journal of Neuroradiology*, 3, 193–5.

Al Rajeh, S., el Mouzan, M.I., Ahlberg, A. & Ozaksoy, D. (1988). The syndrome of osteopetrosis, renal acidosis and cerebral calcification in two sisters. *Neuropediatrics*, 19(3), 162–5.

Beighton, P., Horan, F. & Hamersma, H. (1977). A review of the osteopetroses. *Postgraduate Medical Journal*, 53(622), 507–16.

Benecke, J.E. (1993). Facial nerve dysfunction in osteopetrosis. *Laryngoscope*, 103, 494–7.

Bischel, P., Vandevelde, M. & Lang, J. (1984). Spinal cord infarction following fibrocartilaginous embolism in the dog and cat. *Schweiz Archiv Tierheilkdunde*, 126(8), 387–97.

Boerkoel, C.F., Nowaczyk, M.J., Blaser, S.I., Meschino, W.S. & Weksberg, R. (1998). Schimke immunoosseous dysplasia complicated by moyamoya phenomen. *American Journal of Medical Genetics*, **78**(2), 118–22.

Bollerslev, J. (1987). Osteopetrosis. A genetic and epidemiological study. *Clinical Genetics*, **31**(2), 86–90.

Bollerslev, J., Grodum, E. & Grontved, A. (1987). Autosomal dominant osteopetrosis (a family study). *Journal of Laryngology and Otology*, **101**, 1088–91.

Bots, G.T., Wattendorff, A.R., Buruma, O.J., Roos, R.A. & Endtz, L.J. (1981). Acute myelopathy caused by fibrocartilaginous emboli. *Neurology*, **31**(10), 1250–6.

Chinidia, M.L., Ocholla, T.J. & Imalingat, B. (1991). Osteopetrosis presenting with paroxysmal trigeminal neuralgia. A case report. *International Journal of Oral Maxillofacial Surgery*, **20**, 199–200.

Colonia, A.M., Schaimberg, C.G., Yoshinari, N.H., Santos, M., Jorgetti, V. & Cossermelli, W. (1993). Osteopetrosis: report of 2 cases and review of the literature. *Reviews of Hospital Clinical Faculty of Medicine, Sao Paulo*, **48**(5), 242–7.

Cook, J.R. Jr. (1988). Fibrocartilaginous embolism. *Veterinary Clinics of North America Small Animal Practice*, **18**(3), 581–92.

Cure, J.K., Key, L.L., Shankar, L. & Gross, A.J. (1996). Petrous carotid canal stenosis in malignant osteopetrosis: CT documentation with MR angiographic correlation. *Radiology*, **199**(2), 415–21.

Dahl, N., Holmgren, G., Holmberg, S. & Ersmark, H. (1992). Fracture patterns in malignant osteopetrosis (Albers–Schonberg disease). *Archives of Orthopaedic and Trauma Surgery*, **111**(2), 121–3.

David, L.R., Wilson, J.A., Watson, N.E. & Argenta, L.C. (1996). Cerebral perfusion defects secondary to simple craniosynostosis. *Journal of Craniofacial Surgery*, **7**(3), 177–85.

Eddy, R., Resendes, M. & Genant, H. (1992). Case report 718. Osteopetrosis with carbonic anhydrase II deficiency. *Skeletal Radiology*, **21**(2), 135–6.

Ehrich, J.H., Burchert, W., Schring, E. et al. (1995). Steroid resistant nephrotic syndrome associated with spondyloepiphyseal dysplasia, transient ischemic attacks and lymphopenia. *Clinical Nephrology*, **43**(2), 89–95.

Farre, J.M. & Delcambre, B. (1989). Functional consequences and complications of Paget's disease. *Reviews of Practice*, **39**, 1129–36.

Fournie, A., Fournie, B. & Lassoied, S. (1989). Paget's disease: errors to be avoided. *Reviews of Practice*, **39**, 1143–6.

Friedman, A.C., Orcutt, J. & Madewell, J.E. (1982). Paget disease of the hand: radiographic spectrum. *American Journal of Roentgenology*, **138**(4), 691–3.

Fuentealba, I.C., Weeks, B.R., Martin, M.T., Joyce, J.R. & Wease, G.S. (1991). Spinal cord ischemic necrosis due to fibrocartilaginous embolism in a horse. *Journal of Veterinary Diagnosis and Investigation*, **3**(2), 176–9.

Ginsberg, L.E., Elster, A.D. & Moody, D.M. (1992). MRI of Paget disease with temporal bone involvement presenting with sensorineural hearing loss. *Journal of Computer Assisted Tomography*, **16**(2), 314–16.

Jeffrey, M. & Weels, G.A. (1986). Multifocal ishemic encephalomye-

lopathy associated with fibrocartilaginous emboli in the lamb. *Neuropathology and Applied Neurobiology*, **12**(4), 415–24.

Johnson, R.C., Anderson, W.I. & King, J.M. (1988). Acute pelvic limb paralysis induced by a lumbar fibrocartilaginous embolism in a sow. *Cornell Veterinary*, **78**(3), 231–4.

Kon, M. & de Visser, A.C. (1981). A poly (HEMA) sponge for restoration of articular cartilage defects. *Plastic Reconstructive Surgery*, **63**, 288–94.

Lerman-Sagie, T., Levi, Y., Kidron et al. (1987). Syndrome of osteopetrosis and muscular degeneration associated with cerebrooculo-facio-skeletal changes. *American Journal of Medical Genetics*, **28**, 137–42.

McCleary, L., Rovit, R.I. & Murali, R. (1987). Case report: myelopathy secondary to congenital osteopetrosis of the cervical spine. *Neurosurgery*, **20**(3), 487–9.

Makin, G.J., Coastes, R.K., Pelz, D., Drake, C.G. & Barnett, H.J. (1986). Major cerebral arterial and venous disease in osteopetrosis. *Stroke*, **17**(1), 106–10.

Marcos-Perez, S.M., Montes-Plaza, J.M., Valda-Rodrigo, J. & Rubio-Sanz, M.J. (1992). Paget's disease with temporal involvement, hypoacusis and vertigo. Apropos a case. *Acta Otorrinolaringologica Espana*, **43**(4), 232–4.

Miyamoto, R.T., House, W.F. & Brackmann, D.E. (1980). Neurotologic manifestations of the osteopetroses. *Archives of Otolaryngology*, **106**, 210–14.

Neer, T.M. (1992). Fibrocartilaginous emboli. *Veterinary Clinics of North American Small Animal Practice*, **22**(4), 1017–26.

Ohlsson, A., Stark, G. & Sakati, N. (1980). Marble brain disease: recessive osteopetrosis, renal tubular acidosis and cerebral calcification in three Saudi Arabian families. *Developmental Medicine and Child Neurology*, **22**(1), 72–84.

Pryce, A.P. & Wiener, S.N. (1990). Syringomyelia associated with Paget disease of the skull. *American Journal of Roentgenology*, **155**(4), 881–2.

Renier, J.C. (1989). What is Paget's disease? *Reviews of Practice*, **39**, 1104–8.

Ryan, L.M., Cheung, H.S. & McCarty, D.J. (1981). Release of pyrophosphate by normal mammalian articular hyaline and fibrocartilage in organ culture. *Arthritis and Rheumatism*, **24**, 1522–7.

Schimke, R.N., Horton, W.A. & King, C.R. (1971). Chondroitin-6-sulphaturia, defective cellular immunity, and nephrotic syndrome. *Lancet*, **ii**, 1088–9.

Schubert, T.A. (1980). Fibrocartilaginous infarct in a German Shepherd dog. *Veterinary Medicine Small Animal Clinics*, **75**(5), 839–42.

Scwartz, G.J., Brion, L.P., Corey, H.E. & Dorfman, H.D. (1991). Case report 668. Carbonic anhydrase II deficiency syndrome (osteopetrosis associated with renal tubular acidosis and cerebral calcification. *Skeletal Radiology*, **20**(6), 447–52.

Shapiro, F. (1993). Osteopetrosis. Current clinical considerations. *Clinical Orthopaedics*, **294**, 34–44.

Szappanos, L. & Thomazy, V. (1987). Spondylolysis in osteopetrosis. *Magy Traumatology Orthopaedics Helyreallito Sebesz*, **30**, 72–8.

Toro, G., Roman, G.C., Navarro-Roman, L., Cantillo, J., Serrano, B. &

Vergara, I. (1994). Natural history of spinal cord infarction caused by nucleus pulposus embolism. *Spine*, **19**(3), 360–6.

Toro-Gonzales, G., Havarro-Roman, L., Roman, G.C. et al. (1993). Acute ischemic stroke from fibrocartilaginous embolism to the middle cerebral artery. *Stroke*, **24**(5), 738–40.

Uhthoff, H.K. & Rahn, B.A. (1981). Healing patterns of metaphyseal fractures. *Clinical Orthopaedics*, **160**, 295–303.

Whyte, M.P., Murphy, W.A., Fallon, M.D. et al. (1980). Osteopetrosis, renal tubular acidosis and basal ganglia calcification in three sisters. *American Journal of Medicine*, **69**(1), 64–74.

Wilms, G., Casaer, P., Demaerel, P. et al. (1990). Cerebrovascular occlusive complications in osteopetrosis major. *Neuroradiology*, **32**, 511–13.

48

Other uncommon angiopathies

Serge Blecic[1] and Julien Bogousslavsky[2]

[1]Service de Neurologie, Hôpital Erasme, Brussels, Belgium
[2]Department of Neurology, University of Lausanne, Switzerland

Introduction

Uncommon angiopathies are a heterogeneous group of disorders characterized by involvement of arteries in the absence of an inflammatory process.

They are rarely found to be a cause of stroke. Their frequencies vary between 1 in 5000 and 1 in 200 000 patients. Most of these pathologies are sporadic, but a congenital mode of inheritance is sometimes found for several forms of angiopathies such as the cutaneous vascular syndromes.

We classify the stroke-related uncommon angiopathies discussed in this chapter as either sporadic or congenital.

Sporadic angiopathies

Association of atrial myxoma-lentiginosis and stroke

Facial lentiginosis associated with atrial myxoma is a rare cause of stroke (Carney et al., 1985; Fressinaud et al., 1993). The frequency of atrial myxoma is approximately 1 in 100 000 in different autopsy series. A congenital dominant autosomal form has been described in patient with the association of lentiginosis and myxoma (Carney et al., 1985; Fressinaud et al., 1993).

Embryologically, it is probably an involvement of the mesodermic structures which led to an entity described by Forney et al. in 1966, which combines facial lentiginosis, mitral insufficiency, myxoma, deafness and bone abnormalities. Several different patients were reported and, in all instances, cerebral infarction was probably due to cardiac embolism. Although this syndrome is rare, its congenital origin leads to study of family members who could also have cardiac tumours and neoplasic conversion of skin lesions (Fressinaud et al., 1993).

Cerebral aneurysms

Strokes secondary to subarachnoidal hemorrhage result mainly from vasospasm of the major cerebral arteries. However, other mechanisms such as aneurysm-to-artery emboli can be proposed when aneurysmal sacs are greater then 25 mm (Wolpert & Caplan, 1992; Parenti et al., 1992). In the presence of these giant cerebral aneurysms, ischemic stroke due to emboli arising from the sac can occur. This clinical finding is rare but has to be considered in selected patients in whom no other cause of stroke has been found. The first observation was made by Taptas and Katsiotis in 1968 who reported a patient who had stroke after a sub-arachnoidal hemorrhage and in whom angiography did not show vasospasm (Taptas & Katsiotis, 1968). A subsequent work-up revealed stroke was the consequence of an aneurysm-to-artery embolus.

Four criteria were proposed to confirm this etiology: (i) presence of TIA or stroke, (ii) presence of a thrombus in the aneurysmal sac, (iii) absence of other sources of emboli and (iv) absence of vasospasm on cerebral angiography (Parenti et al., 1992). Currently, the best means of showing this entity is MRI, which can image partially or total thrombosed aneurysms combined to the use of transcranial Döppler which can provide information about the presence of associated vasospasm (Parenti et al., 1992; Kindl et al., 1993; Nakai et al., 1993). Histologically, there is a good correlation between the aneurysmal sac size and the incidence of saccular thrombosis; the larger the aneurysm the greater is the risk of having an intra-aneurysmal thrombus (Taptas & Katsiotis, 1968; Lasjaunias & Berenstein, 1987; Parenti et al., 1992; Kindl et al., 1993; Nakai et al., 1993). Stroke can occur before or perioperatively.

Aneurysm surgery is the treatment and during the surgical dissection one must take care to avoid secondary emboli. In patients in whom surgery is not possible, preventive treatments are still discussed, particularly the use of anticoagulants, which can avoid thrombus formation but could favour fatal subarachnoidal hemorrhage.

Diffuse meningocerebral angiomatosis and leukoencephalopathy: Divry–Van Bogaert syndrome

Diffuse meningocerebral angiomatosis and leukoencephalopathy is a congenital recessive disease, which involves both adults and children (Van Bogaert, 1967; Vonsattel & Hedley-Whyte, 1989).

This syndrome was first described in 1946 by Divry and Van Bogaert who had examined three brothers who had livedo reticularis, and who gradually developed dementia, seizures and pyramidal signs that occurred in all three brothers roughly 15 years after the diagnosis (Van Bogaert, 1967). Autopsy performed at this time disclosed leptomeningeal angiopathies and brain infarcts. Demyelination was also present (Van Bogaert, 1967).

Two forms can be distinguished. The adult form includes skin lesions and neurological disorders. The skin findings consist of the presence of a diffuse symmetrical livedo reticularis, which can increase at the onset of neurological problems. Skin biopsies disclose increased dermal capillaries with focal loss of 'zonulae occludens' between endothelial cells (Van Bogaert, 1967; Alarcon-Segovia et al., 1989). Neurologic disorders include seizures, dementia and motor disturbances. Among these symptoms, dementia is the most frequent manifestation (Van Bogaert, 1967; Vonsattel & Hedley-Whyte, 1989). Motor disturbances are related to the presence of the brain infarcts. Generally, death occurs between 10 and 15 years after the onset of neurological symptoms (Van Bogaert, 1967; Vonsattel & Hedley-Whyte, 1989).

In the infantile form, the onset of symptoms occurs after the age of three (Van Bogaert, 1967). In one patient, a poliomyelitis vaccination was the presumptive cause (Vonsattel & Hedley-Whyte, 1989). This form includes skin anomalies and neurological disorders. In contrast to the adult form, skin lesions can be absent in children but do not differ from these found in the adult form, when present (Van Bogaert, 1967; Vonsattel & Hedley-Whyte, 1989). The neurological signs include seizures, motor involvement and cognitive decline. The duration of the disease is shorter in adults and death occurs generally within the 24 months after onset of neurological signs (Van Bogaert, 1967).

Neuropathologic abnormalities are brain infarcts, demyelination of white matter and cerebromeningeal angiomatosis, which is the most constant and pathognomonic finding of this disease (Van Bogaert, 1967; Vonsattel & Hedley-Whyte, 1989). It is a large corticomeningeal network with vascular congestion, and multiple vessel occlusions. Microscopic examination shows fibrotic changes of the vascular walls with fatty degeneration and amyloid deposits. These abnormalities lead to diffuse cerebral infarctions in the grey and white matters. In addition, demyelination of the central white matter is observed in practically all the cases and consists of axonal and oligodendrocytic loss with astrogliosis (Van Bogaert, 1967) These abnormalities occur mostly predominantly around the vessels.

Eosinophil induced neurotoxicity and cerebral infarction

Hypereosinophilia is usually a secondary process in response to allergic or parasitic diseases (Durack et al., 1979; Fauci, 1982). Although they can have some beneficial effects on the primary disease, eosinophils can exert several non-specific toxic effects, with concomitant damages to tissues. Both the central and peripheral nervous system are frequently involved by this undesirable toxic effect (Durack et al., 1979; Dorfman et al., 1983; Fauci, 1982). According to Weaver and colleagues who described a patient with cerebral involvement due to hypereosinophilic syndrome, the mechanisms of eosinophil-induced neuronal damage are multiple; they are summarized in Table 48.1 (Weaver et al., 1988). In addition, the neurotoxic potential of eosinophil proteins must also be considered. Actually, three basic proteins have been isolated: medial-basic protein (MBP), eosinophil-cationic protein (ECP) and eosinophil-derived neurotoxin (EDN) (Durack et al., 1979). Release of MBP can damage endothelial cells and can be the cause of thrombosis and secondary artery-to-artery emboli (Durack et al., 1979, Fauci, 1982). ECP can increase a hypercoagulable state and contribute to a thrombotic tendency. EDN has a direct toxic action on neuronal tissue and on myelinated axons (Table 48.1).

The three major clinical pictures of eosinophil-induced neurotoxicity are axonal peripheral neuropathy, dementia and stroke (Dorfman et al., 1983; Weaver et al., 1988).

Cerebral infarction is secondary to mainly MBP-mediated endothelial damage and ECP-mediated hypercoagulability and eosinophil-mediated cardiopathy. The patient reported by Weaver et al., first had a left occipital cerebral infarction followed 3 months later by a right parietal cerebral infarction (Weaver et al., 1988). Dementia developed 1 year later and neurophysiological study showed a polyneuropathy (Weaver et al., 1988).

Management consists of the treatment of hypereosino-

Table 48.1. *Mechanisms of eosinophil-induced neurotoxicity*

- Direct neural tissue infiltration
- Damage related to eosinophil function, either by direct cytotoxicity or by antibody-dependent cellular cytotoxicity
- Damage related to eosinophil products, either by secretion into neurons or by secretion of intracytoplasmic granules contained in the circulation, with subsequent damage to neural tissue
- Embolic cerebral infarction related either to thrombus or generalized hypercoagulable state
- Nervous system damage secondary to eosinophil-mediated action in remote organ systems

philia and includes prednisone and hydroxyurea. Concerning embolic cerebral infarctions, Weaver et al. recommended anticoagulation in preference to antiplatelet therapy (Weaver et al., 1988).

Endovascular lymphoma

Also called angiotrophic large cell lymphoma, or malignant angio-endotheliomatosis, endovascular lymphoma is a rare arteriopathy, always lethal, which has a particular predilection for small- and middle-sized vessels of the lung, but can involve all organs such as central nervous system, lymphatic system, skin, spleen and marrow bone (Smadja et al., 1991).

Endothelial proliferation involves exclusively small and middle-sized vessels, either arteries or veins, leading to widening, narrowing and vessel occlusions with tumour cell extravasation (Wick & Mills, 1991). Neoplastic large lymphoid cells are confined to the intravascular compartment and create, in the lung, a pattern akin to cellular interstitial pneumonia (Yousem & Colby, 1990). The atypical cytology, with frequent involvment of central nervous system and immunohistochemical and genotypic studies, confirm its inclusion within the group of pulmonary lymphoma (Yousem & Colby, 1990; Smadja et al., 1991; Wick & Mills, 1991). Immunohistochemistry studies always disclose an endothelial infiltration of type B lymphocytes, with a positive reaction for CD-20, CD-45, CD-75 IgG antibodies (Yousem & Colby, 1990; Smadja et al., 1991; Wick & Mills, 1991; Delplace et al., 1995). Only rare cases of type T-lymphocyte infiltration were reported.

About 1 in 5000 ischemic strokes is the consequence of this rare arteriopathy. At presentation, patients demonstrate fever, dyspnea, cough, hypoxemia and signs of central nervous involvement such as paresis and fre-

quently obtundation. Brain CT scan or MRI discloses small subcortical infarctions (Delplace et al., 1995). Chest X-ray reveals bilateral fine linear infiltrates.

Prognosis is extremely poor, although sporadic responses to steroids have been observed (Yousem & Colby, 1990; Smadja et al., 1991; Wick & Mills, 1991; Delplace et al., 1995).

Epidermal nevus syndrome

The epidermal nevus syndrome is a sporadic neurocutaneous disorder that consists of epidermal nevi and congenital anomalies involving all systems and among them, frequently, the brain (Dobyns & Garg,1991; el Shanti et al., 1992; Pavone et al., 1991).

Two entities are commonly described: the classical form that consist of epidermal naevi and brain infarctions, and the second, often called the neurologic variant, consists of hemimegalencephaly, gyral malformation, mental retardation, seizures and facial hemihypertrophy (Pavone et al., 1991). One-half of the 70 patients previously described, had the hemimegalencephaly variant (Pavone et al., 1991).

Neurologic manifestations result from infarcts due to blood vessel dysplasia. Clinically, the epidermal nevus syndrome is found in young patients and in newborns (el Shanti et al.,1992). In all the patients, the diagnosis is confirmed by angiography which demonstrates vascular dysplasia consisting of segmental beading and dilatation of cerebral arteries. An increase of the vascularity in the capillary field and widening of the posterior portion of the superior sagittal sinus is frequently seen (Dobyns & Garg, 1991). Less often, angiography shows fusiform aneurysms and dilatation of the cavernous part of the carotid arteries (Dobyns & Garg, 1991).

Fibromuscular dysplasia

Fibromuscular dysplasia is an arteriopathy which occurs predominantly in Caucasian women. It is the most frequent arterial dysplasia and represents roughly 1% of autopsy and angiography series (Wolpert & Caplan, 1992). It involves mainly renal, splanchnic and cervicocranial arteries. Middle-sized arteries are most frequently involved. Fibromuscular dysplasia is often discovered by chance, and the relationship with subsequent stroke pathology remains unclear (Josien, 1992; Sandmann et al., 1992; Velkey et al., 1992; Wolpert & Caplan, 1992).

Fibrodysplasia is most often localized to the distal two-thirds of the renal arteries and the segments of the distal extracranial vertebral and carotid arteries adjacent to the second cervical vertebra (Josien, 1992; Watanabe et al.,

1993; Wolpert & Caplan, 1992). More rarely, fibromuscular dysplasia can involved the cavernous part of the carotid arteries and the arteries of the circle of Willis.

Pathologically, each layer of the arterial wall can be involved, but involvement of the medial layer is most commonly encountered (Wolpert & Caplan, 1992; Sandman et al., 1992). The pathological process consists of fibrodysplasia of smooth muscles leading to the formation of rings of fibrous tissue and smooth muscles. These rings alternate with areas of medial thickening and destruction of the elastic layer, leading to alternating narrowing and widening of the arterial lumen. Less frequently, the intimal part is involved and causes proliferation of fibrous cells leading to narrowing of the lumen. This last type of fibrodysplasia is mainly found in children and young adults (Wolpert & Caplan, 1992).

The diagnosis is practically always made on angiography. Duplex imaging of the extracranial carotid and vertebral arteries as well as transcranial Döppler can help to confirm the diagnosis (Edwards et al., 1992; Giller et al., 1992). The typical appearance is alternating zones of widening and narrowing of the arterial lumen leading to the classical pattern of 'string of beads' (Edwards et al., 1992; Giller et al., 1992; Josien, 1992; Sandmann et al., 1992; Velkey et al., 1992; Wolpert & Caplan, 1992; Watanabe et al., 1993). Less frequent features are tubular stenosis, diverticular appearance or aneurysmal dilatation. MR angiography can suggest diagnosis (Ashleigh et al., 1992; Heiserman et al., 1992; Shulze et al., 1992). For patients suspected of having fibromuscular dysplasia after duplex examination, MRA may avoid the need for conventional arteriography.

The mechanism by which fibrous dysplasia causes stroke is unclear. The concomitant use of cigarette smoking and of contraceptive therapy has been proposed to explain the female predominance (Wolpert & Caplan, 1992), but as the fibromuscular dysplasia 'pattern' is a frequent finding after stroke, the relationship with stroke and arterial anomalies remains questionable (Sandmann et al., 1992; Shulze et al., 1992; Wolpert & Caplan, 1992). Nevertheless, several stroke mechanisms have been proposed such as artery-to-artery emboli, local thrombosis, emboli arising from a diverticular or from a pseudoaneurysmal sac. Nevertheless a mechanism leading to stroke in these patients is spontaneous artery dissection (Ashleigh et al., 1992; Bour et al., 1992; Galatica et al., 1992; Nishiyama et al., 1992; Shulze et al., 1992; Watanabe et al., 1992; Baumgartner & Waespe, 1993). In addition, the association of atherosclerosis and fibromuscular dysplasia is frequent but it is uncertain how much the primary condition could favour the development of atherosclerotic disease (Ashleigh et al., 1992; Bour et al., 1992; Galatica et al., 1992; Nishiyama et al., 1992; Shulze, 1992; Watanabe et al., 1993; Baumgartner & Waespe, 1993).

Treatment of fibromuscular dysplasia is unknown and, currently nobody knows if any given treatment is useful. Generally antiplatelet therapy is proposed (Wolpert & Caplan, 1992). Anticoagulants are not recommended because of the risk of bleeding in the presence of cerebral aneurysms (Wolpert & Caplan, 1992; Baumgartner & Waespe, 1993). Several surgical procedures have been proposed, but thromboendarterectomy should be considered only in case of symptomatic carotid stenosis (Bour et al., 1992). Some endovascular radiologists suggested angioplasty in case of carotid or vertebral involvement; however, this procedure should be cautiously proposed since it could favour arterial dissection which is already a frequent complication of fibrous dysplasia (Galatica et al., 1992; Wolpert & Caplan, 1992; Baumgartner & Waespe, 1993).

Kinking, coiling, hypoplasia and dolichoectasia of the cervical arteries

Kinking or coiling of the cervical as well as of the cerebral arteries can be observed in both the carotid or vertebral systems. The origin of these anomalies is probably congenital (Weibel & Fields, 1965; Brachlow et al., 1992). In most patients, kinking is discovered after angiography but Döppler ultrasonography with frequency analysis and B-mode imaging can also suggest the problem, when it concerns cervical arteries (Fig. 48.3). They are rarely known to induce occlusive disease or even symptoms, but transient ischemic attack or stroke can occur in the case of permanent head rotation during surgical procedure. In 1992, Brachlow et al. reported the case of a fatal intra-operative cerebral ischemia due to a kinking of the internal carotid artery (Brachlow et al., 1992).

In other conditions, these anomalies are fortuitous and, in stroke patients, are rarely related to the cerebrovascular event (Weibel & Fields, 1965; Brachlow et al., 1992).

Congenital hypoplasias are rare anomalies and probably congenital. They are defined by segmental narrowing of carotid or vertebral artery. They are practically always associated with either intracranial aneurysm, or anomalies of Circle of Willis vessels or intra–extracranial physiological bypass (Brachlow et al., 1992). Angiography disclosed a sudden narrowing of the internal carotid just after the primitive division (Wolper & Caplan, 1992). Differential diagnosis is difficult with arterial dissection, but computed tomography of the skull basis disclosed in carotid hypoplasia a small carotid canal.

Dolichoectasia of cervical and cerebral arteries consists of segmental narrowing, widening and lengthening of arteries of both vertebro-basilar or carotid systems. Arteries of all sizes can be affected alone or in combination with other arteries. Histologically, a thinning down of the arterial wall, due to a rarefaction of the elastic layer associated with a transformation of the media in a fibrous tissue is observed. Atherosclerosis, the consequence but not the cause of these changes, can be observed in such arteries (Brachlow et al., 1992; Wolpert & Caplan, 1992). Other vascular malformation can be shown such as cerebral sacular aneurysms, aneurysm of the aorta or carotid hypoplasia (Brachlow et al., 1992; Wolpert & Caplan, 1992). Adults in their sixth decade are more frequently involved and a male predominance is observed.

The consequence of this process can be cerebral infarction due either to occlusions of small arteries or to artery emboli. Cranial nerve compressions at the base of the skull can be the consequence of a dolichoectasic artery. Subarachnoidal hemorrhages are rare, but can occur in case of rupture of the dolichoectasic arteries (Brachlow et al., 1992; Wolpert & Caplan, 1992).

Diagnosis is often made by chance in a routine CT scan or MRI. It is confirmed by angiography, which discloses a lengthening of the artery.

Radiation-induced angiopathy

The side effects of radiation on blood vessels have been known since the end of the nineteenth century. Involvement of both extracranial and intracranial arteries can be observed, and both arteries and veins can be involved (Levinson et al., 1973; Murros & Toole, 1989).

Radiation-induced arteriopathy results from therapeutic irradiation of neck tumours such as lymphoma or thyroid tumour or intracranial tumours such as optic tract gliomas.

Pathologically, arterial lesions due to radiation have been studied in both animal and human models. In animal models, Lambrechts and de Boer in 1965 showed that, in hypercholesterolemic rabbits, a 5 gray irradiation induces extensive changes in small and middle-sized arteries. These changes can be summarized as penetration of fat into the arterial walls, deposition of lipophages, formation of atherosclerotic plaques in the intima, and structural changes in the elastic fibres. They concluded that radiation primarily affects the endothelial cells. They emphasized the role of a high cholesterol diet, which activates lysosomal enzymes and favours infiltration of lipid droplets beneath the endothelium (Lambrecht & de Boer, 1965). Further studies using electron microscopy show extensive endothelial changes. The adventitial lesions are due to involvement of the vaso-vasorum (Murros & Toole, 1989).

Extrapolation to human arteries is difficult, but autopsy examinations disclose vacuolization and thickening of the intima, changes in the elastic fibres and, degeneration of the endothelial cells due to the same process seen in animal models (Levinson et al., 1973; Murros & Toole, 1989). Electron microscopy disclosed swelling and detachment of endothelial cells with a splitting of the basement membrane. It also disclosed subintimal foam cells which closely resemble circulating lipid-laden macrophages leading to a process of atherosclerotic-like lesions, and in man, subintimal foam cells in middle and small-sized vessels are stated to be diagnostic of radiation therapy (Murros & Toole, 1989).

Large arteries, such as the carotid or vertebral arteries, are less involved in X-ray therapy. However, few authors have reported rupture of internal carotid artery after subclavian X-ray (Levinson et al., 1973). Autopsy study disclosed intimal necrosis, infiltration of leukocytes and fragmentation of elastic fibres. In addition, Glick in 1972 demonstrated an accumulation of fat-laden macrophages in the arterial media with atheromatous proliferation and calcification of the intima (Lambrecht & de Boer, 1965). Few studies reported the effect of X-ray therapy in large intracranial arteries. In these patients, the same pathological process was demonstrated.

Clinically, the effect of radiation therapy can be observed from 1 week to several decades after radiation therapy (Lambrecht & de Boer, 1965; Glick, 1972; Levinson et al., 1973; Murros & Toole, 1989). The former are rare and generally due to skin necrosis and infection of surgical wounds. Delayed complications are more frequent and occur from 6 months to 10 years (median: 2 years). Clinically, skin radionecrosis is often observed. Cerebral angiography frequently discloses arterial stenosis within the radiation area (Fig. 48.1).

The interval from irradiation to symptomatic cerebrovascular events is directly related to the size of the irradiated arteries and seems longer for larger arteries.

Retinocochleocerebral arteriolopathy

The retinocochleocerebral arteriolopathy is a diffuse encephalopathy with retinal vascular occlusions, hearing loss and absence of systemic disease which was first described by Susac et al. in 1979, in two women with predominant psychiatric symptoms. Both also had retinal artery occlusions and hearing loss. The cognitive signs were predominant and are present in progressive memory troubles and abulia. Blindness was the consequence of multiple retinal artery occlusions.

Bogousslavsky and Caplan together described several patients with this syndrome. In all the patients, laboratory

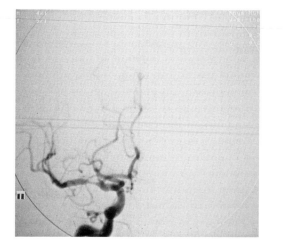

Fig. 48.1. Multiple segmental narrowings found at the proximal part of both middle and cerebral arteries, 15 years after base skull X-ray therapy (arrows).

tests were unremarkable, except in a few patients there was a slight increase of the sedimentation rate, the presence, at low titres, of antinuclear antibodies, and increase of CSF protein content (Bogousslavsky et al., 1989).

Generally, angiography disclosed segmental narrowing, and involvement of small pial and cortical vessels. In one case, biopsy showed 'healed angiitis'. Bogousslavsky's patients also had anomalies of lymphocyte T-cell helpers and suppressors, which was an argument that led to immunosuppresive therapy. One patient improved under this treatment, but another worsened (Bogousslavsky et al., 1989).

Currently, steroid therapy is recommended in the acute phase but benefit from prolonged immunosuppressive therapy is not yet established (Heikala et al., 1988)

Stroke and primitive arteries

In the very early stages of human embryonic life, various anastomotic channels exist into, and between, the carotid and vertebrobasilar systems. Each of them is normally present during the first stages of life and disappears when the embryo is approximately 12 to 14 mm long (Padget, 1954; Lasjaunias et al., 1978).

These anastomotic channels are known as the persistent primitive trigeminal, hypoglossal, otic and, proatlantal arteries (Lasjaunias et al., 1978). They were first named by Padget in 1953 (Padget, 1954) and reviewed by Lasjaunias et al. in 1978. Rarely, some of these channels fail to regress and persist into adult life (Anderson & Sondheimer, 1976; Lasjaunias et al., 1978).

Occlusions of these persistent arteries can lead to cerebral infarctions. In 1993, Bashi et al. described a patient (a 55-year-old woman) with a top of the basilar syndrome, due to persistent primitive proatlantal intersegmental artery, admitted for loss of consciousness due to bilateral mesencephalic and thalamic infarctions. Other rare cases of ischemic stroke in the carotid territory were described after occlusion of persistent trigeminal artery, a collateral of the basilar artery, which reaches the internal carotid artery near the base of the skull (Lasjaunias et al., 1978).

These anastomotic vessel occlusions can be due either to cerebral emboli or more frequently to *in situ* thrombosis (Anderson & Sondheimer, 1976; Lasjaunias et al., 1978; Bashi et al., 1993).

Congenital angiopathies

Congenital cutaneo-vascular syndromes

The congenital cutaneovascular syndromes include several diseases which have in common the presence of cutaneous abnormalities associated to cerebrovascular malformations such as artery occlusions, intracerebral hemorrhages, multiple aneurysms or arteriovenous malformations.

Frequently, the cutaneous abnormality is present at birth and constitutes a clue in the setting for congenital cutaneovascular syndromes.

Sturge–Weber syndrome: encephalo-facial angiomatosis

The frequency of Sturge–Weber syndrome is estimated to be 1 in 5000 to 1 in 10000 births. In the classical form, patients have facial nevi also called 'port-wine lesions' (see colour Fig. 48.2) (Roach, 1988). Normally, the facial nevus is limited to the fifth cranial nerve distribution. The cutaneous lesion is frequently unilateral but can, rarely, involve the whole face and can extend to the trunk and extremities. There is no evidence that the facial lesion is directly associated with intracranial abnormalities but Enjolras et al. in 1985 showed that most of the patients who had intracranial vascular abnormalities, had cutaneous lesions of the upper face especially with involvement of the eye lid (Enjolras et al.,1985). Sturge–Weber syndrome can also be present without facial lesion (Talby et al., 1987; Liang & Liang, 1992).

The clinical manifestations of the Sturge–Weber syndrome are due to the presence of vascular malformations (Fig. 48.3). The most frequent symptom is epilepsy, which

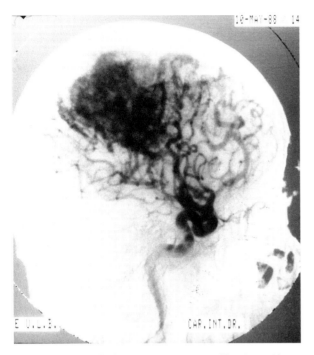

Fig. 48.3. Giant cerebral angioma in a 15-year-old patient with Sturge–Weber syndrome.

generally begins early in life. Epileptic seizures can be accompanied by focal neurological signs such as hemiparesis, hemianopia, aphasia, and other cognitive and behavioral abnormalities, for which the suspected mechanism is localized cerebral hypoxia (Roach, 1988; Kotagal & Rothner, 1993).

Leptomeningeal, intracerebral, cerebellar and spinal cord angiomas can also be present; in these patients neurological manifestations could be the consequence of either epileptic seizures or venous or arterial occlusions (Kennedy et al., 1992; Mizutani et al., 1992). Although intracerebral hemorrhages are relatively rare, subarachnoidal hemorhages are frequent and due to leptomeningeal vessel ruptures.

The diagnosis of Sturge–Weber syndrome is easy because of the presence of port wine angiomas (Fig. 48.2), frequently accompanied by ocular involvement such as cataract or glaucoma. However, as not all patients with facial nevi have brain involvement, it is necessary to perform complementary investigations to detect the patients who are at risk of presenting cerebrovascular complications (Ruby et al., 1992; Wilms et al., 1992; Gillian et al., 1993; Agarwal et al., 1993; Kurtz et al., 1993). Currently, magnetic resonance imaging (MRI) and magnetic resonance arteriography (MRA) are the gold standards for the detection of

vascular malformations. MRI and MRA can also be useful for the preoperative setting of leptomeningeal or intracerebral angioma (Marti-Bonmati et al., 1992; Benedikt et al., 1993; Campistol-Plana et al., 1993; Magauda et al., 1993; Truhan & Filipek, 1993; Vogl et al., 1993).

As the radiographic hallmark of Sturge–Weber's syndrome is the presence of cerebral calcifications close to the leptomeningeal angioma, a brain CT-scan can be helpful for the detection of brain involvement in a newly diagnosed Sturge–Weber syndrome (Marti-Bonmati et al., 1992). However, this investigation is only a first step, and should be completed by MR examinations.

Other technical examinations such as an electroencephalogram, which characteristically shows asymmetrical slower frequency in the affected area, and positron emission tomography, which can show either hypometabolism or hypermetabolism of the affected area, provide little important clinically useful information (Rintahaka et al., 1993). Currently, since the advent of MRI and MRA, conventional arteriography should be considered only in patients considered for surgery.

Pathologically, brain and leptomeningeal vessel calcifications are the most prominent findings. Neuronal loss and gliosis are often found and attributed to ischemic changes due to epileptic seizure. Microscopic examination of brain vessels discloses calcifications in the different arterial layers. Examination of leptomeningeal vessels shows hyalinization and subendothelial proliferations of arterial walls (Kuster & Happle, 1993; Tiacci et al., 1993).

Treatment of Sturge–Weber syndrome consists first of control of seizures. In the case of refractory seizures, hemispherectomy has been recommended early in life, first to improve seizure control and secondly to promote intellectual development (Kuster & Hopple, 1993; Villemure & Rasmussen, 1993). Prophylactic treatment with antiplatelet therapy was proposed, based on the fact that stepwise deterioration could be a consequence of occlusive disease (Roach, 1988; Loevner & Quint, 1992; Kotagal & Rothner, 1993; Kuster & Happle, 1993).

Ehlers–Danlos syndrome

Ehlers–Danlos syndrome is a heterogeneous disorder characterized by joint hypermobility, skin hyperextensibility and fragility of connective tissues and hyperelasticity of the skin (Muyner & Margulis, 1981; Schievink et al., 1990; Tucker, 1992; Sato et al., 1993). Today, 11 types of collagen anomalies have been described.

Ehlers–Danlos syndrome was first described in 1668 by Job van Mekren. He observed a young man with extraordinary elasticity of the skin. Ehlers–Danlos syndrome is, in fact, a congenital disease due to different base mutations in the gene for different types of collagen (Schievink et al., 1990). The most frequent manifestation of Ehlers–Danlos syndrome is attributed to the type IV, which results from abnormality of collagen type III. As Ehlers–Danlos syndrome is a collagen disease, most of the neurological complications are due to arterial malformations (Tucker, 1992; Kivirikko, 1993). The most frequent findings are intracranial aneurysms, carotid-cavernous fistula, and aorta and carotid dissections (Muyner & Margulis, 1981; Adami et al., 1993).

All other organs can be involved, such as eyes, heart, kidneys, gut and skin (Kharsa et al., 1992; Mishra et al., 1992; Majorana & Fachetti, 1992; Wertelecki et al., 1992; Cameron, 1993; Sato et al., 1993). Among them, cerebrovascular complications and mainly carotid or large vessel dissections are the most feared (Wertelecki et al., 1992, Grenko et al., 1993). For this reason, angiography in these patients should be avoided or performed with extreme caution.

Pathologically, Ehlers–Danlos syndrome type IV is caused by mutation in the gene for lysyl hydroxylase which is the enzyme catalysing the metabolism of hydroxylysine in collagen and in other proteins with collagen-like amino acid sequences. Clinically, the diagnosis is made by fibroblast culture, which discloses a decrease in the proportion of type III collagen (Hautala et al., 1993; Johnson et al., 1992; Petty et al., 1993; Smith et al., 1992; Richards et al., 1992; Quentin-Hoffmann et al., 1993; Vandenberg, 1993)

Angiokeratoma corporis diffusum: Fabry's disease

Angiokeratoma corporis diffusum or Fabry's disease is a congenital X-linked disease characterized by abnormality of lyzosomal storage and accumulation of ceramidetrihexoside caused by reduced activity of the enzyme α galactosidase A (Brady et al., 1967).

As the disease is linked to the X chromosome, a complete penetrance in males is observed.

Clinically, the first symptoms of Fabry's disease begin generally in the first decade of life (Brady et al., 1967). First symptoms consist of dysesthesia of the extremities. They always precede skin eruption, constituted by dark red papules of approximately 1–2 mm diameter (see colour Fig. 48.4). Generally, they are found on the trunk, scrotum and on the proximal limbs. They can be rarely observed on the face and distal parts of the limbs. They can vary and occur in clusters. Other organs can be involved such as the eyes, with abnormalities in retinal vessels or, the presence of cataracts. Later in life, renal failure is observed and is due to nephroangiosclerosis (Taaffe, 1977; Zeluff et al., 1978; Thomas, 1988).

Neurologic complications are frequent and due either to vascular occlusions or more rarely to brain hemorrhage. Vascular occlusions are due to involvement of small and medium-sized arteries by glycolipid accumulation in the elastin and in smooth muscle layers. This process leads to progressive occlusion of the vascular lumen. Hemorrhages, particularly in the brain, can be the consequence of arterial hypertension, frequently seen in patients with renal failure. It could also be due to involvement of small and medium-sized arteries due to accumulation of glycolipids (Fig. 48.5).

Pathologically, the disease is caused by deficiency in the lyzosomal enzyme α galactosidase A (Vetrie et al., 1993). The gene encoding for this enzyme is a map to the chromosome X in position q22 (Vetrie et al., 1993). Currently, diagnosis of angiokeratoma corporis diffusum is made by the characteristic skin lesions and measurement of α-galactosidase A activity in leukocytes and fibroblasts and blood dosage of ceramidetrihexoside. Genetic mapping confirms the diagnosis (Vetrie et al., 1993).

Currently, treatment is symptomatic and consists of antiplatelet therapy, treatment of renal failure and treatment for arterial hypertension.

Experimental infusion of α-galactosidase A has not yet proved beneficial. Plasmapheresis to reduce the plasma level of ceramidetrihexoside does not improve the clinical findings (Taaffe, 1977; Vetrie et al., 1993)

Hereditary hemorrhagic telangiectasia: Osler–Weber–Rendu disease

Osler–Weber–Rendu disease or hereditary hemorrhagic telangiectasia (HHT) is an autosomal dominant disease, characterized by telangiectasia disseminated on the skin, nasal and visceral areas, associated with recurrent hemorrhages (Neau et al., 1987; Fisher & Zito, 1983).

The most common feature is recurrent epistaxis. Some patients can have hepatic encephalopathy due to multiple liver telangiectasia. Cerebrovascular events are mainly due to the presence of multiple intracranial arterial and venous malformations, but also to extracranial mechanisms such as aneurysm-to-artery emboli. In 1983, Fisher et al. reported the case of a patient with HHT and recurrent right side paresis due to multiple emboli arising from a carotido-ophthalmic aneurysm (Fisher & Zito, 1983)

Other authors reported patients with pulmonary arteriovenous fistulas and parodoxical emboli and even air emboli in the case of bronchovascular fistulas (Allen et al., 1993; Iwabushi et al., 1993). Other organs can also be involved such as the heart, gut and urogenital system (Humphries et al., 1993).

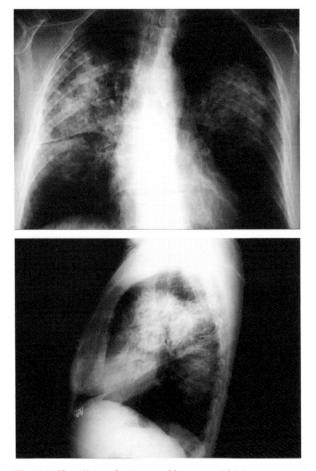

Fig. 48.5. Chest X-ray of a 67-year-old woman with Wegener granulomatosis bilateral pneumonia with alveolar involvement.

Phenotypically, patients can have small stature, mental retardation, sex-developmental retardation with adreno-genital syndrome (Carlborg et al., 1959).

Several different systems can be impaired, but ocular and skin involvements are the most frequent.

Ocular involvement consists of choroidal lesions with exudative macular degeneration and angoid streaks (Fasshauer et al., 1984). Microscopically, the streaks are found in Bruch's membrane with a choroidal capillary proliferation in the subretinal space. Skin lesions are yellowish efflorescence, due to an increase of elastic fibres, with calcifications. The appearance of this pattern has suggested the name 'pseudoxanthoma elasticum' (Fasshauer et al., 1984).

Several other organs can be involved such as the cardiovascular system, endocrine system, frequently with thyroid function impairment.

Neurological symptoms are the consequence of multiple cerebral infarctions, mostly due to small vessel disease but arterial dissections can also be found.

Pathologically, this process involved the elastic layer of large and medium-sized arteries, leading to disruption of the elastic layer and either artery-to-artery emboli, dissection or occlusion.

Recently, Struck and Coll, have conducted a genome-wide screen on a collection of 38 families with two or more affected siblings. Excess allele sharing was found on the short arm of chromosome 16. That was confirmed by a conventional linkage analysis, localizing the disease gene under a recessive model with a maximum of two point score of 21.27 on chromosome 16p13.1 (Struck et al., 1997).

Treatment consists of antiplatelets. Anticoagulants are not recommended in these patients, because of the risk of aneurysm rupture. Surgical therapy is considered only in patients with stroke due to emboli arising from cerebral aneurysm therapy (Allen et al., 1993; Iwabushi et al., 1993; Humphries et al., 1993).

Grönblad–Stranberg syndrome: 'pseudoxanthoma elasticum'

First described by Grönblad in 1932, this entity is a congenital systemic disease involving elastic and connective tissues. The cause of this disease is an inborn anomaly of mucopolysaccharide metabolism, leading to calcifications of collagen and elastic fibres. Clinically, a more common autosomal recessive and a less common autosomal dominant pattern of inheritance, with high penetrance, have been described. The estimated penetrance of this disease is 1 in 70000 to 100000.

Von Recklinghausen's neurofibromatosis

Von Recklinghausen's neurofibromatosis is a congenital disease which can involve any organ system. Currently, two forms are distinguished. Type I, related to a chromosome 17 anomaly, is characterized by the presence of hyperpigmented patches of skin 'café au lait macules', axillary freckles, Lish nodules, sphenoid wing dysplasia and peripheral nerve tumours. Type II, related to a chromosome 22 anomaly, meets some criteria seen in type I, and is characterized by the presence of acoustic neuroma, frequently bilateral (Sobata et al., 1988). Both forms can be accompanied by vascular abnormalities, involving mainly the splanchnic and renal arteries (Green et al. 1974; Gilly et al., 1982).

Involvement of cerebral arteries is uncommon (Lamas et al., 1978; Sobata et al., 1988). It consists of occlusions of the distal part of the internal carotid arteries or of the proximal part of the anterior circulation arising from the circle of

Willis, accompanied by a Moyamoya collateral network (Cano et al., 1992). Cerebral aneurysm can occur alone or accompanied by occlusions. At this day, only about 44 cases have been reported. In the majority of the cases, occlusions alone were found. In addition, most of the patients had arterial hypertension, probably due to renal artery involvement.

Histologically, arterial lesions consist of diffuse hyperplasia of the intimal layer, producing luminal stenosis and, intimal hyperplasia with fragmentation and reduplication of the elastic layer of the intrapetrosal segment of the internal carotid artery or of the proximal part of the anterior and middle cerebral arteries (Sobata et al., 1988; Cano et al., 1992; Hashigushi et al., 1992).

Marfan syndrome

The Marfan syndrome is an inherited, autosomal dominant disorder that affects the skeletal, ocular, cardiovascular and central nervous systems (Bennis et al., 1993; Raftopoulos et al., 1993). There is extreme variability in clinical expression and some patients can have all systems involved, while others can have only one organ impairment. Its frequency varies from 1 in 10000 to 1 in 50000 (Bennis et al., 1993).

Clinical manifestations are the consequence of involvement of eyes, arteries and veins and the skeleton. Cardiovascular impairment is the most frequent finding in Marfan syndrome (Ferreira et al., 1993; Simpson et al., 1993). Involvement of large arteries such as the aorta and carotid arteries is the rule and the cause of death. Actually, it is dissection of the proximal part of the aorta and of the primitive carotid arteries which are the most life-threatening events. Heart involvement is not rare and consists of valvular abnormalities such as mitral and aortic insufficiency (Simpson et al., 1993). Involvement of medium and small-sized arteries is exceptional and in Marfan syndrome cerebral infarctions result from artery-to-artery emboli or carotid occlusion rather than distal local thrombosis (Bennis et al., 1993; Ferreira et al., 1993; Raftopoulos et al., 1993; Simpson et al., 1993).

Ocular manifestations are frequent. They result from anomalies of the connective tissue, which is the support of the different parts of the eye. Dislocation or subluxation of the lens is frequently observed. They occur in approximately 80% of the patients with Marfan syndrome and are preceded by iridonesis, a slight tremor of the iris. Clinical consequences can be glaucoma, uveitis and cataract.

Skeleton anomalies consist of increased length of bones and most of the patients are tall. Disproportion of the different part of the body are characteristic of the syndrome and generally the inferior part of the body (pubic bone to feet) is taller than the upper part (pubis to head) (Bennis et al., 1993). Fingers are extremely long and constitute the so-called 'arachnodactilis syndrome'. Hyperlaxity of joints, especially of the wrist and fingers is also a major finding. Finally the hard palate is abnormal and has an 'arch-like' form.

Pathologically, Marfan syndrome results from defects in the connective tissue protein fibrillin. The disease has been associated with mutations in the fibrillin gene, which is mapped to the chromosome 7 (Foster et al., 1993). Fibrillin is a component of microfibrils, structures found in the extracellular matrices of most tissues and leading to the formation of elastin. The appearance of microfibrils in the matrix produced by Marfan patients' fibroblasts is different from normal cells (Christodoulou et al., 1993; Dietz et al., 1993; Maslen & Glanville, 1993). Microscopically, involvement of the media is observed with dislocation of the elastic layer. Treatment of patients with Marfan syndrome remains symptomatic.

References

Adami, P., Manzoni, P. & Rohmer, P. (1993) Anévrysmes evolutifs au cours d' un syndrome d' Ehlers–Danlos de type IV. A propos d' une observation. *Annales Radiologique Paris*, **36**, (2), 129–33.

Agarwal, H.C., Sandramouli, S., Sihota, R. & Sood, N.N. (1993). Sturge–Weber syndrome: management of glaucoma with combined trabeculotomy-trabeculectomy. *Ophthalmic Surgery*, **24**, 399–402.

Alarcon-Segovia, D., Délézé, M. & Oria, C. (1989). Antiphospholipid antibodies and the antiphospholipid syndrome in systemic lupus erythematosus. A prospective analysis of 500 consecutive patients. *Medicine*, **66**, 353–65.

Allen, S.W., Whitfield, J.M., Clarke, D.R., Sujanski, E. & Wiggins, J.W. (1993). Pulmonary arteriovenous malformation in the newborn: a familial case. *Pediatric cardiology*, **14**, 58–61.

Anderson, R.A. & Sondheimer, F.K. (1976). Rare carotid–vertebrobasilar anastomoses with notes on the differentiation between proatlantal and hypoglossal arteries. *Neuroradiology*, **11**, 113–18.

Ashleigh, R.J., Weller, J.M. & Leggate (1992). Fibromuscular hyperplasia of the internal carotid artery. A further cause of the 'Moyamoya' collateral circulation. *British Journal of Neurosurgery*, **6**, 269–73.

Bashi, Y.Z., Uysal, H., Peker, S. & Yurdakul, M. (1993). Persistant primitive proatlantal intersegmental (Proatlantal artery I) results in top of the basilar syndrome. *Stroke*, **24**, 2114–17.

Baumgartner, R.W. & Waespe, W. (1993). Behandelbare erkrankungen des nervensystems mit kataraktbildung. *Klinik Monatsblatter für Augenheilkunde*, **202**, 89–93.

Benedikt, R.A., Brown, D.C., Walker, R., Ghaed, V.N., Mitchell, M.

Geyer, C.A. (1993). Sturge–Weber syndrome: cranial MR imaging with Gd-DTPA. **14**, 409–15.

Bennis, A., Mehadji, B.A., Soulami, S., Tahiri, A. & Chraibi, N. (1993). Les manifestations cardio-vasculaires des dysplasies héréditaires du tissu conjonctif. *Annales de Cardiologie et d'Angeiologie* (*Paris*) **42**, 173–81.

Bogousslavsky, J., Gaio, J-M., Caplan, L.R., et al. (1989). Encephalopathy, deafness and blindness in young women: a distinct retinocochleocerebral arteriolopathy? *Journal of Neurology, Neurosurgery and Psychiatry*, **52**, 43–6.

Bour, P., Taghavi, I., Bracard, S., Frisch, N. & Fieve, G. (1992). Aneurysms of the extracranial internal carotid artery due to fibromuscular dysplasia: results of surgical management. *Annals of Vascular Surgery*, **6**, 205–8.

Brachlow, J., Schafer, M., Oliveira, F. & Jantzen, J.P. (1992). Todliche intraoperative zerebrale ischamie infolge Kinking der arteria carotis interna ? *Anesthesist*, **41**, 361–4.

Brady, R.O., Gal, A.E., Bradley, R.M., Martensson, E., Warshaw, A.L. & Laster, L. (1967). Enzymatic defects in Fabry's disease–ceramidetrihexosidase deficiency. *New England Journal of Medicine*, **276**, 1163–7.

Cameron, J.A. (1993). Corneal abnormalities in Ehlers–Danlos syndrome type IV. *Cornea*. **12**(1), 54–9.

Campistol-Plana, J., Lopez-Castillo, J., Capdevilla-Cirera, A. & Fernandez-Alvarez, E. (1993). Magnetic resonance with gadolinium in Sturge–Weber syndrome. *Annales Espanoles Pediatrics*, **39**, 33–6.

Cano, A., Roquer, J., Herraiz, J., Rovira, A. & Mirosa, F. (1992). Moyamoya syndrome. Diagnosis with angio-MRI. *Archives Neurobiology Madrid*, **55**(6), 276–9.

Carlborg, U., Ejrup, B., Grönblad, E. & Lund, F. (1959). Vascular studies in pseudoxanthoma elasticum. *Acta Medica Scandinavia*, **166** (Suppl 350), 1–84.

Carney, J.A., Gordon, H., Carpentier, P.C., Shenoy, B.V. & Liang, W.V. (1985). The complex of myxomas, spotty pigmentation and endocrine overactivity. *Medicine*, **64**, 270–83.

Christodoulou, J., Petrova-Benedict, R., Robinson, G.H., Jay, V. & Clarke, J.T. (1993). An unusual patient with the neonatal Marfan phenotype and mitochondrial complex I deficiency. *European Journal of Pediatrics*, **152**, 428–32.

Delplace, J., Van Blercom, N., Dargent, J.L., Blecic, S., & Jacobovitz, D. (1995). Accidents vasculaires cérébraux d' étiologie inhabituelle et d' évolution fatale. *Annals of Pathology*, **15**, 219–20.

Dietz, H.C., McIntosh, I., Sakai, L.Y. et al (1993). Four novel FBN1 mutations: significance for mutant transcript level and EGF-like domain calcium binding in the pathogenesis of Marfan syndrome. *Genomics*, **17**, 468–75.

Dobyns, W.B. & Garg, B.P. (1991). Vascular abnormalities in epidermal nevus syndrome. *Neurology*, **41**, 276–78.

Dorfman, L.J., Ransom, B.R., Formo, L.S. & Klets, A. (1983). Neuropathy in the hypereosinophilic syndrome. *Muscle Nerve*, **6**, 291–8.

Durack, D.T., Sumi, S.M. & Klebanoff, S.J. (1979). Neurotoxicity of human eosinophils. *Proceedings of the National Academy of Sciences, USA*, **76**, 1443–7.

Edwards, J.M., Zaccardi, M.J. & Strandness, D.E. (1992). A preliminary study of the role of duplex scanning in defining the adequacy of patients with renal artery fibromuscular dysplasia. *Journal of Vascular Surgery*, **15**, 604–11.

el Shanti, H., Bell, W.E. & Waziri, M.H. (1992). Epidermal nevus syndrome: subgroup with neuronal migration defects. *Journal of Child Neurology*, **7**, 29–34.

Enjolras, O., Riche, M.C., Merland, J.J. (1985). Facial portwine stains and and Sturge–Weber syndrome. *Pediatrics*, **76**, 48–51.

Fasshauer, K., Reimers, C.D., Gnau, H.J., Strempel, I. & Rossberg, C. (1984). Neurological complications of Grönblad–Strandberg syndrome. *Journal of Neurology*, **231**, 250.

Fauci, A.S. (1982). NIH conference: the idiopathic hypereosinophilic syndrome. *Annals of Internal Medicine*, **97**, 78–92.

Ferreira, A., Fernando, P.M., Macedo, F. & Capuco, R. (1993). Endocardite infecciosa. Forma de apresentacao da sindrome de Marfan. *Reviews of Portuguese Cardiology*, **12**, 571–5.

Fisher, M. & Zito, J. (1983). Focal cerebral ischemia distal to a cerebral aneurysm in hereditary hemorrhagic telangiectasia. *Stroke*, **14**, 419–21.

Forney, W.R., Robinson, S.J. & Pascoe, D.J. (1966). Congenital heart disease, deafness and skeletal malformation: a new syndrome. *Journal of Pediatrics*, **68**, 14–26.

Foster, K., Ferrel, R., King-Underwood, L. et al. (1993). Description of a dinucleotide repeat polymorphism in the human elastin gene and its use to confirm assignment of the gene to chromosone 7. *Annals of Human Genetics*, **57**, 87–96.

Fressinaud, C., Preux, P.M., Milor, A.M., Daunas, I., Dumas, M. & Vallat, J.M. (1993). Complexe familial myxome-lentiginose révélé par un accident ischémique transitoire. *Revue Neurologie*, **149**, 219–21.

Galitica, Z., Gibas, Z. & Martinez-Hernandez, A. (1992). Dissecting aneurysm as a complication of generalized fibromuscular dysplasia. *Human Pathology*, **23**, 568.

Giller, C.A., Mathews, D., Purdy, P., Kopitnik, T.A., Batjer H.H. & Samson, D.S. (1992). The transcranial Doppler appearance of acute carotid artery occlusion. *Annals of Neurology*, **31**, 101–3.

Gillian, A.C., Ragge, N.K., Perez, M.I. & Bolognia, J.L. (1993). Phakomatosis pigmentovascularis type IIb with iris mamillations. *Archives of Dermatology*, **129**, 340–2.

Gilly, R., Erbaz, N., Langue, J. & Raveau, J. (1982). Sténoses artérielles cérébrales multiples et progressives, sténose de l' artère rénale et maladie de Recklinghausen. *Pédiatrie*, **37**, 523–30.

Glick, B. (1972). Bilateral carotid occlusive disease. *Archives of Pathology and Laboratory Medicine*, **93**, 352–5.

Green, J.F., Fitzwater, J.E. & Burgess, J. (1974). Arterial lesion associated with neurofibromatosis. *American Journal of Clinical Pathology*, **62**, 481–7.

Grenko, R.T., Burns, S.L., Golden, E.A., Byers, P.H. & Bovill, E.G. (1993). Type IV Ehlers–Danlos syndrome with aspirin sensitivity. A family study. *Archives of Pathology and Laboratory Medicine*, **117** (10), 989–92.

Grönblad, E. (1932). Pseudoxanthoma elasticum and changes in the eye. *Acta Dermotalogica Venereologica*, **13**, 417–22.

Hashigushi, T., Maruyama, I., Sonoda, K. et al. (1992). Ehlers–Danlos syndrome combined with Von Recklinghausen neurofibromatosis. *Internal Medicine*, **31**(5), 671–3.

Hautala, T., Heikkinen, L., Kivirikko, K.I. & Myllyla, R. (1993). A large duplication in the gene for lysil-hydroxylase accounts for the type VI variant of Ehlers–Danlos syndrome in two siblings. *Genomics*, **15**(2), 399–404.

Heikala, H., Somer, H., Kovanen, J., Poutianen, E., Karli, H. & Haltia, M. (1988). Microangiopathy with encephalopathy, hearing loss and retinal arteriolar occlusions: two new cases. *Journal of Neurological Science*, **86**, 239–50.

Heiserman, J.E., Drayer, B.P., Fram, E.K. & Keller, P.J. (1992). MR angiography of cervical fibromuscular dysplasia. **13**, 1454–7.

Humphries, J.E., Frierson, H.F. Jr & Underwood, P.B. Jr (1993). Vaginal telangiectasia: unusual presentation of the Osler–Weber–Rendu syndrome, *Annals of Dermatology*, **81**, 865–6.

Iwabushi, S., Horikoshi, A., Okada, S., Tanita, T. & Fujimura, S. (1993). Intrapleural rupture of pulmonary fistula occurring just beneath the pleura: report of a case. *Surgery Today*, **23**, 468–70.

Johnson, P.H., Richards, A.J., Pope, F.M. & Hopkinson, D.A. (1992). A COL3 A1 glycine 1006 to glutamic acid substitution in a patient with Ehlers–Danlos syndrome type IV detected by denaturing gradient gel electrophoresis. *Journal of Inheritable Metabolic Diseases*, **15**(3), 426–30.

Josien, E. (1992). Extracranial vertebral artery dissection: nine cases. *Journal of Neurology*, **239**, 327–30.

Kennedy, C., Oranje, A.P., Kaizer, K., van den Heuvel, M.M. & Castan-Berrevoets, C.E. (1992). Cutis marmorata telangiectatica congenita. *International Journal of Dermatology*, **31**, 249–52.

Kharsa, G., Molas, G., Potet, F., Baglin, A.C., Vaudry, P. & Grossin, M. (1992). Elastomes du colon. discussion pathogenique à propos de 7 observations. *Annals of Pathology*, **12**, 362–6.

Kindl, R., Nigbur, H., Horsch, S. (1993). Das extrakranielle Aneurysma der arteria carotis interna. Eine fallbeschreibung. *Vasa*, **22**, 256–9.

Kivirikko, K.I. (1993). Collagens and their abnormalities in a wide spectrum of diseases. *Annals of Medicine*, **25**(2), 113–26.

Kotagal, P. & Rothner, A.D. (1993). Epilepsy in the settings of neurocutaneous syndromes. *Epilepsia*, **34**(Suppl.3), S71–8.

Kurtz, S.N., Melamed, S. & Blumenthal, M. (1993). Cataract and intraocular lens implantation after remote trabeculectomy for Sturge–Weber syndrome. *Journal of Cataract Refractive Surgery*, **19**, 539–41.

Kuster, W. & Happle, R. (1993). Neurocutaneous disorders in children. *Current Opinion in Pediatrics*, **5**, 436–40.

Lamas, E., Rabato, R.D., Cabello, A. & Abad, J.M. (1978). Multiple intracranial occlusions (Moyamoya disease) in patients with neurofibromatosis. One case report with autopsy. *Acta Neurochirurgica*, **445**, 133–45.

Lambrechts, H.D. & de Boer, W.G.R.M. (1965). Contributions to the study of immediate and early x-ray reactions with regard to chemoprotection: VI. X-ray induced atheromatous lesions in the arterial wall of cholesterolemic rabbits. *International Journal of Radiological Biology*, **9**, 165–74.

Lasjaunias, P., Theron, J. & Moret, J. (1978). The occipital artery. *Neuroradiology*, **15**, 31–7.

Lasjaunias, P. & Berenstein, A. (1987). Aneurysms. In *Surgical Neuro-angiography. 2. Endovascular Treatment of Craniofacial Lesion*, ed. A. Berenstein, pp. 235–71. Berlin, Heidelberg, New York, London, Paris, Tokyo: Springer-Verlag.

Levinson, S.A., Close, M.B., Herenfeld, W.K. et al. (1973). Carotid artery of occlusive disease following external cervical irradiation. *Archives of Surgery*, **107**, 395–9.

Liang, C.W. & Liang, K.H. (1992). Sturge–Weber syndrome without facial nevus. *Chinese Medical Journal*, **105**, 964–5.

Loevner, H. & Quint, D.J. (1992). Persistant trigeminal artery in a patient with Sturge–Weber syndrome. *American Journal of Radiology*, **158**, 872–4.

Magauda, A., Dalla-Bernardirna, B., De Marco, P. et al. (1993). Bilateral occipital calcification, epilepsy and coeliac disease: clinical and neuroimaging features of a new syndrome. *Journal of Neurology, Neurosurgery and Psychiatry*, **56**, 885–9.

Majorana, A. & Fachetti, F. (1992). The oro-dental findings in the Ehlers–Danlos syndrome. A report of two clinical cases. *Minerva Stomatology*, **41**(3), 127–33.

Marti-Bonmati, L., Menor, F., Poyatos, C. & Cortina, H. (1992). Diagnosis of Sturge–Weber syndrome: comparison of the efficacy of CT and MR imaging in 14 cases. *American Journal of Radiology*, **158**, 867–71.

Marti-Bonmati, L., Menor, F. & Mulas, F. (1993). The Sturge–Weber syndrome: correlation between the clinical status and radiological CT and MRI findings.*Child Nervous System*, **9**, 107–9.

Maslen, C.L. & Glanville, R.W. (1993). The molecular basis of Marfan syndrome. DNA *Cell Biology*, **12**, 561–72.

Mishra, M., Chambers, J.B. & Grahame, R. (1992). Ventricular septal aneurysms in a case of Ehlers–Danlos syndrome. *International Journal of Cardiology*, **36**(3), 369–70.

Mizutani, T., Tanaka, H. & Aruga, T. (1992). Multiple arterio-venous malformations located in the cerebellum, posterior fossa, spinal cord, dura, and scalp associated port wine stain and supra tentorial venous anomaly. *Neurosurgery*, **31**, 137–40.

Murros, K.E. & Toole, J.F. (1989). The effect of radiation on carotid arteries. *Archives of Neurology*, **46**, 449–55.

Muyner, T.P. & Margulis, A.R. (1981). Pseudoxanthoma with internal carotid artery aneurysm. *American Journal of Roentgenology*, **136**, 1023–6.

Nakai, H., Kawata, Y., Tomabechi, M. et al. (1993). Markedly dilated cervical carotid arteries in a patient with a ruptured aneurysm of the anterior communicating artery: a case report. *No Shinkei Geka*, **21**, 333–9.

Neau, J.P., Boissonot, L., Boutaud, P., Fontanel, J.P., Gil, R. & Lefevre, J.P. (1987). Manifestations neurologiques de la maladie de Rendu–Osler–Weber. A propos de 4 observations. *Revue de Medicine Interne*, **8**, 75–8.

Nishiyama, K., Fuse, S., Shimizu, J., Takeda, K. & Sakuta, M. (1992). A case of fibromuscular dysplasia presenting with Wallenberg syndrome, and developing a giant aneurysm of the internal carotid artery in the cavernous sinus. *Rhinsho Shinkeigaku*, **32**, 1117–20.

Padget, D.H. (1954). Designation of the embryonic intersegmental arteries in references to the vertebral artery and subclavian stem. *Anatomical Record*, **119**, 349–56.

Parenti, G., Fiori, L. & Marconi, F. (1992). Intracranial aneurysm and cerebral embolism. *European Neurology*, **32**, 212–15.

Pavone, L., Curatolo, P., Rizzo, R. et al. (1991). Epidermal nevus syndrome: a neurologic variant with hemimegalencephaly, gyral malformation, mental retardation, seizures and facial hemihypertrophy. *Neurology*, **41**, 266–71.

Petty, E.M., Seahore, M.R., Bravermann, I.M., Spiesel, S.Z., Smith, L.T., Milstone, L.M. (1993). Dermatospraxis in children. A case report and review of the newly recognized phenotype. *Archives in Dermatology*, **129**(10), 1310–15.

Quentin-Hoffmann, E., Harrach, B., Robenek, H. & Kresse, H. (1993). Genetics defects in proteoglycans biosynthesis. *Pediatric Radiology*, **28**(1): 37–41.

Raftopoulos, C., Delecluse, F., Braude, P., Rodesch, G. & Brotchi, J. (1993). Anterior sacral meningocele and Marfan syndrome: a review. *Acta Chirurgie Belgique*, **93**, 1–7.

Richards, A.J., Ward, P.N., Narcisi, P., Nicholls, A.C., Lloyd, J.C. & Popoe, F.M. (1992). A single base mutation in the gene for type III collagen (COL3 A1) converts glycine 847 to glutamic acid in a family with Ehlers–Danlos syndrome type IV. An unaffected family member is mosaic for the mutation. *Human Genetics*, **89**(4), 414–18.

Rintahaka, P.J., Chugani, H.T., Messa, C. & Phelps, M.E. (1993). Hemimegaencephaly: evaluation with positron emission tomography. *Pediatric Neurology*, **9**, 21–8.

Roach, E.S. (1988). Diagnosis and management of neurocutaneous syndromes. *Seminars in Neurology*, **8**, 83–96.

Ruby, A.J., Jampol, L.M., Golberg, M.F., Schroeder, R. & Anderson-Nelson, S. (1992). Choroidal neovascularisation associated with choroidal hemangiomas. *Archives in Ophthamology*, **110**, 658–61.

Sandmann, J., Hojer, C., Bewermeyer, H., Bamborschke, S. & Neufang, K.F. (1992). Die fibromuskulare dysplasie als ursache zerebrale insulte. *Nervenarzt*, **63**, 335–40.

Sato, T., Ito, H., Miyazaki, S., Komine, S. & Hayashida, Y. (1993). Megacystis and megacolon in an infant with Ehlers–Danlos syndrome. *Acta Paediatrica Japan*, **35**(4), 358–60.

Schievink, W.I., Limburg, M., Oorthuys, J.W.E., Fleury, P. & Pope, F.M. (1990). Cerebrovascular disease in Ehlers–Danlos syndrome type IV. *Stroke*, **21**, 626–32.

Smadja, D., Mas, J.L., Fallet-Bianco, C. et al. (1991). Intravascular lymphomatosis (neoplastic angioendotheliosis) of the central nervous system: case report and literature review. *Journal of Neuro-Oncology*, **11**, 171–80.

Shulze, H.E., Ebner, A. & Besinger, U.A. (1992). Report of dissection of the internal carotid artery in three cases. *Neurosurgical Review*, **15**, 61–4.

Simpson, I.A., de-Belder, M.A., Treasure, T., Camm, A.J. & Pumphrey, C.W. (1993). Cardiovascular manifestations of Marfan's syndrome: improved evaluation by transoesophageal echocardiography. *British Heart Journal*, **69**, 104–8.

Smith, L.T., Wertelecki, W., Milstone, L.M. et al. (1992). Human dermatopraxis: a form of Ehlers–Danlos syndrome that results from failure to remove the amino terminal propeptide of type I procollagen. *American Journal of Human Genetics*, **51**(2), 235–44.

Sobata, E., Ohkuma, H. & Suzuki, S. (1988). Cerebrovascular disorders associated with Von Recklinghausen's neurofibromatosis: a case report. *Neurosurgery*, **22**, 544–9.

Struck, B., Neldner, K.H., Rao, V.S., St. Jean, P. & Lindpaintner, K. (1997). Mapping of both autosomal recessive and dominant variants of pseudoxanthoma elasticum to chromosome 16p13.1. *Human Molecular Genetics*, **6**(11), 1323–8.

Susac, J.O., Hardmann, J.M. & Selhorst, J.B. (1979). Microangiopathy of the brain and retina. *Neurology*, **29**, 313–16.

Taaffe, A. (1977). Angiokeratoma corporis diffusum: the evolution of a disease entity. *Postgraduate Medicine*, **53**, 78–81.

Talby, A.B., Nagaraja, D., Shanker, S.K. & Pratibha, N.G. (1987). Sturge–Weber Dimitre disease without facial nevus. *Neurology*, **37**, 1063–4.

Taptas, J.N. & Katsiotis, P.A. (1968). Arterial embolism as a cause of hemiplegia after subarachnoidal hemorrhage from aneurysm. *Progress in Brain Research*, **30**, 357–60.

Thomas, P.K. (1988). Inherited neuropathies related to disorders of lipid metabolism. *Advances in Neurology*, **48**, 133–44.

Tiacci, C., D'Allessandro, P., Cantisani, T.A. et al. (1993). Epilepsy with bilateral occipital calcifications: Sturge–Weber variant or a different encephalopathy? *Epilepsia*, **34**, 528–39.

Truhan, A.P. & Filipek, P.A. (1993). Magnetic resonance imaging. Its role in the neuroradiologic evaluation of neurofibromatosis, tuberous sclerosis, and Sturge–Weber syndrome. *Archives of Dermatology*, **129**, 219–26.

Tucker, L.B. (1992). Heritable disorders of connective tissue and disability and chronic disease in childood. *Current Opinion in Rheumatology*, **4**(5), 731–40.

Van Bogaert, L. (1967). Sur l'angiomatose méningée avec leucodystrophie. *Wien Zeitschrift für Nervenheilkunde Deren Grenzgebieten*, **25**, 131–6.

Vandenberg, P. (1993). Molecular basis of heritable connective tissue disease. *Biochemical Medicine and Metabolic Biology*, **49**(1), 1–12.

Velkey, I., Lombay, B. & Panczel, G. (1992). Obstruction of cerebral arteries in childhood stroke. *Pediatric Radiology*, **22**, 386–7.

Vetrie, D., Bentley, D., Bobrow, M., Harris, A. (1993). Physical mapping shows close linkage between the alpha-galactosidase A gene (GLA) and the DXS178 locus. *Human Genetics*, **92**, 95–7.

Villemure, J.G. & Rasmussen, T. (1993). Functional hemispherectomy in children. *Neuropediatrics*, **23**, 53–5.

Vogl, T.J., Stemmler, J., Bergmann, C., Pfluger, T., Egger, E. & Lissner, J. (1993). MR and MR angiography of Sturge–Weber syndrome. **14**, 417–25.

Vonsattel, J.-P. G. & Hedley-Whyte, T. (1989). Diffuse meningocerebral angiomatosis and leucoencephalopathy. In *Handbook of Clinical Neurology. Vascular Diseases*, ed. P.J. Vinken, G.W. Bruyn & H.L. Klawans. Part III, ed. J.F. Toole, vol. 55, pp. 317–24. The Netherlands: Elsevier Science Publishers.

Watanabe, S., Tanaka, K., Nakayama, T. & Kazneko, M. (1993). Fibromuscular dysplasia at the internal carotid origin: a case of carotid web. *No Shinkei Geka*, **21**, 449–52.

Weaver, D.F., Hefernan, L.P., Purdy, R.A. & Ing, V.W. (1988). Eosinophil-induced neurotoxicity: axonal neuropathy, cerebral infarction and dementia. *Neurology*, **38**, 144–6.

Weibel, J. & Fields, W.S. (1965). Tortuosity, coiling and kinking of the internal carotid artery: etiology, and radiographic anatomy. *Neurology*, **15**, 7–20.

Wertelecki, W., Smith, L.T. & Byers, P. (1992). Initial observation of human dermatopraxis: Ehlers–Danlos syndrome type VII. *Canadian Journal of Pediatrics*, **121**(4), 558–64.

Wick, W.R. & Mills, S.E. (1991). Intravascular lymphomatosis: clinicopathologic features and differential diagnosis. *Seminars in Diagnostic Pathology*, **8**, 91–101.

Wilms, G., Van Wijck, E., Demaerel, P., Smet, M.H., Plets, C. & Brucher, J.M. (1992). Gyriform calcifications in tuberous sclerosis simulating the appearance of Sturge–Weber disease. *American Journal of Neuroradiology*, **13**, 295–7.

Wolpert, S.M. & Caplan, L.R. (1992). Current role of cerebral angiography in the diagnosis of cerebrovascular diseases. *American Journal of Roentgenology*, **159**, 191–7.

Yousem, S.A. & Colby, T.V. (1990). Intravascular lymphomatosis presenting in the lung. *Cancer*, **65**, 349–53.

Zeluff, G.W., Caskey, C.T. & Jackson, D. (1978). Heart attack and stroke in a young man? Think Fabry's disease. *Heart and Lung*, **7**, 1056–61.

Index